Treatment Resistance in Psychiatry

Yong-Ku Kim
Editor

Treatment Resistance in Psychiatry

Risk Factors, Biology, and Management

Springer

Editor
Yong-Ku Kim
Department of Psychiatry
College of Medicine, Korea University
Seoul
South Korea

ISBN 978-981-10-4357-4 ISBN 978-981-10-4358-1 (eBook)
https://doi.org/10.1007/978-981-10-4358-1

Library of Congress Control Number: 2018957846

This Springer imprint is published by the registered company Springer Nature Singapore Pte Ltd.
The registered company address is: 152 Beach Road, #21-01/04 Gateway East, Singapore 189721, Singapore

Preface

Despite its great progress in psychopharmacology, a significant proportion of psychiatric patients do not respond satisfactory to the treatment. Given the lack of consistence for defining criteria, it is difficult to assess the accurate prevalence of treatment-resistant psychiatric disorders. Approximately 30% of psychiatric patients would be considered recovered from the standard treatments, 30–40% of patients would be considered improved, whereas 30% of patients would be barely touched by the contemporary treatments. In spite of the fact that there is no full agreement regarding the definition of treatment resistance of psychiatric disorders, treatment resistance clearly refers to the occurrence of an inadequate response following adequate treatment. Coping with the treatment resistance in psychiatric disorders is an important issue facing psychiatrists and their patients.

The search of potential biological markers for treatment-resistant psychiatric disorders is a current challenge in the field of biological psychiatry. One way to fulfill these challenges would be to investigate molecular and cellular causes responsible for the treatment resistance using blood and cerebrospinal fluid analysis, neuroimaging, and genetic and epigenetic techniques. Then, obtained biological markers would be used for developing clinical risk factors for treatment resistance and for delivering effective treatments to reach complete remission of symptoms. However, the goal is presently out of reach. Therefore, we need to think outside the box and get away from conventional ways of thinking.

Post hoc experimental design can be regarded only as a consequence of having treatment-resistance, rather than being causal risk factors for it. So, we need a paradigm shift toward cause-and-effect relationship. Our lack of information on treatment resistance can start with the misinterpreted post hoc design of many studies. To deal with this situation, untreated patients are enrolled in the study to identify biological markers for treatment resistance.

This book reviews all the important aspects of treatment-resistant psychiatric disorders, covering issues such as definitions, clinical aspects, neurobiological correlates, treatment options, and predictors of treatment response. The book is divided into three parts, the first (Chaps. 1, 2, 3, 4, 5, and 6) of which examines the most recent thinking on treatment resistance in psychiatry, including definition and epidemiology, paradigm shift in the study of the subjects, individual susceptibility and resilience, abnormal structural or functional connectivity, and insights from animal models. The second (Chaps. 7, 8, 9, 10, 11, 12, 13, 14, 15, 16, 17, and 18) part then discusses treatment resistance in each of the major psychiatric disorders, with particular focus on the responsible clinical and biological factors and the available management strategies. Finally, in third (Chaps. 19, 20, 21, 22, 23, 24, and 25) part, more detailed information is presented on diverse pharmacological and nonpharmacological therapeutic interventions. The book, written by leading experts from across the world, will be of value to all who seek a better understanding of the clinical-neurobiological underpinnings and the development of management for treatment resistance in psychiatric disorders.

Chapter 1 highlights a current and available knowledge about definition, epidemiology, risk factors, and improving strategies of treatment resistance in mental disorders. The definition of treatment resistance in psychiatry remains controversial in spite of importance. Most definitions have focused on pharmacotherapy but even these have struggled to capture the complexity of varying response and duration of treatment. This review discusses the importance of treatment resistance and factors affecting its definition in the light of recent advances in knowledge and treatment. The optimization of treatment, such as personalized medicine, measurement-based care, combination and augmentation strategies and experimental treatment strategies, diminishes the occurrence of treatment resistance.

Chapter 2 reviews some methodological considerations to uncover initial risk factors for treatment-resistant psychiatric disorders and propose a better study design for future research by discussing the shortcomings of traditional study design. The post hoc experimental design can be regarded only as a consequence of having treatment resistance, rather than being causal risk factors for it. Data derived from such studies often do not allow for a distinction to be made between cause and effect. To deal with this problem, untreated patients should be enrolled in the study to identify biological markers for treatment resistance. Such information can give a cue to improve the initial diagnosis and provide more effective treatment for treatment resistance.

Chapter 3 focuses on clinical evidences from pharmacogenetic or pharmacogenomic data in major psychiatric disorders in order to better understand potential biomarkers that can be aid in the prediction of therapeutic response. Although the search for genetic biomarkers is facilitated by several approaches including epidemiological studies, molecular methods, genome-wide association studies, transcriptional and microRNA analyses, gene-environment interaction, and epigenetic approaches, no biomarkers have good enough sensitivity and specificity to be applied in clinical practice at present. The majority of available pharmacogenetic studies in psychiatry refers to how a specific gene or a set of genes can influence a patient's response or side effects and only few of them are specifically designed to explore biomarkers underlying treatment resistance.

Chapter 4 illustrates recent study findings regarding clinical application of brain-based biomarkers derived from patients for the prediction of response or resistance to treatment, as well as for improved design of clinical studies, to find more robust brain-based biomarkers of treatment response or resistance. Earlier identification of patients who are prone to treatment resistance can avoid the frustration of a trial-and-error approach and facilitate the design of more optimized treatment regimens and setting of individualized levels of care. In future, more active application of machine-learning and medical bioinformatics frameworks to the brain biomarker-based prediction of treatment response and recommendation of a personalized treatment regimen are warranted.

Chapter 5 suggests ways to develop new drugs that may be effective in the treatment of resistant depression. Animal models of depression have been developed with a focus on those likely to demonstrate useful drugs in resistant depression or associations. Are there animal models for resistant depression? Researchers have proposed models likely to develop drugs that can treat resistant depression. A potential model to discover antidepressants active in resistant depression is based on genetic. To date, the genetic model has not been used in the development of treatments for resistant depression, but it is a path that seems interesting.

Chapter 6 highlights the hypothetical conceptualization of an integrated approach to treatment-resistant psychiatric disorders. The integrated approaches for treatment-resistant psychiatric disorders can be an important issue in the perspective of clinical psychiatry. The synergistic effect of interactions between specific genes and childhood trauma has been identified as a significant factor for defining treatment resistance in psychiatric disorders. A new approach to psychotherapy, inspired by the reconsolidation-updating paradigm, which we refer to as the histone acetylation inhibitor-augmented psychotherapy (plasticity-augmented psychotherapy) is proposed. Combination of psychotherapy and pharmacotherapy can be integrated from the viewpoint of epigenetic regulation and used to manage treatment-resistant psychiatric disorders in the future.

Chapter 7 discusses recent findings on neurobiological mechanisms underlying treatment-resistant depression (TRD) and novel pharmacological treatment strategies. Genetics, along with interactions with environmental factors, and alterations in neural substrates are deeply implicated in TRD. Neuroinflammation, glutamatergic neurotransmission, and glial cell pathology, that in turn influence neurogenesis and neurodegeneration, are all considered to play key roles in the pathophysiology of TRD. Based on the speculated etiological factors, novel treatment agents such as anti-inflammatory drugs and ketamine are suggested as potent candidates that will aid us to treat TRD.

Chapter 8 focuses on the evolution of the concept of treatment-resistant schizophrenia (TRS) and treatment strategies for TRS. Treatment resistance in schizophrenia is a concept that still holds different positions in clinical settings and research areas. Categorical and criteria-based approach with more emphasis on positive symptoms is preferred for research, while individualized and holistic view for treatment resistance seems appropriate for day-to-day clinical situations. Regarding pharmacological treatment of TRS, till now only clozapine has demonstrated conclusive favorable evidence. Current knowledge about these augmentation strategies does not support an evidence-based treatment algorithm, but it can aid clinicians in selecting the best treatment based on psychopathology and side effect profile. Among the various augmentation strategies best level of evidence is for electroconvulsive therapy.

Chapter 9 sheds light on the challenges surrounding the concept of treatment-resistant bipolar disorder (BD), possible pathophysiological factors in the development of resistance, and various therapeutic interventions aiming at the management of treatment-resistant patients. The concept of treatment-resistant BD is not well established and there is not enough evidence to support it as a single construct. Evidence suggests that as the disease progresses, the compensatory mechanisms become overwhelmed, resulting in neuroprogression and, likely, in resistance to treatment. Some alternative pharmacological strategies (including not only novel agents but also different combinations of traditional agents) are currently available. With respect to nonpharmacological biological treatments, electroconvulsive therapy (ECT) seems to display good efficacy in the treatment of resistant case, despite the shortage of controlled studies in treatment-resistant BD. Psychosocial interventions seem to play a prominent role in its management during the maintenance phase in treatment-resistant BD.

Chapter 10 emphasizes the issue of treatment resistance in posttraumatic stress disorder (PTSD). Advances in improving treatment resistance in PTSD requires a more sophisticated classification of PTSD that takes account of the heterogeneity of this condition and the progressions which occur with chronicity that impact on treatment responsiveness. Sensitization, kindling, and allostatic load in PTSD highlight the importance of the biological mechanisms of the onset and chronicity of this disorder. The underlying circuitry neural regions which have been identified as being relevant to the etiology of PTSD are equally those involved in depression and the emergence of treatment resistance. The staging model of PTSD can lead to more systematic research into the treatment of PTSD and assist in strategies to develop treatment resistance such as a personalized medicine approach.

Chapter 11 highlights several factors that can contribute to treatment resistance in obsessive-compulsive disorder (OCD) and current treatment options for treatment-resistant OCD patients. Management options for treatment-resistant OCD should be evaluated based on the level of response the individual demonstrates. Management of partial response to initial first-line treatments can include increasing dose and duration, or augmentation of serotonin reuptake inhibitors (SSRIs) with exposure and response prevention (ERP), a structured psychotherapy that involves two major components: systematic confrontation with feared situations and stimuli and voluntary restriction from engaging in compulsive rituals. For patients with minimal to no response, options include switching medications, or augmenting with an antipsychotic. Patients who continue to see an inadequate response to these treatments can explore novel treatment strategies including new glutamate medications. Only in the most severe cases should neurosurgical approaches be considered.

Chapter 12 focuses current managements for treatment-resistant opioid dependence. Opioid dependence is a chronic, relapsing disorder with high mortality rates with comorbid psychiatric and physical diseases. A broad spectrum of pharmacological and nonpharmacological interventions is now available for treatment-refractory opioid dependence. In addition to opioid maintenance treatment with partial or full opioid agonists, treatment with opioid antagonists is a realistic treatment option. Whether novel dopamine antagonists or partial agonists can be used for treatment of opioid dependence remains to be seen. In contrast to the situation for other substance use disorders such as cocaine, amphetamine, and cannabis use disorder, treatment of opioid dependence is an emerging and promising field with different treatment options.

Chapter 13 discusses definition, biosocial risk factors, underlying pathophysiology, and treatment options in treatment-resistant panic disorder (TRPD). TRPD is defined as the failure to achieve remission according to the previously mentioned criteria after at least 9–12 months of optimal treatment. The five major risk factors for TRPD, including the characteristic essence of panic disorder, personal demographic characteristics, comorbid medical illnesses, comorbid psychiatric disorders, and psychosocial factors, are proposed. A biopsychosocial model in TRPD explains the potential pathophysiology of that illness. The prompt and optimal interventions, especially the combination of medication treatment and cognitive behavioral therapy (CBT) and the well-intervention for psychosocial stresses, benefit TRPD sufferers and reduce the risk of chronic morbidity and disability.

Chapter 14 reviews treatment resistance in generalized anxiety disorder (GAD) and social anxiety disorder (SAD). GAD shares substantial genetic variation with major depression and the personality trait neuroticism, and an alarm reaction mediated by activation of neuronal circuits including amygdale and other limbic structures is most often found in neuroimaging studies of GAD. Abnormalities in the limbic-medial prefrontal circuit shown in functional neuroimaging studies may be critical for the pathophysiology of SAD which has dysfunctional emotion regulation by reappraisal of social criticism. Options for treatment-resistant GAD and SAD include augmentation with other antidepressants, atypical antipsychotics, benzodiazepines, and pregabalin. A partial NMDA agonist D-cycloserine is considered as a newer treatment option with exposure therapy in anxiety disorders.

Chapter 15 discusses conventional and novel pharmacological treatments and neuromodulation therapy in treatment-resistant attention deficit/hyperactivity disorder (ADHD). ADHD is a heterogeneous disorder with a variety of core symptom presentations, degree of severity, and psychiatric comorbidities. Treatment involves a stepwise, systematic approach targeting the predominant clinical symptoms with the goal of minimizing the negative impact on social and academic functioning. For treatment-resistant ADHD patients, well-delivered evidence-based medication management combined with psychosocial interventions may be necessary to see responses to treatment. Other moderating factors may be the presence of co-occurring anxiety disorders and conduct disorder symptoms as these patients have shown significant benefit with behavioral therapy alone or in combination with medication management. Investigational therapies such as cognitive training, noninvasive brain stimulation, and neurofeedback training have limited evidence currently and are not recommended as standard treatment for these patients.

Chapter 16 reviews routine strategies for the management of refractory Tourette syndrome (TS). TS is a complex neurodevelopmental disorder with the presence of multiple motor and phonic tics that begin during childhood and persist for more than 1 year. Although the term "treatment-refractory TS" is commonly used in research and clinical practice, there has been no consensus regarding its definition. However, the presence of comorbidities is also frequently associated with refractory TS. There are currently no guidelines for the treatment of refractory TS, but emerging therapy, including transcranial magnetic stimulation (TMS) and deep brain stimulation (DBS), is recommended for patients with refractory TS.

Chapter 17 provides a comprehensive review of neurobiology and management in treatment-resistant eating disorders such as anorexia nervosa and bulimia nervosa. Treatment-resistant eating disorders are characterized with protracted course; profoundly detrimental impact on social, vocational, psychological, and physical health; and low recovery rates of less than 50%. Neuro-adaptive changes in response to the highly disturbed eating pattern may cause treatment resistance in eating disorders. It can be beneficial to use treatments that directly target some of the dysregulated circuits that maintain the disorder. New interventions targeting the neural changes such as cognitive remediation therapy (CRT), cognitive bias modification (CBM), repetitive transcranial magnetic stimulation (rTMS), and oxytocin therapy may improve the response to treatment in enduring eating disorders.

Chapter 18 addresses sleep and wake problems that are often comorbid in treatment-resistant psychiatric conditions and their causes and managements. In chronic psychiatric disorders, the sleep and wake problems, such as insomnia, sleep apnea, restless legs syndrome, sleepiness, irregular circadian sleep wake cycle, and prolonged and inappropriate hypnotic use, are commonly comorbid and often contribute to a treatment-resistant condition if not properly managed. Insomnia is treated effectively with cognitive behavioral therapy for insomnia (CBT-I), even if it is accompanied by psychiatric illness, but it is better to modify the CBT-I modality for each psychiatric disorder. Patients with psychiatric disorders often do not complain or conceal obstructive sleep apnea (OSA) symptoms themselves, and therapists should be more aggressive in considering the evaluation and management of OSA during pharmacotherapy.

Chapter 19 introduces the concept of creative, person-centered narrative psychopharmacotherapy for treatment resistance in psychiatry. A paradigm shift is needed from the mechanistic, formistic, and reductionistic ways of thinking of technical, nomothetic, and impersonal psychopharmacology to contextual, systemic, and creative thinking with a new treatment paradigm of individualized and person-centered psychopharmacology. The best treatments are those that timely utilize and integrate multiple therapeutic modalities. Creative, person-centered narrative psychopharmacotherapy as a multimodal resilience enhancing concept may significantly contribute to better treatment effectiveness and efficiency in current psychiatry and thus overcome treatment failures and resistance.

Chapter 20 reviews literature describing psychodynamic approaches to treatment resistance and demonstrating the relevance of psychodynamic concepts and the effectiveness of psychodynamic therapies. Despite the growth of neurobiological research in psychiatry, the fundamental clinical problems of psychiatry remain unresolved. Psychodynamic concepts and psychodynamic therapy (PDT) offer opportunities for novel, effective approaches to treatment resistance. Psychodynamic approaches have a value in work with the treatment-resistant patient both in providing a person-centered, biopsychosocial perspective that avoids reductionism and includes awareness of the complex effects of the treatment relationship and contributing psychotherapies that provide an alternative to symptom-focused treatments such as CBT.

Chapter 21 aims to provide an overview about effectiveness and applications of cognitive behavioral therapy (CBT) and behavioral activation (BA) for treatment-resistant depression (TRD). CBT is an evidence-based adjunctive or stand-alone psychological therapy for TRD. In addition to CBT, which has high demands on cognitive functioning, simpler approaches like BA are proven to be effective for TRD. Thus, both CBT and BA appear to be attractive alternatives or supplements for the medication of TRD. Promoting early utilization of professional help and to increasing access to evidence-based interventions can be achieved by the provision of Internet-based and smartphone app-delivered mental health interventions for persons with TRD.

Chapter 22 provides a comprehensive review on neuromodulatory strategies that are either clinically available (electroconvulsive therapy, transcranial magnetic stimulation, vagal nerve stimulation) or under investigation (trigeminal nerve stimulation, transcranial direct current stimulation, deep brain stimulation) for the treatment-resistant psychiatric disorders. This chapter focuses on current state of knowledge on how each modality may contribute to relieving the tremendous suffering of individuals afflicted with refractory psychiatric conditions, anxiety disorders, bipolar disorder, depression, OCD, PTSD, and schizophrenia and what the future may hold.

Chapter 23 focuses on managing strategies of clozapine-resistant schizophrenia with a focus on augmentation strategies aimed to improve efficacy in such devastating condition. It has been estimated that around 40–70% of patients with treatment-resistant schizophrenia (TRS) on clozapine treatment may have an incomplete or absent response or remission and are commonly referred to as "ultra-resistant" or "refractory." The clozapine-refractory schizophrenia represents a challenge for the clinician and a misfortune for the patients, and several strategies have been proposed to overcome this problem.

Chapter 24 introduces its promising application of fecal microbiota transplantation (FMT) in treatment-resistant psychiatric disorders. The bidirectional relationship between gut and brain microbiota has been indicated by numerous preclinical and clinical studies. Dysbiosis, which occurs in the microbiota due to the causes such as nutrition, antibiotic use, stress, and aging, can be restored through FMT. The main purpose of FMT is to restore the dysfunction in the intestines with a healthy bacterial flora transplantation. The potential use of FMT in treatment-resistant psychiatric disorders emerges through the restoration of impaired gut microbiota.

Chapter 25 provides an extensive review on neurosurgical interventions for treatment-resistant psychiatric disorders. Although neurosurgical intervention is best considered for patients with severe, disabling, and chronic psychiatric illness, this important therapeutic option should no longer be relegated to a position of last resort. The advent of MR image-guided high-intensity focused-ultrasound lesioning, stereotactic radiosurgery, deep brain stimulation, and cerebral neuromodulation has been revolutionary. Among other things, DBS offers reversibility and the possibility of implanting closed-loop systems.

I am grateful to all of contributors for their valuable time spending preparing manuscripts. They are leading research scientists with knowledge and expertise in their respective fields. It goes without saying that without their support, this book would not exist. I also wish to thank Mr. Vinoth Kuppan at Springer Nature Publisher, Inc. for his assistance in all aspects of this book. I believe that this book would function as a step on the path toward the ultimate goal of understanding and treating treatment-resistant psychiatric disorders.

Seoul, South Korea Yong-Ku Kim

Contents

Part I Rethinking the Treatment Resistance in Psychiatry

1 **Definition and Epidemiology of Treatment Resistance in Psychiatry** 3
Sanne Y. Smith-Apeldoorn, Jolien K. E. Veraart, and Robert A. Schoevers

2 **Paradigm Shift in Study of Treatment-Resistant Psychiatric Disorder** 25
Sang Won Jeon, Meysam Amidfar, and Yong-Ku Kim

3 **Genetic Factors Underlying Treatment Resistance in Psychiatry** 33
Eduard Maron, Chen-Chia Lan, and David Nutt

4 **Using Neuroimaging and Electroencephalography for Prediction of Treatment Resistance in Psychiatric Disorders** 65
Je-Yeon Yun and Seung-Hwan Lee

5 **Developing Therapies for Treatment-Resistant Depressive Disorder in Animal Models** 79
Michel Bourin

6 **Integrated Approaches for Treatment-Resistant Psychiatric Disorders** 87
Seon-Cheol Park and Yong-Ku Kim

Part II Treatment Resistance in Specific Disorders

7 **Treatment-Resistant Depression: Understandings on the Neurobiological Etiology that Lead to Novel Pharmacological Treatment Options** 99
Eunsoo Won, Byoung-Joo Ham, and Yong-Ku Kim

8 **Treatment-Resistant Schizophrenia: Assessment and Management** 109
Sandeep Grover, Harsh Garekar, and Anisha Agarwal

9 **Treatment Resistance in Bipolar Disorders** 139
Marsal Sanches, João Quevedo, and Jair C. Soares

10 **Treatment Resistance in Post-traumatic Stress Disorder** 151
Alexander Cowell McFarlane

11 **Treatment Resistance in Obsessive-Compulsive Disorder** 165
Rachel Middleton, Michael G. Wheaton, Reilly Kayser, and H. Blair Simpson

12 **Treatment of Opioid Dependence** 179
Michael Soyka

13 **Treatment-Resistant Panic Disorder** 189
Mu-Hong Chen and Shih-Jen Tsai

14 **Treatment Resistance in Anxiety Disorder: Generalized Anxiety Disorder and Social Anxiety Disorder** 207
Kang Soo Lee and Sang Hyuk Lee

15 **Treatment Resistance in Attention-Deficit/Hyperactivity Disorder** 215
Amber D. Hunt, David W. Dunn, Hillary S. Blake, and Jennifer Downs

16 **Treatment Resistance in Tourette Syndrome** 237
Renata Rizzo and Mariangela Gulisano

17 **Treatment-Resistant Eating Disorders** 253
Youl-Ri Kim and Jione Kim

18 **Comorbid Sleep and Wake Problems in Treatment-Resistant Psychiatric Conditions** 261
Seung-Gul Kang, Heon-Jeong Lee, Yong-Ku Kim, and Leen Kim

Part III Therapeutic Intervention for Treatment Resistance

19 **Creative, Person-Centered Psychopharmacology for Treatment Resistance in Psychiatry** 273
Miro Jakovljevic

20 **A Psychodynamic Approach to Treatment Resistance** 295
Elizabeth Weinberg, Erin Seery, and Eric M. Plakun

21 **Cognitive Behavioral Therapy and Behavioral Activation Therapy for Treatment-Resistant Depression: Traditional and Digital Therapy Perspectives** 311
Jennifer Apolinário-Hagen, Lara Fritsche, Liesemarie Albers, and Christel Salewski

22 Novel Neurostimulation Therapeutic Approaches for Treatment-Resistant Psychiatric Disorders 325
Ralph J. Koek, Janine Roach, Nicholas Athanasiou, and Arkady Korotinsky

23 When Clozapine Fails: Augmentation Strategies in the Management of Clozapine-Resistant Schizophrenia. . . . 349
Domenico De Berardis, Michele Fornaro, Annalisa Anastasia, Federica Vellante, Alessandro Valchera, Marilde Cavuto, Giampaolo Perna, Marco Di Nicola, Gianluca Serafini, Alessandro Carano, Maurizio Pompili, Laura Orsolini, Carmine Tomasetti, Gabriella Di Emidio, Giovanni Martinotti, and Massimo Di Giannantonio

24 Fecal Microbiota Transplantation in the Treatment-Resistant Psychiatric Disorders. 369
Alper Evrensel and Mehmet Emin Ceylan

25 Neurosurgical Intervention for Treatment-Resistant Psychiatric Disorders 377
Daniel E. Nijensohn and Teodoro Forcht Dagi

Index. 405

Part I

Rethinking the Treatment Resistance in Psychiatry

Definition and Epidemiology of Treatment Resistance in Psychiatry

1

Sanne Y. Smith-Apeldoorn, Jolien K. E. Veraart, and Robert A. Schoevers

1.1 Prevalence of Mental Disorders and Burden of Disease

Mental and substance use disorders are highly prevalent and account for a large proportion of disability across the world. Comparative epidemiological studies estimated the lifetime prevalence of psychiatric disorders in adults from different European and American countries to range from 12.2% to 48.6% [1]. The World Health Organization (WHO) estimated that 322 million people worldwide are affected by depression. The total estimated number of people having an anxiety disorder is 264 million. Bipolar disorders affect about 60 million people worldwide, and schizophrenia affects approximately 21 million people [2].

Sanne Smith-Apeldoorn and Jolien Veraart contributed equally to this work.

S. Y. Smith-Apeldoorn · J. K. E. Veraart
Department of Psychiatry, University Medical Center Groningen, University of Groningen, Groningen, The Netherlands
e-mail: s.y.apeldoorn@umcg.nl; j.k.e.veraart@umcg.nl

R. A. Schoevers (✉)
Department of Psychiatry, University Medical Center Groningen, University of Groningen, Research School of Behavioural and Cognitive Neurosciences (BCN), Interdisciplinary Center for Psychopathology and Emotion regulation (ICPE), Groningen, The Netherlands
e-mail: r.a.schoevers@umcg.nl

Psychiatric disorders have significant consequences for patients, their families, and communities. They lead to disability and a reduced quality of life and are the most important cause of self-harm, suicide attempts and completed suicides. WHO studies on the global burden of disease of approximately 300 different disorders showed that mental and substance use disorders account for 7.4% of all disability-adjusted life years (DALYs) worldwide. One DALY represents the loss of 1 year of healthy life, and the burden of disease is the sum of these DALYs across the population. A DALY is calculated as the sum of mortality (years of life lost, YLL) and morbidity/disability (years lost due to disability, YLD). Furthermore, mental and substance use disorders are the leading cause of years lost due to disability (YLDs) worldwide and account for no less than 22.9% of all YLDs [3]. In line with this, two mental disorders were in the top ten of leading medical causes of disability (Table 1.1).

The large contribution of mental and substance use disorders to disability is a result of the high prevalence of mental disorders [1], the early age of onset [1], the substantial impairment in people's ability to function [4] and the tendency towards a chronic or recurrent course [5] of illness.

Unfortunately, only a minority of patients suffering from psychiatric disorders receive adequate treatment, and initial treatment is often delayed for years. This treatment gap in mental

Y.-K. Kim (ed.), *Treatment Resistance in Psychiatry*, https://doi.org/10.1007/978-981-10-4358-1_1

Table 1.1 Leading causes of global YLDs 2015

1	Lower back and neck pain
2	Sense organ disease
3	Depressive disorders
4	Iron-deficiency anaemia
5	Skin diseases
6	Diabetes
7	Migraine
8	Other musculoskeletal disorders
9	Anxiety disorders
10	Oral disorders
11	Asthma
12	Schizophrenia
13	Osteoarthritis
14	COPD
15	Falls
16	Autistic spectrum
17	Gynaecological diseases
18	Drug use disorders
19	Other mental and substance
20	Medication overuse headache
21	Bipolar disorder
22	Congenital anomalies
23	Haemoglobinopathies
24	Chronic kidney disease
25	Ischaemic heart disease
26	Alzheimer's disease
27	Alcohol use disorders
28	Epilepsy
29	Other cardiovascular
30	Conduct disorder
31	Other unintentional
32	Diarrhoeal diseases
33	Intestinal nematode

health care is caused by different factors concerning the patients, the mental health system and the health-care providers.

Patients may fail to recognize or underestimate the symptoms of a psychiatric disorder; they could be prevented from seeking psychiatric care due to stigma, or they might be noncompliant to treatment once it has been offered. Other important factors are limited access to care and financial considerations (e.g. lack of insurance coverage).

Provider-based reasons include poor education about psychiatric disorders and the benefits of different supportive, psychotherapeutic and pharmacotherapeutic treatment approaches, having limited time to evaluate and treat mental disorders and prescription of medication in inadequate doses or for inadequate durations [6].

The WHO estimates that in middle- and low-income countries, between 76% and 85% of patients receive no treatment for their mental disorder. This rate is between 35% and 50% in high-income countries. Even in severe and often persistent psychiatric disorders like schizophrenia, approximately one third of patients still remain untreated [2].

1.2 Treatment Outcomes in Psychiatry

Apart from the high prevalence rates of psychiatric disorders and the significant treatment gap in mental health, the efficacy of psychiatric treatment is an important issue to address. Psychiatric treatments, and psychotropic drugs in particular, have been subject of criticism and mistrust, in spite of randomized controlled trials (RCTs) supporting efficacy. This might be partly caused by the fact that the aetiology of many psychiatric disorders and the mechanisms of action of different treatment options are not fully understood. Other reasons could be the lack of diagnostic tests, side effects or a commercial conflict of interest. Critics claim that pharmaceutical industries are corrupted; they would underreport side effects and withhold evidence of clinical drug trials for commercial reasons [7, 8]. Publication bias, the interpretation of efficacy, and the efficacy of psychiatric treatments will be further addressed.

1.2.1 Publication Bias

It has clearly been demonstrated that publication bias plays a role in the reporting of pharmacotherapy treatment outcomes of randomized controlled trials in mental disorders. Turner et al. compared the efficacy of antidepressants derived from published literature with drug efficacy inferred from Food and Drug Administration (FDA) reviews. Drug companies have to preregister all trials they aim to use for marketing approval in an FDA database. In depression, they found a bias towards publication of positive results. The published results in scientific journals overestimated the outcomes of the original studies submitted to the FDA by around 30% [9]. Furthermore, favourable secondary outcomes were sometimes highlighted instead of negative primary outcomes, also giving the impression of higher clinical benefit [10].

In the reporting of trials of second-generation antipsychotics in the treatment of schizophrenia or schizoaffective disorder, Turner et al. also found indications for publication bias [11]. Of the 24 FDA-registered trials, 4 remained unpublished. Three of these trials failed to show superiority of the study drug over placebo, and one trial showed inferiority of the study drug compared to an inexpensive active drug. However, the difference between the point estimate mean effect size (the standardized mean difference) derived from published data and from FDA reviews was smaller in schizophrenia, and it was not statistically significant (8% increase due to publication bias).

In anxiety disorders, reporting bias inflated the effect size of second-generation antidepressants by 15% with differences between individual anxiety disorders, ranging from 6% in generalized anxiety disorder to 25% in panic disorder. RCTs that were deemed positive by the FDA had a five times higher chance of being published than non-positive trials [12].

Furthermore, reports of publication bias were found for aripiprazole, lamotrigine and gabapentin in the treatment of bipolar disorder. The role of sponsorship became clear when it was shown that published efficacy results in industry-sponsored studies are more favourable than the results in studies with other forms of funding [10].

It can be concluded that treatment outcomes of psychotropic drugs have undoubtedly been mispresented in the literature, which is a very serious concern for the whole field. And this is not unique for the results of pharmacotherapy: in psychotherapy there has been a similar overestimation of the effects in meta-analytical studies [13, 14]. Cuijpers et al. assessed the quality of 115 randomized controlled trials examining psychotherapy for depression based on eight criteria. In the high-quality studies, considerably smaller effect sizes (0.22) were found than in other studies (0.74), although the effects of psychotherapy in depression remained statistically significant. In a meta-analytic study of publication bias, Cuijpers et al. examined funnel plots; graphs designed to test for publication bias. Studies are assumed to be spread evenly on both sides of the average, creating a funnel-shaped distribution. Asymmetry in funnel plots is an indication for publication bias. In this meta-analysis, the overall effect size of studies comparing psychotherapy and a control condition was 0.67, and the mean effect size after adjustment for publication bias was 0.42 [13]. Turner et al. identified randomized clinical trials funded by the US National Institutes of Health grants and added the data of the unpublished studies to the published studies. Hereby, the point estimate effect size of psychotherapy when compared to control conditions was reduced by 25% (from Hedges' g = 0.52–0.39). It seems that factors other than the commercial interest of pharmaceutical companies also seem to play a role [10].

Factors implicated in publication bias are a possible reluctance of authors to submit manuscripts with negative or inconclusive results and a similar lack of willingness of journals to accept such manuscripts. Researchers might fear a negative influence on future grant applications or might feel reluctant to submit results that do not support their hypotheses. On the other hand, readers show a preference for positive research findings, and manuscripts with positive results are more likely to be accepted for publication by reviewers [10]. Publication bias is not restricted to psychiatry; it is widespread throughout the medical literature and other areas of science (including chemistry and physics). This is receiving much more attention now than before, and a number of safeguards have been implemented by all major medical journals that should significantly reduce the possibility of bias in published literature. These include publication of detailed trial protocols on websites such as clinicaltrials.gov prior to study start and mandatory reporting of primary outcomes. We fully agree with Ioannidis who stated that "The major strength of science is not in being always perfect, but in correcting mistakes, fallacies, and misconceptions using the best evidence and critical thinking" [15].

1.2.2 Efficacy

Review articles considering the efficacy of antidepressants and antipsychotics show smaller drug-placebo differences than we might intuitively expect [16, 17]. Kirsch et al. [16] found antidepressants to be effective when compared to placebo only in patients suffering from severe depression. This effect was attributed to a decreased responsiveness to placebo among patients with severe depression. However, different studies have refuted this [18–21]. These studies re-analysed the available data and showed no relationship between drug-placebo differences and baseline depression severity. They furthermore concluded that antidepressants are clearly superior to placebo in achieving antidepressant response, also in mildly depressed patients. Leucht et al. [17] found a relatively small absolute difference of 18% in responder rates between placebo and antipsychotics in patients with schizophrenia. In their meta-analysis, the pooled effect size for change of overall symptoms was 0.51.

Different factors contribute to the efficacy found and shown in studies that compare psychopharmacologic drugs to placebo, like outcome variables, reporting methods, placebo effects and nonspecific factors.

1.2.2.1 Outcome Variables

Primary outcomes in psychiatric treatments are not only reduction of disease severity and prevention of future episodes but also, for instance, reduction of suicide rates. As an example, the efficacy of maintenance treatment with lithium in prevention of depression is low (SMD 0.2), whereas the efficacy for preventing any relapse is high (SMD 1.12). Acute treatment of mania with lithium shows average efficacy (SMD 0.41). Furthermore, lithium may reduce suicide rates in mood disorders [22, 23]. With concern to antidepressants and antipsychotics, meta-analyses found higher efficacy of antidepressants [24, 25] and antipsychotics [26] compared to placebo in relapse prevention than in acute treatment. Many psychiatric treatments do not only ameliorate symptoms during the acute episode but also prevent relapses, and only long-term studies can demonstrate this. Therefore, the duration of the study should always be taken into account. Funding issues play a role in the amount of evidence that is available.

1.2.2.2 Reporting Methods

The method of reporting study results is important in the interpretation of the effectiveness (Table 1.2). In studies measuring dichotomous outcomes, commonly used measures to quantify the effect are the relative and absolute risk reductions (RRR, ARR) and the number needed to treat (NNT) to prevent one negative outcome. Absolute risk reduction represents the change in the risk of an outcome as a result of a therapy in relation to a comparison therapy. The relative risk reduction is calculated by dividing the ARR by the risk in the control group (the baseline risk). As an example statins have been shown to reduce the risk for cardiovascular events from 18% to 14%. The absolute risk difference is (18 − 14 =) 4%; however, the relative risk reduction is ((1 − (0.14/0.18)) × 100 =) 22%. Clinicians seem to overestimate therapeutic effectiveness when only the RRR is presented [27]. Therefore, reporting the ARR with the baseline risk is important for clinical decision-making.

In studies with continuous outcomes, the standardized mean difference (SMD) is used to report effectiveness. The SMD is the difference between the new treatment improvement and the comparator treatment improvement, divided by the pooled standard deviation. Cohen's rule states that an SMD of 0.2 is a small effect size, 0.5 medium and 0.8 a large effect size. However, the SMD should be interpreted within the context. As it is relative to the pooled standard deviation,

Table 1.2 Explanation of measures to quantify the effect of interventions

	Experimental group (E)	Control group (C)
Events (E)	EE	CE
Non-events (N)	EN	CN
Total subjects (S)	ES = EE + EN	CS = CE + CN
Events rate (ER)	EER = EE/ES	CER = CE/CS

Abbreviation	Variable	Equation/explanation
ARR	Absolute risk reduction	EER – CER
RRR	Relative risk reduction	(EER – CER)/CER
NNT	Number needed to treat	1/(EER – CER)
RR	Relative risk	EER/CER
OR	Odds ratio	(EE/EN)/(CE/CN)
ES	Effect size	Measures the strength of the relationship between two variables
SMD	Standardized mean difference	Expresses the difference in means in standard deviation units; (mean experimental group – mean control group)/pooled standard deviation

a large variability in scores reduces the SMD. This is often seen in psychiatry, when rating scales are used for heterogeneous diseases such as depression.

1.2.2.3 Placebo Effects

Different factors influencing the size of placebo effects have been identified, such as the manner in which a treatment (active or inactive) is presented. A larger amount of pills shows better effects than fewer pills, intravenous administration is superior to oral administration, and the cost of treatments, elaborate accompanying rituals or invasive sham conditions and the use of a well-known brand name may also be of influence [28].

The expectancy theory states that patients who expect to receive an effective treatment experience a reduction in their symptoms. This was supported by the finding of higher placebo effects in trials with an increased change of receiving active treatment, for instance, in trials comparing two active drug arms with an inert placebo arm. This occurred in different psychiatric disorders such as schizophrenia, psychosis and depression [29]. Additionally, in a trial in which tricyclic antidepressants were compared to an inactive and an active placebo arm, the effect of the active placebo was superior to the effect of the inert placebo [30]. The physiological reaction to active drugs such as side effects might increase the expectation of a positive effect and lead to clinical improvement. On the other hand, when patients do not experience any physiological changes in response to an inert placebo, they are more likely to lower their expectations of the intervention leading to a decrease in effect. In addition, early improvement in patients receiving more effective drugs increases the expectation of receiving an effective treatment and in itself produces additional placebo effects. Via these mechanisms, side effects and symptom reduction lead to unblinding and may inflate the placebo effect in patients receiving active drugs [31].

Another factor influencing the size of the placebo effect is associated with the practitioner administrating the intervention. When the doctors have positive beliefs about the efficacy of the treatment, outcomes are better than when they assume the intervention is ineffective. This was shown in a study of analgesia in which all patients received inactive placebo. Pain scores were significantly lower when the practitioners believed the injection could contain fentanyl in comparison with pain scores when doctors believed the injection might contain naloxone [32]. Doctors who are positive and optimistic increased the effectiveness of a placebo intervention when compared to doctors who were more indifferent [33].

1.2.2.4 Nonspecific Effects

Many psychiatric disorders are self-limiting or show spontaneous variation in symptom severity. These changes are part of the natural course of the disorder and may incorrectly be ascribed to treatment. Furthermore, improved medical care (e.g. increased contact with researchers and examinations) during clinical trials could induce a decrease in symptoms. Moreover, interventions are often initiated when symptoms are most severe. They will then tend to improve over time, independent of the intervention. On the other hand, symptom severity can also be inflated by patients or researchers before study participation, to meet entry criteria. After recruitment for the study, this is no longer required which can cause a decrease in symptoms shortly after treatment initiation. Changes in the circumstances of the patient or seasonal variations can also impact the measurements. Other relevant factors in the course of the study are the learning curves of clinicians and patients. Practitioners become more skilled in performing the interventions and measurements later on in the trial. Patients can become acquainted with the clinical setting and interventions which might influence the way they experience their symptoms. Furthermore, a statistical phenomenon called regression towards the mean occurs when measuring biological variables. If a measurement is extreme, subsequent measurements will tend to be closer to the average. Another relevant phenomenon is the Hawthorne effect, also known as the observer effect, which implies that patients modify an aspect of their behaviour (e.g. smoking, alcohol consumption or exercise) in reaction to receiving medical attention [34].

1.2.3 Efficacy of Psychiatric Treatments

Below, we will summarize the efficacy of different psychiatric treatments for several mental disorders (Table 1.3).

1.2.3.1 Major Depressive Disorder

Recent meta-analyses (conducted in mainly outpatients) show absolute responder differences of 10–15% for selective serotonin reuptake inhibitors (SSRIs) and tricyclic antidepressants (TCAs) versus placebo [35]. Paroxetine, for instance, increases the response percentage from 42% to 53% [36]. Maintenance treatment with antidepressants reduces the relapse rate from 41% in the placebo group to 18% [24, 37]. Cognitive behavioural therapy (CBT) leads to a standardized mean difference (SMD) of 0.7 in depression when compared to treatment as usual control conditions, such as general practitioner management [38].

1.2.3.2 Schizophrenia

Antipsychotics for the acute treatment of psychosis show a response rate of 41%, compared to 24% in the placebo group [17]. For maintenance treatment, the relapse rate is 27% after 1 year, whereas the relapse rate in the placebo group is 64% [39].

1.2.3.3 Bipolar Disorder

Acute mania treatment increases the proportion of patients responding from 34% in the placebo group to 52% with lithium [40] and from 31% with placebo to 50% with antipsychotics [41]. Relapse rates are 36% in maintenance treatment with lithium versus 81% in patients with placebo [42] or from 61% to 40% after the exclusion of studies in which lithium was suddenly discontinued [24]. Acute treatment with antidepressants in bipolar depression increases the response rate from 34% with placebo to 58% [43].

1.2.3.4 Obsessive-Compulsive Disorder (OCD)

In the acute phase, SSRIs are more effective than placebo in patients with OCD in reducing symptoms. They show a response rate of 43% in comparison with 23% with placebo when overall symptoms are measured [44]. A meta-analysis showed that outpatient CBT is also effective in reducing OCD-specific symptoms (SMD 1.46) [45].

1.2.3.5 Panic Disorder

TCAs, SSRIs and benzodiazepines have a SMD of 0.40–0.41 in the acute treatment of panic disorders [46].

1.2.3.6 Attention-Deficit Hyperactivity Disorder

Robust effect sizes in the overall reduction of attention-deficit hyperactivity disorder symptoms are shown in the treatment with methylphenidate (SMD 0.78), amphetamines (SMD 1.00) and atomoxetine (SMD 0.64) [47–49].

1.2.4 Putting Psychiatric Treatment Efficacy in Perspective

Leucht et al. compared the efficacy of psychiatric pharmacotherapy to medical interventions for common diseases in general medicine [50]. It was emphasized that comparison of treatments for different diseases can only be qualitative and should only be used as a way to place psychiatric treatments into perspective. Medication efficacy of common medical and psychiatric disorders were compared using data from 94 meta-analyses (48 drugs in 20 medical diseases and 16 drugs in 8 psychiatric disorders). An arbitrary selection of the general medication discussed in the review of Leucht et al. is listed in Table 1.4. The authors of the review article identified common somatic diseases by consensus, based on frequency, importance and availability of treatment. They identified primary treatments by consulting national and international guidelines.

The effect sizes of psychiatric drugs were found to be in the same range as most drugs in general medicine. However, both in psychiatry and general medicine, there is large variation in the efficacy of interventions. Therefore, the efficacy of treatment should always be evaluated in the context of the severity and duration of the disease, the natural course, outcome measurements, side effects and adverse events.

1.3 The Definition of Treatment Resistance

The term treatment resistance is widely used in the context of psychiatric disorders. But defining it, both conceptually and in practice, has proven to be complex. However, terminology is essential in decision-making in clinical practice, in making meaningful comparisons across studies and in identifying predictors of a variety of outcomes.

Although apparently similar, the terminology used to describe treatment resistance varies. Alternative terms or expressions – like (treatment) refractory and pharmacotherapy resistant – are often used interchangeably. Regarding the word “refractory”, to some authors it suggests a greater degree of resistance or even the inability to respond to any current or novel treatment [52]. For reasons of clarity and because the term “resistant” has been applied more frequently in the literature, we will only use the term treatment resistance in this chapter.

In spite of the fact that there is no full agreement regarding the definition of treatment resistance of psychiatric disorders in general, neither for specific mental disorders, treatment resistance clearly refers to the occurrence of an inadequate response following adequate treatment. These

Table 1.3 Efficacy of psychiatric interventions versus placebo according to systematic reviews

Disorder	Acute versus maintenance	Therapy	Outcome	SMD	95% CI	NNT/H	95% CI
Major depressive disorder	Acute episode	Paroxetine	Response	0.24	0.18–0.30	10	8–14
			HAM-D	0.31	0.22–0.40		
		TCAs	Response	0.35	0.28–0.42	7	5–8
			HAM-D	0.33	0.27–0.39		
		Fluoxetine	Response	0.35	0.26–0.45	7	
			HAM-D	0.30	0.21–0.39		
		New ADs	HAM-D	0.32	0.25–0.40		
		TCAs (low dose)	Response	0.40	0.26–0.54	4	
			Severity	0.40	0.21–0.59		
		CBT	Self-report (e.g. BDI)	0.7	0.49–0.90		
	Maintenance treatment	ADs	Relapse	0.64	0.56–0.71	4	
		New ADs	Recurrence	0.53	0.45–0.61	5	4–6
		Lithium	Relapse	0.92	0.61–1.23	3	
Schizophrenia	Acute treatment	SGAs	Response	0.43	0.36–0.51	6	5–7
			PANSS/BPRS	0.51	0.43–0.58		
		Haloperidol	Response	0.30	0.16–0.43	9	6–15
			PANSS/BPRS	0.53	0.43–0.64		
	Maintenance treatment	Antipsychotics	Relapse	0.92	0.86–0.97	3	2–3
Bipolar disorder	Acute manic episode	Lithium	Response	0.41	0.25–0.57	6	4–13
			YMRS/MRS	0.40	0.28–0.53		
		Valporate	Response	0.66	0.30–1.02	4	3–7
			YMRS/MRS	0.40	0.21–0.66		
		Carbamazepine	Response	0.61	0.39–0.83	4	3–8
			YMRS	0.53	0.31–0.75		
		SGAs and haloperidol	Response	0.44	0.36–0.53	5	4–7
			YMRS/MRS/MS	0.45	0.32–0.57		
	Depressive episode	ADs	Response	0.53	0.36–0.71	4	2–7
	Maintenance treatment	Lithium	AR	1.12	0.88–1.37	2	
		Lithium	AR	0.47	0.31–0.63	5	3–13
			MR	0.36	0.12–0.60	10	5–100
			DR	0.20	0.00–0.40	14	H100-T6
		Valproate	AR	0.37	0.09–0.65	7	4–33
			MR	0.16	−0.16 to 0.49	20	H20 – T7
			DR	0.56	0.12–1.01	10	18–80

Obsessive compulsive disorder		SSRIs	YBOCS	0.44	0.36–0.52		
			Response	0.53	0.44–0.62	5	4–6
		Clomipramine	YBOCS	0.48	0.34–0.62		
		Various SSRIs	YBOCS	0.31	0.21–0.41		
		CBT	YBOCS	1.46	1.17–1.75		
Panic disorder		TCAs	Anxiety	0.41			
		SSRIs	Anxiety	0.41			
		Benzodiazepines	Anxiety	0.40			
Attention-deficit hyperactivity disorder		Methylphenidate	Hyperactivity	0.78	0.64–0.91		
		Amphetamine	ADHD symptoms	1.00	0.91–1.10		

ADs antidepressants, *AR* any relapse, *CBT* cognitive behavioural therapy, *CI* confidence interval, *DR* depressive relapse, *HAM-D* Hamilton Depression Rating Scale for Depression, *MR* manic relapse, *NNT/H* number needed to treat or number needed to harm, *PANSS/BPRS* total score of either the Positive and Negative Syndrome Scale or the Brief Psychiatric Rating Scale, *SDM* standardized difference of means, *SGA* second-generation antipsychotics, *SSRIs* selective serotonin reuptake inhibitors, *TCAs* tricyclic antidepressants, *YBOCS* Yale-Brown Obsessive Compulsive Scale, *YMRS* Young Mania Rating Scale [50, 51]

Table 1.4 Efficacy of medication for somatic disorders, selection from the article of Leucht et al. [50]

Disorder	Therapy	Outcome	SMD	95% CI	NNT	95% CI
Cardiovascular disease	Acetylsalicylic acid	Primary prevention of CV events	0.06	−0.03 to 0. 16	1429/year	Unknown
Hypertension	Beta-blockers	CV events and mortality	0.08	0.02–0.14	100	Unknown
	ACE-inhibitors	CV events and mortality	0.16	0.12–0.21	25	Unknown
Diabetes	Metformin	Fasting glucose (mmol/l)	0.87	0.61–1.13	Unknown	Unknown
	Metformin	Mortality	0.27	0.06–0.47	14	8–50
Reflux oesophagitis	PPI	Clinical remission	1.39	1.18–1.60	2	2–2
Chronic heart failure	Diuretics	Worsening	1.88	0.32–3.44	7	3–100
Chronic hepatitis C	Interferon	Virol. resp.	2.27	1.49–3.04	3	2–4

SMD standardized mean difference, *CI* confidence interval, *NNT* number needed to treat, *CV* cardiovascular, *PPI* proton-pump inhibitors, *virol. resp.* virological response two parts of the definition, (adequate) treatment and (inadequate) response, will be further addressed.

1.3.1 Defining Treatment

1.3.1.1 Pseudo-resistance

When evaluating possible treatment resistance, one first needs to ascertain whether a patient has received adequate treatment. The term pseudo-resistance has been used in reference to nonresponse to inadequate treatment. Patients with pseudo-resistance, for example, did not receive the right form of treatment, the duration and dose (for medication) or intensity (for psychotherapy) may have been insufficient, the way the treatment was delivered may not have been adequate, or the patient was non-adherent. Only after pseudo-resistance has been ruled out, true treatment resistance can be considered.

1.3.1.2 Adequate Treatment

Adequate treatment is often defined as treatment that accords with nationally and internationally developed professional treatment guidelines and standards. But treatment regimens are not static phenomena, as they are subject to substantial changes over time. They also offer limited guidance for making specific choices, for example, when a clinician and patient have the possibility to choose between available drug treatments within one class. Furthermore, they do not take into account the unique pathophysiology and clinical characteristics of each individual patient. So it is clear that adequate treatment for any specific patient remains a combination of scientific evidence, clinical wisdom and patient preference. Nevertheless, current guidelines provide an established foundation for the working definition of adequate treatment.

1.3.1.3 Assessing Treatment Adequacy

First of all, a basic requirement in assessing treatment adequacy is the accuracy of the diagnosis of the patient, to ensure that the treatment that is chosen matches the diagnosis (or diagnoses). Misdiagnosis can be relatively common in clinical practice, and one approach to this problem is that of completing a diagnostic re-evaluation, ideally with a structured clinical interview.

With concern to biological treatment, it is important to assess whether the doses prescribed to the patient were in the therapeutic ranges and to assess the duration of the treatment. Unfortunately, more than half of the patients referred for an evaluation of insufficient therapeutic response are assumed to have had inadequate trials of psychiatric medication [53]. An example is a study by Rasmussen et al. in patients with unipolar depression, who found that among patients with a psychotic depression, 95% had not been given an adequate combination of an antidepressant and antipsychotic agent. Among patients with a nonpsychotic depression, 27% had not had an adequate trial of an antidepressant before being referred for electroconvulsive therapy [54]. But even when a trial meets the criteria for adequacy in terms of dose and duration, there are varying degrees of adequacy. For example, in the treatment of major depressive disorder, the duration of the trial could be barely adequate (e.g. 4 weeks) or more substantial (e.g. 10 weeks). It has been suggested that more prolonged trials, sometimes lasting more than 10 weeks, may lead to a therapeutic response in certain resistant cases [55]. Similarly, the dosing could be the minimum effective dose or the maximum tolerated one. These factors can contribute to a marked variability in the degree of response. For some drugs, efficacy is clearly correlated with the presence of adequate plasma levels. This is the case in, for example, the TCAs imipramine, amitriptyline, nortriptyline and clomipramine [56–58] and for (concomitant) the administration of lithium [59].

Certain pharmacokinetic factors may also contribute to inadequate biological treatment. Given that there is an estimated 30-fold range of drug metabolism among individuals [60], it is not uncommon that patients who fail to respond to treatment may do so as a result of less than optimal plasma drug concentrations. For example, the concomitant use of metabolic inducers (e.g. drugs that may increase the metabolism and elimination rate of co-administered agents) may be associated with a relative reduction in blood levels of psychotropic drugs. Also tobacco reduces the blood levels of a number of psychotropic drugs, like the antipsychotics clozapine and olanzapine and the antidepressant fluvoxamine [61]. A similar problem may occur among patients who are fast metabolizers. The presence of polymorphic alleles for cytochrome P (CYP) 450 may result in lack of expression, altered levels of expression or altered function of CYP450 enzymes. Some of these enzymes, for example, CYP2D6, CYP1A2, and CYP3A4/5, are major enzymes in the metabolism of antipsychotics. Polymorphisms of alleles for these enzymes are associated with altered plasma levels of plasma drug concentrations [62]. Consequently, standard dosing may result in drug plasma concentrations that are subtherapeutic in some patients. Nonresponse in the absence of any side effect should raise the possibility of less than adequate blood levels. In such cases, determining polymorphisms may be warranted, and dosage adjustments may produce a significant treatment improvement. Research shows that clinicians not always consider this. Furthermore, doctors and pharmacists are not always aware of relevant polymorphisms, even if they are known [63].

With concern to psychological treatment, it is important to assess the type and quality of the treatment [64] and the number of sessions attended [65]. Unfortunately, patients in primary care as well as in general psychiatry clinics most often do not receive adequate psychological treatment [64]. While, for example, CBT is well known and taught in some psychology graduate programmes, many more provide inadequate training. At the same time, many therapists may purport to "do CBT", when all they do is provide basic education and skills [64].

Another important step towards the assessment of treatment adequacy concerns the level of treatment adherence. Estimates of the extent of non-adherence vary between 20% and 72% (Table 1.5). These numbers do not differ significantly from those in patients with somatic medical conditions (66).

Factors related to medication non-adherence may be patient-related (e.g. younger age, male gender, lower education level and comorbid substance dependence), psychological (e.g. poor insight, denial of illness and negative attitude towards medication), medication-related (e.g. side effects and more complex dosing schedule) and social and environmental (e.g. lower quality of therapeutic alliance, fewer outpatient visits and lack of family support) [66].

Table 1.5 Rates of non-adherence by psychiatric diagnosis, from the article of Julius et al.

Diagnosis	Rates of non-adherence
Major depressive disorder	28–52%
Bipolar disorder	20–50%
Schizophrenia	20–72%
Anxiety disorders	57%

Unfortunately clinicians are not always very accurate in estimating whether their patients actually follow their advice. Therefore, a check to establish treatment adequacy needs to be carried out to rule out the possibility of pseudo-resistance. An assessment of adherence may allow for systematic monitoring through a variety of methods, e.g. patients' self-report, pill count, measuring blood levels or a diary.

1.3.2 Defining Response

It is important to specify response, in order to understand treatment resistance as an inability to attain it. But what constitutes (in)adequate response has been an object of considerable debate in the field, and moreover, it is different in a clinical context compared to a research context.

1.3.2.1 Treatment Outcome in Clinical Context

In clinical practice, response is used to gauge decision-making, such as when to modify, augment and switch treatment strategy. Response can be considered as a continuum that ranges from nonresponse to partial response, to remission and finally to full recovery.

The more traditional view of treatment resistance has focused on nonresponse, e.g. patients who have reported minimal or no improvement. Nowadays, most clinicians focus on remission and recovery. The rationale for this approach is that symptom remission, as opposed to response with residual symptoms, is consistently shown to be associated with better outcome. For example, currently most experts would argue that inadequate response in major depressive disorder is the failure to achieve remission [67, 68]. The definitions of inadequate response in schizophrenia and anxiety disorders comprise the failure to achieve symptomatic remission as well; additionally, also functional criteria are often integrated [53, 69, 70].

Remission, unlike response, entails an absolute allowable ceiling level of symptoms. Several operational definitions of remission have been proposed over the years. One of the definitions that still stands is of Frank et al. [71]. They conceptualized remission of depression as a "relatively brief (> E days but < F days) period during which an improvement of sufficient magnitude is observed that the individual is asymptomatic (i.e. no longer meets syndromal criteria for the disorder and has no more than minimal symptoms)". They furthermore added that a "declaration of remission implies that no increase in the intensity of the treatment regimen is required". In line with this definition, according to Jakovljevic [53], remission in general typically implies the attainment of an asymptomatic stage or at least very substantial improvements in symptom severity.

If remission is sustained, it may transmute to recovery. However, the absence of symptoms does not always mean recovery. One has to make a distinction between syndromal recovery (e.g. "no longer fulfilling the formal criteria of a disorder") and functional recovery (e.g. "return to the pre-illness level of functioning"). A psychiatric disorder by definition affects functioning, but also over time mental disorders are associated with substantial impairment in functioning and quality of life, even after recovery from the syndromal episodes. For example, remission of major depressive disorder, bipolar disorder or anxiety disorders is not associated with full restoration of health-related quality of life, even among those without comorbid disorders [72]. And besides, even a year after syndromal recovery, patients with major depressive disorder or bipolar disorder still experience more functional impairments than healthy controls [73].

1.3.2.2 Treatment Outcome in Research Context

In contrast with the clinical context, in research inadequate response is rarely defined as failure to achieve remission or recovery. Maybe because remission and recovery may occur weeks, months or even years after response, it is more practical to use either lack of response or the persistence of clinically significant levels of symptoms, rather than the lack of remission or recovery [55, 68].

Response in research context is conventionally a reduction in baseline symptomatology of 50% or more, as measured on standard rating scales. A symptom reduction of 25–49% can be called a partial response. Given the persistent and severe nature of some cases of treatment resistance, even a 25–49% reduction in baseline symptom severity can provide a clinically meaningful benefit.

It is interesting that when response is determined in research, no real distinction is drawn between the various symptoms of a disorder. This means that a quantitatively similar response can reflect improvement across very different symptom domains. However, these domains can clinically be very different [74].

1.3.2.3 Measuring Treatment Outcome

The use of measures of outcome is a necessary aspect of ascertaining (in)adequate response. We cannot be sure that response to treatment is (in) adequate, unless we have a careful and systematic assessment of symptoms. Both in clinical practice and research, the use of reliable and valid measures of outcome is advised [67].

There are several well-established clinician-rated and self-rating instruments, which have shown good sensitivity to assess the degree of response following treatment in patients with mental disorders. With concern to clinician-rated instruments, it should be noted though that they are subject to clinicians' biases, that clinicians are often quite inconsistent in using instruments and that residual symptoms are not always adequately measured.

Self-rating instruments may eliminate these aspects. They also provide a useful tool to gain insight into patients' perceptions, their use allows patients to become actively involved in treatment, and they provide the advantage of taking less clinician time. However, these instruments also have some limitations. Their use might be limited in patients with significant cognitive impairment, poor motivation and limited reading skills. They also could be less suited to measure some aspects of behaviour and symptoms associated with poor insight.

Another aspect concerns the timing of gathering of information, especially in research. Prospective gathering of information eliminates the confounding effect of the patients' recall bias, but patients who are currently symptomatic may underestimate the degree of improvement experienced [67].

1.3.3 When Does Inadequate Response Become Treatment Resistance?

How many and which steps of adequate treatment render an individual "treatment resistant"? The number and sort of failed adequate steps may range from one to countless. And what role does non-biological treatment play? Definitions of treatment resistance focus predominantly on failures of pharmacotherapy and physical treatments, with only modest consideration given to outcomes following psychological therapies and social interventions, perhaps because the latter can be less reliably quantified [74]? However, since there is good evidence that psychological and social interventions are effective in the treatment of several mental disorders [75–77], one can argue that a definition of treatment resistance without paying attention to non-biological treatment is too narrow.

There is no consensus on when inadequate response becomes treatment resistance. For example, concerning the mood disorders, treatment-resistant depression has many different definitions. There is no clear agreement regarding either the minimum number of previous antidepressant trials required or of the need for medication to be of similar or different classes. Neither is there consensus about the trials that should be considered in the definition (i.e. those administered only during the current episode or those given as part of previous episodes too). Furthermore, definitions differ regarding the minimum duration necessary for a previous treatment to be considered as unsuccessful, ranging from 4 to 8 weeks, and in terms of the minimum required dose(s). For example, some studies require 200–300 mg/day of imipramine for considering a previous treatment as adequate, whereas others require 100 mg/day. Additionally, some authors use blood levels to determine the adequacy of imipramine treatment. And the same holds for treatment outcome: many authors use "lack of response" or "failure" as their main outcome, and some use "nonremission" or terms such as "refractoriness" or "absence of significant clinical improvement" [68].

To cater for this lack of consensual operational criteria, several authors have proposed staging models to conceptualize treatment resistance in depression. These models range from single antidepressant adequacy ratings to multidimensional and more continuous models, the latter basically considering greater and lesser degrees of resistance. Some of these models also take into consideration the intensity and optimization of each trial, augmentation and combination strategies and psychotherapy [78, 79].

1.3.3.1 Relapse and Recurrences During Continued Treatment

A special form of treatment resistance is represented by the return of symptoms during treatment. This is a common clinical occurrence. In fact, relapses and recurrences during continued treatment appear to occur at rates between 10% and 67% in depression [55], between 10% and 40% in anxiety disorders [80, 81] and in 27% of patients with schizophrenia [39]. Typically, relapses and recurrences during treatment are not included in the most definitions of treatment resistance, maybe because the pathophysiology of these two clinical events is suggested to be distinct [55, 67].

1.4 Prevalence of Treatment Resistance and Risk Factors

Given the lack of consistence in defining criteria, it is difficult to give a reliable figure for the prevalence of treatment resistance in mental disorders. But despite this difficulty, and although some disorders generally show a better response to currently available treatments than others, the overall prevalence of treatment resistance is substantial.

In the largest treatment for depression study to date, the Sequenced Treatment Alternatives to Relieve Depression (STAR*D), 49% of patients showed response, and 37% showed remission after the first treatment with an antidepressant. Remission rates gradually declined with each sequential step thereafter. After four treatment trials, 33% of patients had not achieved remission [82].

Around 98% of the patients with bipolar disorder achieve syndromal recovery from their initial manic or mixed episode within 2 years. Almost 20% of these patients switch directly into an episode of depression, mixed state or psychosis [83, 84]. Nonresponse in bipolar depression is highly prevalent and occurs in more than 40% of patients after treatment with a mood stabilizer. The addition of antidepressants to an ongoing treatment with mood stabilizers is helpful in only a quarter of patients with bipolar depression [85]. By 2 years, 72% of patients with bipolar disorder achieve symptomatic recovery, and around 40% achieve functional recovery [83, 84].

Of patients with a first-episode psychosis, 10–50% show long-term incomplete remission or treatment resistance [70]. Depending on the definition, 20–60% of patients with schizophrenia do not respond to treatment with conventional antipsychotics [86].

In the field of anxiety, one can assume that approximately 30% of patients would be considered recovered from the standard treatments, and 30–40% of patients would be considered improved. Still 30% of the patients would barely have any benefits from contemporary treatments [64, 69].

1.4.1 Risk Factors

Many studies have attempted to analyse predictors of response or conversely nonresponse and treatment resistance. Treatment may be completely or partially unsuccessful for a number of reasons. Knowledge of these reasons is important in the development of an adequate treatment plan for reducing the appearance of treatment resistance, for early detection of treatment resistance and for appropriate adaption of interventions in case of treatment resistance. Without intending to oversimplify this issue, we can divide these risk factors into factors related to psychiatric and medical comorbidity, symptomatic factors, biological factors, environmental factors and demographic factors. The following enumeration is non-exhaustive.

1.4.1.1 Psychiatric Comorbidity

Comorbidity among psychiatric disorders is very common. In patients with a first-episode psychosis, comorbidity with other psychiatric disorders is evident in 90% [70]. In patients with an anxiety disorder, for example, in the generalized anxiety disorder, more than 70% have at least one comorbid psychiatric diagnosis [87]. In major depressive disorder, overall comorbidity rates of more than 50% are reported [88].

The presence of a comorbid psychiatric disorder increases the likelihood of the development of treatment resistance [60, 67, 69, 70, 89–91]. Comorbidity between different psychiatric disorders renders each individual disorder more difficult to treat. Overall, patients with comorbid psychiatric disorders have response rates that are 25–30% lower compared to patients without comorbidity [70].

1.4.1.2 Medical Comorbidity

General medical conditions and their treatments can cause and worsen mental disorders. In patients with treatment-resistant psychiatric disorders, it is crucial to rule out the presence of an underlying medical disorder, for example, from an endocrinologic or neurological origin. Several types of medications for medical disorders may also precipitate or contribute to resistance. In depression, for example, immunosuppressants, steroids and sedatives are associated with treatment resistance [60].

1.4.1.3 Symptomatic Factors

Various symptomatic factors have been discussed in relation to treatment resistance. A greater severity and number of symptoms, early onset of symptoms and certain symptom dimensions are, for example, risk factors of poor outcome in major depressive disorder [60, 67, 70, 89], bipolar disorder [70, 91], schizophrenia [70] and anxiety disorders [90]. Furthermore, it is known that treatment resistance becomes increasingly likely as the duration of a mental disorder lengthens and episodes accumulate [60, 67, 70, 89–91].

1.4.1.4 Biological Factors

There is accumulating evidence for biological markers predicting response to treatment. In psychosis, genetic predisposition appears to confer a 2.2-fold higher risk of treatment resistance [92]. Furthermore, some of the structural and functional imaging abnormalities that are identified in patients with psychosis have also been associated with a reduced response to treatment, for example, decreases in the grey matter volume and enlargement of the lateral and third ventricles [70].

Also in anxiety disorders and mood disorders, genetic predispositions appear to confer a higher risk of treatment resistance. In major depressive disorder, for example, polymorphisms within the 5-HT1a C1019G gene, the NTRK2 gene and the BDNF G196A (Val66Met) gene, are found to be associated with an increased risk of treatment resistance [89]. Another factor that is associated with treatment resistance, via influencing psychotropic drug effects, is P-glycoprotein, which is produced by the multidrug-resistant gene ABCB1 [93].

1.4.1.5 Environmental Factors

Models of mental disorders underscore the interplay between biological and environmental factors. However, stressors are not always recognized by patients and their physicians. Psychosocial stressors include social support problems, social environment problems, occupational problems, economic problems, personal loss, legal problems and childhood adversities. Even severe and/or persistent stressors may go undetected and may impact treatment response [64, 67, 69, 70, 90].

1.4.1.6 Demographic Factors

There is some evidence to support the idea that gender is a risk factor for treatment resistance in psychotic and anxiety disorders [90, 92], and some evidence also suggests that gender is associated with the responsiveness to certain treatment strategies in depression [60].

Ethnic minorities and individuals with a low social economic status may also have an increased risk of treatment resistance, for example, in anxiety disorders [90]. This is in line with environmental factors (stressors) influencing treatment outcome.

1.4.1.7 Treatment Factors

Many state that treatment related factors can be associated with treatment resistance. Although they are clearly associated with outcome, one can question if they are related to well-defined treatment resistance. Factors like delay in treatment initiation, incorrect choice, dose and duration of psychotropic treatment, poor therapeutic alliance and noncompliance are mentioned as risk factors for treatment resistance, while they would be better grouped as risk factors of pseudo-resistance.

1.5 Impact of Treatment Resistance

Treatment resistance is responsible for tremendous individual suffering and is associated with vast losses in quality of life for both patients and those close to them [94–96], impaired social and functional functioning [95–98], an increased risk of somatic morbidity and mortality [98–100], increased rates of alcohol and drug misuse [101] and an increased risk of suicidal ideation [94] and suicide [52, 100].

The impact of treatment resistance is also illustrated by the impressive financial burden to society, due to patients' more extensive and costly use of medical services, both illness-related and general medical, as well as to their loss of productivity associated with their functional impairment. Patients with treatment-resistant depression, for example, have a higher number of medical visits, are at least twice as likely to be hospitalized, impose significantly higher annual costs and have twice the economic costs for employers compared to nontreatment-resistant depressed patients [94, 95, 102–104].

Furthermore, treatment resistance can lead clinicians to feel helpless and burnt out, facilitating high rates of staff turnover and a desire to "throw everything" at treatment-resistant patients hoping for a response. Individuals with treatment-resistant illness might receive complex treatments where the balance of risks and benefits shifts perceptibly [101].

1.6 Strategies for Improvement

The main proposed strategy in diminishing the occurrence of treatment resistance is the optimization of treatment, for example, by the use of more personalized medicine, measurement-based care, combination and augmentation strategies and experimental treatment strategies.

1.6.1 Personalized Medicine

Among the difficulties in mental health is a lack of consensus surrounding diagnostic categories that stems from an incomplete understanding of the processes underlying mental disorders. Field trials raise serious questions about the reliability of the currently used categories [105]. By gaining more understanding of what lies behind the clinical symptoms of patients with (treatment-resistant) psychiatric disorders, we might be able to develop specific targeted therapies that are more effective.

Furthermore, treatment outcomes would likely be improved by the discovery of homogeneous subtypes within and across diagnostic categories, by which treatments could be stratified. Global initiatives are in progress to delineate functional subtypes and improve the accuracy with which patients are categorized and treated [106]. It has been posited that, for example, biological markers are suitable candidates for subtyping mental disorders [107].

Another framework that might be useful in the treatment of mental disorders is clinical staging. Clinical staging tries to define the extent of progression of a disease at a particular point in time and consequently places greater emphasis on detailed description of where a person lies currently along the continuum of the course of an illness. The fundamental assumptions of clinical staging are twofold: patients in the early sates have a better response to treatment and a better prognosis than those in later stages, and the treatments offered in the early stages should be more benign as well as more effective [108].

1.6.2 Measurement-Based Care

Measurement-based care can be defined as the practise of basing clinical care on client data collected throughout treatment. It provides insight into treatment progress and highlights ongoing treatment targets. Research has shown that measurement-based care can result in significant improvement in clinical outcomes, especially for clients identified as likely to experience treatment failure [109, 110]. Moreover, as a framework to guide treatment, measurement-based care has transtheoretical and transdiagnostic relevance with a broad reach [111].

1.6.3 Combination and Augmentation Strategies

One may combine treatment strategies rationally to achieve a greater success. These include combination strategies and augmentation strategies. In major depressive disorder, for example, combination strategies involve the use of two or more different antidepressant treatments together. The aim of combining antidepressant treatments is to combine two or more mechanisms of action in an attempt to obtain enhancement of efficacy or tolerability. This requires some understanding of the targets of different treatments and flexibility in administration. Different antidepressants can be combined, but also combinations with electroconvulsive therapy and psychotherapy can be made. Combinations are found to enhance the rate of remission for patients suffering from treatment-resistant depression [112], although not all combinations are found effective [113, 114]. Augmentation strategies in depression consist of the addition of a non-antidepressant therapy to an antidepressant. For example, mood stabilizers and antipsychotics have been proven to be effective adjuncts to standard antidepressants, also in subjects who are unresponsive to conventional antidepressant therapy [112].

In case of comorbidity, one may target the comorbid condition at the same time when possible. This as well will lead to the use of multiple treatments at the same time.

1.6.4 Experimental Treatment Strategies

Nonresponse to current treatment strategies also calls for the development of new treatment modalities. For example, a relative novel intervention that has shown rapid and robust effects in patients with treatment-resistant unipolar and bipolar depression [115, 116], and possibly anxiety disorders [117], is the administration of the N-methyl-D-aspartate (NMDA) receptor antagonist ketamine. However, despite highly favourable results, several important difficulties remain. Ketamine's therapeutic benefit quickly dissipates. Achieving sustained remission of illness may require repeated doses of ketamine, but there are currently not enough data on the efficacy and safety of continuation or maintenance treatment. Furthermore, there is paucity of information about other routes of administration for ketamine, such as the oral or intranasal routes. Given the high prevalence of treatment-resistant disorders and the foreseeable need for repeated doses of ketamine, this issue is of high importance to facilitate the practical utility of ketamine on a day-to-day basis. Therefore, ongoing studies focus on central concerns like elucidating ketamine's mechanism of action, understanding the administration profile necessary to provide (sustained) therapeutic benefit and examining ketamine's safety profile, particularly with repeated administration [118].

In schizophrenia, accumulating data suggests that inflammatory processes play an important role in the pathophysiology of the disorder. The attractiveness of the inflammatory hypothesis lies in the possibility that the shift towards a pro-inflammatory status in the brain can potentially be corrected with anti-inflammatory agents. Therefore, several trials have been conducted to investigate the potential of (augmentation with) anti-inflammatory agents to improve symptoms of schizophrenia. So far, there is some preliminary evidence for the efficacy of some of the studied anti-inflammatory agents, like aspirin and N-acetylcysteine [119]. At this point however, it is too early to make conclusions on the benefits of this strategy.

1.7 Final Considerations

It is clear that much remains to be done to reduce the high level of treatment resistance in mental disorders. First of all early detection of potential treatment resistance is important, as is the possibility to provide appropriate adaption of interventions. This includes the possibility to offer a range of treatments, something that unfortunately is not the case for many patients. Furthermore, clear definitions are needed, as terminology is essential in decision-making in clinical practice, in making comparisons across studies and in identifying risk factors. Furthermore, we need to improve our diagnostic accuracy using established instruments to measure and confirm primary and comorbid mental and somatic disorders. We also need to ensure that our patients receive adequate treatment, and we need to respond to risk factors of treatment resistance. And finally, we need to optimize our interventions, for example, by the use of more personalized medicine and measurement-based care. Lastly and in line with the aim of developing individualized treatments, our fields need to invest in deepening our understanding of the neurobiology of psychiatric disorders through scientific research. When compared to cancer, mental disorders have received far less funding over the years, which is not consistent with their impact on the lives of a great many patients and those around them [120, 121].

References

1. Kessler RC, Berglund P, Demler O, Jin R, Merikangas KR, Walters EE. Lifetime prevalence and age-of-onset distributions of DSM-IV disorders in the National Comorbidity Survey Replication. Arch Gen Psychiatry. 2005;62(6):593–602.
2. Funk M, Ivbijaro G, editors. Integrating mental health into primary care: a global perspective. Geneva: WHO Press; 2008.
3. World Health Organization. Health statistics and information systems [Internet]. Geneva: World Health Organization; 2018. http://www.who.int/healthinfo/global_burden_disease/en/.
4. Bijl RV, Ravelli A. Current and residual functional disability associated with psychopathology: findings from the Netherlands Mental Health Survey and Incidence Study (NEMESIS). Psychol Med. 2000;30(3):657–68.
5. WHO International Consortium in Psychiatric Epidemiology. Cross-national comparisons of the prevalences and correlates of mental disorders. Bull World Health Organ. 2000;78(4):413–26.
6. Hirschfeld RM, Keller MB, Panico S, Arons BS, Barlow D, Davidoff F, et al. The national depressive and manic-depressive association consensus statement on the undertreatment of depression. JAMA. 1997;277(4):333–40.
7. Gøtzsche PC. Deadly medicines and organised crime: how big pharma has corrupted healthcare. London: Radcliffe Publishing; 2013.
8. Gøtzsche PC. Antidepressants are addictive and increase the risk of relapse. BMJ. 2016;352:i574.
9. Turner EH, Matthews AM, Linardatos E, Tell RA, Rosenthal R. Selective publication of antidepressant trials and its influence on apparent efficacy. N Engl J Med. 2008;358(3):252–60.
10. Turner EH. Publication bias, with a focus on psychiatry: causes and solutions. CNS Drugs. 2013;27(6):457–68.
11. Turner EH, Knoepflmacher D, Shapley L. Publication bias in antipsychotic trials: an analysis of efficacy comparing the published literature to the US Food and Drug Administration database. PLoS Med. 2012;9(3):e1001189.
12. Roest AM, de Jonge P, Williams CD, de Vries YA, Schoevers RA, Turner EH. Reporting bias in clinical trials investigating the efficacy of second-generation antidepressants in the treatment of anxiety disorders: a report of 2 meta-analyses. JAMA Psychiatry. 2015;72(5):500–10.
13. Cuijpers P, van Straten A, van Schaik A, Andersson G. Psychological treatment of depression in primary care: a meta-analysis. Br J Gen Pract. 2009;59(559):e51–60.
14. Driessen E, Hollon SD, Bockting CL, Cuijpers P, Turner EH. Does publication bias inflate the apparent efficacy of psychological treatment for major depressive disorder? A systematic review and meta-analysis of US National Institutes of Health-funded trials. PLoS One. 2015;10(9):e0137864.
15. Ioannidis JP. Defending biomedical science in an era of threatened funding. JAMA. 2017;317(24):2483–4.
16. Kirsch I, Deacon BJ, Huedo-Medina TB, Scoboria A, Moore TJ, Johnson BT. Initial severity and antidepressant benefits: a meta-analysis of data submitted to the Food and Drug Administration. PLoS Med. 2008;5(2):e45.
17. Leucht S, Arbter D, Engel RR, Kissling W, Davis JM. How effective are second-generation antipsychotic drugs? A meta-analysis of placebo-controlled trials. Mol Psychiatry. 2009;14(4):429–47.
18. Rabinowitz J, Werbeloff N, Mandel FS, Menard F, Marangell L, Kapur S. Initial depression severity and response to antidepressants v. placebo: patient-level data analysis from 34 randomised controlled trials. Br J Psychiatry. 2016;209(5):427–8.
19. Fountoulakis KN, Veroniki AA, Siamouli M, Möller HJ. No role for initial severity on the efficacy of antidepressants: results of a multi-meta-analysis. Ann Gen Psychiatry. 2013;12(1):26.
20. Gibbons RD, Hur K, Brown CH, Davis JM, Mann JJ. Benefits from antidepressants: synthesis of 6-week patient-level outcomes from double-blind placebo-controlled randomized trials of fluoxetine and venlafaxine. Arch Gen Psychiatry. 2012;69(6):572–9.
21. Melander H, Salmonson T, Abadie E, Van Zwieten-Boot B. A regulatory Apologia – a review of placebo-controlled studies in regulatory submissions of new-generation antidepressants. Eur Neuropsychopharmacol. 2008;18(9):623–7.
22. Baldessarini RJ, Tondo L. Suicide risk and treatments for patients with bipolar disorder. JAMA. 2003;290(11):1517–9.
23. Cipriani A, Pretty H, Hawton K, Geddes JR. Lithium in the prevention of suicidal behavior and all-cause mortality in patients with mood disorders: a systematic review of randomized trials. Am J Psychiatry. 2005;162(10):1805–19.
24. Geddes JR, Carney SM, Davies C, Furukawa TA, Kupfer DJ, Frank E, et al. Relapse prevention with antidepressant drug treatment in depressive disorders: a systematic review. Lancet. 2003;361(9358):653–61.
25. Hansen R, Gaynes B, Thieda P, Gartlehner G, Deveaugh-Geiss A, Krebs E, et al. Meta-analysis

of major depressive disorder relapse and recurrence with second-generation antidepressants. Psychiatr Serv. 2008;59(10):1121–30.
26. Komossa K, Depping AM, Heres S, Kissling W, Davis JM, Leucht S. Maintenance treatment with antipsychotic drugs for schizophrenia. Cochrane Database Syst Rev. 2009;4:CD008016.
27. Naylor CD, Chen E, Strauss B. Measured enthusiasm: does the method of reporting trial results alter perception of therapeutic effectiveness? Ann Intern Med. 1992;117(11):916–21.
28. Goldacre B. Bad science. London: Fourth Estate; 2008.
29. Weimer K, Colloca L, Enck P. Placebo effects in psychiatry: mediators and moderators. Lancet Psychiatry. 2015;2(3):246–57.
30. Thomson R. Side effects and placebo amplification. Br J Psychiatry. 1982;140:64–8.
31. Gaudiano BA, Herbert JD. Methodological issues in clinical trials of antidepressant medications: perspectives from psychotherapy outcome research. Psychother Psychosom. 2005;74(1):17–25.
32. Gracely RH, Dubner R, Deeter WR, Wolskee PJ. Clinicians' expectations influence placebo analgesia. Lancet. 1985;1(8419):43.
33. Gryll SL, Katahn M. Situational factors contributing to the placebos effect. Psychopharmacology (Berlin). 1978;57(3):253–61.
34. McQueen D, Cohen S, St. John-Smith P, Rampes H. Rethinking placebo in psychiatry: the range of placebo effects. BJPsych Adv. 2013;19(3):162–70.
35. Storosum JG, Elferink AJ, van Zwieten BJ, van den Brink W, Gersons BP, van Strik R, et al. Short-term efficacy of tricyclic antidepressants revisited: a meta-analytic study. Eur Neuropsychopharmacol. 2001;11(2):173–80.
36. Barbui C, Furukawa TA, Cipriani A. Effectiveness of paroxetine in the treatment of acute major depression in adults: a systematic re-examination of published and unpublished data from randomized trials. CMAJ. 2008;178(3):296–305.
37. Hansen RA, Gartlehner G, Lohr KN, Gaynes BN, Carey TS. Efficacy and safety of second-generation antidepressants in the treatment of major depressive disorder. Ann Intern Med. 2005;143(6):415–26.
38. Watts SE, Turnell A, Kladnitski N, Newby JM, Andrews G. Treatment-as-usual (TAU) is anything but usual: a meta-analysis of CBT versus TAU for anxiety and depression. J Affect Disord. 2015;175:152–67.
39. Leucht S, Tardy M, Komossa K, Heres S, Kissling W, Salanti G, et al. Antipsychotic drugs versus placebo for relapse prevention in schizophrenia: a systematic review and meta-analysis. Lancet. 2012;379(9831):2063–71.
40. Storosum JG, Wohlfarthe T, Schene A, Elferink A, van Zwieten BJ, van den Brink W. Magnitude of effect of lithium in short-term efficacy studies of moderate to severe manic episode. Bipolar Disord. 2007;9(8):793–8.
41. Scherk H, Pajonk FG, Leucht S. Second-generation antipsychotic agents in the treatment of acute mania: a systematic review and meta-analysis of randomized controlled trials. Arch Gen Psychiatry. 2007;64(4):442–55.
42. Davis JM, Janicak PG, Hogan DM. Mood stabilizers in the prevention of recurrent affective disorders: a meta-analysis. Acta Psychiatr Scand. 1999;100(6):406–17.
43. Gijsman HJ, Geddes JR, Rendell JM, Nolen WA, Goodwin GM. Antidepressants for bipolar depression: a systematic review of randomized, controlled trials. Am J Psychiatry. 2004;161(9):1537–47.
44. Soomro GM, Altman D, Rajagopal S, Oakley-Browne M. Selective serotonin re-uptake inhibitors (SSRIs) versus placebo for obsessive compulsive disorder (OCD). Cochrane Database Syst Rev. 2008;1:CD001765.
45. Hans E, Hiller W. A meta-analysis of nonrandomized effectiveness studies on outpatient cognitive behavioral therapy for adult anxiety disorders. Clin Psychol Rev. 2013;33(8):954–64.
46. Mitte K. A meta-analysis of the efficacy of psycho- and pharmacotherapy in panic disorder with and without agoraphobia. J Affect Disord. 2005;88(1):27–45.
47. Schachter HM, Pham B, King J, Langford S, Moher D. How efficacious and safe is short-acting methylphenidate for the treatment of attention-deficit disorder in children and adolescents? A meta-analysis. CMAJ. 2001;165(11):1475–88.
48. Faraone SV, Biederman J. Efficacy of Adderall for attention-deficit/hyperactivity disorder: a meta-analysis. J Atten Disord. 2002;6(2):69–75.
49. Cheng JY, Chen RY, Ko JS, Ng EM. Efficacy and safety of atomoxetine for attention-deficit/hyperactivity disorder in children and adolescents – meta-analysis and meta-regression analysis. Psychopharmacology. 2007;194(2):197–209.
50. Leucht S, Hierl S, Kissling W, Dold M, Davis JM. Putting the efficacy of psychiatric and general medicine medication into perspective: review of meta-analyses. Br J Psychiatry. 2012;200(2):97–106.
51. Bijkersma-Pot LM, Cuijpers P, Beekman AT, Schoevers RA. Comparison of efficacy of psychiatric treatment versus treatment in general medicine. Tijdschr Psychiatry. 2016;58:751–8.
52. Nemeroff CB, editor. Management of treatment-resistant major psychiatric disorders. Oxford: Oxford University Press; 2012.
53. Jakovljevic M. Creative, person-centered and narrative psychopharmacotherapy or how to prevent and overcome treatment resistance in psychiatry. Psychiatr Danub. 2015;27(3):291–301.
54. Rasmussen KG, Mueller M, Kellner CH, Knapp RG, Petrides G, Rummans TA, et al. Patterns of psychotropic medication use among patients with severe depression referred for electroconvulsive therapy: data from the Consortium for

Research on Electroconvulsive Therapy. J ECT. 2006;22(2):116–23.
55. Rush AJ, Thase ME, Dubé S. Research issues in the study of difficult-to-treat depression. Biol Psychiatry. 2003;53(8):743–53.
56. Breyer-Pfaff U, Gaertner HJ, Giedke H. Plasma levels, psychophysiological variables, and clinical response to amitriptyline. Psychiatry Res. 1982;6(2):223–34.
57. Faravelli C, Ballerini A, Ambonetti A, Broadhurst AD, Das M. Plasma levels and clinical response during treatment with clomipramine. J Affect Disord. 1984;6(1):95–107.
58. Moleman P. Praktische psychofarmacologie. Houten: Bohn Stafleu van Loghum; 1998.
59. Crossley NA, Bauer M. Acceleration and augmentation of antidepressants with lithium for depressive disorders: two meta-analyses of randomized, placebo-controlled trials. J Clin Psychiatry. 2007;68(6):935–40.
60. Berlim MT, Turecki G. Definition, assessment, and staging of treatment-resistant refractory major depression: a review of current concepts and methods. Can J Psychiatry. 2007;52(1):46–54.
61. Zevin S, Benowitz NL. Drug interactions with tobacco smoking. An update. Clin Pharmacokinet. 1999;36(6):425–38.
62. Ravyn D, Ravyn V, Lowney R, Nasrallah HA. CYP450 pharmacogenetic treatment strategies for antipsychotics: a review of the evidence. Schizophr Res. 2013;149(1–3):1–14.
63. Simoons M, Mulder H, Schoevers RA, Ruhé HG, van Roon EN. Availability of CYP2D6 genotyping results in general practitioner and community pharmacy medical records. Pharmacogenomics. 2017;18(9):843–51.
64. Roy-Byrne P. Treatment-refractory anxiety; definition, risk factors, and treatment challenges. Dialogues Clin Neurosci. 2015;17(2):191–206.
65. Craske MG, Roy-Byrne P, Stein MB, Sullivan G, Hazlett-Stevens H, Bystritsky A, et al. CBT intensity and outcome for panic disorder in a primary care setting. Behav Ther. 2006;37(2):112–9.
66. Julius RJ, Novitsky MA Jr, Dublin WR. Medication adherence: a review of the literature and implications for clinical practice. J Psychiatr Pract. 2009;15(1):34–44.
67. Fava M. Diagnosis and definition of treatment-resistant depression. Biol Psychiatry. 2003;53(8):649–59.
68. Berlim MT, Turecki G. What is the meaning of treatment resistant/refractory major depression (TRD)? A systematic review of current randomized trials. Eur Neuropsychopharmacol. 2007;17(11):696–707.
69. Bystritsky A. Treatment-resistant anxiety disorders. Mol Psychiatry. 2006;11(9):805–14.
70. Huber CG, Naber D, Lambert M. Incomplete remission and treatment resistance in first-episode psychosis: definition, prevalence and predictors. Expert Opin Pharmacother. 2008;9(12):2027–38.
71. Frank E, Prien RF, Jarrett RB, Keller MB, Kupfer DJ, Lavori PW, et al. Conceptualization and rationale for consensus definitions of terms in major depressive disorder. Remission, recovery, relapse, and recurrence. Arch Gen Psychiatry. 1991;48(9):851–5.
72. Rubio JM, Olfson M, Villegas L, Pérez-Fuentes G, Wang S, Blanco C. Quality of life following remission of mental disorders: findings from the National Epidemiologic Survey on Alcohol and Related Conditions. J Clin Psychiatry. 2013;74(5):e445–50.
73. van der Voort TY, Seldenrijk A, van Meijel B, Goossens PJ, Beekman AT, Penninx BW, et al. Functional versus syndromal recovery in patients with major depressive disorder and bipolar disorder. J Clin Psychiatry. 2015;76(6):e809–14.
74. Malhi GS, Byrow Y. Is treatment-resistant depression a useful concept? Evid Based Ment Health. 2016;19(1):1–3.
75. Hollon SD, Ponniah K. A review of empirically supported psychological therapies for mood disorders in adults. Depress Anxiety. 2010;27(10):891–932.
76. Hunot V, Churchill R, Silva de Lima M, Teixeira V. Psychological therapies for generalised anxiety disorder. Cochrane Database Syst Rev. 2007;1:CD001848.
77. Marazziti D, Carlini M, Dell'Osso L. Treatment strategies of obsessive-compulsive disorder and panic disorder/agoraphobia. Curr Top Med Chem. 2012;12(4):238–53.
78. Fekadu A, Wooderson S, Donaldson C, Markopoulou K, Masterson B, Poon L, et al. A multidimensional tool to quantify treatment resistance in depression: the Maudsley staging method. J Clin Psychiatry. 2009;70(2):177–84.
79. Ruhé HG, van Rooijen G, Spijker J, Peeters FP, Schene AH. Staging methods for treatment resistant depression. A systematic review. J Affect Disord. 2012;137(1–3):35–45.
80. Ferguson JM, Khan A, Mangano R, Entsuah R, Tzanis E. Relapse prevention of panic disorder in adult outpatient responders to treatment with venlafaxine extended release. J Clin Psychiatry. 2007;68(1):58–68.
81. Mochcovitch MD, Da Rocha Freire RC, Garcia RF, Nardi AE. Can long-term pharmacotherapy prevent relapses in generalized anxiety disorder? A systematic review. Clin Drug Investig. 2017;37(8):737–43.
82. Rush AJ, Trivedi MH, Wisniewsky SR, Nierenberg AA, Stewart JW, Warden D, et al. Acute and longer-term outcomes in depressed outpatients requiring one or several treatment steps: a STAR*D report. Am J Psychiatry. 2006;163(11):1905–17.
83. Tohen M, Hennen J, Zarate CM Jr, Baldessarini RJ, Strakowski SM, Stoll AL, et al. Two-year syndromal and functional recovery in 219 cases of first-episode major affective disorder with psychotic features. Am J Psychiatry. 2000;157(2):220–8.
84. Tohen M, Zarate CA Jr, Hennen J, Khalsa HM, Strakowski SM, Gebre-Medhin P, et al. The McLean-Harvard First-Episode Mania Study: prediction

of recovery and first recurrence. Am J Psychiatry. 2003;160(12):2099–107.
85. Sienaert P, Lambrichts L, Dols A, De Fruyt J. Evidence-based treatment strategies for treatment-resistant bipolar depression: a systematic review. Bipolar Disord. 2013;15(1):61–9.
86. Solanki RK, Singh P, Munshi D. Current perspectives in the treatment of resistant schizophrenia. Indian J Psychiatry. 2009;51(4):254–60.
87. Ruscio AM, Hallion LS, Lim CC, Aguilar-Gaxiola S, Al-Hamzawi A, Alonso J, et al. Cross-sectional comparison of the epidemiology of DSM-5 generalized anxiety disorder across the globe. JAMA Psychiatry. 2017;74(5):465–75.
88. Kornstein SG, Schneider RK. Clinical features of treatment-resistant depression. J Clin Psychiatry. 2001;62(Suppl 16):18–25.
89. Bennabi D, Aouizerate B, El-Hage W, Doumy O, Moliere F, Courtet P, et al. Risk factors for treatment resistance in unipolar depression: a systematic review. J Affect Disord. 2015;171:137–41.
90. Chen MH, Tsai SJ. Treatment-resistant panic disorder: clinical significance, concept and management. Prog Neuro-Psychopharmacol Biol Psychiatry. 2016;70:219–26.
91. Treuer T, Tohen M. Predicting the course and outcome of bipolar disorder: a review. Eur Psychiatry. 2010;25(6):328–33.
92. Murray RM, van Os J. Predictors of outcome in schizophrenia. J Clin Psychopharmacol. 1998;18(2 Suppl 1):2S–4S.
93. Brückl TM, Urh M. ABCB1 genotyping in the treatment of depression. Pharmacogenomics. 2016;17(18):2039–69.
94. Mrazek DA, Hornberger JC, Altar CA, Degtiar I. A review of the clinical, economic, and societal burden of treatment-resistant depression: 1996–2013. Psychiatr Serv. 2014;65(8):977–87.
95. Mauskopf JA, Simon GE, Kalsekar A, Nimsch C, Dunayevich E, Cameron A. Nonresponse, partial response, and failure to achieve remission: humanistic and cost burden in major depressive disorder. Depress Anxiety. 2009;26(1):83–97.
96. Qiao J, Qian LJ, Zhao HF, Gong GH, Geng DQ. The relationship between quality of life and clinical phenotype in patients with treatment resistant and non-treatment resistant depression. Eur Rev Med Pharmacol Sci. 2017;21(10):2432–6.
97. Paykel ES. Achieving gains beyond response. Acta Psychiatr Scand Suppl. 2002;415:12–7.
98. Greden JF. The burden of disease for treatment-resistant depression. J Clin Psychiatry. 2001;62(Suppl 16):26–31.
99. Carney RM, Freedland KE. Treatment-resistant depression and mortality after acute coronary syndrome. Am J Psychiatry. 2009;166(4):410–7.
100. Fekadu A, Rane LJ, Wooderson SC, Markopoulou K, Poon L, Cleare AJ. Prediction of longer-term outcome of treatment-resistant depression in tertiary care. Br J Psychiatry. 2012;201(5):369–75.
101. Berk M, Berk L, Udina M, Moylan S, Stafford L, Hallam K, et al. Palliative models of care for later stages of mental disorder: maximizing recovery, maintaining hope, and building morale. Aust N Z J Psychiatry. 2012;46(2):92–9.
102. Lepine BA, Moreno RA, Campos RN, Couttolenc BF. Treatment-resistant depression increases health costs and resource utilization. Rev Bras Psiquiatr. 2012;34(4):379–88.
103. Crown WH, Finkelstein S, Berndt ER, Ling D, Poret AW, Rush AJ, et al. The impact of treatment-resistant depression on health care utilization and costs. J Clin Psychiatry. 2002;63(11):963–71.
104. Ivanova JI, Birnbaum HG, Kidolezi Y, Subramanian G, Khan SA, Stensland MD. Direct and indirect costs of employees with treatment-resistant and non-treatment-resistant major depressive disorder. Curr Med Res Opin. 2010;26(10):2475–84.
105. Regier DA, Narrow WE, Clarke D, Kraemer HC, Kuramoto SJ, Kuhl EA, et al. DSM-5 field trials in the United States and Canada, part II: test-retest reliability of selected categorical diagnoses. Am J Psychiatry. 2013;170(1):59–70.
106. Insel TR, Medicine CBN. Brain disorders? Precisely Sci. 2015;348(6234):499–500.
107. Strawbridge R, Young AH, Cleare AJ. Biomarkers for depression: recent insights, current challenges and future prospects. Neuropsychiatr Dis Treat. 2017;13:1245–62.
108. McGorry PD, Hickie IB, Yung AR, Pantelis C, Jackson HJ. Clinical staging of psychiatric disorders: a heuristic framework for choosing earlier, safer and more effective interventions. Aust N Z J Psychiatry. 2006;40(8):616–22.
109. Guo T, Xiang YT, Xiao L, Hu CQ, Chiu HF, Ungvari GS, et al. Measurement-based care versus standard care for major depression: a randomized controlled trial with blind raters. Am J Psychiatry. 2015;172:1004–13.
110. Lambert MJ, Whipple JL, Hawkins EJ, Vermeersch DA, Nielsen SL, Smart DW. Is it time for clinicians to routinely track patient outcome? A meta-analysis. Clin Psychol Sci Pract. 2003;10(3):288–301.
111. Scott K, Lewis CC. Using measurement-based care to enhance any treatment. Cogn Behav Pract. 2015;22(1):49–59.
112. Moret C. Combination/augmentation strategies for improving the treatment of depression. Neuropsychiatr Dis Treat. 2005;1(4):301–9.
113. Gaynes BN, Dusetzina SB, Ellis AR, Hansen RA, Farley JF, Miller WC, et al. Treating depression after initial treatment failure. Directly comparing switch and augmenting strategies in STAR*D. J Clin Psychopharmacol. 2012;32(1):114–9.
114. Rush AJ, Trivedi MH, Stewart JW, Nierenberg AA, Fava M, Kurian BT, et al. Combining medications to enhance depression outcomes (CO-MED): acute and long-term outcomes of a single-blind randomized study. Am J Psychiatry. 2011;168(7):689–701.

115. Han Y, Chen J, Zou D, Zheng P, Li Q, Wang H, et al. Efficacy of ketamine in the rapid treatment of major depressive disorder: a meta-analysis of randomized, double-blind, placebo-controlled studies. Neuropsychiatr Dis Treat. 2016;12:2859–67.
116. Kishimoto T, Chawla JM, Hagi K, Zarate CA, Kane JM, Bauer M, et al. Single-dose infusion ketamine and non-ketamine N-methyl-D-aspartate receptor antagonist for unipolar and bipolar depression: a meta-analysis of efficacy, safety and time trajectories. Psychol Med. 2016;46(7):1459–72.
117. Rodriguez CI, Kegeles LS, Levinson A, Feng T, Marcus SM, Vermes D, et al. Randomized controlled crossover trial of ketamine in obsessive-compulsive disorder: proof-of-concept. Neuropsychopharmacology. 2013;38(12):2475–83.
118. Sanacora G, Frye MA, McDonald W, Mathew SJ, Turner MS, Schatzberg AF, et al. A consensus statement on the use of ketamine in the treatment of mood disorders. JAMA Psychiatry. 2017;74(4):399–405.
119. Sommer IE, van Westrhenen R, Begemann MJ, de Witte LD, Leucht S, Kahn RS. Efficacy of anti-inflammatory agents to improve symptoms in patients with schizophrenia: an update. Schizophr Bull. 2014;40(1):181–91.
120. Collins PY, Patel V, Joestl SS, March D, Insel TR, Daar AS, et al. Grand challenges in global mental health. Nature. 2011;475(7354):27–30.
121. Ledford H. Medical research: if depression were cancer. Nature. 2014;515(7526):82–4.

2 Paradigm Shift in Study of Treatment-Resistant Psychiatric Disorder

Sang Won Jeon, Meysam Amidfar, and Yong-Ku Kim

2.1 Introduction

Treatment-resistant psychiatric disorder (TRP) is an important new frontier area in medical and psychological services [12, 13]. On the one hand, several therapeutic approaches are tried to achieve a complete remission of TRP. On the other hand, if biological risk factors of TRP are identified, individuals with a TRP risk factor can be detected early and provided with more concentrated management [3, 15]. To do so, recent studies have focused on the development and use of a biomarker to identify individuals "at risk of TRP." The premise of those studies is that biological causes exist which clearly differentiate treatment-resistant and treatment-responsive patient groups [9]. However, a review of biomarker studies conducted to identify TRP risk factors reveals a few problems.

First, treatment-resistant patients are defined as a group of patients not responsive to adequate treatments known so far [5]. The definition of TRP is not based on objective observation, but is a result of subjective phenomenological observation. Hence, as treatment approaches are updated and developed, the definition of TRP also changes [4]. Also, one may question what an adequate, optimal treatment is. So far, numerous treatment algorithms and strategies have been suggested for the treatment of psychiatric illnesses, and they continue to be under discussion. For potential TRP risk factors, several biological markers have been investigated, but if the definition of TRP is not solidly established, the outcomes of all such research efforts will lack a foundation.

Second, most of the aforementioned studies were designed as a post hoc experimental study [8, 16]. In other words, they were sort of a case-control study, in that after treatments were administered (clinical and experimental trials), patients were divided into treatment-resistant and treatment-responsive groups in accordance with a known definition and the two groups were retrospectively examined to identify risk factors. Here, the treatment-resistant group is a case group, and the treatment-responsive group is a control group. To search for biological risk factors, it is necessary to analyze such data as imaging studies and specimens collected in a baseline study [7]. In the post hoc experimental study design, a baseline study is performed after

S. W. Jeon
Department of Psychiatry, Kangbuk Samsung Hospital, Sungkyunkwan University School of Medicine, Jongno-gu, Seoul, Republic of Korea

M. Amidfar
Fasa University of Medical Sciences, Fasa, Iran

Y.-K. Kim (✉)
Department of Psychiatry, College of Medicine, Korea University Ansan Hospital, Ansan-si, Gyeonggi-do, Republic of Korea
e-mail: yongku@korea.ac.kr

Y.-K. Kim (ed.), *Treatment Resistance in Psychiatry*, https://doi.org/10.1007/978-981-10-4358-1_2

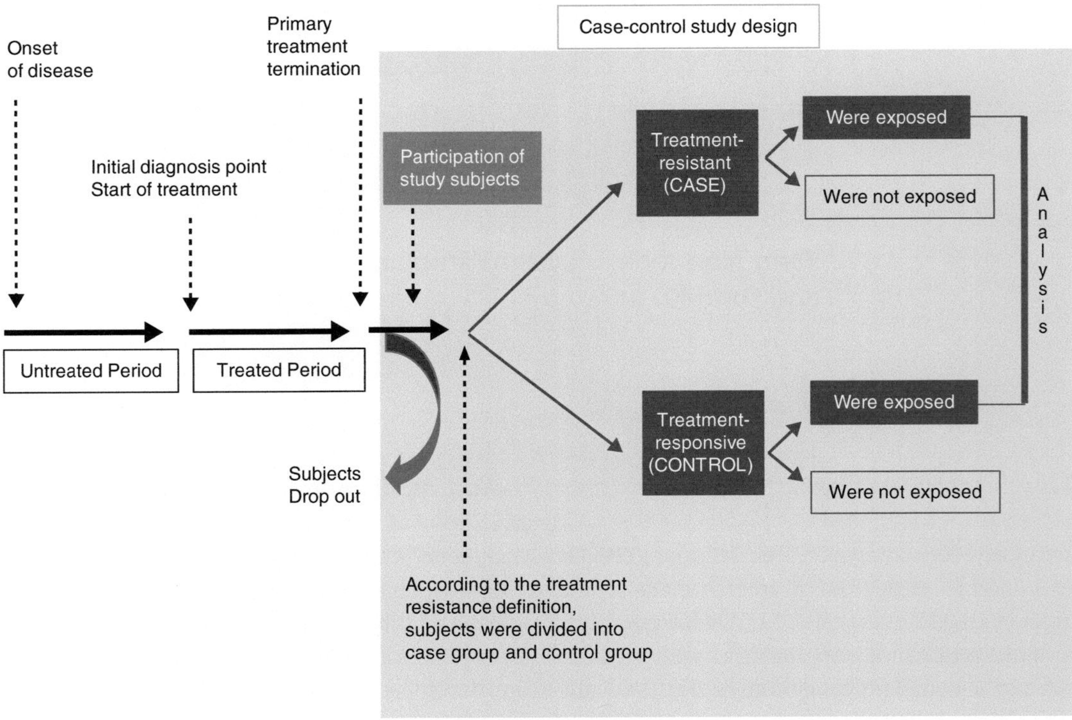

Fig. 2.1 An illustration of traditional study design in TRP research

treatment is given because subjects are enrolled into study after treatment has already been administered (Fig. 2.1). Biomarkers discovered in such baseline study are not the initial risk factors for TRP. And it is possible for initial biomarkers to be altered during the treatment process. If the study objective is to identify initial biological risk factors, it is most ideal to enroll untreated patients (those who were diagnosed but have not yet undergone treatment) as study subjects.

In this chapter, the authors will review methodological considerations to uncover initial biological risk factors for TRP and propose a better study design for future research by discussing the shortcomings of the traditional study design.

2.2 Definition and Variables for TRP

Most researchers who study TRP feel the lack of standardized definitions and operational criteria from the start. For example, just focusing on treatment-resistant depression (TRD), numerous definitions were proposed in the past few decades [11]. It is widely accepted that TRP does not represent a diagnosis or syndrome per se. Therefore, it is critical at the start of TRP research to determine which of the definitions to apply. Important factors to consider when defining TRP are (i) correct diagnosis and comorbidity, (ii) adequate treatment, (iii) treatment response, and (iv) the number and type of failed trials [1, 18].

Most common confounding factors in the post hoc analysis done in TRP research are misdiagnosis, suboptimal treatments, and illness duration [1, 18]. To collect data regarding treatment duration and treatment dose, direct interviews are conducted and medical records reviewed. But, if these processes are inaccurate, a problem arises in which a high degree of heterogeneity is observed among subjects.

In TRP research, many variables are involved prior to the determination of treatment resistance or treatment responsiveness [10, 19]. Among those, treatment variables are the most important. The most critical among treatment variables are undertreatment of psychiatric disease, delay in initiating treatment predominant, and long-lasting untreated illness [19]. Subject compliance and tolerance should also be considered. Additionally, patient variables should be considered and analyzed. For example, people of older age and females show a higher risk for TRD. Another factor to be considered is illness characteristics. In TRD, for example, unipolar depression vs. bipolar depression, psychotic depression, premorbid personality, and comorbid physical illness (e.g., thyroid dysfunction) should be considered [19]. The consideration of all such variables as above will exclude pseudo-resistant cases.

2.3 Limitation of Traditional Study Design

After the definition of TRP and variables are under control to some extent, a study can be designed to uncover TRP risk factors. Recent biomarker research studies utilize multimodal approaches such as neuroimaging, genetics, proteomics, and metabolomics [6]. Most traditional studies conducted to find biological risk factors of TRP use the case-control study design, which is a retrospective experimental study design [2, 14]. In traditional TRP studies, patient samples are obtained according to some definition of treatment-resistant patients (case) and treatment-responsive patients (control), and the levels of predictor variables are compared between the two samples to examine which predictor variables are associated with the outcome (resistance vs. responsiveness) (Fig. 2.1). Conducting a study designed in this fashion is safe with low risk and relatively less expensive, and thus, many studies are designed this way. However, there are fatal flaws in studies using the design.

First, there is a sampling problem known as separate sampling. The ratio between subjects selected for treatment resistance and treatment responsiveness does not follow the corresponding ratio in the population, because the researcher artificially determines the sampling of cases and controls. For case sampling, subjects have to be selected among those who have already been determined as treatment resistant and are available for study. Such a sample, however, may not represent all patients resistant to treatment, because those whose illness is not diagnosed or misdiagnosed, who are not treated, who do not consent to register for study, and who are deceased (e.g., by committing suicide) are not included in the study.

Second, as shown above, the definition of TRP changes with time, and furthermore, several definitions are present at a given point. Hence, instability exists in that case groups differ depending on which definition the researcher uses to define a case. To complement the shortcomings, the researcher should be careful when sampling so that the sampling ratio may be close to the ratio in the population of all patients with the illness of interest and have extensive background knowledge and confidence in regard to the current definitions of TRP.

Third, there is a problem of differential measurement bias. This problem is caused by the use of a retrospective approach in measuring a predictor variable. Case and control groups are asked to recall past exposures. Recall of, and retrospective analysis on, whether or not study subjects had sufficiently received adequate treatment before determined to be treatment resistant is nothing but incomplete. In a case like this, problems of non-differential or differential misclassification and recall bias arise, making it more difficult to find associations that are being measured in the study. To overcome the shortcomings, a prospective study should be conducted [17]. The aforementioned problems such as recall bias are not present in a cohort study, because the entire treatment process of subjects is exposed and recorded before the diagnosis of treatment resistance is made. Moreover, with an application of an experimental study design in a cohort study, the treatment process will be controlled most completely, and the involvement of extraneous variables will be minimized. If a prospective study is impossible to conduct, the level of comparability between case and control should be improved by increasing the level of accuracy in recall of the treatment process before a patient is determined as treatment resistant or treatment responsive, and a pair matching or frequency matching method should be appropriately utilized.

Finally, the most problematic in a study conducted to find TRP risk factors that is designed as a post hoc experimental study is the point in time at which the baseline study is performed [17]. In most existing studies, patients were registered for study after intervened with treatment, at which point a case-control study begins. Thus, baseline data needed for risk factor analysis are obtained after the primary treatment is complete. Could biological markers like images and specimens obtained at this point be initial risks for the TRP patients? Definitely not. In biological research, a baseline study should be performed on the images or specimens obtained in the past. It is highly likely that the initial and unique characteristics of the illness itself are lost in several biological markers due to the treatment intervention. To resolve this problem, the time of study registration should be when "patients are diagnosed but have not yet begun treatment." That is, the timing of a baseline study to be performed should be prior to the first treatment intervention, when the subjects are untreated patients. Data gathered at this point have the value as true initial risk factors of TRP.

2.4 Overcoming of Traditional Study Design

To overcome the shortcomings of the traditional study design, a prospective study like cohort research should be conducted. There are difficulties in conducting cohort research. Namely, it requires many subjects and a long period of observation, it is expensive to conduct, and it is difficult to follow up subjects. However, of all observational research methods, cohort research provides the most critical information on a causal relationship, and most clearly shows the temporal precedence relationship between factor and illness. In conclusion, it is necessary to design a cohort study with the strengths of case-control studies that is economical and fast to perform. The nested case-control study design is a representative case of such methodological approach (Fig. 2.2).

A nested case-control study costs less by investigating only selected cases and controls, while enjoying many advantages of cohort research. It is a case-control study, but has many positives of cohort research because it is designed to survey risk factors before an outcome variable. But, a nested case-control study is possible only if the images and specimens obtained in the baseline study are well preserved. In TRP research, the starting point for a cohort should be at a time when study subjects have not yet begun treatment, and a cross-sectional study should have been conducted by obtaining specimens and images prior to the initiation of treatment (baseline study).

There may be a cohort in whom a study objective has been minimally determined. For example, patients diagnosed with depression for the first time may register for a study before undergoing treatment. In such case, the objectives of cohort research are to study depressed patients only and investigate patients with TRD.

Below, an illustration of the nested case-control study design to uncover initial biomarkers of TRD is provided (Fig. 2.2).

2.4.1 Identification of a Cohort

Recruit and enroll patients who are diagnosed with depression and have not yet begun treatment. Descriptive information, specimens, and images are obtained from the registered patients (baseline study). Patients who already started treatment and those who do not have specimens, images, and other data prior to treatment are excluded from the cohort.

2.4.2 Follow-Up: Observational or Experimental

After the baseline study is completed, treatment for depression is initiated in accordance

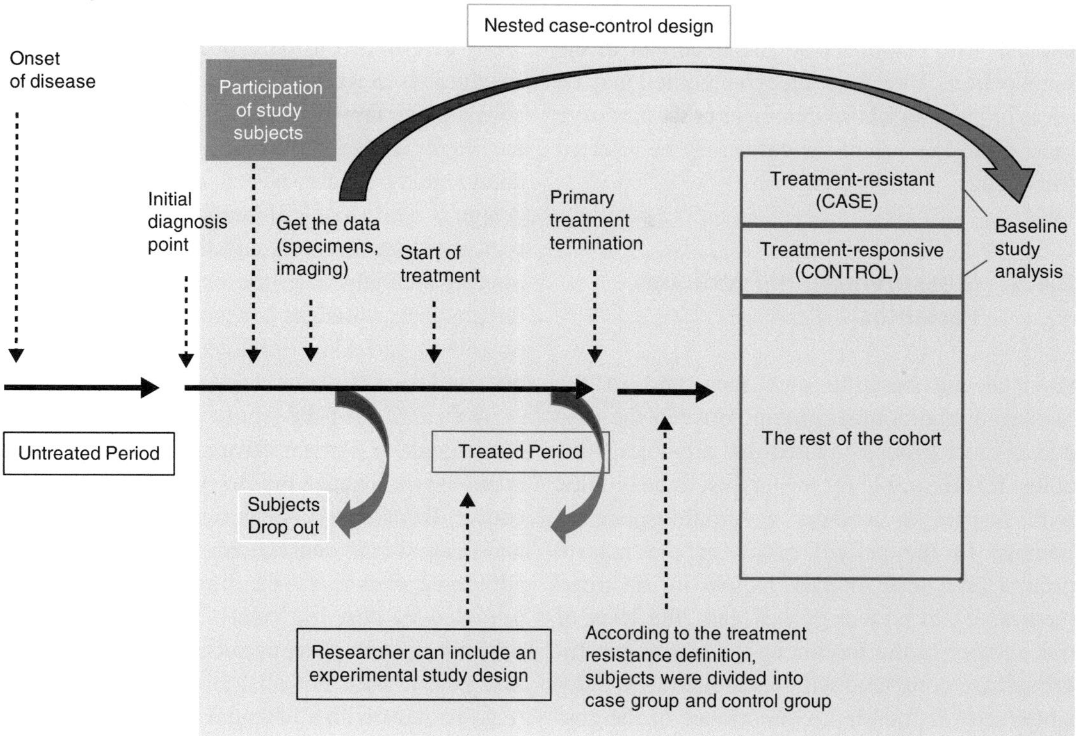

Fig. 2.2 An illustration of the nested case-control study design in TRP research. (1) Determining the cohort whose specimens are obtained during the baseline study. (2) An experimental study design can be included. Experimental control is provided for subjects to receive similar treatments during the cohort follow-up. (3) Determining patients during a follow-up period (treatment-resistant patients). Sampling of the experimental (treatment-resistant patient) and control (treatment-responsive patient) groups. (4) Investigating risk factors from the specimens obtained in the past

with the treatment algorithm. The researcher follows up and records the depression treatment process (exposure variables). During the follow-up of a cohort, an experimental study design may be applied. For instance, when selecting appropriate treatments for depression, the researcher may decide to experimentally administer only the predetermined antidepressants. Also, the type, frequency, and duration of psychotherapy administered in combination of antidepressant therapy may be manipulated to be the same across all subjects. If such experimental intervention is administered within a cohort, the treatment process is the most completely controlled for all subjects to minimize the confounding by intermediate variables involved in the case-control analysis to be conducted later.

2.4.3 Identification of the Patient Group Upon the Completion of Follow-Up

At the end of the follow-up period for a given cohort, examine patients whose treatment is completed according to a "treatment algorithm (observational)" or an "operational intervention (experimental)," and select those patients determined to have TRD based on the definition chosen by the researcher.

2.4.4 Selection of the Control Group

For an appropriate control group, select patients who belong to the same cohort and are determined to be responsive to treatment for depression. Here, the control group consists of patients who responded to the treatment in the same cohort. A random selection method may be used, or patients whose treatment processes were most close to those of the cases may be selected (matching).

2.4.5 Measurement of Predictor Variables

Analyze the baseline data measured in the beginning and compare them between the case and control groups to measure predictor variables. It is desirable for the analyst to be blinded with respect to whether a sample specimen belongs to the patient group or the control group. "The level of risk factors in the treatment-resistant patient group" and "the level of risk factors in the treatment-responsive patient group" are compared with each other. If a plausible factor is found, the importance of the possible causal factor is finally measured. It is known as influence measure. It measures "the size of additionally occurring treatment-resistant illness if the causal factor is entered" or "the benefit obtained if the causal factor is removed." If the result is significant, the factor is a powerful candidate as an initial biological risk factor for TRD which only treatment-resistant patients have.

It is relatively expensive to test serum and other specimens and conduct imaging studies in order to confirm biological causes of TRP patients. The nested case-control study design is particularly useful if the cost is high in conducting tests at the beginning of the study and storing the biological data for later analysis. The cost reduction effect is greater if the measurements are made just on the samples determined as cases and controls, rather than in the entire cohort, spending a large sum of cost. The cost issue may have been the most important reason why until now the case-control study design was preferred in TRP research. The time issue was probably not so critical, because it is highly likely that it takes a few years, not decades, for a patient to be eventually determined to be treatment resistant after an illness is diagnosed and treated. As discussed above, if the aim of a study is to find initial risk factors for TRP, the study must be designed as a cohort study. If the nested case-control study design is used, cost will be reduced compared to typical cohort research, and the study will have the very strengths of a cohort study, in which data on predictor variables are collected before the outcome variable (treatment resistance) is observed.

A weakness of this study design is that it is fundamentally a prospective study, and hence, it is not easy to change the study design during the course. If a study is not designed with accuracy and in detail, the consequence is irreversible. An additional weakness is that limited information is provided in post hoc analysis conducted after follow-up is complete, because the study population begins with not all individuals of interest (e.g., patients with a potential to develop depression) but those whose range is narrowed in accordance with the study objective (e.g., patients diagnosed with depression but having not yet begun treatment).

2.5 Other Considerations

A researcher planning to conduct a large-scale prospective study should keep in mind conducting analysis for a nested case-control study at a later time and consider storing biological specimens, images, records, etc. which are expensive to measure. If not all subjects in a cohort cannot be tested, the researcher should make an effort to save the data of only those who could potentially be used in the analysis for a nested case-control study and ensure that the materials and image data of interest are saved until the analysis is performed and pay close attention. In addition, during a cohort follow-up period, the researcher should frequently collect new specimens and information which can be used in case-control comparison.

Conclusion

Psychiatric patients with many episodes that do not respond satisfactorily numerous sequential treatment regimens were included in the treatment resistance studies. Such post hoc experimental design can be regarded only as a consequence of having treatment resistance, rather than being a causal risk factor for it. Although informative, data derived from such studies often do not allow for a distinction to be made between cause and effect. So, we should shift paradigm toward examining the risk for developing treatment resistance in untreated psychiatric patients. To deal with this problem, untreated patients should be enrolled in the study to identify biological markers for treatment resistance. Such information could give a cue to improve the initial diagnosis and provide more effective treatment for treatment resistance.

References

1. Berlim MT, Turecki G. Definition, assessment, and staging of treatment-resistant refractory major depression: a review of current concepts and methods. Can J Psychiatr. 2007;52(1):46–54.
2. Cepeda MS, Reps J, Fife D, Blacketer C, Stang P, Ryan P. Finding treatment-resistant depression in real-world data: how a data-driven approach compares with expert-based heuristics. Depress Anxiety. 2017;35:220–8.
3. Conley RR, Kelly DL. Management of treatment resistance in schizophrenia. Biol Psychiatry. 2001;50(11):898–911.
4. Conway CR, George MS, Sackeim HA. Toward an evidence-based, operational definition of treatment-resistant depression: when enough is enough. JAMA Psychiat. 2017;74(1):9–10.
5. Holtzmann J, Richieri R, Saba G, Allaili N, Bation R, Moliere F, et al. How to define treatment-resistant depression? Presse Med. 2016;45(3):323–8.
6. Kalia M, Costa E Silva J. Biomarkers of psychiatric diseases: current status and future prospects. Metabolism. 2015;64(3 Suppl 1):S11–5.
7. Liu C, Cripe TP, Kim MO. Statistical issues in longitudinal data analysis for treatment efficacy studies in the biomedical sciences. Mol Ther. 2010;18(9):1724–30.
8. Liu Y, Zhou X, Qin B, Del Giovane C, Zhang Y, Xie P. Efficacy, quality of life, and acceptability outcomes of atypical antipsychotic augmentation treatment for treatment-resistant depression: protocol for a systematic review and network meta-analysis. Syst Rev. 2014;3:133.
9. Lucas N, Hubain P, Loas G, Jurysta F. Treatment resistant depression: actuality and perspectives in 2017. Rev Med Brux. 2017;38(1):16–25.
10. Malhi GS, Byrow Y. Is treatment-resistant depression a useful concept? Evid Based Ment Health. 2016;19(1):1–3.
11. McIntyre RS, Filteau MJ, Martin L, Patry S, Carvalho A, Cha DS, et al. Treatment-resistant depression: definitions, review of the evidence, and algorithmic approach. J Affect Disord. 2014;156:1–7.
12. Miyamoto S, Jarskog LF, Fleischhacker WW. New therapeutic approaches for treatment-resistant schizophrenia: a look to the future. J Psychiatr Res. 2014;58:1–6.
13. Mrazek DA, Hornberger JC, Altar CA, Degtiar I. A review of the clinical, economic, and societal burden of treatment-resistant depression: 1996–2013. Psychiatr Serv. 2014;65(8):977–87.
14. Murphy JA, Sarris J, Byrne GJ. A review of the conceptualisation and risk factors associated with treatment-resistant depression. Depress Res Treat. 2017;2017:4176825.
15. Perlis RH. A clinical risk stratification tool for predicting treatment resistance in major depressive disorder. Biol Psychiatry. 2013;74(1):7–14.
16. Samara MT, Dold M, Gianatsi M, Nikolakopoulou A, Helfer B, Salanti G, et al. Efficacy, acceptability, and tolerability of antipsychotics in treatment-resistant schizophrenia: a network meta-analysis. JAMA Psychiat. 2016;73(3):199–210.
17. Smith DF. Quest for biomarkers of treatment-resistant depression: shifting the paradigm toward risk. Front Psych. 2013;4:57.
18. Souery D, Amsterdam J, de Montigny C, Lecrubier Y, Montgomery S, Lipp O, et al. Treatment resistant depression: methodological overview and operational criteria. Eur Neuropsychopharmacol. 1999;9(1–2):83–91.
19. Trevino K, McClintock SM, McDonald Fischer N, Vora A, Husain MM. Defining treatment-resistant depression: a comprehensive review of the literature. Ann Clin Psychiatry. 2014;26(3):222–32.

Genetic Factors Underlying Treatment Resistance in Psychiatry

3

Eduard Maron, Chen-Chia Lan, and David Nutt

3.1 Introduction

There are vast numbers of pharmacogenetic studies aiming at identifying genetic biomarkers that can aid in the prediction of therapeutic response in psychiatric disorders. The biomarkers would give impetus to the precision or even personalized medicine approach by guiding decision-making and the selection of the most suitable medication for individual patients. Moreover, the incorporation of predicting biomarkers into treatment algorithms could speed up the recovery process by shortening or eliminating lengthy and ineffective trials. Although the search for genetic biomarkers is facilitated by several approaches including epidemiological (family and twin) studies, molecular (linkage and association) methods, and more recently genome-wide association (GWA) studies, transcriptional and microRNA analyses, gene–environment interaction, and epigenetic approaches, no biomarkers have good enough sensitivity and specificity to be applied in clinical practice at present. In addition, the majority of available pharmacogenetic studies in psychiatry usually refer to how a specific gene or a set of genes can influence a patient's response or intolerance (e.g., side effects) to particular medicine(s), and only few of them have been specifically designed to explore biomarkers underlying treatment resistance, where nonresponse to at least two trials of medication of adequate dose and duration has been well-documented. In this chapter we reviewed large amount of available data and particularly focused on clinical evidence from pharmacogenetic data in major psychiatric disorders, in order to better understand the potential biomarkers involved in their treatment.

Two strategies are used for the exploration of treatment response-related genetic variability: pharmacogenetics and pharmacogenomics. Pharmacogenetics uses existing information and knowledge-based hypotheses for the selection of candidate genes to investigate their relation to

E. Maron (✉)
Department of Medicine, Centre for Neuropsychopharmacology, Division of Brain Sciences, Imperial College London, London, UK

Department of Psychiatry, University of Tartu, Tartu, Estonia

Department of Psychiatry, North Estonia Medical Centre, Tallinn, Estonia
e-mail: e.maron@imperial.ac.uk

C.-C. Lan
Department of Medicine, Centre for Neuropsychopharmacology, Division of Brain Sciences, Imperial College London, London, UK

Department of Psychiatry, Taichung Veterans General Hospital, Taichung, Taiwan
e-mail: c.lan16@imperial.ac.uk

D. Nutt
Department of Medicine, Centre for Neuropsychopharmacology, Division of Brain Sciences, Imperial College London, London, UK
e-mail: d.nutt@imperial.ac.uk

Y.-K. Kim (ed.), *Treatment Resistance in Psychiatry*, https://doi.org/10.1007/978-981-10-4358-1_3

response phenotypes, whereas pharmacogenomic studies conduct genome-wide investigations that are not based on previous knowledge or specific hypotheses. Although most studies use one or the other strategy, they are complementary and can be conducted in parallel or sequentially on the same cohorts. Often, the sample size determines the chosen analysis strategy. Small sample sizes should not be used for genome-wide studies of complex traits as the false-positive rate is significantly increased, and a candidate-gene approach is preferred. Large cohorts (in excess of $n = 1000$) are normally used for genome-wide investigations but are prone to producing false negatives after the stringent multiple analysis corrections are applied. The preferred strategy, sample size permitting, is the genome-wide approach followed by or in parallel to candidate gene studies, thus producing information on novel gene associations and simultaneously validating hypotheses.

3.2 Autism Spectrum Disorder (ASD)

The main diagnostic features of autism spectrum disorders (ASD) are stereotyped interests, impaired social communication, and repetitive behaviors. Although the precise etiology of ASD is still unknown, it is thought to be caused by abnormal neurodevelopment [104, 245]. There is no specific treatment for the core social deficits of ASD; however several clinical evidences indicate the efficacy of antipsychotics in the treatment of ASD-associated interfering behavior and irritability [213, 321, 348]. Although selective serotonin reuptake inhibitors (SSRIs) have often been used to control aggression, self-injury, repetitive behaviors, and anxiety in ASD [40], a Cochrane Database Systematic Review showed no evidence supporting the use of SSRIs for children with ASD and limited evidence of benefits in adults [347]. Furthermore, stimulant medications such as methylphenidate or mixed amphetamine salts are used for inattention and hyperactivity in ASD patients, although with higher side effects and lower response rates as compared to attention-deficit hyperactivity disorder (ADHD) patients without comorbid ASD [348].

Two available studies have explored pharmacogenomic effects of SSRIs, including fluvoxamine [322] and escitalopram [232] in ASD. Sugie et al. [322] evaluated whether variants in the promoter of a serotonin transporter gene (5-HTTLPR) influence the treatment response of 12-week fluvoxamine medication in very small sample of 19 Japanese youth with ASD. The authors reported that carriers of the L allele had greater response on the Clinical Global Impression – Improvement (CGI-I) subscale to fluvoxamine than those with the S variant (LL/LS versus SS); however, these data should be interpreted with caution due to limited sample size. Owley et al. [232] demonstrated in a larger sample of 58 children and adolescents diagnosed with ASD that subjects with the S/S genotype had the smallest reduction in the Aberrant Behavior Checklist–Irritability (ABC-I) scores after 10-week escitalopram treatment as compared to L-allele carriers.

In terms of pharmacogenetics of atypical antipsychotics in ASD, several neurotransmitter genes involved in the metabolism of risperidone were investigated in 45 children and adolescents with ASD to explore genetic variations associated with risperidone efficacy and safety [78]. In particular, polymorphisms in four genes were associated with clinical improvement, as measured by the Autism Treatment Evaluation Checklist (ATEC), including three neurotransmitter receptor genes [serotonin receptors HTR2A and HTR2C and dopamine receptor D3 (DRD3a)] and ABCB1, the gene encoding P-glycoprotein which is largely responsible for risperidone absorption in the small intestine [78]. Additionally, polymorphisms in three serotonin receptor genes (HTR2A, HTR2C, and HTR6) and brain-derived neurotrophic factor (BDNF) were associated with drug-associated change in prolactin levels. An open-label, flexible-dose trial among 32 children and adolescents with pervasive developmental disorder, not otherwise specified (PDD-NOS), demonstrated that T allele of HTR2C polymorphism rs3813929 was associated with reduced weight gain following 8-week risperidone treatment [112]. In a later report combining 181 young patients aged 4–17 years from 2 previous trials evaluating genetic effects of risperidone-induced side effects, at least 2 variants in cannabinoid receptor 1 (CNR1) and 1 variant in leptin (LEP) were significantly associated with weight gain [228]. The predictive impact of peripheral blood gene expressions of all exons on the behavioral responses to risperidone was explored in 42 children with ASD [189]. It was reported that mRNA levels of a total of 89 exons significantly differentiated high responders from low responders to risperidone, as evaluated by changes in ABC-I subscale scores. In particular, there were five genes significantly ($p < 0.001$) correlated with ABC-I percent change including guanylate-binding protein family member 6 (GBP6), RAB member RAS oncogene family-like 5 (RABL5), ring finger protein 213 (RNF213), nuclear factor of kappa light polypeptide gene enhancer in B-cell inhibitor delta (NFKBID), and ring finger protein 40 E3 ubiquitin-protein ligase (RNF40, which is located on 16p11.2, a region implicated in ASD). While the genes identified in this study did not corroborate prior pharmacogenetic findings from Correia et al. [78], the authors assume that the gene expression may reflect convergent downstream mechanisms from multiple genetic backgrounds [189].

Finally, the single pharmacogenetic study of stimulants so far has implicated monoaminergic genes in the therapeutic effect of methylphenidate on ASD-related behavioral problems [212]. As was demonstrated among children diagnosed with autistic disorder or PDD-NOS, several genes, including the dopamine receptor DRD1 ($p = 0.006$), adrenoceptor alpha 2A (ADRA2A) ($p < 0.02$), COMT ($p < 0.04$), DRD3 ($p < 0.05$), and DRD4 ($p < 0.05$), modify the reduction of hyperactive–impulsive symptoms [212]. Furthermore, the variants in two solute carrier family 6 (SLC6A) genes demonstrated borderline significant differences between responders and nonresponders, SLC6A4 ($p < 0.05$) and SLC6A3 ($p < 0.05$) [212]. Additionally, the minor allele of DRD2 ($p < 0.01$) was associated with a protective effect toward treatment intolerability, and rs6280 of DRD3 increased the risk for intolerability ($p < 0.04$), whereas DRD5, MAOB, and MAOA had no effect on treatment response or tolerability [212].

3.3 Attention-Deficit Hyperactivity Disorder (ADHD)

Attention-deficit hyperactivity disorder is characterized by excessive inattention and/or hyperactivity and impulsivity as well as executive dysfunction and lack of emotional self-control and motivation.

Pharmacotherapy with methylphenidate is generally suggested as the first-line treatment of choice in both children and adults with ADHD. A review of ADHD pharmacogenetics in children demonstrated significant effects of genes associated with neurodevelopment and noradrenergic systems in methylphenidate (MPH) response, whereas negative or inconsistent results were found in dopaminergic and serotonergic signaling, synaptosomal-associated protein 25 (SNAP25), and various metabolic enzymes [48]. In particular, the gene that encodes dopamine transporter (DAT) has been considered a promising candidate for pharmacogenetic research due to the major role of the transporter in stimulant's action. The most studied polymorphism is the 40-base pair (bp) variable number of tandem repeats in the 3′ untranslated region (3′-VNTR) at the dopamine transporter gene (DAT1 or SLC6A3) where the 10-repeat allele (10R) was associated with higher expression levels of the transporter [221, 257]. However, the pharmacogenetic effects of DAT1 VNTR on MPH responses were inconsistent. Several studies reported decreased MPH response in both adult and children homozygous with either 9-repeat allele (9R) [130, 318] or 10R [257, 267, 349], while other reports showed better MPH response in 10R homozygotes [154, 236], and still others reported no pharmacogenetic effect of the DAT1 VNTR [76, 174, 214, 219, 337, 375]. Two meta-analyses demonstrated no significant effect for the DAT1 VNTR on both methylphenidate treatment response and specific symptom dimensions [38, 134] Thus, DAT1 VNTR was considered to be a non-reliable predictor of methylphenidate treatment outcome (see for review Bruxel et al. [48]). Although there are some evidences showing that responsiveness to methylphenidate is affected by certain DRD4 gene polymorphisms, the available data are insufficient and limited to children samples (see for review Bruxel et al. [48].

The other good gene candidate is catechol-O-methyltransferase (COMT), which modulates catecholamine balance in the prefrontal cortex under methylphenidate action [65]. However, no strong evidence for the involvement of COMT in treatment response to MPH has been showed so far. Previous pharmacogenetic studies suggested a positive association between Val allele and response to methylphenidate [67, 144]; however no effect was found in an adult sample [74], and only a trend level improvement of hyperactive–impulsive symptoms with increasing doses of MPH in COMT Val homozygous was demonstrated in a children sample [100].

In terms of noradrenaline gene candidates, Kim et al. [148] explored the possible association between two single nucleotide polymorphisms (SNPs) at the norepinephrine transporter gene (NET1 or SLC6A2) and response to MPH treatment in Korean children with ADHD. Improvement in CGI-I following MPH treatment was observed among 61.4% of T-allele carriers as compared to 37.9% of A allele homozygous for the A-3081T (rs28386840) SNP ($P = 0.03$). However, no significant gene over-dose interaction effect for this SNP on MPH response was detected. Additionally, G1287A (rs5569) polymorphism showed no significant association with MPH response. Notably, the same research group did not replicate the association between MPH response and NET1 polymorphisms in their next study [180], and no effect was found in an adult sample [159]. Nevertheless, Yang et al. [362] reported that rs3785143 in NET1 had a nominally significant association with response rate to atomoxetine treatment in 111 Chinese ADHD children. In particular, the C allele was present in 77.1% of responders, whereas T allele was observed in 55.8% ($P = 0.005$). Regarding the pharmacogenetic effects of the adrenergic alpha 2A gene (ADRA2A), the G allele at SNP C-1291G (rs1800544) was associated with greater MPH response in children and adolescent [82, 100, 249], but again no effect of ADRA2A was found in an adult sample [75].

No association was observed between therapeutic response to methylphenidate and several serotonergic gene variations, including 5-HTTLPR, HTR1B (rs11568817, rs6296, and 13212041), tryptophan hydroxylase 2 (TPH2), and dopamine beta-hydroxylase (DBH) genes [74, 328]. Therefore, the serotonergic genes seem to be not major players in the therapeutic response either in children or adults with ADHD.

As was earlier showed, the functional polymorphism of BDNF gene (Val66Met), involved in intracellular trafficking and BDNF activity-dependent secretion, may have promising predictive effect on methylphenidate therapeutic outcome in ADHD. For example, recent study showed in 102 children with ADHD that those homozygous to Val/Val genotype achieve higher proportion of symptom remission (95.2%) than Met-carrier children (74.1%) ($p = 0.013$). Moreover, Val-allele homozygous patients were more frequently (81%) assessed as "not ill" or "very mild" according to CGI-I compared to 37% of Met-allele carriers ($P = 0.0002$), as well as more than 50% reduction in ADHD severity was observed in 95.2% of the Val-allele homozygous patients and in contrast to 74.1% of Met-allele carriers ($P = 0.018$) [147]. It was suggested that better methylphenidate response in Val/Val genotype carriers may probably be explained by a lower degree of brain anatomical anomaly and functional impairment in these individuals [147]. The other interesting candidate is the latrophilin 3 gene (LPHN3), which plays an important role in the regulation of neurotransmitter exocytosis [259]. In a study with large sample of children with ADHD ($n = 416$), four of the six investigated LPHN3 SNPs (rs1947274, rs2345039, rs6551655, and rs6858066) showed significant difference between responders and nonresponders

[167]. Moreover, the authors found that the rs6858066 G allele confers both risk to ADHD and better treatment response. LPHN3 polymorphism was also associated with combined-type ADHD in an independent adult sample [263]. However, the G allele of LPHN3 SNP rs6551665 has been paradoxically reported to be associated with better treatment response in the hyperactive dimension [12] and poorer treatment response in inattentive dimension [167]. It is possible that the differences in sample subtype composition and symptom dimension might be responsible for these divergent results observed in LPHN3 pharmacogenetic studies.

3.4 Panic Disorder with Agoraphobia (PDA)

Panic disorder is characterized by recurrent panic attacks, which are discrete periods of intense fear or discomfort, accompanied by at least 4 of 13 somatic and psychic symptoms [6]. About two-thirds of all patients with panic disorder suffer from comorbid agoraphobia, which is defined as fear in places or situations (e.g., crowds, public transport) from which escape might be difficult or in which help may not be available in the event of having unexpected panic attacks.

Although the data from twin and family studies suggest an involvement of genetic factors in the familial transmission of PD with the heritability estimate close to 48% [108], the genetic substrate underlying treatment response is still underinvestigated. Two available reports indicate that better response to selective serotonin reuptake inhibitor (SSRI) treatment is predicted by the L-form of 5-HTTLPR [243] and the 5-HT1A receptor -1019C/G polymorphism [366]. Additionally, the COMT 158Val allele was associated with greater symptom relief during exposure-based CBT [193], while carriers of the long MAOA-uVNTR alleles showed significantly worse response to CBT [262]. Recently, Trautmann et al. [330] reported preliminary evidence for poorer CBT treatment outcomes in a subgroup of female traumatized individuals carrying the low-active variant of the MAOA gene.

3.5 Generalized Anxiety Disorder (GAD)

The main feature of this anxiety disorder is excessive and persistent worry, accompanied by somatic anxiety symptoms as well as difficulty concentrating, muscle tension, sleep disturbances, restlessness, irritability, and fatigue.

Promising data have been reported by pharmacogenetic initiatives, where intensive search for genetic treatment predictors has revealed a few genes, including the pituitary adenylate cyclase-activating peptide (PACAP), the serotonin transporter (5-HTT), and the serotonin 2A receptor gene (HTR2A), as potential markers predicting treatment response to serotonin–norepinephrine reuptake inhibitors (SNRI) in patients with GAD [191]. Particularly, the Asp54Gly (rs2856966) variant in the PACAP gene was associated with better treatment outcome in 156 patients with GAD who have received 6 months of open-label venlafaxine XR flexible-dose treatment (75–225 mg/day) [77]. The involvement of HTR2A rs7997012 SNP in venlafaxine XR treatment response was also confirmed by individual analysis, showing that G allele predicts better treatment response being more prevalent among responders (70%) as compared to nonresponders (56%) at 6 months ($P = 0.05$) of medication [191]. In the same sample, they also examined a possible interaction between the serotonin transporter gene (SLC6A4) 5-HTTLPR/rs25531 haplotype and the HTR2A SNP rs7997012. The results show that subjects with 5-HTTLPR/rs25531 genotypes La/La+G/G or La/La+G/A ($n = 28$) had significantly lower Hamilton Anxiety Scale (HAM-A) scores than those with genotypes La/S+A/A or S/S+A/A ($n = 12$) at 6 months of treatment (HAM-A difference = 10.7; $P < 0.0001$) [192]. This difference was larger than the single marker analysis of either gene alone and demonstrated a gene–gene interaction effect. In contrast, none of the investigated polymorphisms within dopamine receptor D2 or dopamine transporter DAT1 genes showed impact on venlafaxine XR treatment response in the same sample of patients with GAD [278]. Earlier, Perlis et al.

[241] examined associations between 825 SNPs in 61 candidate genes and therapeutic response in patients with GAD receiving duloxetine 60–120 mg (N = 164) or placebo (N = 95). Variants in corticotropin-releasing hormone receptor 1 (CRHR1), dopamine receptor D3 (DRD3), nuclear receptor subfamily group C member 1 (NR3C1), and phosphodiesterase 1A (PDE1A) were associated with duloxetine response in GAD in their study.

3.6 Social Phobia (Social Anxiety Disorder, SAD)

SAD is characterized by persistent and unreasonable fear of being observed or evaluated negatively by others in social performance or interaction situations (e.g., speaking in public or being exposed to possible scrutiny by others) and is associated with somatic and cognitive anxiety symptoms.

Only few pharmacogenetic studies have ever been conducted in SAD so far. Small study reported that 5-HTTLPR genotype is associated with reduction in social anxiety symptoms during SSRI treatment [320]. However, in another study with a larger sample, none of the three gene candidates including 5-HTT, COMT, and TPH2 predicted CBT response [7]. The most powerful study to date with 346 patients with SAD has found that two of the four regulators of G-protein signaling 2 (RGS2) SNPs predicted remission to sertraline treatment and suggested this gene may be a genetic predictor of SSRI treatment response in social phobia [319].

3.7 Obsessive–Compulsive and Related Disorders (OCRDs)

OCD is characterized by recurrent obsessions (concerns involving contamination, harm, or sexual and religious preoccupations) or compulsions (e.g., behaviors or mental acts such as washing, checking, repeating, ordering, counting, hoarding), or both, that cause significant distress, interference with functioning, or time consumption by symptoms.

Several pharmacogenetic studies have been reported in OCD, but no definitive results support a single genetic variation or gene that determines SSRI response in OCD. However, the most intriguing pharmacogenetic findings involving both pharmacokinetics and pharmacodynamics have been reviewed in more details in very comprehensive review by Zai et al. [372]. As the authors summarized, only two cytochrome P450 liver enzyme genes, CYP2D6 and CYP2C19, have been studied in relation to the SSRI response in OCD. Nonresponders appear to be more common among non-extensive metabolizers according to genetic status of CYP2D6, suggesting that genes regulating drug metabolism may play an important role in treatment efficacy [43]. Regarding the pharmacodynamic studies in OCD, available data are still preliminary, either inconsistent or not, yet replicated in independent and well-powered samples. Among various candidates, a number of genes in the serotonin, glutamate, and dopamine systems and neurotrophic factors have been identified as promising genetic predictors of treatment response to antidepressants in OCD [372]. Furthermore, many new loci, including GRIN2B, glypican 6 (GPC6), dispatched homologue 1 (*Drosophila*) (DISP1), ankyrin repeat and fibronectin type III domain-containing protein 1, and arrestin domain-containing protein 4 (T-cell lymphoma invasion and metastasis 1, protocadherin 10 (PCDH10), and LOCT30101), have been showed as top hits associated with SSRI response in OCD patients [258]. However, a further research is required to clarify their functional status and their potential role in the treatment response.

3.8 Post-traumatic Stress Disorder (PTSD)

PTSD develops after a terrifying event that involved physical harm or the threat of physical harm and is characterized by recurrent and intrusive distressing recollections of the event, nightmares, dissociative flashbacks, distress at exposure to cues that resemble the trauma cause, avoidance of stimuli associated with the trauma, isolation from others, disturbed sleep, difficulty concentrating, exaggerated startle response, irritability, and hypervigilance.

Only few studies have been looking at the genetics of treatment response in PTSD. In particular, the LL genotype of 5-HTTLPR was related to greater response and lower dropouts due to adverse events to sertraline treatment among PTSD patients [224]. Additionally, Bryant et al. [49] demonstrated that the S allele of 5-HTTLPR may be associated with poorer long-term response to imaginal exposure-based CBT in individuals with PTSD. Two small studies indicate the possible predictive role of BDNF and glucocorticoid receptor gene BCLI polymorphisms on CBT treatment outcome in PTSD; however due to limited sample size, these data need further replication [97, 365].

3.9 Substance Use Disorders (SUDs)

Substance use disorders (SUDs), including abuse (harmful use) and dependence, are characterized by somatic or psychiatric problems caused by pathological patterns of the use of one or more substances.

3.10 Alcohol

Several pharmacogenetic studies have investigated the impact of opioid receptor mu subunit (OPRM1) gene on the response to the opioid antagonist naltrexone. The first report from a placebo-controlled treatment trial demonstrated that the Asp40 allele of Asn40Asp, encoded by an A118G SNP, predicted a significantly lower relapse rate of heavy drinking in naltrexone-treated patients [231]. Furthermore, under naltrexone treatment, European-American Asp40-allele carriers (n = 141) had a reduced likelihood of relapse to heavy drinking than Asn40-allele homozygotes, whereas no genotype effect was observed in the placebo groups [231]. Subsequently, in a larger sample of alcoholics (n = 604), Anton et al. [9] found that Asp40-allele carriers treated with naltrexone (100 mg/day) had a greater percentage of abstinent days and a lower percentage of heavy drinking days than Asn40-allele homozygotes. In an uncontrolled naltrexone trial (50 mg/day), Kim et al. [150] reported that alcohol-dependent individuals with one or two copies of the Asp40 allele maintained abstinence longer than Asn40-allele homozygotes, whose risk of relapse was 10.6 times that of the Asp40-allele carrier group, but due to the small sample size (n = 66), this effect did not reach statistically significant level. Additionally, heavy drinkers carrying Asp40 G allele showed a significantly greater percentage of non-hazardous drinking days following treatment with 100 mg/day of naltrexone when compared to placebo controls or carriers of A-allele homozygotes in either treatment group [63]. Regarding other opioid candidate genes, Krystal et al. [165] demonstrated earlier that not only polymorphisms in OPRD1 and OPRK1, but also OPRM1, failed to influence the effects of naltrexone (50 mg/day) in alcohol-dependent male subjects. Despite the inconsistent findings for Asn40Asp impact on naltrexone efficacy, a meta-analysis conducted by Chamorro et al. [60] has concluded that alcohol-dependent Asp40-allele carriers are approximately half as likely to relapse when treated with naltrexone as compared with placebo. However, no main effect of either naltrexone or the Asn40Asp SNP was demonstrated in the first prospective study of the Asn40Asp SNP as a moderator of naltrexone's effects among 221 alcohol-dependent individuals [230]. Finally, a number of OPRM1, OPRD1, and OPRK1 polymorphisms did not moderate any effect on the response to nalmefene 20 mg/day in a large sample of individuals (n = 272) with alcohol problems [13].

Among dopaminergic genes, DBH showed moderating effects of naltrexone medication on the primary outcome of abstinence from heavy drinking in alcohol-dependent individuals (n = 107). Carriers of the DBH rs1611115 T allele were significantly more likely to not drink heavily than C-allele homozygotes under naltrexone treatment but responded poorer to disulfiram treatment [14]. Earlier, Lawford et al. [177] found that the greatest reductions in craving were achieved in 83 alcohol-dependent inpatients with bromocriptine (7.5 mg/day), who were C-allele carriers (i.e., A1/A1 or A1/A2 genotype) of the ankyrin repeat and kinase domain-containing protein 1 (ANKK1; adjacent to DRD2) Taq1A polymorphism. Furthermore, the impact of several polymorphisms at ANKK1 (Taq1A), GABRB2 (C1412T), and GABRA6 (T1519C) on naltrexone (50 mg/day) and acamprosate (1.3–2.0 g/day) treatment was reported by Ooteman et al. [229] in alcohol-dependent patients ($n = 126$), although most findings failed to reach the conventional significance level of <0.05 and there was no effort to correct for multiple testing, leaving the findings uninterpretable. Additionally, 12 weeks of treatment with topiramate or placebo in heavy drinkers ($n = 122$) revealed that only homozygote carriers of rs2832407 C allele in the kainate GluK1 receptor subunit gene (GRIK1) had greater reduction of heavy drinking days as compared to placebo [162]. Earlier, Ray et al. [261] reported that this SNP moderated topiramate's adverse effects in non-treatment-seeking heavy drinkers. In a 3-month acamprosate trial in a relatively large sample of alcohol-dependent subjects ($n = 225$), the length of abstinence was significantly associated with two polymorphisms (rs2058878, rs2300272) in GRIN2B, which encode the GluN2B subunit of the NMDA receptor. Among acamprosate-treated alcoholics, the minor A allele of rs2058878 was associated with a longer duration of abstinence, while the minor rs2300272 G allele was associated with a shorter duration of abstinence [137].

Kranzler et al. [161] examined the effects of the 5-HTTLPR tri-allelic genotype on the response to sertraline (200 mg/day) in 134 individuals with early-onset or late-onset alcohol dependence. In L′ homozygotes, later age of onset was significantly associated with better treatment response to sertraline, while younger age of onset demonstrated poorer response. Johnson et al. [126] studied the effect of ondansetron, a 5-HT-3 antagonist, on reducing the severity of alcohol drinking and its genetic association. They reported that 5-HTTLPR L-allele homozygotes treated with ondansetron had fewer heavy drinking days and more abstinent days than those receiving placebo. In addition, individuals who were also rs1042173*T-allele (a SNP in the 3′ untranslated region of SLC6A4) homozygotes showed the greatest reductions in drinking outcomes compared to the remaining genotype by medication groups combined. In a secondary analysis of the same trial, Johnson et al. [127] revealed that individuals with one or more of the following genotypes, rs1150226-AG and rs1176713-GG in HTR3A, or rs17614942-AC in HTR3B, had significantly greater response to ondansetron than placebo. They calculated that the use of these three genotypes plus the two SLC6A4 polymorphisms would identify 34% of European Americans with alcohol dependence who are likely to respond very favorably to ondansetron treatment.

3.11 Nicotine

To date, available pharmacogenetic studies on nicotine dependence have focused mainly on the impact of genetic variation on the subjective response to the drug and on treatment outcome in smoking cessation trials [128]. Perkins et al. [237] found that during negative mood states, Taq1A T-allele carriers reported greater "liking" and consumed greater amount of nicotine cigarettes than C-allele homozygotes. Similarly, DRD2 C957T*C-allele homozygotes also smoked more nicotine cigarettes during negative mood states than during positive mood states [238]. However, no association between smoking cessation and variation in a number of dopaminergic genes, including COMT, DRD2, DRD3, DRD4, SLC6A3, and TH, was demonstrated in another prospective outcome trial in women. Furthermore, mixed results have also been reported regarding the involvement of ANKK1 polymorphisms on pharmacological treatment outcome in smokers. Cinciripini et al. [70] reported that smokers without the Taq1 A1 allele treated with venlafaxine had a substantial reduction in negative affect following smoking cessation. A1-allele carriers also quit significantly less often than A2 homozygotes; however, no genotype by treatment interaction was revealed on abstinence rates. In contrast, Taq1 A1 allele was not associated with withdrawal or with daily smoking abstinence rates during the 6-week treatment following smoking cessation [266]. Nevertheless, the effect of ANKK1 gene was observed on bupropion efficacy for smoking cessation in 577 heavy smokers. In particular, A1 homozygotes treated with bupropion had a 28% greater likelihood of smoking cessation, compared to a 12% greater likelihood of cessation among A2-allele carriers [44]. However, the opposite effect was observed by another large randomized, placebo-controlled study (722 smokers) in which A2 homozygotes treated with bupropion were more than 3 times as likely as placebo-treated individuals to be abstinent at the end of the treatment and at 6-month follow-up [85]. Earlier, Yudkin et al. [371] found that A1-allele carriers had less therapeutic benefit from the nicotine patch than A2-allele homozygotes, but no significant mediating effect of the Taq1A genotype on the efficacy of nicotine replacement therapy (NRT) in smoking cessation was demonstrated by other studies [30, 86, 316]. In addition, smokers with at least one copy of the DRD2 141C Del allele and two copies of the neuronal calcium sensor-1 protein FREQ A allele (rs1054879) had a significantly higher abstinence rate with NRT compared to other smokers (62% vs. 29–38%) [83].

3.12 Opioids

A number of pharmacogenetic trials have examined the impact of genetic variations on methadone and buprenorphine treatment response in opioid dependence. For example, exploring 95 treatment-seeking opioid users, Lawford et al. [176] reported a significant association between the Taq1 A1 allele and poor response to methadone treatment. However, no significant differences in A1-allele frequency were found between methadone- and buprenorphine-treated patients with poor and successful treatment outcomes in a later study with 116 subjects [25]. Crettol et al. [79] also failed to confirm any association between the Taq1 A1 allele, the D1 dopamine common variant (Ddel, −48A>G), and mu opioid Asn40Asp (A118G) receptor gene and the response to methadone treatment in a sample of 238 methadone-maintained patients, but they did find an association with the C/C genotype of DRD2 polymorphism C957T and poor response to methadone treatment.

Regarding opioid receptor genes, no association between OPRM1 alleles and methadone treatment response was revealed [99]. The effect of the delta opioid receptor gene (OPRD1) SNPs on the response to opioid substitution therapy was investigated in 643 patients who were randomized to receive 24 weeks of buprenorphine/naloxone or methadone maintenance treatment [80]. As demonstrated, an intronic OPRD1 SNP (rs678849) predicted treatment outcome for both pharmacotherapies among African-American participants ($N = 77$). In a more recent study, researchers found that two other intronic OPRD1 SNPs (rs581111 and rs529520) predicted buprenorphine treatment outcomes, but in females only. Particularly, females with the AA or AG genotypes at rs581111 had significantly worse outcomes compared to carriers of the GG genotype, while females with rs529520 AA genotype had a significantly worse outcome as compared to females with the CC genotype [71].

3.13 Cocaine

Only few pharmacogenetic studies have been published so far on cocaine dependence. Disulfiram treatment has been reported to reduce the number of cocaine-positive urines significantly, but the effect was only seen among subjects with the dopamine β-hydroxylase (DβH) gene variant that is associated with normal DβH levels [160]. Other dopamine-related genes, such as the ANKK1 (rs1800497) and DRD2 (rs2283265) polymorphisms, seem to be associated with disulfiram treatment response [309]. The α-1 adrenergic receptor (ADRA1A) polymorphism (rs1048101) was also associated with disulfiram treatment response [303]. In particular, the minor T allele had a significantly lower percentage of cocaine-positive urines, while no treatment effect was observed among those homozygous for the major C allele.

3.14 Dementia

Dementia is a syndrome of progressive cognitive decline, characterized by various central neurodegenerative or ischemic processes, sufficient to interfere with the activities of daily living.

It should be noted that pharmacogenetic trials of dementia are still in a very early stage. To date, apolipoprotein-E (APOE) has been the main candidate gene, and the presence of the APOE-4 allele has been reported to differentially influence drug response in Alzheimer's disease patients treated with cholinergic enhancers (such as donepezil, galantamine, rivastigmine), endogenous nucleotides, neuroprotective compounds, rosiglitazone, immunotrophins, neurotrophic factors, or their combinations [50–53, 55, 56, 265, 268, 269]. Controversial results are frequently observed due to methodological problems, study design, and patient recruitment in clinical trials. Nevertheless, APOE-4/4 carriers have been demonstrated to be associated with the worst treatment outcome in long-term open clinical trials with multifactorial treatment [50–53, 55, 56]. Similarly, the presenilin gene has also been reported to interact with multifactorial treatment response that PSEN1-1/1 homozygotes are the worst responders and PSEN1-2/2 carriers are the better responders [53]. In addition, angiotensin-converting enzyme (ACE) genotype also influences multifactorial treatment response as the ACE-D/D patients showed the poorest response, ACE-I/I carriers had intermediate response, and ACE-I/D carriers had the most positive treatment response [51, 54].

The genetic variations in drug-metabolizing enzymes, including CYP2D6 and CYP3A4, were the other promising candidates for pharmacogenetic research in dementia. In a prospective study including 127 Caucasian Alzheimer' patients treated with donepezil for 6 months, the nonresponders had a significantly higher frequency of the G allele of the CYP2D6 rs1080985 SNP [248]. Since it has been demonstrated that the G allele is associated with a higher enzyme activity and, therefore, a faster metabolism, it is suggested that the poorer response to donepezil is due to lower plasma concentrations of the drug [248]. However, another clinical trial exploring treatment response to three cholinesterase inhibitors (ChEIs) including donepezil, galantamine, or rivastigmine found no significant associations between CYP2D6 and BCHE (the gene coding for butyrylcholinesterase) genotypes and response to treatment after 1 year for all three ChEIs [68]. The controversial results might be explained by the difference in follow-up periods and the definition of treatment response. However, since higher plasma concentrations could be associated with a higher response rate but possibly also with a higher frequency of adverse effects, further research is needed to clarify the impact of polymorphisms in CYP2D6 on plasma concentrations of donepezil and the clinical response. To date, no major role in the variability in donepezil metabolism has been observed for CYP3A4 and CYP3A5 genes [197].

3.15 Schizophrenia (SCH)

Schizophrenia is a chronic, severe, and debilitating mental disorder, which is affecting about 1% of the population in the world and characterized by psychotic or "positive" symptoms, including hallucinations and delusions, as well as negative symptoms and various deficits, including inability to pay attention, the loss of sense of pleasure, and social withdrawal.

A number of pharmacogenetic studies have investigated either the drug class or specific antipsychotics (e.g., clozapine, olanzapine, and risperidone); however, most of the findings have not been clearly replicated in independent studies; therefore the results should be interpreted with caution [23]. Numerous studies suggest the involvement of dopaminergic candidate genes in the efficacy of clozapine. The finding that a 48 bp repeat in exon III of the dopamine receptor 4 (DRD4) gene was associated with clozapine treatment response indicates that this receptor might be important in clozapine's efficacy [297, 299, 376]. The five-repeat allele was more frequently found in clozapine nonresponders; however this evidence was not replicated in two later studies [260, 264]. The DRD3 Ser9Gly functional polymorphism has been demonstrated to be associated with clozapine efficacy in several studies. The D3 Gly9 variant, which codes for a higher-affinity dopamine receptor, was related to better improvement of psychotic symptom following clozapine treatment [280, 298]. A meta-analysis concluded that although not statistically significant, a trend level of this D3 Gly9 variant association was found, and the small effect may be explained by differences in the clinical characteristics of different studies [120]. Dopamine D1 and D2 genetic variants have also been shown to be associated with clozapine treatment response [117–119, 253]. Finally, dopamine transporter (DAT) genetic variants have been associated with clozapine response [356], although a previous study did not find an association in a cohort of patients treated with a variety of second-generation antipsychotics [326].

Evidence suggesting an involvement of serotonergic receptor gene variants in clozapine efficacy has also been reported. Several 5-HT2A polymorphisms have been associated with clozapine response [15, 16, 21, 22, 205, 369], although these associations have not been clearly replicated [19, 22]. Insufficient clozapine effect on psychotic symptoms has been associated with the HTR2A 102-C and −1438-G variants, which cause reduced receptor expression, and Tyr452, and as consequence decreased receptor functioning [18]. In addition, 5-HT2C [20, 306], 5-HT6 [368] receptor, and serotonin transporter (5-HTT or SLC6A4) variants [20, 157] have also been reported to be associated with clozapine treatment effect, although negative findings also exist (please see Arranz et al. [23]).

In single reports clozapine efficacy has also been associated with histamine H2 receptor (H2) [199], COMT [351], CYP1A2 [93], G-protein subunit 3 (GNB3) [158], and dysbindin (DTNPB1) [380], oxytocin (OXT) [307], and GDNF family receptor α2 (GFRA2) [308] gene variants; however further replications in independent studies are needed. In the contrary, clozapine-targeted adrenergic and glutamatergic receptor variants [36, 37, 332] and CYP2D6 functional variants [17] were not associated with clozapine response.

In terms of pharmacogenetics of olanzapine efficacy, once again the main target genes belong to dopaminergic and serotonergic systems. An association between the DRD3 Gly9 variant with greater improvement of positive symptoms during olanzapine treatment was observed [2, 312] although this association was not found in Indian patients [329]. The long allele (L) of the 5-HTTLPR polymorphism [42] and several 5-HT6 polymorphisms [115] were associated with better response to olanzapine. In addition, olanzapine efficacy has also been associated with COMT [31], glutamate receptor type 3 (GRM3) [35], multidrug resistance transporter (MDR1 or ABCB1) [41], adrenergic receptor 1A (ADRA1A) [115], noradrenaline transporter (SLC6A2) [216], and melacortin 2 receptor (MC2R) [115] variants. No positive association was demonstrated between the efficacy of olanzapine and CYP2D6 and CYP1A2 gene polymorphisms [329].

Lower risperidone efficacy has been reported to be associated with several DRD2 polymorphisms including the D2 Ser311 allele [171] and the D2 −241-G allele [122, 355]. Patients who are D2 Taq1 polymorphism A1 variant homozygotes also showed superior improvement in psychotic symptoms with risperidone treatment [122]. Additionally, the DRD3 Ser9Gly polymorphism has been associated with the efficacy of risperidone in a study of Chinese patients [170], but this finding was not replicated in another independent study [359]. Finally, no association was found with D4 variants in a small cohort of Israeli patients [373].

Significant associations with the efficacy of risperidone have also been demonstrated for serotonergic polymorphisms. In particular, the 5-HT2A 102-C variant has been associated with better risperidone efficacy in Chinese [169] and

Korean [145] patients but poorer response in Caucasian patients [18]. In Japanese patients, 5-HT2A haplotypes also showed a trend of association with risperidone efficacy [360]. Several 5-HT2C polymorphisms were associated with risperidone efficacy in Chinese patients [190]. In addition, better risperidone efficacy has been shown in patients with the 5-HT6 267-T/T [172], 5-HT3A rs14396-G/G [106], and 5-HT1A 1019--C/C [340] genotypes, while no association was observed for 5-HT7 gene variants [344]. Finally, the L allele of the 5-HTTLPR polymorphism has been associated with greater response to risperidone [341].

In terms of other candidate genes, risperidone efficacy, similar to that of clozapine and olanzapine, has been associated with COMT [98, 107] and MDR1 [354] variants. In addition, CYP3A4 1G variant has been demonstrated to be associated with the degree of improvement in psychotic symptoms [92]. Finally, BDNF repeat [357], GRM3 rs724226 polymorphism [98], and several SNPs in RGS4 [173] were reported to be associated with the efficacy of risperidone treatment.

There have been fewer studies of other antipsychotics where all the patients in the cohort have been treated with the same medication. Chlorpromazine and haloperidol are two first-generation antipsychotics with high dopamine receptor binding affinity, and the efficacy of these two antipsychotics was associated with DRD2 gene [279, 353]. Haloperidol efficacy was also associated with the number of active alleles of CYP2D6 gene [47]. Aripiprazole is a dopamine D2 receptor partial agonist with high affinity for dopamine and relatively low affinity for serotonin receptors. Dopamine D2 Taq1 genotypes seem to moderate aripiprazole efficacy in Chinese and Korean patients [166, 300], but no significant effect was observed between D3 variants and aripiprazole efficacy [66]. Finally, a single report associated MDR1 variants with the efficacy of the first-generation antipsychotic bromperidol [363].

The first genome-wide association (GWA) studies on both first-generation and second-generation antipsychotics identified a region in chromosome 12 hypothesized to contain genes associated with antipsychotic-induced weight gain [59] and GABA pathway genes related to drug-induced tardive dyskinesia [124], but these results needed to be interpreted with caution due to small sample sizes. Several GWA studies were conducted on a subgroup of 750 subjects from the CATIE (Clinical Antipsychotic Trials of Intervention Effectiveness) study, and the results showed association of polymorphisms in the ankyrin repeat and sterile α-motif domain containing 1B (ANKS1B) and contactin-associated protein-like 5 (CNTNAP5) and the treatment efficacy of olanzapine and risperidone in resolving negative symptoms [210]. Polymorphisms in the proximity of ETS homologous factor (EHF), solute carrier family 26 member 9 (SLC26A9), D2, G-protein-coupled receptor 137B (GPR137B), carbohydrate sulfotransferase 8 (CHST8), and interleukin-1α (IL1A) have also been demonstrated to be associated with neurocognition improvement during treatment [211]. In terms of treatment-associated side effects, polymorphisms in the nitric oxide synthase 1 adaptor protein (NOS1AP) and in the nucleotide-binding protein-like (NUBPL) genes were linked to QT interval prolongation [1]. A Meis homeobox 2 (MEIS2) gene polymorphism was found to mediate risperidone's effect on hip and waist circumference [3]. Finally, EPF1, NOVA1, and FIGN underlined antipsychotic-induced parkinsonism [5]. However all these reported associations need further confirmation in independent samples.

Two GWA studies performed in a sample of 457 patients treated with the relatively new antipsychotic iloperidone revealed polymorphisms in the neuronal PAS domain protein 3 (NPAS3) and Kell blood group complex subunit-related family member 4 (XKR4) genes associated with treatment response [175], and polymorphisms in the ceramide kinase-like (CERKL) and solute carrier organic anion transporter 3A1 (SLCO3A1) genes associated with QT interval prolongation [339]. Implementing parallel in vivo transcriptomic studies and GWA studies on patient cohorts, several genes in neurodevelopment and neurogenesis were demonstrated to be involved in risperidone action [121].

Several gene association studies have focused on the association with treatment-resistant status in patients with schizophrenia, although all of these studies involved white participants only and none of these findings have survived multiple-testing correction. Treatment resistance has been associated with fewer long alleles of the BDNF dinucleotide repeat polymorphism [163] but not associated with either the BDNF G169A polymorphism (Val66Met) or the C270T polymorphism [10]. In addition, the C/C genotype of the 5-HT2A T102C polymorphism has been associated with treatment resistance [129], and this result was replicated in another sample (but only in females) [11]. A significantly higher frequency of the C/A genotype for the TPH1 gene in treatment-resistant patients was also shown, but the guanine nucleotide-binding protein (GNB3) gene did not differ between treatment-resistant and good-response patients [11].

The dopamine receptor 3 (DRD3) gene, specifically the Bal I polymorphism, demonstrated significantly less homozygosity in treatment-resistant patients [164]. In a study focusing on the 5′UTR (ccG repeat) polymorphism of the reelin gene, a significantly higher frequency of ccG10 alleles in treatment-resistant patients was found [105]. No group differences between treatment-resistant and treatment-responsive patients in terms of RGS4 gene were observed [135]. Finally, the human leukocyte antigen (HLA) A1 allele was significantly more prevalent in treatment-resistant patients [168], but another study showed no group difference in terms of HLA genotype [217].

Finally, one study attempted to probe into the association of genetic loading and the prevalence of schizophrenia spectrum disorders, cluster A personality disorders, and long-term psychiatric care in relatives [131]. The authors reported that first- and second-degree relatives of treatment-resistant patients demonstrated a significantly higher morbidity risk of schizophrenia spectrum disorders as compared to relatives of treatment-responsive patients, and a significantly higher familial-loading score was observed for treatment-resistant patients.

3.16 Unipolar Depression

Unipolar depression, or major depressive disorder (MDD), is characterized by the persistence of low mood, lack of motivation or energy, and negative thoughts that disrupt cognition and behavior.

The serotonergic system has been the most extensively explored system in pharmacogenetics of antidepressant response to date due to the fact that all major antidepressants act on 5-HT signaling and that serotonin transporter is one of the main genetic targets. Several meta-analyses [139, 252, 286] and later studies [270, 276, 302, 313] reported that the 5-HTTLPR L or L(A) carriers have higher response and remission rates, but one meta-analysis [327] and two later studies [8, 250] found no association between 5-HTTLPR and antidepressant response. Ethnical differences in involved samples may explain the discrepancy in evidences as most associations with treatment response were found in Caucasians but not in other ethnicities [39, 222]. However, the S allele has been associated with better response in elderly and Asian patients with MDD [149, 225, 255, 282, 350]. Furthermore, the S allele has been linked to higher rates of side effects [251, 313] and antidepressant-induced mania [32, 84, 101]. SLC6A4 variable number tandem repeat (VNTR) polymorphism within intron 2 (STin2) has also been investigated regarding its association with antidepressant response, and the 12/12 genotype was related to a better response in individuals of Asian descent [139, 226] but a poorer response in Caucasian patients with MDD [222, 346]. However, several studies did not confirm an association of this polymorphism with antidepressant response [91, 125, 305]. Other polymorphisms in SCL6A4 have been studied less extensively, but the rs8076005 AA genotype and A allele were associated with response rate of antidepressant medication [208].

The study focusing on serotonin receptor gene produced more divergent results. Three meta-analyses have looked into HTR1A rs6295 (−1019C/G) polymorphism but found no significant effect of rs6295 on antidepressant response or side effects [139, 226, 377]. Inconsistent findings were also reported regarding the associations of HTR1A rs10042486, rs1364043, and rs180042 [61, 138, 370]. The HTR1B rs6296 and rs6298 polymorphisms were associated with antidepressant response in two studies [338, 358], but negative results were demonstrated by another study [346]. The A allele of the HTR2A rs7997012 polymorphism has been associated with superior treatment response in the Sequenced Treatment Alternatives to Relieve Depression (STAR*D) trial [215]. However, two meta-analyses found mixed results in terms of the association of rs7997012 polymorphism and treatment response [188, 226]. In addition, mixed results have also been noted regarding HTR2A rs6311 (−1438 A/G) [26, 96, 123, 141, 155, 188, 226, 227] or rs6313 (102C/T) [188, 226] polymorphisms and treatment response.

TPH1 and TPH2 are two genes coding for the enzyme responsible for 5-hydroxytryptamine synthesis but have been associated with antidepressant response inconsistently [123, 151, 246, 247, 270, 294, 295, 358, 367]. While TPH1 rs1800532 C/C carriers have been reported to have better response to medication by an earlier meta-analysis [139], a later meta-analysis could not confirm this association [226].

Most genetic studies on BDNF have focused on the rs6265 (Val66Met, G196A), and meta-analyses have found that Val homozygotes are associated with poorer antidepressant response [139] and that Val/Met heterozygotes had superior overall response, remission, and SSRI response [226, 361]. Furthermore, drug-specific genotype associations [72], better response with the Met allele receiving paroxetine in elderly with depression [223], and duration until SSRI response [203] have been associated with rs6265 polymorphism, but other studies reported negative results (please see [183]).

The FKBP5 gene is involved in the inhibition of glucocorticoid receptors in the hypothalamus–pituitary–adrenal axis. Its several polymorphisms, including rs1360780, rs4713916, and rs3800373, have been associated with antidepressant response [34]. Interactive effects between rs1360780 polymorphism and SNPs in GRIK4 and HTR2A on remission during antidepressant treatment have also been observed [113]. Overall, associations between rs1360780 and antidepressant response have been replicated in other samples [152, 315], but negative findings were also reported [46, 235, 277, 331]. Associations of other variants with treatment response such as rs4713916 and rs352428 have also been demonstrated [94, 182]. Notably, association of FKBP5 variants with treatment-emergent suicide ideation has been earlier detected [46, 244]. Finally, meta-analyses have shown association with antidepressant response with FKBP5 rs4713916, rs1360780, and rs3800373 polymorphisms and suggested FKBP5 may be one of the most promising candidate genes in major depression [226, 379]. Other genes involved in the HPA axis, such as corticotrophin-releasing hormone (CRH), CRH-binding protein, and CRH receptor 1, as well as glucocorticoid receptors, have also been implicated in antidepressant treatment response [33, 62, 185].

A number of other genes have been investigated in relation to antidepressant response. The guanine nucleotide-binding protein beta polypeptide 3 (GNB3) gene C825T polymorphism (rs5443) has been associated with antidepressant response [143, 178, 186, 290, 345, 378], but negative or contradictory findings are also reported [132, 136, 140]. Moreover, meta-analyses showed inconsistent findings as better antidepressant response in T-allele carriers was shown in participants of Asian descent [116, 226], but no such association was found in another studies [139]. The GRIK4 rs1954787 C allele and other GRIK4 variants have been linked to antidepressant response [113, 220, 233, 256], although again negative findings are also reported so far [240, 284]. Recently, a meta-analysis showed that rs1954787 C allele was associated with better treatment response [142]. The COMT, DAT, DRD2, or DRD4 gene showed contradictory and mostly negative results in terms of the association with antidepressant response [183]. Several inflammation-related genes have been linked to antidepressant response, including cyclic AMP-responsive element-binding protein 1 (CREB1)

[57, 223], tumor necrosis factor, interleukin 11 [254], interleukin 1 beta [28], and melanocortin 1 receptor [352]. Finally, although the association of CYP2D6 or CYP2C19 on antidepressant response has been demonstrated [183], the combination of genotyping with therapeutic drug monitoring in certain cases has been earlier recommended when exploring these genes [111]. In addition, there are also recommendations for the initial dosage of antidepressant treatment based on genetic information [109, 110, 153].

Several GWAS have investigated genetic effects on antidepressant response, but no variants with genome-wide significance were identified so far [183]. A meta-analysis utilizing the data from the Genome-Based Therapeutic Drugs for Depression (GENDEP) project, the Munich Antidepressant Response Signature (MARS) project, and the Sequenced Treatment Alternatives to Relieve Depression (STAR*D) study samples revealed no variant associated with treatment response at a genome-wide level of significance [103]. Future investigations conducting more in-depth analyses of gene–gene and gene–environment interactions, pathway analyses, and machine learning techniques may advance our understandings of genetic variants associated with antidepressant response [187].

3.17 Bipolar Disorder

Bipolar disorder is a debilitating mental disorder characterized by the recurrence of depressive and hypomanic or manic episodes alternating with intervals of partial or full recovery.

Pharmacogenetic research in bipolar disorder is still in a relative nascent stage, and further large cohorts of patients with well-characterized treatment regimen and response profiles are needed to advance our understanding in this important field. So far, most of the pharmacogenetic research in bipolar disorder focused on lithium.

The serotonergic system is one of the most explored by pharmacogenetics in bipolar disorder. The 5-HTTLPR polymorphism has been associated with lithium response but with controversial results. The heterozygous L/S genotype was associated with superior lithium response [293], while the S/S genotype has been associated with both good and poor responses to lithium [87, 273]. The 5-HTTLPR S allele alone was associated with poor response to lithium in patients with bipolar disorder [271], but no association was found by other studies [201, 218]. In addition, patients with both the S allele and the BDNF Val/Val genotype were significantly more frequent among the poor lithium responders [275]. Association studies on serotonin receptor gene did not show association between genetic variants and lithium prophylaxis response, excluding a major involvement of serotonin genes in response to lithium prophylaxis in bipolar disorder [89, 201, 292]. Finally, an association between the TPH1 rs1800532 A/A genotype and poor response to lithium was earlier demonstrated [287].

Regarding the dopaminergic systems, the G allele of the DRD1 rs4532 polymorphism predicted a poor response to treatment in patients with bipolar disorder [272]. Additionally, no associations between other dopamine receptors and dopamine-metabolizing enzyme (including MAOA and COMT) gene polymorphism were reported by several studies [288, 289, 291, 333]. In terms of genetic variants of the glutamatergic system, several studies found no association with lithium response [69, 271, 324]. However, two other genes coding for protein that interacts with the glutamatergic receptors, the CACNG2 gene [304] and the FYN gene rs3730353 [325] and rs6916861 [271] polymorphism, were associated with lithium response.

In regard to BDNF gene variants and lithium response, some studies have suggested that the Val allele of the functional polymorphism rs6265 (Val66Met) predicts a poor response to lithium [89, 274]. Interestingly, Wang et al. demonstrated association between the Val/Met and Met/Met genotypes and a good lithium response in bipolar I disorder patients, while the same genotypes were associated with a poor response in bipolar II disorder patients [343]. Furthermore, no association between five BDNF polymorphisms (including Val66Met) and lithium response was observed in a Korean sample [234]. Finally, divergent results were found in regard to the association between the NTRK2 gene and lithium response [45, 90].

Lithium has been shown to be involved in the inositol pathway [301], and several genetic variants related to this pathway and their association with lithium response were explored. Two polymorphisms of the IMPA2 gene showed a trend to significant association with good lithium response [88]. An association between the INNP1 C937A polymorphism and response to lithium was found in Norwegian bipolar patients but not in an independent Israeli sample [317]. In addition, INNP1 rs2067421 polymorphism was linked to lithium response in patients with bipolar disorder [45], but this result was not replicated in another sample [218]. A dinucleotide repeat allele of the PLCG1 gene related was associated with lithium-responsive bipolar disorder [195, 334], but other markers within the coding region of PLCG1 did not give such evidence of a major role for this gene in lithium response [102]. Finally, an Asn796Ser SNP in the BCR gene was found to be significantly associated with lithium response [206].

The modulation of GSK3B activity has been demonstrated to be pivotal in the action of mood stabilizers [184]. Lithium inhibits GSK3B by a magnesium-competitive mechanism [156, 314]. Significant association between the C/C genotype of -50T/C GSK3B (rs334558) polymorphism and good lithium response was reported [4, 29]. On the contrary, no association of GSK3B SNPs with lithium response was found in several other studies [218, 271, 323], although a trend for association between the rs6438552 SNP of the GSK3B [4, 29] gene and good response to lithium was reported [209].

A few studies have investigated circadian clock genes in relation to lithium response. The T allele of the Rev-Erb-α rs2314339 polymorphism was linked to poor lithium response [58], but another study failed to detect such association [202]. In addition, the NR1D1 rs2071427 and CRY1 rs8192440 polymorphisms were associated with good response to lithium [209]. Notably, the rs2071427 of NR1D1 and rs6438552 of GSK3B had significant additive effects in predicting lithium response [209].

Moreover, lithium interacts with the PKC pathway, which plays a crucial role in mediating a number of intracellular responses to neurotransmitters [204]. However, PKC pathway-related gene variants showed mostly no association with lithium response [45, 310].

The involvement of lithium in the regulation of various gene expressions makes the transcription factor genes interesting targets for pharmacogenomic studies in lithium response. An association between the G/G genotype of the XBP1 rs2269577 polymorphism and reduced response to lithium has been demonstrated [133, 207]. A significant association between the CREB1 rs6740584 and rs2551710 SNPs and good response to lithium was showed [198]. The AP2B gene association study with lithium response performed to date led to negative results [218].

Linkage studies carried out thus far have suggested over 40 susceptibility regions in bipolar disorder (see for review [81]), but available meta-analyses have failed to provide strong evidence for any of the loci [24]. To sum up, chromosome 18 [95], 18q22.3 [335], 7q11.2 [336], 3p25 and 3p14 [194], and 14q11 [194] were identified in these linkage studies focusing on lithium response. In terms of the GWAS, two did not report any genome-wide significant findings [242, 311]. In another GWAS conducted in a sample of 294 Han patients with bipolar disorder from Taiwan, a GADL1 SNP reached genome-wide significance [64]. However, this finding could not be replicated in independent samples from Taiwan and Japan so far [73, 122]. Finally, the largest GWAS to date on lithium response totaling 2563 uniformly phenotyped bipolar patients from more than 20 sites across 4 continents has been published very recently by the Consortium on Lithium Genetics. Four linked SNPs of a single locus located on chr21q21.1, where two genes for long, non-coding RNAs, AL157359.3 and AL157359.4, are located, reached genome-wide significance [114, 200, 281].

Antidepressant monotherapy for acute bipolar depression is generally not recommended given the concern for mood switching [27, 364]. The majority of the pharmacogenetic studies of clinical response to antidepressants in bipolar patients have focused on the serotonergic pathway. An association of the S allele of the 5-HTTLPR with insufficient response to SSRI antidepressant treatment in bipolar disorder has been observed [285, 374]. The HTR1A rs6295 C/C genotype has also been reported to be associated with favorable response to fluvoxamine [283]. In addition, there was an association between HTR2A SNP rs7997012 and response to antidepressant therapy in a Caucasian sample of MDD [196]. Limited evidence is available for the genes encoding dopamine and glutamate receptors (please see for review [296]). Some research efforts have focused on the Gβ3 gene which played a role in signal transduction and found an association between the T/T genotype of the rs5443 functional polymorphism and good response to treatment with antidepressant [290, 378].

Regarding the genetic variants associated with antipsychotic response in bipolar disorder, no association between the COMT rs4680 polymorphism and olanzapine response in bipolar I disorder patients was observed. Polymorphisms in the DRD3, HRH1, and MC2R were linked to the response to an olanzapine/fluoxetine combination [239]. Several studies have probe into the association of various genetic variants the response to anticonvulsant. The A1/A1 DRD2/ANKK1 genotype had been reported to be associated with significantly better clinical response to valproate than those who were A2/A2 homozygous [181]. The 116G allele of the XBP1 rs2269577 polymorphism demonstrated better response to valproate in bipolar patients [146]. In addition, an association of the BDNF and NTRK2 genes and the response to valproate was showed [342, 343]; however there was reported significant association between the Met/Met COMT genotype and poor response to valproate and carbamazepine [179]. Finally, seven genes including ANKK1, DRD2, DRD4, DBH, HRH1, MC2R, and NR3C1 were linked to lamotrigine response [239].

References

1. Aberg K, Adkins DE, Liu Y, et al. Genome-wide association study of antipsychotic-induced QTc interval prolongation. Pharmacogenomics J. 2012;12:165–72.
2. Adams DH, Close S, Farmen M, et al. Dopamine receptor D3 genotype association with greater acute positive symptom remission with olanzapine therapy in predominately Caucasian patients with chronic schizophrenia or schizoaffective disorder. Hum Psychopharmacol. 2008;23:267–74.
3. Adkins DE, Aberg K, McClay JL, et al. Genomewide pharmacogenomic study of metabolic side effects to antipsychotic drugs. Mol Psychiatry. 2011;16:321–32.
4. Adli M, Hollinde DL, Stamm T, et al. Response to lithium augmentation in depression is associated with the glycogen synthase kinase 3-beta –50T/C single nucleotide polymorphism. Biol Psychiatry. 2007;62:1295–302.
5. Alkelai A, Greenbaum L, Rigbi A, et al. Genome-wide association study of antipsychotic-induced parkinsonism severity among schizophrenia patients. Psychopharmacology. 2009;206:491–9.
6. American Psychiatric Association. Diagnostic and statistical manual of mental disorders, vol. 716. 5th ed. Arlington: American Psychiatric Association; 2013.
7. Andersson E, Rück C, Lavebratt C, et al. Genetic polymorphisms in monoamine systems and outcome of cognitive behavior therapy for social anxiety disorder. PLoS One. 2013;8:e79015.
8. Andre K, Kampman O, Illi A, et al. SERT and NET polymorphisms, temperament and antidepressant response. Nord J Psychiatry. 2015;69:531–8.
9. Anton RF, Oroszi G, O'Malley S, et al. An evaluation of mu-opioid receptor (OPRM1) as a predictor of naltrexone response in the treatment of alcohol dependence: results from the Combined Pharmacotherapies and Behavioral Interventions for Alcohol Dependence (COMBINE) study. Arch Gen Psychiatry. 2008;65:135–44.

10. Anttila S, Illi A, Kampman O, et al. Lack of association between two polymorphisms of brain-derived neurotrophic factor and response to typical neuroleptics. J Neural Transm. 2005;112:885–90.
11. Anttila S, Kampman O, Illi A, et al. Association between 5-HT2A, TPH1 and GNB3 genotypes and response to typical neuroleptics: a serotonergic approach. BMC Psychiatry. 2007;7:22.
12. Arcos-Burgos M, Jain M, Acosta MT, et al. A common variant of the latrophilin 3 gene, LPHN3, confers susceptibility to ADHD and predicts effectiveness of stimulant medication. Mol Psychiatry. 2010;15:1053–66.
13. Arias AJ, Armeli S, Gelernter J, et al. Effects of opioid receptor gene variation on targeted nalmefene treatment in heavy drinkers. Alcohol Clin Exp Res. 2008;32:1159–66.
14. Arias AJ, Gelernter J, Gueorguieva R, et al. Pharmacogenetics of naltrexone and disulfiram in alcohol dependent, dually diagnosed veterans. Am J Addict. 2014;23:288–93.
15. Arranz M, Collier D, Sodhi M, et al. Association between clozapine response and allelic variation in 5-HT2A receptor gene. Lancet. 1995a;346:281–2.
16. Arranz MJ, Collier DA, Munro J, et al. Analysis of a structural polymorphism in the 5-HT2A receptor and clinical response to clozapine. Neurosci Lett. 1996;217:177–8.
17. Arranz MJ, Dawson E, Shaikh S, et al. Cytochrome P4502D6 genotype does not determine response to clozapine. Br J Clin Pharmacol. 1995b;39:417–20.
18. Arranz MJ, de Leon J. Pharmacogenetics and pharmacogenomics of schizophrenia: a review of last decade of research. Mol Psychiatry. 2007;12:707–47.
19. Arranz MJ, Kapur S. Pharmacogenetics in psychiatry: are we ready for widespread clinical use? Schizophr Bull. 2008;34:1130–44.
20. Arranz MJ, Munro J, Birkett J, et al. Pharmacogenetic prediction of clozapine response. Lancet. 2000;355:1615–6.
21. Arranz MJ, Munro J, Owen MJ, et al. Evidence for association between polymorphisms in the promoter and coding regions of the 5-HT2A receptor gene and response to clozapine. Mol Psychiatry. 1998a;3:61–6.
22. Arranz MJ, Munro J, Sham P, et al. Meta-analysis of studies on genetic variation in 5-HT2A receptors and clozapine response. Schizophr Res. 1998b;32:93–9.
23. Arranz MJ, Rivera M, Munro JC. Pharmacogenetics of response to antipsychotics in patients with schizophrenia. CNS Drugs. 2011;25:933–69.
24. Badner JA, Gershon ES. Meta-analysis of whole-genome linkage scans of bipolar disorder and schizophrenia. Mol Psychiatry. 2002;7:405–11.
25. Barratt DT, Coller JK, Somogyi AA. Association between the DRD2 A1 allele and response to methadone and buprenorphine maintenance treatments. Am J Med Genet B Neuropsychiatr Genet. 2006;141B:323–31.
26. Basu A, Chadda RK, Sood M, et al. Association of serotonin transporter (SLC6A4) and receptor (5HTR1A, 5HTR2A) polymorphisms with response to treatment with escitalopram in patients with major depressive disorder: a preliminary study. Indian J Med Res. 2015;142:40–5.
27. Bauer M, Ritter P, Grunze H, Pfennig A. Treatment options for acute depression in bipolar disorder. Bipolar Disord. 2012;14(Suppl 2):37–50.
28. Baune BT, Dannlowski U, Domschke K, et al. The interleukin 1 beta (IL1B) gene is associated with failure to achieve remission and impaired emotion processing in major depression. Biol Psychiatry. 2010;67:543–9.
29. Benedetti F, Serretti A, Pontiggia A, et al. Long-term response to lithium salts in bipolar illness is influenced by the glycogen synthase kinase 3-beta -50 T/C SNP. Neurosci Lett. 2005;376:51–5.
30. Berlin I, Covey LS, Jiang H, Hamer D. Lack of effect of D2 dopamine receptor TaqI A polymorphism on smoking cessation. Nicotine Tob Res. 2005;7:725–8.
31. Bertolino A, Caforio G, Blasi G, et al. Interaction of COMT (Val(108/158)Met) genotype and olanzapine treatment on prefrontal cortical function in patients with schizophrenia. Am J Psychiatry. 2004;161:1798–805.
32. Biernacka JM, McElroy SL, Crow S, et al. Pharmacogenomics of antidepressant induced mania: a review and meta-analysis of the serotonin transporter gene (5HTTLPR) association. J Affect Disord. 2012;136:e21–9.
33. Binder EB, Owens MJ, Liu W, et al. Association of polymorphisms in genes regulating the corticotropin-releasing factor system with antidepressant treatment response. Arch Gen Psychiatry. 2010;67:369–79.
34. Binder EB, Salyakina D, Lichtner P, et al. Polymorphisms in FKBP5 are associated with increased recurrence of depressive episodes and rapid response to antidepressant treatment. Nat Genet. 2004;36:1319–25.
35. Bishop JR, Ellingrod VL, Moline J, Miller D. Association between the polymorphic GRM3 gene and negative symptom improvement during olanzapine treatment. Schizophr Res. 2005;77:253–60.
36. Bolonna AA, Arranz MJ, Munro J, et al. No influence of adrenergic receptor polymorphisms on schizophrenia and antipsychotic response. Neurosci Lett. 2000;280:65–8.
37. Bolonna AA, Kerwin RW, Munro J, et al. Polymorphisms in the genes for mGluR types 7 and 8: association studies with schizophrenia. Schizophr Res. 2001;47:99–103.
38. Bonvicini C, Faraone SV, Scassellati C. Attention-deficit hyperactivity disorder in adults: a systematic review and meta-analysis of genetic, pharmacogenetic and biochemical studies. Mol Psychiatry. 2016;21:1643.

39. Bousman CA, Sarris J, Won E-S, et al. Escitalopram efficacy in depression: a cross-ethnicity examination of the serotonin transporter promoter polymorphism. J Clin Psychopharmacol. 2014;34:645–8.
40. Bowers K, Lin P-I, Erickson C. Pharmacogenomic medicine in autism: challenges and opportunities. Paediatr Drugs. 2015;17:115–24.
41. Bozina N, Kuzman MR, Medved V, et al. Associations between MDR1 gene polymorphisms and schizophrenia and therapeutic response to olanzapine in female schizophrenic patients. J Psychiatr Res. 2008;42:89–97.
42. Bozina N, Medved V, Kuzman MR, et al. Association study of olanzapine-induced weight gain and therapeutic response with SERT gene polymorphisms in female schizophrenic patients. J Psychopharmacol (Oxford). 2007;21:728–34.
43. Brandl EJ, Tiwari AK, Zhou X, et al. Influence of CYP2D6 and CYP2C19 gene variants on antidepressant response in obsessive-compulsive disorder. Pharmacogenomics J. 2014;14:176–81.
44. Breitling LP, Twardella D, Hoffmann MM, et al. Prospective association of dopamine-related polymorphisms with smoking cessation in general care. Pharmacogenomics. 2010;11:527–36.
45. Bremer T, Diamond C, McKinney R, et al. The pharmacogenetics of lithium response depends upon clinical co-morbidity. Mol Diagn Ther. 2007;11:161–70.
46. Brent D, Melhem N, Ferrell R, et al. Association of FKBP5 polymorphisms with suicidal events in the Treatment of Resistant Depression in Adolescents (TORDIA) study. Am J Psychiatry. 2010;167:190–7.
47. Brockmöller J, Kirchheiner J, Schmider J, et al. The impact of the CYP2D6 polymorphism on haloperidol pharmacokinetics and on the outcome of haloperidol treatment. Clin Pharmacol Ther. 2002;72:438–52.
48. Bruxel EM, Akutagava-Martins GC, Salatino-Oliveira A, et al. ADHD pharmacogenetics across the life cycle: new findings and perspectives. Am J Med Genet B Neuropsychiatr Genet. 2014;165B:263–82.
49. Bryant RA, Felmingham KL, Falconer EM, et al. Preliminary evidence of the short allele of the serotonin transporter gene predicting poor response to cognitive behavior therapy in posttraumatic stress disorder. Biol Psychiatry. 2010;67:1217–9.
50. Cacabelos R. Pharmacogenetic basis for therapeutic optimization in Alzheimer's disease. Mol Diagn Ther. 2007a;11:385–405.
51. Cacabelos R. Molecular pathology and pharmacogenomics in Alzheimer's disease: polygenic-related effects of multifactorial treatments on cognition, anxiety and depression. Methods Find Exp Clin Pharmacol. 2007b;29(Suppl A):1–91.
52. Cacabelos R. Pharmacogenomics and therapeutic prospects in dementia. Eur Arch Psychiatry Clin Neurosci. 2008a;258(Suppl 1):28–47.
53. Cacabelos R. Pharmacogenomics and therapeutic strategies for dementia. Expert Rev Mol Diagn. 2009;9:567–611.
54. Cacabelos R. Pharmacogenomics in Alzheimer's disease. Methods Mol Biol. 2008b;448:213–357.
55. Cacabelos R, Fernandez-Novoa L, Lombardi V, et al. Molecular genetics of Alzheimer's disease and aging. Methods Find Exp Clin Pharmacol. 2005;27(Suppl A):1–573.
56. Cacabelos R, Llovo R, Fraile C, Fernández-Novoa L. Pharmacogenetic aspects of therapy with cholinesterase inhibitors: the role of CYP2D6 in Alzheimer's disease pharmacogenetics. Curr Alzheimer Res. 2007;4:479–500.
57. Calati R, Crisafulli C, Balestri M, et al. Evaluation of the role of MAPK1 and CREB1 polymorphisms on treatment resistance, response and remission in mood disorder patients. Prog Neuro-Psychopharmacol Biol Psychiatry. 2013;44:271–8.
58. Campos-de-Sousa S, Guindalini C, Tondo L, et al. Nuclear receptor rev-erb-{alpha} circadian gene variants and lithium carbonate prophylaxis in bipolar affective disorder. J Biol Rhythm. 2010;25:132–7.
59. Chagnon YC, Mérette C, Bouchard RH, et al. A genome wide linkage study of obesity as secondary effect of antipsychotics in multigenerational families of eastern Quebec affected by psychoses. Mol Psychiatry. 2004;9:1067–74.
60. Chamorro A-J, Marcos M, Mirón-Canelo J-A, et al. Association of μ-opioid receptor (OPRM1) gene polymorphism with response to naltrexone in alcohol dependence: a systematic review and meta-analysis. Addict Biol. 2012;17:505–12.
61. Chang HS, Lee H-Y, Cha J-H, et al. Interaction of 5-HTT and HTR1A gene polymorphisms in treatment responses to mirtazapine in patients with major depressive disorder. J Clin Psychopharmacol. 2014;34:446–54.
62. Chang HS, Won E, Lee H-Y, et al. Association analysis for corticotropin releasing hormone polymorphisms with the risk of major depressive disorder and the response to antidepressants. Behav Brain Res. 2015;292:116–24.
63. Chen AC, Morgenstern J, Davis CM, et al. Variation in mu-opioid receptor gene (OPRM1) as a moderator of naltrexone treatment to reduce heavy drinking in a high functioning cohort. J Alcohol Drug Depend. 2013;1:101.
64. Chen C-H, Lee C-S, Lee M-TM, et al. Variant GADL1 and response to lithium therapy in bipolar I disorder. N Engl J Med. 2014;370:119–28.
65. Chen J, Lipska BK, Halim N, et al. Functional analysis of genetic variation in catechol-O-methyltransferase (COMT): effects on mRNA, protein, and enzyme activity in postmortem human brain. Am J Hum Genet. 2004;75:807–21.
66. Chen S-F, Shen Y-C, Chen C-H. Effects of the DRD3 Ser9Gly polymorphism on aripiprazole efficacy in schizophrenic patients as modified by clinical factors. Prog Neuro-Psychopharmacol Biol Psychiatry. 2009;33:470–4.

67. Cheon K-A, Jun J-Y, Cho D-Y. Association of the catechol-O-methyltransferase polymorphism with methylphenidate response in a classroom setting in children with attention-deficit hyperactivity disorder. Int Clin Psychopharmacol. 2008;23:291–8.
68. Chianella C, Gragnaniello D, Maisano Delser P, et al. BCHE and CYP2D6 genetic variation in Alzheimer's disease patients treated with cholinesterase inhibitors. Eur J Clin Pharmacol. 2011;67:1147–57.
69. Chiesa A, Crisafulli C, Porcelli S, et al. Influence of GRIA1, GRIA2 and GRIA4 polymorphisms on diagnosis and response to treatment in patients with major depressive disorder. Eur Arch Psychiatry Clin Neurosci. 2012;262:305–11.
70. Cinciripini P, Wetter D, Tomlinson G, et al. The effects of the DRD2 polymorphism on smoking cessation and negative affect: evidence for a pharmacogenetic effect on mood. Nicotine Tob Res. 2004;6:229–39.
71. Clarke TK, Crist RC, Ang A, et al. Genetic variation in OPRD1 and the response to treatment for opioid dependence with buprenorphine in European-American females. Pharmacogenomics J. 2014;14:303–8.
72. Colle R, Gressier F, Verstuyft C, et al. Brain-derived neurotrophic factor Val66Met polymorphism and 6-month antidepressant remission in depressed Caucasian patients. J Affect Disord. 2015;175:233–40.
73. Consortium on Lithium Genetics, Hou L, Heilbronner U, et al. Variant GADL1 and response to lithium in bipolar I disorder. N Engl J Med. 2014;370:1857–9.
74. Contini V, Victor MM, Bertuzzi GP, et al. No significant association between genetic variants in 7 candidate genes and response to methylphenidate treatment in adult patients with ADHD. J Clin Psychopharmacol. 2012;32:820–3.
75. Contini V, Victor MM, Cerqueira CCS, et al. Adrenergic α2A receptor gene is not associated with methylphenidate response in adults with ADHD. Eur Arch Psychiatry Clin Neurosci. 2011;261:205–11.
76. Contini V, Victor MM, Marques FZC, et al. Response to methylphenidate is not influenced by DAT1 polymorphisms in a sample of Brazilian adult patients with ADHD. J Neural Transm. 2010;117:269–76.
77. Cooper AJ, Rickels K, Lohoff FW. Association analysis between the A118G polymorphism in the OPRM1 gene and treatment response to venlafaxine XR in generalized anxiety disorder. Hum Psychopharmacol. 2013;28:258–62.
78. Correia CT, Almeida JP, Santos PE, et al. Pharmacogenetics of risperidone therapy in autism: association analysis of eight candidate genes with drug efficacy and adverse drug reactions. Pharmacogenomics J. 2010;10:418–30.
79. Crettol S, Besson J, Croquette-Krokar M, et al. Association of dopamine and opioid receptor genetic polymorphisms with response to methadone maintenance treatment. Prog Neuro-Psychopharmacol Biol Psychiatry. 2008;32:1722–7.
80. Crist RC, Clarke T-K, Ang A, et al. An intronic variant in OPRD1 predicts treatment outcome for opioid dependence in African-Americans. Neuropsychopharmacology. 2013;38:2003–10.
81. Cruceanu C, Alda M, Turecki G. Lithium: a key to the genetics of bipolar disorder. Genome Med. 2009;1:79.
82. da Silva TL, Pianca TG, Roman T, et al. Adrenergic alpha2A receptor gene and response to methylphenidate in attentiondeficit/hyperactivity disorder-predominantly inattentive type. J Neural Transm. 2008;115:341–5.
83. Dahl JP, Jepson C, Levenson R, et al. Interaction between variation in the D2 dopamine receptor (DRD2) and the neuronal calcium sensor-1 (FREQ) genes in predicting response to nicotine replacement therapy for tobacco dependence. Pharmacogenomics J. 2006;6:194–9.
84. Daray FM, Thommi SB, Ghaemi SN. The pharmacogenetics of antidepressant-induced mania: a systematic review and meta-analysis. Bipolar Disord. 2010;12:702–6.
85. David SP, Strong DR, Munafò MR, et al. Bupropion efficacy for smoking cessation is influenced by the DRD2 Taq1A polymorphism: analysis of pooled data from two clinical trials. Nicotine Tob Res. 2007;9:1251–7.
86. De Ruyck K, Nackaerts K, Beels L, et al. Genetic variation in three candidate genes and nicotine dependence, withdrawal and smoking cessation in hospitalized patients. Pharmacogenomics. 2010;11:1053–63.
87. Del Zompo M, Ardau R, Palmas MA, et al. Lithium response: association study with two candidate genes. Mol Psychiatry. 1999;4:S66–7.
88. Dimitrova A, Milanova V, Krastev S, et al. Association study of myo-inositol monophosphatase 2 (IMPA2) polymorphisms with bipolar affective disorder and response to lithium treatment. Pharmacogenomics J. 2005;5:35–41.
89. Dmitrzak-Weglarz M, Rybakowski JK, Suwalska A, et al. Association studies of 5-HT2A and 5-HT2C serotonin receptor gene polymorphisms with prophylactic lithium response in bipolar patients. Pharmacol Rep. 2005;57:761–5.
90. Dmitrzak-Weglarz M, Rybakowski JK, Suwalska A, et al. Association studies of the BDNF and the NTRK2 gene polymorphisms with prophylactic lithium response in bipolar patients. Pharmacogenomics. 2008;9:1595–603.
91. Dogan O, Yuksel N, Ergun MA, et al. Serotonin transporter gene polymorphisms and sertraline response in major depression patients. Genet Test. 2008;12:225–31.
92. Du J, Zhang A, Wang L, et al. Relationship between response to risperidone, plasma concentrations of risperidone and CYP3A4 polymorphisms in schizophrenia patients. J Psychopharmacol (Oxford). 2010;24:1115–20.

93. Eap CB, Bender S, Jaquenoud Sirot E, et al. Nonresponse to clozapine and ultrarapid CYP1A2 activity: clinical data and analysis of CYP1A2 gene. J Clin Psychopharmacol. 2004;24:214–9.
94. Ellsworth KA, Moon I, Eckloff BW, et al. FKBP5 genetic variation: association with selective serotonin reuptake inhibitor treatment outcomes in major depressive disorder. Pharmacogenet Genomics. 2013;23:156–66.
95. Ewald H, Wang AG, Vang M, et al. A haplotype-based study of lithium responding patients with bipolar affective disorder on the Faroe Islands. Psychiatr Genet. 1999;9:23–34.
96. Falkenberg VR, Gurbaxani BM, Unger ER, Rajeevan MS. Functional genomics of serotonin receptor 2A (HTR2A): interaction of polymorphism, methylation, expression and disease association. NeuroMolecular Med. 2011;13:66–76.
97. Felmingham KL, Dobson-Stone C, Schofield PR, et al. The brain-derived neurotrophic factor Val66Met polymorphism predicts response to exposure therapy in posttraumatic stress disorder. Biol Psychiatry. 2013;73:1059–63.
98. Fijal BA, Kinon BJ, Kapur S, et al. Candidate-gene association analysis of response to risperidone in African-American and white patients with schizophrenia. Pharmacogenomics J. 2009;9: 311–8.
99. Fonseca F, Gratacòs M, Escaramís G, et al. Response to methadone maintenance treatment is associated with the MYOCD and GRM6 genes. Mol Diagn Ther. 2010;14:171–8.
100. Froehlich TE, Epstein JN, Nick TG, et al. Pharmacogenetic predictors of methylphenidate dose-response in attention-deficit/hyperactivity disorder. J Am Acad Child Adolesc Psychiatry. 2011;50:1129–39.e2.
101. Frye MA, McElroy SL, Prieto ML, et al. Clinical risk factors and serotonin transporter gene variants associated with antidepressant-induced mania. J Clin Psychiatry. 2015;76:174–80.
102. Ftouhi-Paquin N, Alda M, Grof P, et al. Identification of three polymorphisms in the translated region of PLC-gamma1 and their investigation in lithium responsive bipolar disorder. Am J Med Genet. 2001;105:301–5.
103. GENDEP Investigators, MARS Investigators, STAR*D Investigators. Common genetic variation and antidepressant efficacy in major depressive disorder: a meta-analysis of three genome-wide pharmacogenetic studies. Am J Psychiatry. 2013;170:207–17.
104. Geschwind DH. Advances in autism. Annu Rev Med. 2009;60:367–80.
105. Goldberger C, Gourion D, Leroy S, et al. Population-based and family-based association study of 5'UTR polymorphism of the reelin gene and schizophrenia. Am J Med Genet B Neuropsychiatr Genet. 2005;137B:51–5.
106. Gu B, Wang L, Zhang A-P, et al. Association between a polymorphism of the HTR3A gene and therapeutic response to risperidone treatment in drug-naive Chinese schizophrenia patients. Pharmacogenet Genomics. 2008;18:721–7.
107. Gupta M, Bhatnagar P, Grover S, et al. Association studies of catechol-O-methyltransferase (COMT) gene with schizophrenia and response to antipsychotic treatment. Pharmacogenomics. 2009;10:385–97.
108. Hettema JM, Neale MC, Kendler KS. A review and meta-analysis of the genetic epidemiology of anxiety disorders. Am J Psychiatry. 2001;158: 1568–78.
109. Hicks JK, Bishop JR, Sangkuhl K, et al. Clinical pharmacogenetics implementation consortium (CPIC) guideline for CYP2D6 and CYP2C19 genotypes and dosing of selective serotonin reuptake inhibitors. Clin Pharmacol Ther. 2015;98:127–34. https://doi.org/10.1002/cpt.147.
110. Hicks JK, Swen JJ, Thorn CF, et al. Clinical Pharmacogenetics Implementation Consortium guideline for CYP2D6 and CYP2C19 genotypes and dosing of tricyclic antidepressants. Clin Pharmacol Ther. 2013;93:402–8. https://doi.org/10.1038/clpt.2013.2.
111. Hiemke C, Baumann P, Bergemann N, et al. AGNP consensus guidelines for therapeutic drug monitoring in psychiatry: update 2011. Pharmacopsychiatry. 2011;44:195–235. https://doi.org/10.1055/s-0031-1286287.
112. Hoekstra PJ, Troost PW, Lahuis BE, et al. Risperidone-induced weight gain in referred children with autism spectrum disorders is associated with a common polymorphism in the 5-hydroxytryptamine 2C receptor gene. J Child Adolesc Psychopharmacol. 2010;20:473–7. https://doi.org/10.1089/cap.2009.0071.
113. Horstmann S, Lucae S, Menke A, et al. Polymorphisms in GRIK4, HTR2A, and FKBP5 show interactive effects in predicting remission to antidepressant treatment. Neuropsychopharmacology. 2010;35: 727–40. https://doi.org/10.1038/npp.2009.180.
114. Hou L, Heilbronner U, Degenhardt F, et al. Genetic variants associated with response to lithium treatment in bipolar disorder: a genome-wide association study. Lancet. 2016;387:1085–93. https://doi.org/10.1016/S0140-6736(16)00143-4.
115. Houston JP, Adams DH, Kirkwood SC, et al. Neuroreceptor gene polymorphisms and olanzapine depressive symptom response in schizophrenia. J Clin Psychopharmacol. 2007;27:520–3. https://doi.org/10.1097/JCP.0b013e31814f4d82.
116. Hu Q, Zhang S-Y, Liu F, et al. Influence of GNB3 C825T polymorphism on the efficacy of antidepressants in the treatment of major depressive disorder: a meta-analysis. J Affect Disord. 2015;172:103–9. https://doi.org/10.1016/j.jad.2014.09.039.
117. Hwang R, Shinkai T, De Luca V, et al. Association study of 12 polymorphisms spanning the dopamine D(2) receptor gene and clozapine treatment response

in two treatment refractory/intolerant populations. Psychopharmacology. 2005;181:179–87. https://doi.org/10.1007/s00213-005-2223-5.
118. Hwang R, Shinkai T, De Luca V, et al. Association study of four dopamine D1 receptor gene polymorphisms and clozapine treatment response. J Psychopharmacol (Oxford). 2007;21:718–27. https://doi.org/10.1177/0269881106072341.
119. Hwang R, Shinkai T, Deluca V, et al. Dopamine D2 receptor gene variants and quantitative measures of positive and negative symptom response following clozapine treatment. Eur Neuropsychopharmacol. 2006;16:248–59. https://doi.org/10.1016/j.euroneuro.2005.09.004.
120. Hwang R, Zai C, Tiwari A, et al. Effect of dopamine D3 receptor gene polymorphisms and clozapine treatment response: exploratory analysis of nine polymorphisms and meta-analysis of the Ser9Gly variant. Pharmacogenomics J. 2010;10:200–18. https://doi.org/10.1038/tpj.2009.65.
121. Ikeda M, Tomita Y, Mouri A, et al. Identification of novel candidate genes for treatment response to risperidone and susceptibility for schizophrenia: integrated analysis among pharmacogenomics, mouse expression, and genetic case-control association approaches. Biol Psychiatry. 2010;67:263–9. https://doi.org/10.1016/j.biopsych.2009.08.030.
122. Ikeda M, Yamanouchi Y, Kinoshita Y, et al. Variants of dopamine and serotonin candidate genes as predictors of response to risperidone treatment in first-episode schizophrenia. Pharmacogenomics. 2008;9:1437–43. https://doi.org/10.2217/14622416.9.10.1437.
123. Illi A, Setälä-Soikkeli E, Viikki M, et al. 5-HTR1A, 5-HTR2A, 5-HTR6, TPH1 and TPH2 polymorphisms and major depression. Neuroreport. 2009;20:1125–8. https://doi.org/10.1097/WNR.0b013e32832eb708.
124. Inada T, Koga M, Ishiguro H, et al. Pathway-based association analysis of genome-wide screening data suggest that genes associated with the gamma-aminobutyric acid receptor signaling pathway are involved in neuroleptic-induced, treatment-resistant tardive dyskinesia. Pharmacogenet Genomics. 2008;18:317–23. https://doi.org/10.1097/FPC.0b013e3282f70492.
125. Ito K, Yoshida K, Sato K, et al. A variable number of tandem repeats in the serotonin transporter gene does not affect the antidepressant response to fluvoxamine. Psychiatry Res. 2002;111:235–9.
126. Johnson BA, Ait-Daoud N, Seneviratne C, et al. Pharmacogenetic approach at the serotonin transporter gene as a method of reducing the severity of alcohol drinking. Am J Psychiatry. 2011;168: 265–75.
127. Johnson BA, Seneviratne C, Wang X-Q, et al. Determination of genotype combinations that can predict the outcome of the treatment of alcohol dependence using the 5-HT(3) antagonist ondansetron. Am J Psychiatry. 2013;170:1020–31.
128. Jones JD, Comer SD. A review of pharmacogenetic studies of substance-related disorders. Drug Alcohol Depend. 2015;152:1–14.
129. Joober R, Benkelfat C, Brisebois K, et al. T102C polymorphism in the 5HT2A gene and schizophrenia: relation to phenotype and drug response variability. J Psychiatry Neurosci. 1999;24:141–6.
130. Joober R, Grizenko N, Sengupta S, et al. Dopamine transporter 3′-UTR VNTR genotype and ADHD: a pharmaco-behavioural genetic study with methylphenidate. Neuropsychopharmacology. 2007;32:1370–6.
131. Joober R, Rouleau GA, Lal S, et al. Increased prevalence of schizophrenia spectrum disorders in relatives of neuroleptic-nonresponsive schizophrenic patients. Schizophr Res. 2005;77:35–41.
132. Joyce PR, Mulder RT, Luty SE, et al. Age-dependent antidepressant pharmacogenomics: polymorphisms of the serotonin transporter and G protein beta3 subunit as predictors of response to fluoxetine and nortriptyline. Int J Neuropsychopharmacol. 2003;6:339–46.
133. Kakiuchi C, Kato T. Lithium response and -116C/G polymorphism of XBP1 in Japanese patients with bipolar disorder. Int J Neuropsychopharmacol. 2005;8:631–2.
134. Kambeitz J, Romanos M, Ettinger U. Meta-analysis of the association between dopamine transporter genotype and response to methylphenidate treatment in ADHD. Pharmacogenomics J. 2014;14:77–84.
135. Kampman O, Illi A, Hänninen K, et al. RGS4 genotype is not associated with antipsychotic medication response in schizophrenia. J Neural Transm. 2006;113:1563–8.
136. Kang R-H, Hahn S-W, Choi M-J, Lee M-S. Relationship between G-protein beta-3 subunit C825T polymorphism and mirtazapine responses in Korean patients with major depression. Neuropsychobiology. 2007;56:1–5.
137. Karpyak VM, Biernacka JM, Geske JR, et al. Genetic markers associated with abstinence length in alcohol-dependent subjects treated with acamprosate. Transl Psychiatry. 2014;4:e462.
138. Kato M, Fukuda T, Wakeno M, et al. Effect of 5-HT1A gene polymorphisms on antidepressant response in major depressive disorder. Am J Med Genet B Neuropsychiatr Genet. 2009;150B:115–23.
139. Kato M, Serretti A. Review and meta-analysis of antidepressant pharmacogenetic findings in major depressive disorder. Mol Psychiatry. 2010;15:473–500.
140. Kato M, Wakeno M, Okugawa G, et al. Antidepressant response and intolerance to SSRI is not influenced by G-protein beta3 subunit gene C825T polymorphism in Japanese major depressive patients. Prog Neuro-Psychopharmacol Biol Psychiatry. 2008;32:1041–4.
141. Kautzky A, Baldinger P, Souery D, et al. The combined effect of genetic polymorphisms and clinical parameters on treatment outcome in treatment-resistant depression. Eur Neuropsychopharmacol. 2015;25:441–53.

142. Kawaguchi DM, Glatt SJ. GRIK4 polymorphism and its association with antidepressant response in depressed patients: a meta-analysis. Pharmacogenomics. 2014;15:1451–9.
143. Keers R, Bonvicini C, Scassellati C, et al. Variation in GNB3 predicts response and adverse reactions to antidepressants. J Psychopharmacol (Oxford). 2011;25:867–74.
144. Kereszturi E, Tarnok Z, Bognar E, et al. Catechol-O-methyltransferase Val158Met polymorphism is associated with methylphenidate response in ADHD children. Am J Med Genet B Neuropsychiatr Genet. 2008;147B:1431–5.
145. Kim B, Choi EY, Kim CY, et al. Could HTR2A T102C and DRD3 Ser9Gly predict clinical improvement in patients with acutely exacerbated schizophrenia? Results from treatment responses to risperidone in a naturalistic setting. Hum Psychopharmacol. 2008;23:61–7.
146. Kim B, Kim CY, Lee MJ, Joo YH. Preliminary evidence on the association between XBP1-116C/G polymorphism and response to prophylactic treatment with valproate in bipolar disorders. Psychiatry Res. 2009a;168:209–12.
147. Kim B-N, Cummins TDR, Kim J-W, et al. Val/Val genotype of brain-derived neurotrophic factor (BDNF) Val Met polymorphism is associated with a better response to OROS-MPH in Korean ADHD children. Int J Neuropsychopharmacol. 2011;14:1399–410.
148. Kim B-N, Kim J-W, Hong SB, et al. Possible association of norepinephrine transporter −3081(A/T) polymorphism with methylphenidate response in attention deficit hyperactivity disorder. Behav Brain Funct. 2010;6:57.
149. Kim H, Lim S-W, Kim S, et al. Monoamine transporter gene polymorphisms and antidepressant response in Koreans with late-life depression. JAMA. 2006;296:1609–18.
150. Kim S-G, Kim C-M, Choi S-W, et al. A micro opioid receptor gene polymorphism (A118G) and naltrexone treatment response in adherent Korean alcohol-dependent patients. Psychopharmacology. 2009b;201:611–8.
151. Kim Y-G, Chang H-S, Won E-S, et al. Serotonin-related polymorphisms in TPH1 and HTR5A genes are not associated with escitalopram treatment response in Korean patients with major depression. Neuropsychobiology. 2014;69:210–9.
152. Kirchheiner J, Lorch R, Lebedeva E, et al. Genetic variants in FKBP5 affecting response to antidepressant drug treatment. Pharmacogenomics. 2008;9:841–6.
153. Kirchheiner J, Nickchen K, Bauer M, et al. Pharmacogenetics of antidepressants and antipsychotics: the contribution of allelic variations to the phenotype of drug response. Mol Psychiatry. 2004;9:442–73.
154. Kirley A, Lowe N, Hawi Z, et al. Association of the 480 bp DAT1 allele with methylphenidate response in a sample of Irish children with ADHD. Am J Med Genet B Neuropsychiatr Genet. 2003;121B:50–4.
155. Kishi T, Yoshimura R, Kitajima T, et al. HTR2A is associated with SSRI response in major depressive disorder in a Japanese cohort. NeuroMolecular Med. 2010;12:237–42.
156. Klein PS, Melton DA. A molecular mechanism for the effect of lithium on development. Proc Natl Acad Sci U S A. 1996;93:8455–9.
157. Kohlrausch FB, Salatino-Oliveira A, Gama CS, et al. Influence of serotonin transporter gene polymorphisms on clozapine response in Brazilian schizophrenics. J Psychiatr Res. 2010;44:1158–62.
158. Kohlrausch FB, Salatino-Oliveira A, Gama CS, et al. G-protein gene 825C>T polymorphism is associated with response to clozapine in Brazilian schizophrenics. Pharmacogenomics. 2008;9:1429–36.
159. Kooij JS, Boonstra AM, Vermeulen SH, et al. Response to methylphenidate in adults with ADHD is associated with a polymorphism in SLC6A3 (DAT1). Am J Med Genet B Neuropsychiatr Genet. 2008;147B:201–8.
160. Kosten TR, Wu G, Huang W, et al. Pharmacogenetic randomized trial for cocaine abuse: disulfiram and dopamine β -hydroxylase. Biol Psychiatry. 2013;73:219–24.
161. Kranzler HR, Armeli S, Tennen H, et al. A double-blind, randomized trial of sertraline for alcohol dependence: moderation by age of onset [corrected] and 5-hydroxytryptamine transporter-linked promoter region genotype. J Clin Psychopharmacol. 2011;31:22–30.
162. Kranzler HR, Covault J, Feinn R, et al. Topiramate treatment for heavy drinkers: moderation by a GRIK1 polymorphism. Am J Psychiatry. 2014;171:445–52.
163. Krebs MO, Guillin O, Bourdell MC, et al. Brain derived neurotrophic factor (BDNF) gene variants association with age at onset and therapeutic response in schizophrenia. Mol Psychiatry. 2000;5:558–62.
164. Krebs MO, Sautel F, Bourdel MC, et al. Dopamine D3 receptor gene variants and substance abuse in schizophrenia. Mol Psychiatry. 1998;3:337–41.
165. Krystal JH, Cramer JA, Krol WF, et al. Naltrexone in the treatment of alcohol dependence. N Engl J Med. 2001;345:1734–9.
166. Kwon JS, Kim E, Kang D-H, et al. Taq1A polymorphism in the dopamine D2 receptor gene as a predictor of clinical response to aripiprazole. Eur Neuropsychopharmacol. 2008;18:897–907.
167. Labbe A, Liu A, Atherton J, et al. Refining psychiatric phenotypes for response to treatment: contribution of LPHN3 in ADHD. Am J Med Genet B Neuropsychiatr Genet. 2012;159B:776–85.

168. Lahdelma L, Ahokas A, Andersson LC, et al. Association between HLA-A1 allele and schizophrenia gene(s) in patients refractory to conventional neuroleptics but responsive to clozapine medication. Tissue Antigens. 2008;51:200–3.
169. Lane H-Y, Chang Y-C, Chiu C-C, et al. Association of risperidone treatment response with a polymorphism in the 5-HT(2A) receptor gene. Am J Psychiatry. 2002;159:1593–5.
170. Lane H-Y, Hsu S-K, Liu Y-C, et al. Dopamine D3 receptor Ser9Gly polymorphism and risperidone response. J Clin Psychopharmacol. 2005;25:6–11.
171. Lane H-Y, Lee C-C, Chang Y-C, et al. Effects of dopamine D2 receptor Ser311Cys polymorphism and clinical factors on risperidone efficacy for positive and negative symptoms and social function. Int J Neuropsychopharmacol. 2004a;7:461–70.
172. Lane H-Y, Lin C-C, Huang C-H, et al. Risperidone response and 5-HT6 receptor gene variance: genetic association analysis with adjustment for nongenetic confounders. Schizophr Res. 2004b;67:63–70.
173. Lane H-Y, Liu Y-C, Huang C-L, et al. RGS4 polymorphisms predict clinical manifestations and responses to risperidone treatment in patients with schizophrenia. J Clin Psychopharmacol. 2008;28:64–8.
174. Langley K, Turic D, Peirce TR, et al. No support for association between the dopamine transporter (DAT1) gene and ADHD. Am J Med Genet B Neuropsychiatr Genet. 2005;139B:7–10.
175. Lavedan C, Licamele L, Volpi S, et al. Association of the NPAS3 gene and five other loci with response to the antipsychotic iloperidone identified in a whole genome association study. Mol Psychiatry. 2009;14:804–19.
176. Lawford BR, Young RM, Noble EP, et al. The D(2) dopamine receptor A(1) allele and opioid dependence: association with heroin use and response to methadone treatment. Am J Med Genet. 2000;96:592–8.
177. Lawford BR, Young RM, Rowell JA, et al. Bromocriptine in the treatment of alcoholics with the D2 dopamine receptor A1 allele. Nat Med. 1995;1:337–41.
178. Lee HJ, Cha JH, Ham BJ, et al. Association between a G-protein beta 3 subunit gene polymorphism and the symptomatology and treatment responses of major depressive disorders. Pharmacogenomics J. 2004;4:29–33.
179. Lee H-Y, Kim Y-K. Catechol-O-methyltransferase Val158Met polymorphism affects therapeutic response to mood stabilizer in symptomatic manic patients. Psychiatry Res. 2010;175:63–6.
180. Lee SH, Kim SW, Lee MG, et al. Lack of association between response of OROS-methylphenidate and norepinephrine transporter (SLC6A2) polymorphism in Korean ADHD. Psychiatry Res. 2011;186:338–44.
181. Lee S-Y, Chen S-L, Chang Y-H, et al. The DRD2/ANKK1 gene is associated with response to add-on dextromethorphan treatment in bipolar disorder. J Affect Disord. 2012;138:295–300.
182. Lekman M, Laje G, Charney D, et al. The FKBP5-gene in depression and treatment response – an association study in the Sequenced Treatment Alternatives to Relieve Depression (STAR*D) Cohort. Biol Psychiatry. 2008;63:1103–10.
183. Lett TA, Walter H, Brandl EJ. Pharmacogenetics and imaging-pharmacogenetics of antidepressant response: towards translational strategies. CNS Drugs. 2016;30:1169–89.
184. Li X, Jope RS. Is glycogen synthase kinase-3 a central modulator in mood regulation? Neuropsychopharmacology. 2010;35:2143–54.
185. Licinio J, O'Kirwan F, Irizarry K, et al. Association of a corticotropin-releasing hormone receptor 1 haplotype and antidepressant treatment response in Mexican-Americans. Mol Psychiatry. 2004;9:1075–82.
186. Lin E, Chen PS, Chang HH, et al. Interaction of serotonin-related genes affects short-term antidepressant response in major depressive disorder. Prog Neuro-Psychopharmacol Biol Psychiatry. 2009;33:1167–72.
187. Lin E, Lane H-Y. Genome-wide association studies in pharmacogenomics of antidepressants. Pharmacogenomics. 2015;16:555–66.
188. Lin J-Y, Jiang M-Y, Kan Z-M, Chu Y. Influence of 5-HTR2A genetic polymorphisms on the efficacy of antidepressants in the treatment of major depressive disorder: a meta-analysis. J Affect Disord. 2014;168:430–8.
189. Lit L, Sharp FR, Bertoglio K, et al. Gene expression in blood is associated with risperidone response in children with autism spectrum disorders. Pharmacogenomics J. 2012;12:368–71.
190. Liu B-C, Zhang J, Wang L, et al. HTR2C promoter polymorphisms are associated with risperidone efficacy in Chinese female patients. Pharmacogenomics. 2010;11:685–92.
191. Lohoff FW, Aquino TD, Narasimhan S, et al. Serotonin receptor 2A (HTR2A) gene polymorphism predicts treatment response to venlafaxine XR in generalized anxiety disorder. Pharmacogenomics J. 2013a;13:21–6.
192. Lohoff FW, Narasimhan S, Rickels K. Interaction between polymorphisms in serotonin transporter (SLC6A4) and serotonin receptor 2A (HTR2A) genes predict treatment response to venlafaxine XR in generalized anxiety disorder. Pharmacogenomics J. 2013b;13:464–9.
193. Lonsdorf TB, Rück C, Bergström J, et al. The COMTval158met polymorphism is associated with symptom relief during exposure-based cognitive-behavioral treatment in panic disorder. BMC Psychiatry. 2010;10:99.

194. Lopez de Lara C, Jaitovich-Groisman I, Cruceanu C, et al. Implication of synapse-related genes in bipolar disorder by linkage and gene expression analyses. Int J Neuropsychopharmacol. 2010;13:1397–410.
195. Løvlie R, Berle JO, Stordal E, Steen VM. The phospholipase C-gamma1 gene (PLCG1) and lithium-responsive bipolar disorder: re-examination of an intronic dinucleotide repeat polymorphism. Psychiatr Genet. 2001;11:41–3.
196. Lucae S, Ising M, Horstmann S, et al. HTR2A gene variation is involved in antidepressant treatment response. Eur Neuropsychopharmacol. 2010;20:65–8.
197. Magliulo L, Dahl M-L, Lombardi G, et al. Do CYP3A and ABCB1 genotypes influence the plasma concentration and clinical outcome of donepezil treatment? Eur J Clin Pharmacol. 2011;67:47–54.
198. Mamdani F, Alda M, Grof P, et al. Lithium response and genetic variation in the CREB family of genes. Am J Med Genet B Neuropsychiatr Genet. 2008;147B:500–4.
199. Mancama D, Arranz MJ, Munro J, et al. Investigation of promoter variants of the histamine 1 and 2 receptors in schizophrenia and clozapine response. Neurosci Lett. 2002;333:207–11.
200. Manchia M, Adli M, Akula N, et al. Assessment of response to lithium maintenance treatment in bipolar disorder: a consortium on lithium genetics (ConLiGen) report. PLoS One. 2013;8:e65636.
201. Manchia M, Congiu D, Squassina A, et al. No association between lithium full responders and the DRD1, DRD2, DRD3, DAT1, 5-HTTLPR and HTR2A genes in a Sardinian sample. Psychiatry Res. 2009a;169:164–6.
202. Manchia M, Squassina A, Congiu D, et al. Interacting genes in lithium prophylaxis: preliminary results of an exploratory analysis on the role of DGKH and NR1D1 gene polymorphisms in 199 Sardinian bipolar patients. Neurosci Lett. 2009b;467:67–71.
203. Mandelli L, Emiliani R, Porcelli S, et al. Genes involved in neuroplasticity and stressful life events act on the short-term response to antidepressant treatment: a complex interplay between genetics and environment. Hum Psychopharmacol. 2014;29:388–91.
204. Manji HK, Lenox RH. Protein kinase C signaling in the brain: molecular transduction of mood stabilization in the treatment of manicdepressive illness. Biol Psychiatry. 1999;46:1328–51.
205. Masellis M, Basile V, Meltzer HY, et al. Serotonin subtype 2 receptor genes and clinical response to clozapine in schizophrenia patients. Neuropsychopharmacology. 1998;19:123–32.
206. Masui T, Hashimoto R, Kusumi I, et al. A possible association between missense polymorphism of the breakpoint cluster region gene and lithium prophylaxis in bipolar disorder. Prog Neuro-Psychopharmacol Biol Psychiatry. 2008;32:204–8.
207. Masui T, Hashimoto R, Kusumi I, et al. A possible association between the -116C/G single nucleotide polymorphism of the XBP1 gene and lithium prophylaxis in bipolar disorder. Int J Neuropsychopharmacol. 2006;9:83–8.
208. Matsumoto Y, Fabbri C, Pellegrini S, et al. Serotonin transporter gene: a new polymorphism may affect response to antidepressant treatments in major depressive disorder. Mol Diagn Ther. 2014;18:567–77.
209. McCarthy MJ, Nievergelt CM, Shekhtman T, et al. Functional genetic variation in the Rev-Erbα pathway and lithium response in the treatment of bipolar disorder. Genes Brain Behav. 2011;10:852–61.
210. McClay JL, Adkins DE, Aberg K, et al. Genome-wide pharmacogenomic analysis of response to treatment with antipsychotics. Mol Psychiatry. 2011a;16:76–85.
211. McClay JL, Adkins DE, Aberg K, et al. Genome-wide pharmacogenomic study of neurocognition as an indicator of antipsychotic treatment response in schizophrenia. Neuropsychopharmacology. 2011b;36:616–26.
212. McCracken JT, Badashova KK, Posey DJ, et al. Positive effects of methylphenidate on hyperactivity are moderated by monoaminergic gene variants in children with autism spectrum disorders. Pharmacogenomics J. 2014;14:295–302.
213. McCracken JT, McGough J, Shah B, et al. Risperidone in children with autism and serious behavioral problems. N Engl J Med. 2002;347:314–21.
214. McGough JJ, McCracken JT, Loo SK, et al. A candidate gene analysis of methylphenidate response in attention-deficit/hyperactivity disorder. J Am Acad Child Adolesc Psychiatry. 2009;48:1155–64.
215. McMahon FJ, Buervenich S, Charney D, et al. Variation in the gene encoding the serotonin 2A receptor is associated with outcome of antidepressant treatment. Am J Hum Genet. 2006;78:804–14.
216. Méary A, Brousse G, Jamain S, et al. Pharmacogenetic study of atypical antipsychotic drug response: involvement of the norepinephrine transporter gene. Am J Med Genet B Neuropsychiatr Genet. 2008;147B:491–4.
217. Meged S, Stein D, Sitrota P, et al. Human leukocyte antigen typing, response to neuroleptics, and clozapine-induced agranulocytosis in Jewish Israeli schizophrenic patients. Int Clin Psychopharmacol. 1999;14:305–12.
218. Michelon L, Meira-Lima I, Cordeiro Q, et al. Association study of the INPP1, 5HTT, BDNF, AP-2beta and GSK-3beta GENE variants and retrospectively scored response to lithium prophylaxis in bipolar disorder. Neurosci Lett. 2006;403:288–93.
219. Mick E, Biederman J, Spencer T, et al. Absence of association with DAT1 polymorphism and response to methylphenidate in a sample of adults with

ADHD. Am J Med Genet B Neuropsychiatr Genet. 2006;141B:890–4.
220. Milanesi E, Bonvicini C, Congiu C, et al. The role of GRIK4 gene in treatment-resistant depression. Genet Res (Camb). 2015;97:e14.
221. Mill J, Asherson P, Browes C, et al. Expression of the dopamine transporter gene is regulated by the 3′ UTR VNTR: evidence from brain and lymphocytes using quantitative RT-PCR. Am J Med Genet. 2002;114:975–9.
222. Mrazek DA, Rush AJ, Biernacka JM, et al. SLC6A4 variation and citalopram response. Am J Med Genet B Neuropsychiatr Genet. 2009;150B:341–51.
223. Murphy GM, Sarginson JE, Ryan HS, et al. BDNF and CREB1 genetic variants interact to affect antidepressant treatment outcomes in geriatric depression. Pharmacogenet Genomics. 2013;23:301–13.
224. Mushtaq D, Ali A, Margoob MA, et al. Association between serotonin transporter gene promoter-region polymorphism and 4- and 12-week treatment response to sertraline in posttraumatic stress disorder. J Affect Disord. 2012;136:955–62.
225. Myung W, Lim S-W, Kim S, et al. Serotonin transporter genotype and function in relation to antidepressant response in Koreans. Psychopharmacology. 2013;225:283–90.
226. Niitsu T, Fabbri C, Bentini F, Serretti A. Pharmacogenetics in major depression: a comprehensive meta-analysis. Prog Neuro-Psychopharmacol Biol Psychiatry. 2013;45:183–94.
227. Noordam R, Direk N, Sitlani CM, et al. Identifying genetic loci associated with antidepressant drug response with drug-gene interaction models in a population-based study. J Psychiatr Res. 2015;62:31–7.
228. Nurmi EL, Spilman SL, Whelan F, et al. Moderation of antipsychotic-induced weight gain by energy balance gene variants in the RUPP autism network risperidone studies. Transl Psychiatry. 2013;3:e274.
229. Ooteman W, Naassila M, Koeter MWJ, et al. Predicting the effect of naltrexone and acamprosate in alcohol-dependent patients using genetic indicators. Addict Biol. 2009;14:328–37.
230. Oslin DW. Prospective study of the Asn40Asp SNP as a moderator of naltrexone treatment of alcohol dependence. Oral presentation at the annual meeting of the Research Society on Alcoholism, Bellevue, WA, 21–25 June 2014.
231. Oslin DW, Berrettini W, Kranzler HR, et al. A functional polymorphism of the mu-opioid receptor gene is associated with naltrexone response in alcohol-dependent patients. Neuropsychopharmacology. 2003;28:1546–52.
232. Owley T, Brune CW, Salt J, et al. A pharmacogenetic study of escitalopram in autism spectrum disorders. Autism Res. 2010;3:1–7.
233. Paddock S, Laje G, Charney D, et al. Association of GRIK4 with outcome of antidepressant treatment in the STAR*D cohort. Am J Psychiatry. 2007;164:1181–8.
234. Pae C-U, Chiesa A, Porcelli S, et al. Influence of BDNF variants on diagnosis and response to treatment in patients with major depression, bipolar disorder and schizophrenia. Neuropsychobiology. 2012;65:1–11.
235. Papiol S, Arias B, Gastó C, et al. Genetic variability at HPA axis in major depression and clinical response to antidepressant treatment. J Affect Disord. 2007;104:83–90.
236. Pasini A, Sinibaldi L, Paloscia C, et al. Neurocognitive effects of methylphenidate on ADHD children with different DAT genotypes: a longitudinal open label trial. Eur J Paediatr Neurol. 2013;17:407–14.
237. Perkins KA, Lerman C, Coddington S, et al. Gene and gene by sex associations with initial sensitivity to nicotine in nonsmokers. Behav Pharmacol. 2008a;19:630–40.
238. Perkins KA, Lerman C, Grottenthaler A, et al. Dopamine and opioid gene variants are associated with increased smoking reward and reinforcement owing to negative mood. Behav Pharmacol. 2008b;19:641–9.
239. Perlis RH, Adams DH, Fijal B, et al. Genetic association study of treatment response with olanzapine/fluoxetine combination or lamotrigine in bipolar I depression. J Clin Psychiatry. 2010a;71:599–605.
240. Perlis RH, Fijal B, Dharia S, et al. Failure to replicate genetic associations with antidepressant treatment response in duloxetine-treated patients. Biol Psychiatry. 2010b;67:1110–3.
241. Perlis RH, Fijal B, Dharia S, Houston JP. Pharmacogenetic investigation of response to duloxetine treatment in generalized anxiety disorder. Pharmacogenomics J. 2013;13:280–5.
242. Perlis RH, Smoller JW, Ferreira MAR, et al. A genomewide association study of response to lithium for prevention of recurrence in bipolar disorder. Am J Psychiatry. 2009;166:718–25.
243. Perna G, Favaron E, Di Bella D, et al. Antipanic efficacy of paroxetine and polymorphism within the promoter of the serotonin transporter gene. Neuropsychopharmacology. 2005;30:2230–5.
244. Perroud N, Bondolfi G, Uher R, et al. Clinical and genetic correlates of suicidal ideation during antidepressant treatment in a depressed outpatient sample. Pharmacogenomics. 2011;12:365–77.
245. Pescosolido MF, Yang U, Sabbagh M, Morrow EM. Lighting a path: genetic studies pinpoint neurodevelopmental mechanisms in autism and related disorders. Dialogues Clin Neurosci. 2012;14:239–52.
246. Peters EJ, Slager SL, Jenkins GD, et al. Resequencing of serotonin-related genes and association of tagging SNPs to citalopram response. Pharmacogenet Genomics. 2009;19:1–10.
247. Peters EJ, Slager SL, McGrath PJ, et al. Investigation of serotonin-related genes in antidepressant response. Mol Psychiatry. 2004;9:879–89.
248. Pilotto A, Franceschi M, D'Onofrio G, et al. Effect of a CYP2D6 polymorphism on the efficacy of donepezil in patients with Alzheimer disease. Neurology. 2009;73:761–7.

249. Polanczyk G, Zeni C, Genro JP, et al. Association of the adrenergic alpha2A receptor gene with methylphenidate improvement of inattentive symptoms in children and adolescents with attention-deficit/hyperactivity disorder. Arch Gen Psychiatry. 2007;64:218–24.
250. Poland RE, Lesser IM, Wan Y-JY, et al. Response to citalopram is not associated with SLC6A4 genotype in African-Americans and Caucasians with major depression. Life Sci. 2013;92:967–70.
251. Popp J, Leucht S, Heres S, Steimer W. Serotonin transporter polymorphisms and side effects in antidepressant therapy – a pilot study. Pharmacogenomics. 2006;7:159–66.
252. Porcelli S, Fabbri C, Serretti A. Meta-analysis of serotonin transporter gene promoter polymorphism (5-HTTLPR) association with antidepressant efficacy. Eur Neuropsychopharmacol. 2012;22:239–58.
253. Potkin SG, Basile VS, Jin Y, et al. D1 receptor alleles predict PET metabolic correlates of clinical response to clozapine. Mol Psychiatry. 2003;8:109–13.
254. Powell TR, Schalkwyk LC, Heffernan AL, et al. Tumor necrosis factor and its targets in the inflammatory cytokine pathway are identified as putative transcriptomic biomarkers for escitalopram response. Eur Neuropsychopharmacol. 2013;23:1105–14.
255. Proft F, Kopf J, Olmes D, et al. SLC6A2 and SLC6A4 variants interact with venlafaxine serum concentrations to influence therapy outcome. Pharmacopsychiatry. 2014;47:245–50.
256. Pu M, Zhang Z, Xu Z, et al. Influence of genetic polymorphisms in the glutamatergic and GABAergic systems and their interactions with environmental stressors on antidepressant response. Pharmacogenomics. 2013;14:277–88.
257. Purper-Ouakil D, Wohl M, Orejarena S, et al. Pharmacogenetics of methylphenidate response in attention deficit/hyperactivity disorder: association with the dopamine transporter gene (SLC6A3). Am J Med Genet B Neuropsychiatr Genet. 2008;147B:1425–30.
258. Qin H, Samuels JF, Wang Y, et al. Whole-genome association analysis of treatment response in obsessive-compulsive disorder. Mol Psychiatry. 2016;21:270–6.
259. Rahman MA, Ashton AC, Meunier FA, et al. Norepinephrine exocytosis stimulated by alpha-latrotoxin requires both external and stored Ca2+ and is mediated by latrophilin, G proteins and phospholipase C. Philos Trans R Soc Lond Ser B Biol Sci. 1999;354:379–86.
260. Rao PA, Pickar D, Gejman PV, et al. Allelic variation in the D4 dopamine receptor (DRD4) gene does not predict response to clozapine. Arch Gen Psychiatry. 1994;51:912–7.
261. Ray LA, Miranda R, MacKillop J, et al. A preliminary pharmacogenetic investigation of adverse events from topiramate in heavy drinkers. Exp Clin Psychopharmacol. 2009;17:122–9.
262. Reif A, Richter J, Straube B, et al. MAOA and mechanisms of panic disorder revisited: from bench to molecular psychotherapy. Mol Psychiatry. 2014;19:122–8.
263. Ribasés M, Ramos-Quiroga JA, Sánchez-Mora C, et al. Contribution of LPHN3 to the genetic susceptibility to ADHD in adulthood: a replication study. Genes Brain Behav. 2011;10:149–57.
264. Rietschel M, Naber D, Oberländer H, et al. Efficacy and side-effects of clozapine: testing for association with allelic variation in the dopamine D4 receptor gene. Neuropsychopharmacology. 1996;15:491–6.
265. Risner ME, Saunders AM, Altman JFB, et al. Efficacy of rosiglitazone in a genetically defined population with mild-to-moderate Alzheimer's disease. Pharmacogenomics J. 2006;6:246–54.
266. Robinson JD, Lam CY, Minnix JA, et al. The DRD2 TaqI-B polymorphism and its relationship to smoking abstinence and withdrawal symptoms. Pharmacogenomics J. 2007;7:266–74.
267. Roman T, Szobot C, Martins S, et al. Dopamine transporter gene and response to methylphenidate in attention-deficit/hyperactivity disorder. Pharmacogenetics. 2002;12:497–9.
268. Roses AD. The medical and economic roles of pipeline pharmacogenetics: Alzheimer's disease as a model of efficacy and HLA-B(*)5701 as a model of safety. Neuropsychopharmacology. 2009;34:6–17.
269. Roses AD, Saunders AM, Huang Y, et al. Complex disease-associated pharmacogenetics: drug efficacy, drug safety, and confirmation of a pathogenetic hypothesis (Alzheimer's disease). Pharmacogenomics J. 2007;7:10–28.
270. Rotberg B, Kronenberg S, Carmel M, et al. Additive effects of 5-HTTLPR (serotonin transporter) and tryptophan hydroxylase 2 G-703T gene polymorphisms on the clinical response to citalopram among children and adolescents with depression and anxiety disorders. J Child Adolesc Psychopharmacol. 2013;23:117–22.
271. Rybakowski JK, Czerski P, Dmitrzak-Weglarz M, et al. Clinical and pathogenic aspects of candidate genes for lithium prophylactic efficacy. J Psychopharmacol (Oxford). 2012;26:368–73.
272. Rybakowski JK, Dmitrzak-Weglarz M, Suwalska A, et al. Dopamine D1 receptor gene polymorphism is associated with prophylactic lithium response in bipolar disorder. Pharmacopsychiatry. 2009;42:20–2.
273. Rybakowski JK, Suwalska A, Czerski PM, et al. Prophylactic effect of lithium in bipolar affective illness may be related to serotonin transporter genotype. Pharmacol Rep. 2005a;57:124–7.
274. Rybakowski JK, Suwalska A, Skibinska M, et al. Prophylactic lithium response and polymorphism of the brain-derived neurotrophic factor gene. Pharmacopsychiatry. 2005b;38:166–70.

275. Rybakowski JK, Suwalska A, Skibinska M, et al. Response to lithium prophylaxis: interaction between serotonin transporter and BDNF genes. Am J Med Genet B Neuropsychiatr Genet. 2007;144B:820–3.
276. Sahraian S, Babashams M, Reza-Soltani P, et al. Serotonin transporter polymorphism (5-HTTLPR) and citalopram effectiveness in Iranian patients with major depressive disorder. Iran J Psychiatry. 2013;8:86–91.
277. Sarginson JE, Lazzeroni LC, Ryan HS, et al. FKBP5 polymorphisms and antidepressant response in geriatric depression. Am J Med Genet B Neuropsychiatr Genet. 2010;153B:554–60.
278. Saung WT, Narasimhan S, Lohoff FW. Lack of influence of DAT1 and DRD2 gene variants on antidepressant response in generalized anxiety disorder. Hum Psychopharmacol. 2014;29:316–21.
279. Schäfer M, Rujescu D, Giegling I, et al. Association of short-term response to haloperidol treatment with a polymorphism in the dopamine D(2) receptor gene. Am J Psychiatry. 2001;158:802–4.
280. Scharfetter J, Chaudhry HR, Hornik K, et al. Dopamine D3 receptor gene polymorphism and response to clozapine in schizophrenic Pakistani patients. Eur Neuropsychopharmacol. 1999;10:17–20.
281. Schulze TG, Alda M, Adli M, et al. The International Consortium on Lithium Genetics (ConLiGen): an initiative by the NIMH and IGSLI to study the genetic basis of response to lithium treatment. Neuropsychobiology. 2010;62:72–8.
282. Seripa D, Pilotto A, Paroni G, et al. Role of the serotonin transporter gene locus in the response to SSRI treatment of major depressive disorder in late life. J Psychopharmacol (Oxford). 2015;29:623–33.
283. Serretti A, Artioli P, Lorenzi C, et al. The C(−1019) G polymorphism of the 5-HT1A gene promoter and antidepressant response in mood disorders: preliminary findings. Int J Neuropsychopharmacol. 2004a;7:453–60.
284. Serretti A, Chiesa A, Crisafulli C, et al. Failure to replicate influence of GRIK4 and GNB3 polymorphisms on treatment outcome in major depression. Neuropsychobiology. 2012;65:70–5.
285. Serretti A, Cusin C, Rossini D, et al. Further evidence of a combined effect of SERTPR and TPH on SSRIs response in mood disorders. Am J Med Genet B Neuropsychiatr Genet. 2004b;129B:36–40.
286. Serretti A, Kato M, De Ronchi D, Kinoshita T. Meta-analysis of serotonin transporter gene promoter polymorphism (5-HTTLPR) association with selective serotonin reuptake inhibitor efficacy in depressed patients. Mol Psychiatry. 2007;12:247–57.
287. Serretti A, Lilli R, Lorenzi C, et al. Tryptophan hydroxylase gene and response to lithium prophylaxis in mood disorders. J Psychiatr Res. 1999a;33:371–7.
288. Serretti A, Lilli R, Lorenzi C, et al. Dopamine receptor D2 and D4 genes, GABA(A) alpha-1 subunit genes and response to lithium prophylaxis in mood disorders. Psychiatry Res. 1999b;87:7–19.
289. Serretti A, Lilli R, Lorenzi C, et al. Dopamine receptor D3 gene and response to lithium prophylaxis in mood disorders. Int J Neuropsychopharmacol. 1998;1:125–9.
290. Serretti A, Lorenzi C, Cusin C, et al. SSRIs antidepressant activity is influenced by G beta 3 variants. Eur Neuropsychopharmacol. 2003;13:117–22.
291. Serretti A, Lorenzi C, Lilli R, et al. Pharmacogenetics of lithium prophylaxis in mood disorders: analysis of COMT, MAO-A, and Gbeta3 variants. Am J Med Genet. 2002;114:370–9.
292. Serretti A, Lorenzi C, Lilli R, Smeraldi E. Serotonin receptor 2A, 2C, 1A genes and response to lithium prophylaxis in mood disorders. J Psychiatr Res. 2000;34:89–98.
293. Serretti A, Malitas PN, Mandelli L, et al. Further evidence for a possible association between serotonin transporter gene and lithium prophylaxis in mood disorders. Pharmacogenomics J. 2004c;4: 267–73.
294. Serretti A, Zanardi R, Cusin C, et al. Tryptophan hydroxylase gene associated with paroxetine antidepressant activity. Eur Neuropsychopharmacol. 2001a;11:375–80.
295. Serretti A, Zanardi R, Rossini D, et al. Influence of tryptophan hydroxylase and serotonin transporter genes on fluvoxamine antidepressant activity. Mol Psychiatry. 2001b;6:586–92.
296. Severino G, Squassina A, Costa M, et al. Pharmacogenomics of bipolar disorder. Pharmacogenomics. 2013;14:655–74.
297. Shaikh S, Collier D, Kerwin RW, et al. Dopamine D4 receptor subtypes and response to clozapine. Lancet. 1993;341:116.
298. Shaikh S, Collier DA, Sham PC, et al. Allelic association between a Ser-9-Gly polymorphism in the dopamine D3 receptor gene and schizophrenia. Hum Genet. 1996;97:714–9.
299. Shaikh S, Makoff A, Collier D, Kerwin R. Dopamine D4 receptors. CNS Drugs. 1997;8:1–11.
300. Shen Y-C, Chen S-F, Chen C-H, et al. Effects of DRD2/ANKK1 gene variations and clinical factors on aripiprazole efficacy in schizophrenic patients. J Psychiatr Res. 2009;43:600–6.
301. Sherman WR, Gish BG, Honchar MP, Munsell LY. Effects of lithium on phosphoinositide metabolism in vivo. Fed Proc. 1986;45:2639–46.
302. Shiroma PR, Drews MS, Geske JR, Mrazek DA. SLC6A4 polymorphisms and age of onset in late-life depression on treatment outcomes with citalopram: a Sequenced Treatment Alternatives to Relieve Depression (STAR*D) report. Am J Geriatr Psychiatry. 2014;22:1140–8.
303. Shorter D, Nielsen DA, Huang W, et al. Pharmacogenetic randomized trial for cocaine abuse: disulfiram and α1A-adrenoceptor gene variation. Eur Neuropsychopharmacol. 2013;23:1401–7.
304. Silberberg G, Levit A, Collier D, et al. Stargazin involvement with bipolar disorder and response to lithium treatment. Pharmacogenet Genomics. 2008;18:403–12.

305. Smits KM, Smits LJM, Peeters FPML, et al. The influence of 5-HTTLPR and STin2 polymorphisms in the serotonin transporter gene on treatment effect of selective serotonin reuptake inhibitors in depressive patients. Psychiatr Genet. 2008;18:184–90.
306. Sodhi MS, Arranz MJ, Curtis D, et al. Association between clozapine response and allelic variation in the 5-HT2C receptor gene. Neuroreport. 1995;7:169–72.
307. Souza RP, de Luca V, Meltzer HY, et al. Schizophrenia severity and clozapine treatment outcome association with oxytocinergic genes. Int J Neuropsychopharmacol. 2010a;13:793–8.
308. Souza RP, Romano-Silva MA, Lieberman JA, et al. Genetic association of the GDNF alpha-receptor genes with schizophrenia and clozapine response. J Psychiatr Res. 2010b;44:700–6.
309. Spellicy CJ, Kosten TR, Hamon SC, et al. ANKK1 and DRD2 pharmacogenetics of disulfiram treatment for cocaine abuse. Pharmacogenet Genomics. 2013;23:333–40.
310. Squassina A, Congiu D, Manconi F, et al. The PDLIM5 gene and lithium prophylaxis: an association and gene expression analysis in Sardinian patients with bipolar disorder. Pharmacol Res. 2008;57:369–73.
311. Squassina A, Manchia M, Borg J, et al. Evidence for association of an ACCN1 gene variant with response to lithium treatment in Sardinian patients with bipolar disorder. Pharmacogenomics. 2011;12:1559–69.
312. Staddon S, Arranz MJ, Mancama D, et al. Clinical applications of pharmacogenetics in psychiatry. Psychopharmacology. 2002;162:18–23.
313. Staeker J, Leucht S, Laika B, Steimer W. Polymorphisms in serotonergic pathways influence the outcome of antidepressant therapy in psychiatric inpatients. Genet Test Mol Biomarkers. 2014;18:20–31.
314. Stambolic V, Ruel L, Woodgett JR. Lithium inhibits glycogen synthase kinase-3 activity and mimics wingless signalling in intact cells. Curr Biol. 1996;6:1664–8.
315. Stamm TJ, Rampp C, Wiethoff K, et al. The FKBP5 polymorphism rs1360780 influences the effect of an algorithm-based antidepressant treatment and is associated with remission in patients with major depression. J Psychopharmacol (Oxford). 2016;30:40–7.
316. Stapleton JA, Sutherland G, O'Gara C, et al. Association between DRD2/ANKK1 Taq1A genotypes, depression and smoking cessation with nicotine replacement therapy. Pharmacogenet Genomics. 2011;21:447–53.
317. Steen VM, Løvlie R, Osher Y, et al. The polymorphic inositol polyphosphate 1-phosphatase gene as a candidate for pharmacogenetic prediction of lithium-responsive manic-depressive illness. Pharmacogenetics. 1998;8:259–68.
318. Stein MA, Waldman ID, Sarampote CS, et al. Dopamine transporter genotype and methylphenidate dose response in children with ADHD. Neuropsychopharmacology. 2005;30:1374–82.
319. Stein MB, Keshaviah A, Haddad SA, et al. Influence of RGS2 on sertraline treatment for social anxiety disorder. Neuropsychopharmacology. 2014;39:1340–6.
320. Stein MB, Seedat S, Gelernter J. Serotonin transporter gene promoter polymorphism predicts SSRI response in generalized social anxiety disorder. Psychopharmacology. 2006;187:68–72.
321. Stigler KA, Diener JT, Kohn AE, et al. Aripiprazole in pervasive developmental disorder not otherwise specified and Asperger's disorder: a 14-week, prospective, open-label study. J Child Adolesc Psychopharmacol. 2009;19:265–74.
322. Sugie Y, Sugie H, Fukuda T, et al. Clinical efficacy of fluvoxamine and functional polymorphism in a serotonin transporter gene on childhood autism. J Autism Dev Disord. 2005;35:377–85.
323. Szczepankiewicz A, Rybakowski JK, Suwalska A, et al. Association study of the glycogen synthase kinase-3beta gene polymorphism with prophylactic lithium response in bipolar patients. World J Biol Psychiatry. 2006;7:158–61.
324. Szczepankiewicz A, Skibińska M, Suwalska A, et al. No association of three GRIN2B polymorphisms with lithium response in bipolar patients. Pharmacol Rep. 2009a;61:448–52.
325. Szczepankiewicz A, Skibinska M, Suwalska A, et al. The association study of three FYN polymorphisms with prophylactic lithium response in bipolar patients. Hum Psychopharmacol. 2009b;24:287–91.
326. Szekeres G, Kéri S, Juhász A, et al. Role of dopamine D3 receptor (DRD3) and dopamine transporter (DAT) polymorphism in cognitive dysfunctions and therapeutic response to atypical antipsychotics in patients with schizophrenia. Am J Med Genet B Neuropsychiatr Genet. 2004;124B:1–5.
327. Taylor MJ, Sen S, Bhagwagar Z. Antidepressant response and the serotonin transporter gene-linked polymorphic region. Biol Psychiatry. 2010;68:536–43.
328. Thakur GA, Grizenko N, Sengupta SM, et al. The 5-HTTLPR polymorphism of the serotonin transporter gene and short term behavioural response to methylphenidate in children with ADHD. BMC Psychiatry. 2010;10:50.
329. Thomas P, Srivastava V, Singh A, et al. Correlates of response to Olanzapine in a North Indian Schizophrenia sample. Psychiatry Res. 2008;161:275–83.
330. Trautmann S, Richter J, Muehlhan M, et al. Does prior traumatization affect the treatment outcome of CBT for panic disorder? The potential role of the MAOA gene and depression symptoms. Eur Arch Psychiatry Clin Neurosci. 2017;15.

331. Tsai S-J, Hong C-J, Chen T-J, Yu YW-Y. Lack of supporting evidence for a genetic association of the FKBP5 polymorphism and response to antidepressant treatment. Am J Med Genet B Neuropsychiatr Genet. 2007;144B:1097–8.
332. Tsai SJ, Wang YC, Yu Younger WY, et al. Association analysis of polymorphism in the promoter region of the alpha2a-adrenoceptor gene with schizophrenia and clozapine response. Schizophr Res. 2001;49:53–8.
333. Turecki G, Grof P, Cavazzoni P, et al. MAOA: association and linkage studies with lithium responsive bipolar disorder. Psychiatr Genet. 1999a;9:13–6.
334. Turecki G, Grof P, Cavazzoni P, et al. Evidence for a role of phospholipase C-gamma1 in the pathogenesis of bipolar disorder. Mol Psychiatry. 1998;3:534–8.
335. Turecki G, Grof P, Cavazzoni P, et al. Lithium responsive bipolar disorder, unilineality, and chromosome 18: a linkage study. Am J Med Genet. 1999b;88:411–5.
336. Turecki G, Grof P, Grof E, et al. Mapping susceptibility genes for bipolar disorder: a pharmacogenetic approach based on excellent response to lithium. Mol Psychiatry. 2001;6:570–8.
337. van der Meulen EM, Bakker SC, Pauls DL, et al. High sibling correlation on methylphenidate response but no association with DAT1-10R homozygosity in Dutch sibpairs with ADHD. J Child Psychol Psychiatry. 2005;46:1074–80.
338. Villafuerte SM, Vallabhaneni K, Sliwerska E, et al. SSRI response in depression may be influenced by SNPs in HTR1B and HTR1A. Psychiatr Genet. 2009;19:281–91.
339. Volpi S, Heaton C, Mack K, et al. Whole genome association study identifies polymorphisms associated with QT prolongation during iloperidone treatment of schizophrenia. Mol Psychiatry. 2009;14:1024–31.
340. Wang L, Fang C, Zhang A, et al. The – 1019 C/G polymorphism of the 5-HT(1) A receptor gene is associated with negative symptom response to risperidone treatment in schizophrenia patients. J Psychopharmacol (Oxford). 2008;22:904–9.
341. Wang L, Yu L, He G, et al. Response of risperidone treatment may be associated with polymorphisms of HTT gene in Chinese schizophrenia patients. Neurosci Lett. 2007;414:1–4.
342. Wang Z, Fan J, Gao K, et al. Neurotrophic tyrosine kinase receptor type 2 (NTRK2) gene associated with treatment response to mood stabilizers in patients with bipolar I disorder. J Mol Neurosci. 2013;50:305–10.
343. Wang Z, Li Z, Chen J, et al. Association of BDNF gene polymorphism with bipolar disorders in Han Chinese population. Genes Brain Behav. 2012;11:524–8.
344. Wei Z, Wang L, Xuan J, et al. Association analysis of serotonin receptor 7 gene (HTR7) and risperidone response in Chinese schizophrenia patients. Prog Neuro-Psychopharmacol Biol Psychiatry. 2009;33:547–51.
345. Wilkie MJV, Smith D, Reid IC, et al. A splice site polymorphism in the G-protein beta subunit influences antidepressant efficacy in depression. Pharmacogenet Genomics. 2007;17:207–15.
346. Wilkie MJV, Smith G, Day RK, et al. Polymorphisms in the SLC6A4 and HTR2A genes influence treatment outcome following antidepressant therapy. Pharmacogenomics J. 2009;9:61–70.
347. Williams K, Brignell A, Randall M, et al. Selective serotonin reuptake inhibitors (SSRIs) for autism spectrum disorders (ASD). Cochrane Database Syst Rev. 2013;8:CD004677.
348. Wink LK, Erickson CA, McDougle CJ. Pharmacologic treatment of behavioral symptoms associated with autism and other pervasive developmental disorders. Curr Treat Options Neurol. 2010;12:529–38.
349. Winsberg BG, Comings DE. Association of the dopamine transporter gene (DAT1) with poor methylphenidate response. J Am Acad Child Adolesc Psychiatry. 1999;38:1474–7.
350. Won E-S, Chang H-S, Lee H-Y, et al. Association between serotonin transporter-linked polymorphic region and escitalopram antidepressant treatment response in Korean patients with major depressive disorder. Neuropsychobiology. 2012;66:221–9.
351. Woodward ND, Jayathilake K, Meltzer HY. COMT val108/158met genotype, cognitive function, and cognitive improvement with clozapine in schizophrenia. Schizophr Res. 2007;90:86–96.
352. Wu G-S, Luo H-R, Dong C, et al. Sequence polymorphisms of MC1R gene and their association with depression and antidepressant response. Psychiatr Genet. 2011;21:14–8.
353. Wu S, Xing Q, Gao R, et al. Response to chlorpromazine treatment may be associated with polymorphisms of the DRD2 gene in Chinese schizophrenic patients. Neurosci Lett. 2005;376:1–4.
354. Xing Q, Gao R, Li H, et al. Polymorphisms of the ABCB1 gene are associated with the therapeutic response to risperidone in Chinese schizophrenia patients. Pharmacogenomics. 2006;7:987–93.
355. Xing Q, Qian X, Li H, et al. The relationship between the therapeutic response to risperidone and the dopamine D2 receptor polymorphism in Chinese schizophrenia patients. Int J Neuropsychopharmacol. 2007;10:631–7.
356. Xu M, Xing Q, Li S, et al. Pharacogenetic effects of dopamine transporter gene polymorphisms on response to chlorpromazine and clozapine and on extrapyramidal syndrome in schizophrenia. Prog Neuro-Psychopharmacol Biol Psychiatry. 2010;34:1026–32.
357. Xu M-Q, St Clair D, Feng G-Y, et al. BDNF gene is a genetic risk factor for schizophrenia and is related to the chlorpromazine-induced extrapyramidal syndrome in the Chinese population. Pharmacogenet Genomics. 2008;18:449–57.
358. Xu Z, Zhang Z, Shi Y, et al. Influence and interaction of genetic polymorphisms in the serotonin system and life stress on antidepressant drug response. J Psychopharmacol (Oxford). 2012;26:349–59.

359. Xuan J, Zhao X, He G, et al. Effects of the dopamine D3 receptor (DRD3) gene polymorphisms on risperidone response: a pharmacogenetic study. Neuropsychopharmacology. 2008;33:305–11.
360. Yamanouchi Y, Iwata N, Suzuki T, et al. Effect of DRD2, 5-HT2A, and COMT genes on antipsychotic response to risperidone. Pharmacogenomics J. 2003;3:356–61.
361. Yan T, Wang L, Kuang W, et al. Brain-derived neurotrophic factor Val66Met polymorphism association with antidepressant efficacy: a systematic review and meta-analysis. Asia Pac Psychiatry. 2014;6:241–51.
362. Yang L, Qian Q, Liu L, et al. Adrenergic neurotransmitter system transporter and receptor genes associated with atomoxetine response in attention-deficit hyperactivity disorder children. J Neural Transm. 2013;120:1127–33.
363. Yasui-Furukori N, Saito M, Nakagami T, et al. Association between multidrug resistance 1 (MDR1) gene polymorphisms and therapeutic response to bromperidol in schizophrenic patients: a preliminary study. Prog Neuro-Psychopharmacol Biol Psychiatry. 2006;30:286–91.
364. Yatham LN, Kennedy SH, Parikh SV, et al. Canadian Network for Mood and Anxiety Treatments (CANMAT) and International Society for Bipolar Disorders (ISBD) collaborative update of CANMAT guidelines for the management of patients with bipolar disorder: update 2013. Bipolar Disord. 2013;15:1–44.
365. Yehuda R, Pratchett LC, Elmes MW, et al. Glucocorticoid-related predictors and correlates of post-traumatic stress disorder treatment response in combat veterans. Interface Focus. 2014;4:20140048.
366. Yevtushenko OO, Oros MM, Reynolds GP. Early response to selective serotonin reuptake inhibitors in panic disorder is associated with a functional 5-HT1A receptor gene polymorphism. J Affect Disord. 2010;123:308–11.
367. Yin L, Zhang YY, Zhang X, et al. TPH, SLC6A2, SLC6A3, DRD2 and DRD4 polymorphisms and neuroendocrine factors predict SSRIs treatment outcome in the Chinese population with major depression. Pharmacopsychiatry. 2015;48:95–103.
368. Yu YW, Tsai SJ, Lin CH, et al. Serotonin-6 receptor variant (C267T) and clinical response to clozapine. Neuroreport. 1999;10:1231–3.
369. Yu YW, Tsai SJ, Yang KH, et al. Evidence for an association between polymorphism in the serotonin-2A receptor variant (102T/C) and increment of N100 amplitude in schizophrenics treated with clozapine. Neuropsychobiology. 2001;43:79–82.
370. Yu YW-Y, Tsai S-J, Liou Y-J, et al. Association study of two serotonin 1A receptor gene polymorphisms and fluoxetine treatment response in Chinese major depressive disorders. Eur Neuropsychopharmacol. 2006;16:498–503.
371. Yudkin P, Munafò M, Hey K, et al. Effectiveness of nicotine patches in relation to genotype in women versus men: randomised controlled trial. BMJ. 2004;328:989–90.
372. Zai G, Brandl EJ, Müller DJ, et al. Pharmacogenetics of antidepressant treatment in obsessive-compulsive disorder: an update and implications for clinicians. Pharmacogenomics. 2014;15:1147–57.
373. Zalsman G, Frisch A, Lev-Ran S, et al. DRD4 exon III polymorphism and response to risperidone in Israeli adolescents with schizophrenia: a pilot pharmacogenetic study. Eur Neuropsychopharmacol. 2003;13:183–5.
374. Zanardi R, Serretti A, Rossini D, et al. Factors affecting fluvoxamine antidepressant activity: influence of pindolol and 5-HTTLPR in delusional and nondelusional depression. Biol Psychiatry. 2001;50:323–30.
375. Zeni CP, Guimarães AP, Polanczyk GV, et al. No significant association between response to methylphenidate and genes of the dopaminergic and serotonergic systems in a sample of Brazilian children with attention-deficit/hyperactivity disorder. Am J Med Genet B Neuropsychiatr Genet. 2007;144B:391–4.
376. Zhao A-L, Zhao J-P, Zhang Y-H, et al. Dopamine D4 receptor gene exon III polymorphism and interindividual variation in response to clozapine. Int J Neurosci. 2005;115:1539–47.
377. Zhao X, Huang Y, Li J, et al. Association between the 5-HT1A receptor gene polymorphism (rs6295) and antidepressants: a meta-analysis. Int Clin Psychopharmacol. 2012;27:314–20.
378. Zill P, Baghai TC, Zwanzger P, et al. Evidence for an association between a G-protein beta3-gene variant with depression and response to antidepressant treatment. Neuroreport. 2000;11:1893–7.
379. Zou Y-F, Wang F, Feng X-L, et al. Meta-analysis of FKBP5 gene polymorphisms association with treatment response in patients with mood disorders. Neurosci Lett. 2010;484:56–61.
380. Zuo L, Luo X, Krystal JH, et al. The efficacies of clozapine and haloperidol in refractory schizophrenia are related to DTNBP1 variation. Pharmacogenet Genomics. 2009;19:437–46.

Using Neuroimaging and Electroencephalography for Prediction of Treatment Resistance in Psychiatric Disorders

4

Je-Yeon Yun and Seung-Hwan Lee

4.1 Introduction

Up to 20% of individuals with schizophrenia show minimal or no response to medication and are considered to have "treatment-resistant" schizophrenia [1]. Likewise, treatment outcomes for pharmacotherapy with antidepressants vary markedly across patients [2]; about one-third of patients suffering from major depressive disorder do not respond adequately to conventional treatment [3] and are classified as having treatment-resistant depression (TRD) [3]. Data-driven decision-making holds that patients diagnosed with depression, who have received at least one antidepressant, will have TRD if they have received ≥3 antidepressants or ≥1 antipsychotic in the last year [4]. Moreover, the longitudinal course of bipolar disorder is highly variable, and a subset of patients seems to suffer a progressive course of multiple-repetitive episodes and associated progressive brain changes; accordingly, there seems to be an association between the number of mood (especially manic) episodes and treatment resistance in patients with bipolar disorder [5–7]. Likewise, pharmacotherapy with serotonin reuptake inhibitors does not attain sufficient symptomatic improvement in 40–60% of patients diagnosed with obsessive–compulsive disorder. Therefore, earlier identification of patients who are prone to treatment resistance could avoid the frustration of a trial-and-error approach and might facilitate the design of more optimized treatment regimens and setting of individualized levels of care [2, 8].

Thus, this chapter illustrates recent (primarily 2015–2018) study findings regarding clinical application of brain-based biomarkers derived from patients for the prediction of response or resistance to treatment, as well as for improved design of clinical studies, to find more robust brain-based biomarkers of treatment response or resistance. The chapter is comprised of three parts. First, for patients diagnosed with psychotic disorders, mood disorders, or anxiety disorders, changing patterns of structural–functional brain characteristics that result from treatment with pharmacotherapy, cognitive behavioral therapy, as well as direct brain stimulation will be reviewed. Second, we will show the brain-based predictors of treatment response at baseline. Third, we will turn from exploration based on groupwise predictive power to the individual-level

J.-Y. Yun
Seoul National University Hospital,
Seoul, Republic of Korea

Yeongeon Student Support Center, Seoul National University College of Medicine,
Seoul, Republic of Korea

S.-H. Lee (✉)
Clinical Emotion and Cognition Research Laboratory, Inje University, Goyang, Republic of Korea

Department of Psychiatry, Inje University, Ilsan-Paik Hospital, Goyang, Republic of Korea
e-mail: lshpss@paik.ac.kr

Y.-K. Kim (ed.), *Treatment Resistance in Psychiatry*, https://doi.org/10.1007/978-981-10-4358-1_4

prediction of treatment response and focus on the recent trends in machine learning-based studies in which brain-based biomarkers are applied as explanatory or predictive features.

4.1.1 Treatment-Related Changes in Brain MRI Measurements (State Markers)

4.1.1.1 Psychotic Disorders

Treatment with antipsychotics for patients diagnosed with schizophrenia could be associated with a decreased volume of the parietal lobe and an increased volume of the basal ganglia [9], as well as reduction of the brain Glx (combined glutamate and glutamine signaling), measured using proton magnetic resonance spectroscopy (^{1}H-MRS) in the fronto-thalamo-temporal brain regions [10]. After pharmacotherapy with olanzapine, the long-range functional connectivity strength of the default mode network and sensorimotor network were restored (from reduced to increased strength); on the other hand, pharmacotherapy-related reduction of the short-range functional connectivity strength in the right inferior parietal lobule (initially elevated prior to pharmacotherapy) and left superior temporal gyrus appears to be associated with better and worse treatment outcome, respectively [11]. In addition, 16 weeks of pharmacotherapy with ziprasidone in patients diagnosed with schizophrenia has been associated with increased functional activation of brain regions, including the anterior cingulate and ventrolateral prefrontal cortices (related to cognitive control) during the performance of a task involving selecting stimuli based on their emotional valence [12]. On the other hand, cognitive behavioral therapy (16–20 biweekly sessions) for patients diagnosed with schizophrenia, who suffer from persistent auditory hallucinations, resulted in reduced functional brain activation in the bilateral amygdalae and left superior temporal and right superior frontal cortices in response to an emotional auditory paradigm, as compared to non-treated schizophrenia patients and healthy controls. This difference was seen even 14 months after the completion of cognitive behavioral therapy [13].

4.1.1.2 Mood Disorders

Depression is associated with diverse structural and functional changes in brain circuits related to emotion processing and mood regulation; some (but not all) of these circuitry changes occur in response to pharmacological/nonpharmacological treatments for depression [14]. At the neurotransmitter level, greater elevation (or smaller reduction) of gamma-aminobutyric acid levels in the pregenual anterior cingulate cortex from baseline to after 3–7 days of citalopram treatment, measured using proton magnetic resonance spectroscopy (^{1}H-MRS), could predict treatment response after 6 weeks of citalopram pharmacotherapy [15]. In relation to task performance, treatment with antidepressants reduces functional brain activation in response to a painful electrical stimulation task in the medial thalamic nuclei of the pulvinar in patients diagnosed with depression. Moreover, the strength of the functional activation at the perigenual anterior cingulate cortex after pharmacotherapy correlated with the degree of symptomatic improvement [16] (Fig. 4.1). Moreover, pharmacotherapy with amisulpride [a D_2/D_3 receptor antagonist] for patients diagnosed with depression increases the functional activation of striatum, as well as the functional connectivity between the nucleus accumbens and midcingulate cortex in response to monetary rewards during the monetary incentive delay task [17]. In terms of cognitive behavioral therapy for depression, longitudinal enhancement of the downregulated blood oxygenation level-dependent (BOLD) signal in the subgenual anterior cingulate–medial prefrontal–lingual cortices for tasks that require a voluntary emotional regulation strategy while recalling negative autobiographical memories was related to a better treatment response [18]. Likewise, treatment response for 5-Hz repetitive transcranial magnetic stimulation (rTMS) to the left dorsolateral prefrontal cortex in patients diagnosed with major depressive disorder or posttraumatic

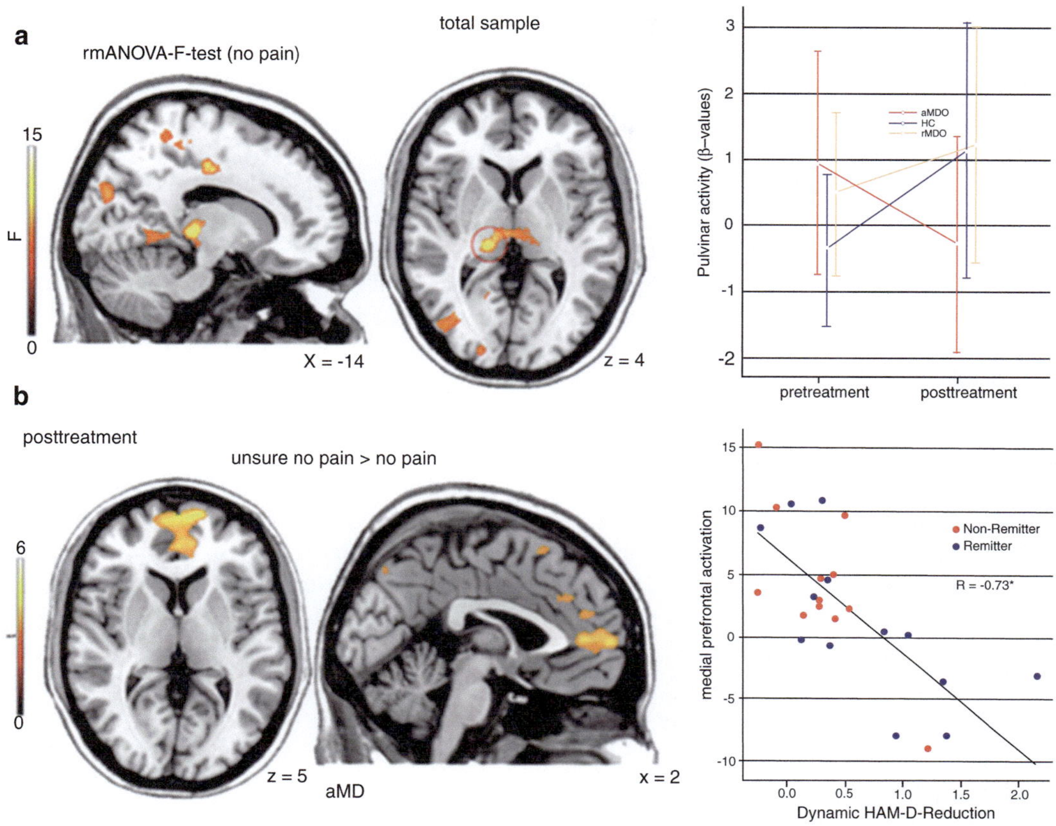

Fig. 4.1 (**a**) Reversal of thalamic hyperactivity after antidepressant treatment. Repeated measures analysis of variance (rmANOVA) comparisons between fMRI-1 and fMRI-2 within healthy controls (HC), remitted depressed patients (rMD), and acute depressed patients (aMD). Acute patients were treated with escitalopram or venlafaxine for 12 weeks. (**a**) *F*-test results depict elevated activation of thalamic pulvinar nuclei in acute patients, which reversed to baseline values of HC after treatment. Activations represent difference in *F*-test between fMRI-2 and. fMRI-1. (**b**) Dynamic response to antidepressant treatment: a significant negative correlation ($p < 0.001$, FWE, cluster-level) between dynamic HAM-D_{24} reduction and perigenual cingulate and medial prefrontal activation was found at fMRI-2. Non-remitter (=HAM-D_{24} >8) exhibited higher activation after treatment. Activations represent t-tests between remitter and non-remitter at fMRI-2. (**a** and **b** are referenced from Figure 4.2a and Figure 4.3c and d of original article by [16] http://creativecommons.org/licenses/by-nc-sa/4.0/)

stress disorder was related to the degree of reduction in the resting-state functional connectivity strength between the subgenual anterior cingulate and the default mode network, left dorsolateral prefrontal cortex, and insula [19].

4.1.1.3 Anxiety Disorders

After pharmacotherapy with the serotonin-related antidepressant paroxetine, the strength of the condition-dependent functional connectivity between the left hippocampus and the left temporal pole during the emotional face perception tasks in patients diagnosed with social anxiety disorder or panic disorder was increased [20]. In addition, the long-term effect of cognitive behavioral therapy in social anxiety disorder is associated with a reduced amygdalar volume at 1 year after the treatment in responders, as compared to nonresponders [21]. On the other hand, treatment response to 10-Hz rTMS at the dorsomedial prefrontal cortex in treatment-resistant patients diagnosed with obsessive–compulsive disorder was proportional to the reduction of resting-state functional connectivity between the dorsomedial prefrontal cortex and the ventral striatum (which was initially elevated prior to the rTMS treatment) [22]. In fact, regardless of the treatment modality, posttreatment improvement of obsessive–compulsive symptoms is accompanied by decreased functional activation of the ventral circuits of the cortico-striato-thalamo-cortical loop during symptom provocation, as well as increased functional recruitment of the dorsal circuit during performance of cognitive processing tasks [23].

4.1.2 Treatment-Related Changes in EEG Measurements (State Markers)

4.1.2.1 Psychotic Disorders

Electroencephalography (EEG) is a noninvasive, inexpensive, and useful tool for investigating the neurobiology of schizophrenia and for biotyping [24]. When patterns of the cortical oscillatory activity in schizophrenia patients were explored using the auditory steady-state response, restoration of the reduced amplitude and intertrial phase coherence of response in the lower gamma (30–50 Hz) range seen in non-medicated schizophrenia was found in patients prescribed with atypical antipsychotics; these findings were comparable to those observed in healthy controls [25]. Moreover, in first-episode psychosis patients prior to pharmacotherapy, the effective connectivity from the right middle frontal gyrus to the left superior temporal gyrus during the eyes-open resting state was decreased as compared to healthy controls. In contrast, first-episode psychosis patients on pharmacotherapy showed improved effective connectivity strength between these regions, comparable to that observed in healthy controls [26]. For patients diagnosed with schizophrenia who showed a treatment response to pharmacotherapy with clozapine, a set of cross-power spectral density (CPSD) features (comprised of a combination of brain regional source activity and connectivity measures derived from the source localization of oddball auditory evoked potential), which spatially overlap with the default mode network, changed after pharmacotherapy [27].

4.1.2.2 Mood Disorders

Treatment-related changes in the EEG profile could be used to predict treatment nonresponders. When depressive patients who have been prescribed antidepressants for 2 weeks show hemispheric asymmetries of reduced absolute beta power and increased delta power in the left hemisphere relative to the right hemisphere, they tend to show less sufficient symptomatic improvement after 8 weeks of pharmacotherapy with antidepressants [28]. From the perspective of resting-state functional connectivity, the significantly decreased alpha connectivity among the dorsolateral prefrontal, dorsomedial prefrontal, and subgenual anterior cingulate cortices after antidepressant pharmacotherapy—observed in male treatment responders—was not detected in nonresponders [29]. On the other hand, treatment with bilateral or unilateral rTMS in the left (10 Hz) and right (1 Hz) dorsolateral prefrontal cortices resulted in a significant reduction in alpha, beta, and gamma frequencies in the medial-superior frontal-cingulate cortices only in responders [30]. Of note, in patients diagnosed with depressive disorder who experienced suicidal ideation, a reduction in the suicidal ideation after magnetic seizure therapy (MST) was strongly correlated with two baseline measures of cortical inhibition, including the N100 amplitude for frontal electrodes (maximum at FC4; $R = -0.64$; $P < 0.001$) and with long-interval cortical inhibition (LICI) values for frontal electrodes (maximum at FC6; $R = 0.58$; $P = 0.002$) [31].

4.1.2.3 Anxiety Disorders

After cognitive behavioral therapy, patients diagnosed with social anxiety disorder (SAD), who tend to exhibit hypervigilance toward facial cues and show enhanced early facial processing as compared to healthy controls, demonstrated reduced hypervigilance for facial stimuli as reflected in the reduced N170 responses to faces, in proportion to the Interaction Anxiousness Scale (IAS) score [32]. In patients diagnosed with obsessive–compulsive disorder, typical cognitive symptoms of overactive performance monitoring are reflected in enhanced error-related negativity (ERN; a negative deflection in the event-related potential after an incorrect response), which has been suggested to arise from the anterior cingulate cortex. The ERN amplitude does not change after pharmacotherapy with antidepressant or cognitive behavioral therapy in obsessive–compulsive disorder [33, 34].

4.1.3 Baseline MRI Measurement Markers of Treatment Response or Resistance (Trait Markers)

4.1.3.1 Psychotic Disorders

Among the patients diagnosed with schizophrenia, the biological underpinnings of the treatment-resistant subgroup could be characterized using structural and functional brain imaging studies. First, a larger total gray matter volume predicts better treatment response, as measured using the Brief Psychiatric Rating Scale (BPRS), after 24 weeks of paliperidone palmitate long-acting injectable treatment in patients diagnosed with schizophrenia [35]. Moreover, treatment resistance in patients diagnosed with schizophrenia has been associated with reduced global network efficiency, in addition to the widespread reductions in resting-state functional connectivity strength predominantly in the frontotemporal, fronto-occipital, and temporo-occipital connections [1]. Of note, the resting-state functional connectivity network of ultra-treatment-resistant schizophrenia patients (with a history of treatment failure of at least two trials of antipsychotics and a trial of clozapine), as compared to other schizophrenia patients who are more responsive to antipsychotic-based pharmacotherapy as well as to healthy controls, demonstrated attenuated functional communication among the cerebellar-parietal-frontal regions. This is thought to underlie the severe treatment resistance [36]. In regard to the dopamine system, during performance of a probabilistic reinforcement learning task utilizing emotionally valenced face stimuli, treatment-resistant schizophrenia patients, but not treatment-responsive patients, showed a positive relationship between emotional bias and reward prediction error-related activation of the bilateral thalamus and caudate during negative feedback [37].

4.1.3.2 Mood Disorders

In patients diagnosed with depressive disorder, the strength of the resting-state functional connectivity in the reward network (between the nucleus accumbens and left superior frontal gyrus/parahippocampus), in addition to the lower variable coefficient of the global brain signal derived from the resting-state functional connectivity network at baseline, could successfully predict poor response to antidepressant pharmacotherapy [38, 39]. On the other hand, lowered nodal efficiency of the left hippocampus in the resting-state functional connectivity network at baseline could predict a better treatment response of depressive symptoms to 2 weeks' antidepressant pharmacotherapy [40]. From the perspective of brain white matter-based structural connectivity, reduced tract integrity measured with fractional anisotropy, especially in the frontoparietal regions at baseline, is associated with a worse treatment response to lurasidone pharmacotherapy in patients suffering from bipolar depression [41]. In terms of brain morphology-based markers of treatment response to antidepressant pharmacotherapy, a decreased gray matter volume in the bilateral anterior cingulate and right superior frontal cortices could predict treatment nonresponse before pharmacotherapy [42]. Furthermore, possibly in relation to cognitive distortions, such as adaptive rumination, a larger gray matter volume in the anterior cingulate cortex prior to treatment could predict a better treatment response and symptomatic improvement after cognitive behavioral therapy for depression [43, 44]. Interestingly, thinner cortical thickness of the left rostral anterior cingulate cortex could predict better improvement of depressive symptoms in response to the rTMS over the left dorsolateral prefrontal cortex [45]. On the other hand, patterns of functional brain activation in response to tasks provide clinicians with useful information for predicting the treatment response; for example, functional activation of the temporoparietal junction during a painful electrical stimulation task (at baseline) predicted non-remission of depressive symptoms even after two antidepressant trials [16].

4.1.3.3 Anxiety Disorders

In patients suffering from social anxiety disorder, task-related functional co-activation patterns of the dorsal anterior cingulate cortex and amygdala for self-referential criticism could predict the degree of treatment response for Internet-delivered cognitive behavioral therapy [46]; likewise, reduced functional activation of the amygdala and rostral anterior cingulate during attentional control over negative distractors, as well as more functional recruitment in the dorsolateral prefrontal cortex during cognitive reappraisal of a negative affective state, were all associated with poor treatment response to cognitive behavioral therapy in patients with social anxiety disorder [47, 48]. On the other hand, poorer treatment response to cognitive behavioral therapy in children or adolescents diagnosed with anxiety disorder is related to the abnormal functional connectivity between the amygdala and insula during the threat-attention task; however, augmentation of attention-bias modification therapy (targeting rapid, implicit threat reactions) with cognitive behavioral therapy resolved these connectivity-related differences in symptomatic improvement [49]. For patients with obsessive–compulsive disorder, the degree centrality values for the amygdala basolateral nuclei (implicated in fear processing) in the resting-state functional connectivity network at baseline show a positive relationship with symptom improvement after cognitive behavioral therapy [50].

4.1.4 Baseline EEG Measurement Markers of Treatment Response or Resistance (Trait Markers)

4.1.4.1 Psychotic Disorders

As one of the trait-like electrophysiological characteristics, a reduction of mismatch negativity (MMN; a pre-attentive event-related potential component) amplitude could predict the development of psychosis in high-risk individuals; on the other hand, patients diagnosed with schizophrenia who show similar MMN amplitude as that of healthy controls have been associated with a better treatment response to pharmacotherapy or cognitive training [51].

4.1.4.2 Mood Disorders

Given the high prevalence of TRD and the long delays in finding effective treatments, finding valid biomarkers of treatment outcome in resting-state EEGs or evoked potentials, with the ability to guide treatment selection for mood disorders, is crucial [52]. Occurrence of any EEG abnormalities, including an epileptiform EEG or EEG slowing, is related to the response to pharmacotherapy with escitalopram and venlafaxine for depression; a slow alpha peak frequency is related to the response to sertraline treatment in depression [53]. Among the various event-related potential parameters of brain activity, male depressive patients with a treatment nonresponse to 8-week pharmacotherapy with venlafaxine revealed significantly smaller N1 amplitudes (generated in a standard two-tone oddball paradigm) than treatment responders [54]. Of note, the loudness dependency of the auditory evoked potentials (LDAEP) and resting EEG alpha and theta power might be biological markers predicting the response to antidepressants with good-to-excellent test–retest reliability [55, 56]. For instance, reduced absolute alpha power and increased relative delta power in the left hemisphere, as well as the absence of parietal cortical asymmetry at baseline, could predict a nonresponse (<50% reduction of Montgomery–Asberg Depression Rating Scale score) at 8 weeks for antidepressant pharmacotherapy [28]. In addition, using a logistic regression classifier, features of resting-state functional brain activities at the frontal and temporal regions, constructed by way of wavelet transform analysis-based time–frequency decomposition, could classify nonresponders from responders to serotonin selective reuptake inhibitor (SSRI) pharmacotherapy with an 87.5% accuracy [57]. From the perspective of brain signal variability, a propensity toward global brain processing, as reflected in the reduced local multiscale entropy at fronto-central regions, in addition to increased global multiscale entropy, could indicate a sufficient treatment response to 12-weeks' antidepressant pharmacotherapy [58]. On the other hand, patients diagnosed with depression who showed lower levels of fronto-midline theta (4–8 Hz) power and theta connectivity during a working memory task did not show sufficient relief from depressive symptoms after 5–8 weeks of rTMS treatment [59]. Furthermore, weaker coupling between a faster reaction time and a smaller late positive potential (LPP; an index of enhanced attention toward aversive stimuli) at the preceding trial, revealed in single-trial level analyses, could predict a poor treatment response to cognitive behavioral therapy for depressive symptoms [60].

4.1.4.3 Anxiety Disorders

For patients diagnosed with obsessive–compulsive disorder, a reduced amount of time spent at the highest level of CNS arousal, assessed using the Vigilance Algorithm Leipzig (VIGILL) during the resting state, could be an indicator of a better treatment response to SSRIs, cognitive behavioral therapy, or both [61].

4.1.5 Machine Learning and Prediction of Treatment Response or Resistance

As psychiatric diseases are extremely heterogeneous, both in clinical manifestation and etiology, their treatment requires a more precise definition of the underlying neurobiology, since different biological origins of the same disorder may require different treatments [62]. In contrast to the conventional brain MRI studies that showed group-level differences, a machine-learning approach allows individual-level classifications from the perspective of diagnosis and treatment response [63]. Application of machine-learning techniques to neuroimaging might uncover more robust and reliable biomarkers of psychiatric disorders, currently under the syndrome-based diagnostic criteria, that could be used at an individual level [64].

4.1.5.1 Psychotic Disorders

Response to treatment for reducing the negative symptoms of schizophrenia using 10-Hz rTMS applied to the left dorsolateral prefrontal cortex could be successfully predicted by way of neuroanatomical pattern recognition for gray matter density reductions in the prefrontal, insular, medio-temporal, and cerebellar cortices and increments in parietal and thalamic regions [65] (Fig. 4.2). To predict the treatment response to pharmacotherapy with antipsychotics only or a combination of electroconvulsive therapy and pharmacotherapy, the similarity score calculated from the schizophrenia vs. healthy controls classifier based on the selected feature of the resting-state functional connectivity network, including the default mode network, the temporal lobe network, the language network, the cortico-striatal network, and the cerebellum network, was used. As the similarity score derived from the resting-state functional connectivity network at baseline is higher, a better treatment response was found for schizophrenia patients [66]. Furthermore, treatment response to pharmacotherapy with amisulpride in alleviating the negative symptoms of schizophrenia differed according to patient subgroups (identified by means of probabilistic principal component analysis), biotyped using the electrophysiological features of pre-pulse inhibition (PPI), mismatch negativity (MMN), and P50 suppression (in addition to clinical and neurocognitive variables) [67].

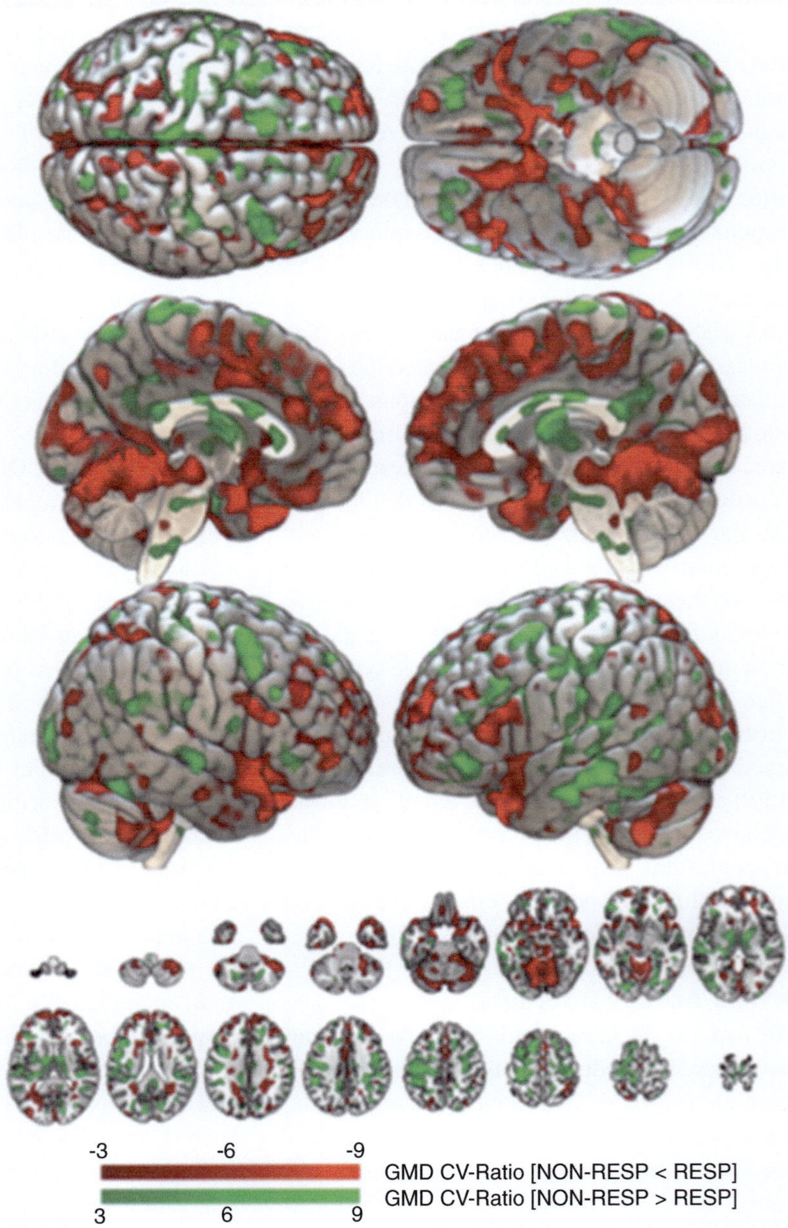

Fig. 4.2 Reliability of the baseline gray matter density pattern predicting subsequent response vs nonresponse to active repetitive transcranial magnetic stimulation (rTMS). The reliability of the gray matter density (GMD) pattern elements was measured in terms of a cross-validation ratio (CVR) map [CVR = mean(**w**)/standard error(**w**), where **w** are the weight vectors of the 5111 support vector machine (SVM) models generated in the study's repeated nested cross-validation setup]. The CVR map was thresholded at a CVR of ±3, corresponding to an alpha level of 0.01; reliable areas of GMD reduction in nonresponders (NON-RESP) vs responders (RESP) are shaded in red colors, whereas areas of GMD increments are painted in green [65]

4.1.5.2 Mood Disorders

Prediction of TRD per individual using brain T1-weighted imaging, at least as quantified by the Massachusetts General Hospital (MGH-S) clinical staging, was not successful [64]. On the other hand, as classified using the alternating decision-tree framework, among the patients diagnosed with late-life depression, patients with more intact white matter tract integrity of the anterior salience network and better preserved resting-state functional connectivity strength for the dorsal default mode network showed less improvement of depressive symptoms in response to pharmacotherapy with antidepressants [68]. Additionally, using the support vector regression model, the pretreatment volume of the subgenual anterior cingulate cortex in patients diagnosed with depression could be successfully applied to predict the degree of relative reduction in the Hamilton Depression Rating Scale score after the ECT [69].

4.1.5.3 Anxiety Disorders

Several trials aiming to predict the response to pharmacotherapy or cognitive behavioral therapy in patients with anxiety disorders, using baseline brain characteristics, have been reported. Using the support vector machine with a radial basis functional kernel, an optimal set of features among the top 12 individualized structural covariance (ISC) features (which reflect a dysfunctional cortical maturation process), including a cortical thickness-based ISC between the dorsolateral prefrontal cortex and precuneus, a cortical surface area-based ISC between the anterior insula versus the intraparietal sulcus, as well as the perisylvian area-related ISCs, could predict the initial prognosis of patients with obsessive–compulsive disorder as responders or nonresponders with 89.0% accuracy [70]. Additionally, the treatment response to cognitive behavioral therapy in obsessive–compulsive disorder patients could be predicted using a multivariate pattern-recognition classifier, in which the resting-state functional connectivity patterns within the default mode network and visual network are implemented [71]. For panic disorder with agoraphobia, a multivariate whole-brain Gaussian process classifier model, comprised of the precentral, fusiform, orbitofrontal, middle temporal, temporo-occipital, paracingulate, and supramarginal cortices, as well as the putamen (using BOLD-dependent signal changes for differential fear-conditioning tasks, at baseline), showed an 82% accuracy in predicting the treatment response to cognitive behavioral therapy [72].

4.2 Future Research Suggestion

Future studies of treatment response-related brain biomarkers need to combine the disease-staging model [73–77] and a mental functioning domain-based approach [78–82], in addition to the classical syndrome-based diagnostic system. Although current candidate biomarkers for psychiatric disorders await further validation, knowledge on candidate genomic and brain-based biomarkers is increasing rapidly. More active application of machine-learning and medical bioinformatics frameworks to the brain biomarker-based prediction of treatment response and recommendation of a personalized treatment regimen are warranted [83].

Acknowledgment This work was supported by a grant from the Korea Science and Engineering Foundation (KOSEF), funded by the Korean government (NRF-2018R1A2A2A05018505), and by the Ministry of Science, ICT and Future Planning (NRF-2015M3C7A1028252).

References

1. Ganella EP, Bartholomeusz CF, Seguin C, Whittle S, Bousman C, Phassouliotis C, et al. Functional brain networks in treatment-resistant schizophrenia. Schizophr Res. 2017;184:73–81.
2. Iniesta R, Malki K, Maier W, Rietschel M, Mors O, Hauser J, et al. Combining clinical variables to optimize prediction of antidepressant treatment outcomes. J Psychiatr Res. 2016;78:94–102.
3. Kautzky A, Baldinger-Melich P, Kranz GS, Vanicek T, Souery D, Montgomery S, et al. A new prediction model for evaluating treatment-resistant depression. J Clin Psychiatry. 2017;78(2):215–22.
4. Cepeda MS, Reps J, Fife D, Blacketer C, Stang P, Ryan P. Finding treatment-resistant depression in real-world data: how a data-driven approach compares with expert-based heuristics. Depress Anxiety. 2018;35(3):220–8.
5. da Costa SC, Passos IC, Lowri C, Soares JC, Kapczinski F. Refractory bipolar disorder and neuroprogression. Prog Neuro-Psychopharmacol Biol Psychiatry. 2016;70:103–10.
6. Kapczinski NS, Mwangi B, Cassidy RM, Librenza-Garcia D, Bermudez MB, Kauer-Sant'anna M, et al. Neuroprogression and illness trajectories in bipolar disorder. Expert Rev Neurother. 2017;17(3):277–85.
7. Passos IC, Mwangi B, Vieta E, Berk M, Kapczinski F. Areas of controversy in neuroprogression in bipolar disorder. Acta Psychiatr Scand. 2016;134(2):91–103.
8. Perlis RH. A clinical risk stratification tool for predicting treatment resistance in major depressive disorder. Biol Psychiatry. 2013;74(1):7–14.
9. Huhtaniska S, Jaaskelainen E, Hirvonen N, Remes J, Murray GK, Veijola J, et al. Long-term antipsychotic

use and brain changes in schizophrenia – a systematic review and meta-analysis. Hum Psychopharmacol. 2017;32(2):e2574.
10. Egerton A, Bhachu A, Merritt K, McQueen G, Szulc A, McGuire P. Effects of antipsychotic administration on brain glutamate in schizophrenia: a systematic review of longitudinal 1H-MRS studies. Front Psychiatry. 2017;8:66.
11. Guo W, Liu F, Chen J, Wu R, Li L, Zhang Z, et al. Olanzapine modulation of long- and short-range functional connectivity in the resting brain in a sample of patients with schizophrenia. Eur Neuropsychopharmacol. 2017;27(1):48–58.
12. Stip E, Cherbal A, Luck D, Zhornitsky S, Bentaleb LA, Lungu O. A neuroimaging study of emotion-cognition interaction in schizophrenia: the effect of ziprasidone treatment. Psychopharmacology. 2017;234(7):1045–58.
13. Aguilar EJ, Corripio I, Garcia-Marti G, Grasa E, Marti-Bonmati L, Gomez-Anson B, et al. Emotional fMR auditory paradigm demonstrates normalization of limbic hyperactivity after cognitive behavior therapy for auditory hallucinations. Schizophr Res. 2018;193:304–12.
14. Wise T, Cleare AJ, Herane A, Young AH, Arnone D. Diagnostic and therapeutic utility of neuroimaging in depression: an overview. Neuropsychiatr Dis Treat. 2014;10:1509–22.
15. Brennan BP, Admon R, Perriello C, LaFlamme EM, Athey AJ, Pizzagalli DA, et al. Acute change in anterior cingulate cortex GABA, but not glutamine/glutamate, mediates antidepressant response to citalopram. Psychiatry Res. 2017;269:9–16.
16. Kraus C, Klobl M, Tik M, Auer B, Vanicek T, Geissberger N, et al. The pulvinar nucleus and antidepressant treatment: dynamic modeling of antidepressant response and remission with ultra-high field functional MRI. Mol Psychiatry. 2018.
17. Admon R, Kaiser RH, Dillon DG, Beltzer M, Goer F, Olson DP, et al. Dopaminergic enhancement of striatal response to reward in major depression. Am J Psychiatry. 2017;174(4):378–86.
18. Rubin-Falcone H, Weber J, Kishon R, Ochsner K, Delaparte L, Dore B, et al. Longitudinal effects of cognitive behavioral therapy for depression on the neural correlates of emotion regulation. Psychiatry Res. 2018;271:82–90.
19. Philip NS, Barredo J, van't Wout-Frank M, Tyrka AR, Price LH, Carpenter LL. Network mechanisms of clinical response to transcranial magnetic stimulation in posttraumatic stress disorder and major depressive disorder. Biol Psychiatry. 2018;83(3):263–72.
20. Pantazatos SP, Talati A, Schneier FR, Hirsch J. Reduced anterior temporal and hippocampal functional connectivity during face processing discriminates individuals with social anxiety disorder from healthy controls and panic disorder, and increases following treatment. Neuropsychopharmacology. 2014;39(2):425–34.
21. Mansson KNT, Salami A, Carlbring P, Boraxbekk CJ, Andersson G, Furmark T. Structural but not functional neuroplasticity one year after effective cognitive behaviour therapy for social anxiety disorder. Behav Brain Res. 2017;318:45–51.
22. Dunlop K, Woodside B, Olmsted M, Colton P, Giacobbe P, Downar J. Reductions in cortico-striatal hyperconnectivity accompany successful treatment of obsessive-compulsive disorder with dorsomedial prefrontal rTMS. Neuropsychopharmacology. 2016;41(5):1395–403.
23. Thorsen AL, van den Heuvel OA, Hansen B, Kvale G. Neuroimaging of psychotherapy for obsessive-compulsive disorder: a systematic review. Psychiatry Res. 2015;233(3):306–13.
24. Hasey GM, Kiang M. A review of recent literature employing electroencephalographic techniques to study the pathophysiology, phenomenology, and treatment response of schizophrenia. Curr Psychiatry Rep. 2013;15(9):388.
25. Alegre M, Molero P, Valencia M, Mayner G, Ortuno F, Artieda J. Atypical antipsychotics normalize low-gamma evoked oscillations in patients with schizophrenia. Psychiatry Res. 2017;247:214–21.
26. Zheng L, Liu W, He W, Yu S, Zhong G. Altered effective brain connectivity at early response of antipsychotics in first-episode schizophrenia with auditory hallucinations. Clin Neurophysiol. 2017;128(6):867–74.
27. Ravan M, Hasey G, Reilly JP, MacCrimmon D, Khodayari-Rostamabad A. A machine learning approach using auditory odd-ball responses to investigate the effect of Clozapine therapy. Clin Neurophysiol. 2015;126(4):721–30.
28. Baskaran A, Farzan F, Milev R, Brenner CA, Alturi S, Pat McAndrews M, et al. The comparative effectiveness of electroencephalographic indices in predicting response to escitalopram therapy in depression: a pilot study. J Affect Disord. 2018;227:542–9.
29. Iseger TA, Korgaonkar MS, Kenemans JL, Grieve SM, Baeken C, Fitzgerald PB, et al. EEG connectivity between the subgenual anterior cingulate and prefrontal cortices in response to antidepressant medication. Eur Neuropsychopharmacol. 2017;27(4):301–12.
30. Kazemi R, Rostami R, Khomami S, Horacek J, Brunovsky M, Novak T, et al. Electrophysiological correlates of bilateral and unilateral repetitive transcranial magnetic stimulation in patients with bipolar depression. Psychiatry Res. 2016;240:364–75.
31. Sun Y, Farzan F, Mulsant BH, Rajji TK, Fitzgerald PB, Barr MS, et al. Indicators for remission of suicidal ideation following magnetic seizure therapy in patients with treatment-resistant depression. JAMA Psychiat. 2016;73(4):337–45.
32. Cao J, Liu Q, Li Y, Yang J, Gu R, Liang J, et al. Cognitive behavioural therapy attenuates the enhanced early facial stimuli processing in social anxiety disorders: an ERP investigation. Behav Brain Funct. 2017;13(1):12.

33. Carrasco M, Hong C, Nienhuis JK, Harbin SM, Fitzgerald KD, Gehring WJ, et al. Increased error-related brain activity in youth with obsessive-compulsive disorder and other anxiety disorders. Neurosci Lett. 2013;541:214–8.
34. Riesel A, Endrass T, Auerbach LA, Kathmann N. Overactive performance monitoring as an endophenotype for obsessive-compulsive disorder: evidence from a treatment study. Am J Psychiatry. 2015;172(7):665–73.
35. Altamura AC, Delvecchio G, Paletta S, Di Pace C, Reggiori A, Fiorentini A, et al. Gray matter volumes may predict the clinical response to paliperidone palmitate long-acting in acute psychosis: a pilot longitudinal neuroimaging study. Psychiatry Res. 2017;261:80–4.
36. McNabb CB, Tait RJ, McIlwain ME, Anderson VM, Suckling J, Kydd RR, et al. Functional network dysconnectivity as a biomarker of treatment resistance in schizophrenia. Schizophr Res. 2017; https://doi.org/10.1016/j.schres.2017.10.015.
37. Vanes LD, Mouchlianitis E, Collier T, Averbeck BB, Shergill SS. Differential neural reward mechanisms in treatment-responsive and treatment-resistant schizophrenia. Psychol Med. 2018;1–10.
38. Zhu J, Cai H, Yuan Y, Yue Y, Jiang D, Chen C, et al. Variance of the global signal as a pretreatment predictor of antidepressant treatment response in drug-naive major depressive disorder. Brain Imaging Behav. 2018; https://doi.org/10.1007/s11682-018-9845-9.
39. Hou Z, Gong L, Zhi M, Yin Y, Zhang Y, Xie C, et al. Distinctive pretreatment features of bilateral nucleus accumbens networks predict early response to antidepressants in major depressive disorder. Brain Imaging Behav. 2017; https://doi.org/10.1007/s11682-017-9773-0.
40. Gong L, Hou Z, Wang Z, He C, Yin Y, Yuan Y, et al. Disrupted topology of hippocampal connectivity is associated with short-term antidepressant response in major depressive disorder. J Affect Disord. 2018;225:539–44.
41. Lan MJ, Rubin-Falcone H, Motiwala F, Chen Y, Stewart JW, Hellerstein DJ, et al. White matter tract integrity is associated with antidepressant response to lurasidone in bipolar depression. Bipolar Disord. 2017;19(6):444–9.
42. Liu J, Xu X, Luo Q, Luo Y, Chen Y, Lui S, et al. Brain grey matter volume alterations associated with antidepressant response in major depressive disorder. Sci Rep. 2017;7(1):10464. https://doi.org/10.1038/s41598-017-10676-5.
43. Webb CA, Olson EA, Killgore WDS, Pizzagalli DA, Rauch SL, Rosso IM. Rostral anterior cingulate cortex morphology predicts treatment response to internet-based cognitive behavioral therapy for depression. Biol Psychiatry Cogn Neurosci Neuroimaging. 2018;3(3):255–62.
44. Sambataro F, Doerig N, Hanggi J, Wolf RC, Brakowski J, Holtforth MG, et al. Anterior cingulate volume predicts response to psychotherapy and functional connectivity with the inferior parietal cortex in major depressive disorder. Eur Neuropsychopharmacol. 2018;28(1):138–48.
45. Boes AD, Uitermarkt BD, Albazron FM, Lan MJ, Liston C, Pascual-Leone A, et al. Rostral anterior cingulate cortex is a structural correlate of repetitive TMS treatment response in depression. Brain Stimul. 2018; https://doi.org/10.1016/j.brs.2018.01.029.
46. Mansson KN, Frick A, Boraxbekk CJ, Marquand AF, Williams SC, Carlbring P, et al. Predicting long-term outcome of Internet-delivered cognitive behavior therapy for social anxiety disorder using fMRI and support vector machine learning. Transl Psychiatry. 2015;5:e530.
47. Klumpp H, Fitzgerald JM, Kinney KL, Kennedy AE, Shankman SA, Langenecker SA, et al. Predicting cognitive behavioral therapy response in social anxiety disorder with anterior cingulate cortex and amygdala during emotion regulation. NeuroImage Clin. 2017;15:25–34.
48. Klumpp H, Roberts J, Kennedy AE, Shankman SA, Langenecker SA, Gross JJ, et al. Emotion regulation related neural predictors of cognitive behavioral therapy response in social anxiety disorder. Prog Neuro-Psychopharmacol Biol Psychiatry. 2017;75:106–12.
49. White LK, Sequeira S, Britton JC, Brotman MA, Gold AL, Berman E, et al. Complementary features of attention bias modification therapy and cognitive-behavioral therapy in pediatric anxiety disorders. Am J Psychiatry. 2017;174(8):775–84.
50. Gottlich M, Kramer UM, Kordon A, Hohagen F, Zurowski B. Resting-state connectivity of the amygdala predicts response to cognitive behavioral therapy in obsessive compulsive disorder. Biol Psychol. 2015;111:100–9.
51. Light GA, Swerdlow NR. Future clinical uses of neurophysiological biomarkers to predict and monitor treatment response for schizophrenia. Ann N Y Acad Sci. 2015;1344(1):105–19.
52. Wade EC, Iosifescu DV. Using electroencephalography for treatment guidance in major depressive disorder. Biol Psychiatry Cogn Neurosci Neuroimaging. 2016;1(5):411–22.
53. Arns M, Gordon E, Boutros NN. EEG abnormalities are associated with poorer depressive symptom outcomes with escitalopram and venlafaxine-XR, but not sertraline: results from the multicenter randomized iSPOT-D study. Clin EEG Neurosci. 2017;48(1):33–40.
54. van Dinteren R, Arns M, Kenemans L, Jongsma ML, Kessels RP, Fitzgerald P, et al. Utility of event-related potentials in predicting antidepressant treatment response: an iSPOT-D report. Eur Neuropsychopharmacol. 2015;25(11):1981–90.
55. Tenke CE, Kayser J, Pechtel P, Webb CA, Dillon DG, Goer F, et al. Demonstrating test-retest reliability of electrophysiological measures for healthy adults in a multisite study of biomarkers of antidepressant treatment response. Psychophysiology. 2017;54(1):34–50.

56. Lee BH, Park YM, Lee SH, Shim M. Prediction of long-term treatment response to selective serotonin reuptake inhibitors (SSRIs) using scalp and source loudness dependence of auditory evoked potentials (LDAEP) analysis in patients with major depressive disorder. Int J Mol Sci. 2015;16(3):6251–65.
57. Mumtaz W, Xia L, Mohd Yasin MA, Azhar Ali SS, Malik AS. A wavelet-based technique to predict treatment outcome for Major Depressive Disorder. PLoS One. 2017;12(2):e0171409.
58. Jaworska N, Wang H, Smith DM, Blier P, Knott V, Protzner AB. Pre-treatment EEG signal variability is associated with treatment success in depression. NeuroImage Clin. 2018;17:368–77.
59. Bailey NW, Hoy KE, Rogasch NC, Thomson RH, McQueen S, Elliot D, et al. Responders to rTMS for depression show increased fronto-midline theta and theta connectivity compared to non-responders. Brain Stimul. 2018;11(1):190–203.
60. Stange JP, MacNamara A, Kennedy AE, Hajcak G, Phan KL, Klumpp H. Brain-behavioral adaptability predicts response to cognitive behavioral therapy for emotional disorders: a person-centered event-related potential study. Neuropsychologia. 2017; https://doi.org/10.1016/j.neuropsychologia.2017.06.027.
61. Dohrmann AL, Stengler K, Jahn I, Olbrich S. EEG-arousal regulation as predictor of treatment response in patients suffering from obsessive compulsive disorder. Clin Neurophysiol. 2017;128(10):1906–14.
62. Schnack HG. Improving individual predictions: machine learning approaches for detecting and attacking heterogeneity in schizophrenia (and other psychiatric diseases). Schizophr Res. 2017; https://doi.org/10.1016/j.schres.2017.10.023.
63. Kim YK, Na KS. Application of machine learning classification for structural brain MRI in mood disorders: critical review from a clinical perspective. Prog Neuro-Psychopharmacol Biol Psychiatry. 2018;80(Pt B):71–80.
64. Johnston BA, Steele JD, Tolomeo S, Christmas D, Matthews K. Structural MRI-based predictions in patients with treatment-refractory depression (TRD). PLoS One. 2015;10(7):e0132958.
65. Koutsouleris N, Wobrock T, Guse B, Langguth B, Landgrebe M, Eichhammer P, et al. Predicting response to repetitive transcranial magnetic stimulation in patients with Schizophrenia using structural magnetic resonance imaging: a multisite machine learning analysis. Schizophr Bull. 2017; https://doi.org/10.1093/schbul/sbx114.
66. Li P, Jing RX, Zhao RJ, Ding ZB, Shi L, Sun HQ, et al. Electroconvulsive therapy-induced brain functional connectivity predicts therapeutic efficacy in patients with schizophrenia: a multivariate pattern recognition study. NPJ Schizophr. 2017;3(1):21.
67. Bak N, Ebdrup BH, Oranje B, Fagerlund B, Jensen MH, Düring SW, et al. Two subgroups of antipsychotic-naive, first-episode schizophrenia patients identified with a Gaussian mixture model on cognition and electrophysiology. Transl Psychiatry. 2017;7(4):e1087.
68. Patel MJ, Andreescu C, Price JC, Edelman KL, Reynolds CF, Aizenstein HJ. Machine learning approaches for integrating clinical and imaging features in LLD classification and response prediction. Int J Geriatr Psychiatry. 2015;30(10):1056–67.
69. Redlich R, Opel N, Grotegerd D, Dohm K, Zaremba D, Burger C, et al. Prediction of individual response to electroconvulsive therapy via machine learning on structural magnetic resonance imaging data. JAMA Psychiat. 2016;73(6):557–64.
70. Yun JY, Jang JH, Kim SN, Jung WH, Kwon JS. Neural correlates of response to pharmacotherapy in obsessive-compulsive disorder: individualized cortical morphology-based structural covariance. Prog Neuro-Psychopharmacol Biol Psychiatry. 2015;63:126–33.
71. Reggente N, Moody TD, Morfini F, Sheen C, Rissman J, O'Neill J, et al. Multivariate resting-state functional connectivity predicts response to cognitive behavioral therapy in obsessive-compulsive disorder. Proc Natl Acad Sci U S A. 2018;115(9):2222–7.
72. Hahn T, Kircher T, Straube B, Wittchen HU, Konrad C, Strohle A, et al. Predicting treatment response to cognitive behavioral therapy in panic disorder with agoraphobia by integrating local neural information. JAMA Psychiat. 2015;72(1):68–74.
73. Berk M, Post R, Ratheesh A, Gliddon E, Singh A, Vieta E, et al. Staging in bipolar disorder: from theoretical framework to clinical utility. World Psychiatry. 2017;16(3):236–44.
74. Dragioti E, Wiklund T, Siamouli M, Moutou K, Fountoulakis KN. Could PANSS be a useful tool in the determining of the stages of schizophrenia? A clinically operational approach. J Psychiatr Res. 2017;86:66–72.
75. Duffy A, Malhi GS, Grof P. Do the trajectories of bipolar disorder and schizophrenia follow a universal staging model? Can J Psychiatry. 2017;62(2):115–22.
76. Kupfer DJ, Frank E, Ritchey FC. Staging bipolar disorder: what data and what models are needed? Lancet Psychiatry. 2015;2(6):564–70.
77. Li T, Wang Q, Zhang J, Rolls ET, Yang W, Palaniyappan L, et al. Brain-wide analysis of functional connectivity in first-episode and chronic stages of schizophrenia. Schizophr Bull. 2017;43(2):436–48.
78. Anderzhanova E, Kirmeier T, Wotjak CT. Animal models in psychiatric research: the RDoC system as a new framework for endophenotype-oriented translational neuroscience. Neurobiol Stress. 2017;7:47–56.
79. Carcone D, Ruocco AC. Six years of research on the National Institute of Mental Health's Research Domain Criteria (RDoC) initiative: a systematic review. Front Cell Neurosci. 2017;11:46.

80. Cohen AS, Le TP, Fedechko TL, Elvevag B. Can RDoC help find order in thought disorder? Schizophr Bull. 2017;43(3):503–8.
81. Luyten P, Fonagy P. The stress-reward-mentalizing model of depression: an integrative developmental cascade approach to child and adolescent depressive disorder based on the research domain criteria (RDoC) approach. Clin Psychol Rev. 2017; https://doi.org/10.1016/j.cpr.2017.09.008.
82. Nusslock R, Alloy LB. Reward processing and mood-related symptoms: an RDoC and translational neuroscience perspective. J Affect Disord. 2017;216:3–16.
83. Bzdok D, Meyer-Lindenberg A. Machine learning for precision psychiatry: opportunities and challenges. Biol Psychiatry Cogn Neurosci Neuroimaging. 2018;3(3):223–30.

Developing Therapies for Treatment-Resistant Depressive Disorder in Animal Models

5

Michel Bourin

5.1 Introduction

The definition of resistant depression, although described in other chapters of this book, should be repeated here to better understand the challenge of psychopharmacologists in developing therapies using animal models [1]. Today, the management of depression is well codified with a proven effectiveness of the use of antidepressants. However, when one makes a balance after 8 weeks of treatment, one finds oneself in several cases of figure: for 1/3 of the patients, there is a correct answer to the treatment, for another third, one observes a partial answer, and for the last third, no response is observed (STAR*D study). From this observation follows a certain definition of the resistant depression which, nevertheless, still varies a lot today. In any case, the consensus is that a depression is said to be resistant when the depressive episode persists despite two well-managed antidepressant treatments (that is to say, at the right dose and on the right duration). And, therefore, despite its frequency, it appears that resistant depression is a poorly understood concept, with little evaluated therapeutic strategies. The treatment of resistant depression has been codified as the addition of two or three antidepressants of different mode of action without therapeutic success [2]. On the other hand, it can be said that its prognosis is bleak as it is accompanied by a profound deterioration of the quality of life, as well as excess mortality and overmorbidity. It seems important to define one or more strategies to develop drugs that can be effective in treating resistant depressions.

M. Bourin
Neurobiology of Anxiety and Mood Disorders,
University of Nantes, Nantes, France
e-mail: michel.bourin@univ-nantes.fr

5.2 Genesis of Animal Models of Depression

It is necessary before considering the development of drugs in the treatment of resistant depression to define the animal models used to find antidepressants [3] to see if they can be used in other conditions to answer the question of resistant depression.

Animal models represent "the backbone" of the preclinical research of psychiatric disorders [4]; they allow a better understanding of the mechanisms involved. Biological behavioral tests model a physiological action. Most often they are used to study the mechanisms responsible for changes in brain function, such as those resulting from chronic drug delivery, brain damage. The sensitivity of the dopaminergic receptors of the nuclei accumbens and striatum is, for example, measured by the increase in locomotor activity and stereotyped behavior induced by psychomotor stimulants. The object of these tests is to measure a physiological activity; one can wonder

Y.-K. Kim (ed.), *Treatment Resistance in Psychiatry*, https://doi.org/10.1007/978-981-10-4358-1_5

about the use of behavioral methods. There are at least four reasons for advocating the use of behavioral tests rather than biochemical tests. First, behavioral methods are not invasive and destructive. Second, the behavioral test is a guarantee that the agents tested actually act on the brain. Third, behavioral measures are functional measures. Indeed, many biochemical indices are not reliable indices of functional changes. Fourth, behavior integrates brain activity and takes into account any changes occurring beyond the measurement point. So a behavioral test is less accurate to appreciate a change in functioning of the brain than a biochemical test, but however it gives a clearer indication of its functional significance. But in this case, he must demonstrate that the behavior taken into account is actually sensitive to changes in the underlying physiological variable (see using the behavior difficulties). Measurements taken at the behavioral level are often carried out at the level of an ordinal scale (storage by rank); plus such measures cannot be processed validly only by nonparametric statistics.

Consider a model of experimental analysis of brain mechanisms underlying the initiation of aggressive driving [5], the muricide test: some rats put in the presence of mouse kill them while other rats will kill them. At that time, the relationship between behavior and brain was apprehended in terms of nervous substrates underlying closely specifically a category of behavior, the behavior of aggression, for example, considered a natural entity. However, some experimental manipulations do not have the same effect, depending on whether they are applied to a "naive rat," which is confronted for the first time with the intrusion of a mouse in his cage, a "non-killer" rat confirmed who is familiar with the presence of a mouse in his environment, or even a "killer" rat which has a long experience of the behavior of interspecific aggression and its consequences. Indeed, the mouse has not the same meaning for all three to type of rats. The fact that a same behavioral strategy be implemented does not imply that game mechanisms are identical. We therefore consider that the behavior is a means of expression and action which enables an individual to master the relationship he establishes with its environment and then to analyze the situation facing the individual, the way he sees and the interpreter and the way he strives to control through the implementation of an appropriate behavioral strategy. This approach presents an additional advantage that focuses on processes and mechanisms that are less closely related to a given species. The research then provides data with validity more general and likely to be extrapolated, with all the caution which applies to the analysis of the biological foundations of human behavior. The muricide model is among the oldest models of depression. With this model the ability of antidepressant drugs to prevent the lethal activity of rats on the mouse is tested. It has been widely used, although it proved inefficient for detecting antidepressant activity and it poses ethical problems [6]. This clearly isn't a good model because it is difficult to find a resemblance between this model and the depression: men do not kill mice, and it is difficult to see any connection between killing a mouse and depression. This could be a test of screening (screening test) for antidepressant drugs. But that would amount to implicitly consider the screening test is a type of animal model of depression. This conceptual confusion may lead us to extrapolate the results to this test outside its field of application and to produce spurious assertions. It is therefore clear that must be examined with care, in each case, the field for which the use of a particular model is justified.

Models are tools whose validity must be estimated. This evaluation is more a matter of judgment than of measurement. However, this judgment can be based on three categories of elements: predictive validity, validity, and construction validity [7]. Animal models are open to criticism, but this critique may be an encouragement to clinicians to apply the same rigor to the analysis of human behavioral disorders [8].

One must keep in mind the following reflection: technique, method, experience, and theory are indissolubly linked; the great danger is that a strict method provides by itself numerous and precise quantitative results. Considering construct animal models of depression, one must consider the biological hypothesis of depression where one or more genetic factors predisposing to the disease exist.

Finally, there are new pathways such as neuroendocrinology (regulation of the hypothalamo-hypophysis axis) and biorhythms (sleep, temperature). Neurochemical theories explore the biochemical imbalance induced or preexisting to the disease, which is on the dosage of neurotransmitters in the blood, urine, and CSF of depressed and/or suicidal depressed patients, as well as the measurement of neurotransmitters in blood, urine, and CSF before and after administration of antidepressants (patients and experimental animals).

5.3 Classical Models of Depression

Before considering strategies for developing therapies for treatment-resistant depressive disorder in animal models, it should be remembered which are the animal models of depression that exist [9]. Some of them may be better suited than others for therapies of resistant depression.

The earliest animal models of depression are models of pharmacological interactions:

- Reserpine: measurement of antagonism of hypothermia and ptosis and measurement of antagonism of reduction of locomotor activity by potential antidepressants in mice [10].
- Oxotremorine: measures the antagonism of hypothermia, akinesia, and tremor with potential antidepressants in mice [11].
- Apomorphine at high dose: hypothermia induced by 16 mg/kg is antagonized by antidepressants, whereas at 1 mg/kg it is antagonized by neuroleptics [12].
- Amphetamine: potentiation of the effects of amphetamine in the presence of antidepressants [13].
- Yohimbine: potentiation of the induced mortality of yohimbine by antidepressants [14].

These models may be interesting to develop in order to obtain one or more models of resistant depression.

The most used models today are behavioral models:

- The muricide model has been described above.
- The forced swimming test: the immobility observed after 2 min of swimming is antagonized by the antidepressants in doses which often decrease the motor activity in a free situation [15].
- Tail suspension test: The behavioral desperate test is a rapid method of evaluating the psychotropic effects of antidepressants on the behavior of a rodent trying to escape an uncomfortable situation. It is a simple and fast test (6 min maximum per cycle), causing no pain in the animal. The principle is based on the measure of the force deployed during the movements and the duration of these movements [16].
- Chronic mild stress: The protocol for unpredictable chronic mild stress takes place over 6 weeks during which animals are subjected to a succession of stressful events that take place so unpredictable, with two to three events per day. The disturbances applied are of a low intensity and without food or dipsic deprivation, the interest of the protocol being the repetition of weak events, in an unpredictable way [17].
- Olfactory bulbectomy in rats is described as a procedure aiming to reproduce anhedonia, a cardinal symptom of depression. It causes various biochemical, cellular, and behavioral changes similar to those of the depressive state that can be reversed by chronic antidepressant treatment [18].

5.4 Are There Models of Resistant Depression?

A model of resistant depression suggests that classic depression models have been modified for this purpose. These simulations of normal human behavior are rare in the face of simulations of abnormal behavior. An animal model of abnormal behavior tries to reproduce a symptom of a disorder, a group of symptoms and even a syndrome. The construction of such a model may include various manipulations including brain injury, selective breeding, selection of particular individuals, and the application of a variety of factors that are assumed to be involved in etiology of the disorder considered such as social isolation and aging. These manipulations lead to the achievement of a behavioral state that is used as a tool to study the different aspects of the modeled disorder: its etiology, its treatment, its physiological bases, and the physiological mechanisms underlying an effective treatment. A given model may be suitable for the study of all or only some of them.

5.4.1 Researchers Have Proposed Models Likely to Develop Drugs That Can Treat Resistant Depression, for Example, Using Telomeres

Telomeres are protective DNA-protein complexes at the ends of each chromosome, maintained primarily by the enzyme telomerase. The shortening of blood leukocyte telomeres is associated with aging, several chronic diseases, and stress, for example, major depression [19]. The hippocampus is essential in the regulation of cognition and mood and in the main brain region of telomerase activity. It was unknown that there was telomere dysfunction in the hippocampus of depressed subjects. Lithium, used in the treatment and prevention of relapse of mood disorders, has been shown to protect against shortening of leukocyte telomeres in humans, but the mechanism has not been elucidated [20]. To answer the questions, if the telomeres are shortened and if the telomerase activity has changed in the hippocampus and if lithium could reverse the process, it used a genetic model of depression, the Flinders sensitive line rat, and treated animals with lithium. The naive Flinders sensitive line has shorter telomere length, restricted TERT expression [21], reduced brain-derived neurotrophic factor levels, and reduced telomerase activity compared to Flinders resistance line controls. Lithium treatment normalized TERT expression and telomerase activity in the Flinders sensitive line and upregulated β-catenin. This is the first report showing dysregulation of telomeres in the hippocampus of a well-defined pattern of depression and the restorative effects of lithium treatment. If replicated in other models of mood disorders, the results will help to understand both the telomere function and the mechanism of action of lithium in the hippocampus in depressed patients. It must be a path to discover new drugs active in resistant depression.

5.4.2 Another Potential Model to Discover Antidepressants Active in Resistant Depression Is Based on Genetic

A model was developed by a directed reproduction of mice with remarkably different responses in the tail suspension test, a stress paradigm used to screen for potential antidepressants [22]. Thus, the “resigned” mice are essentially immobile in the tail suspension test, as well as in the Porsolt forced swimming test; they have a reduced consumption of a sucrose solution (2%) palatable [23]. In addition, “resigned” mice exhibit sleep-wake cycle changes. Compared to “non-resigned” mice, they have higher basal serum corticosterone levels and a lower serotonin turnover rate in the hippocampus. Remarkably, stimulation of the serotonergic 5-HT1A autoreceptor induces greater hypothermia and stronger inhibition of electrical activity of the dorsal raphe nucleus serotonergic neuron in “resigned” mice than in “non-resigned.” Thus, “resigned” mice show a decrease in serotoninergic tone, which evokes that associated with human endogenous depression. Finally, both behavioral alterations and serotonergic dysfunction can be improved by chronic administration of the antidepressant fluoxetine. The line of “depressive mice” may provide an opportunity to approach the genes influencing susceptibility to depression and to search for the neurophysiological and neurochemical substrates underlying antidepressant effects.

For this, the authors used a genetic model of depression in mice, the model of H/Rouen mice. These mice were selected, by directed reproduction, based on their immobility behavior in the tail suspension test, much longer than in non-resected (NH/Rouen) or control mice (I/Rouen) having an intermediate phenotype. H/Rouen mice also have many features reflecting a depressive phenotype [24]. The phenotypic characterization of these three mouse lines was continued, and it was shown that the H/Rouen mice also exhibited more pronounced anxiety behavior than the other two lines in a battery of standard behavioral tests. This observation led to the search for the neural mechanisms involved in the increased vulnerability to cocaine observed in female H/Rouen mice. The neuroanatomical study, based on the expression of the Fos protein during the CPP test, showed stronger activation of the cingulate part of the prefrontal cortex, the accumbens shell core, the basolateral amygdala, and the ventral subiculum in H/Rouen female mice compared to NH/ and I/Rouen mice, which might reflect their higher propensity to drug-conditioned research. The influence of this mixed phenotype of anxiety and depression was studied on cocaine vulnerability. We have shown that H/I and Rouen mice are less sensitive to the acute psychomotor effects of cocaine than NH/Rouen mice; however, all mouse lines express a similar cocaine behavioral sensitization, indicating that the neuroadaptative changes that develop during repeated cocaine injections blur initial differences in reactivity.

On the other hand, H/Rouen female mice exhibit a robust, durable, and higher cocaine-induced conditioned place preference (CPP) than in NH/ and I/Rouen mice, indicating greater sensitivity to background clues associated with effects of this drug. Finally, as the BDNF (brain-derived neurotrophic factor) present at the nucleus accumbens could be involved in both depression and drug vulnerability, the study of its expression was evaluated by the Western blot technique in the three mouse lines, under basal conditions and after cocaine conditioning. To date, this genetic model has not been used in the development of treatments for resistant depression, but it is a path that seems interesting.

5.4.3 Another Approach to the Treatment of Resistant Depression Is Co-administration of Drugs

The biological hypothesis of depression is generally based on the insufficiency of one or more monoamines. Historically, it has been attributed to a noradrenaline deficiency and then to a cerebral serotonin deficiency. Animal models of depression also suggest a dopamine involvement in pathophysiology of depression [25]. So in order to answer the question of the treatment of resistant depression, it is useful to study models of depression if the combination of antidepressants with more or less marked dopaminergic activity could have potentiating effects. Thus in my laboratory, we obtained convincing results by increasing the effect/size of SSRS by associating them with each other or especially with products with dopaminergic components. The most important results were obtained by co-administration of bupropion with SSRIs and SNRIs in forced swimming test in mice, predictive of efficacy in resistant depression [26]. Another very productive work points out the augmentation of aripiprazole with antidepressants on forced swimming test [27].

It has been proven that SSRIs become ineffective in the FST after the animals' brains have been depleted in dopamine by 6-OHDA [28]. It is as well another path using various strains of mice, to understand which are the "resistant" strains according to the studied antidepressants [29]. Considering the role of dopamine in treating resistant depression, this kind of "dopamine depression" could be of interest to develop new drugs. Repeated administration of reserpine which induced in animal a more complete depletion could be an interesting model of resistant depression [30].

5.5 The Way of Ketamine and Glutamatergic Compounds

The literature reports relationships at different levels between glutamate and depressions. Imaging data found an increase in glutamatergic activity in patients with EDM in the occipital cortex, while anterior cortex activity was decreased. Postmortem findings suggest the following: glutamate in the frontal cortex and decreased glutamate receptors 2 and 3 in patients with major depressive episodes and a decrease in the expression of glutamatergic receptor transcripts in the hippocampus of bipolar patients. Genetic data highlight the decreased expression of SAP102, NR1, and glutamate synthetase in EDM patients. In bipolar patients, polymorphisms of genes encoding GRIN1, GRIN2A, and GRIN2B [31] are found to be associated with a higher prevalence of suicidal ideation.

One of the most successful research pathways is that of ketamine, an NMDA receptor antagonist currently used as anesthetic, analgesic, and recreational compound. Recent work has shown that an infusion of this N-methyl-D-aspartate (NMDA) antagonist triggers an antidepressant action within a few hours, whereas oral antidepressants have a much longer onset of action [32]. Other studies, in small groups of patients, have shown that repeated infusions of ketamine in cases of depression resistant to usual treatments may also be effective in the short-term, or even in the medium term in some patients, study conducted without comparison control group [33]. In a meta-analysis [34], the researchers reviewed 21 baseline studies to determine if ketamine actually had an immediate antidepressant effect, if this effect was prolonged over time despite the short half-life of the molecule (3 h), and if repeated injections could be more effective than a single injection. After analysis of these trials, which totaled 437 patients with major depressive episodes, with or without bipolar disorder (with 8–47 subjects each), the authors confirmed that ketamine significantly reduced depressive symptoms during assessments from 4 h to 14 days after a single or repeated infusion. Beyond this duration, the data do not show any significant residual effect of intravenous initial treatment. This work also revealed that the effect varied little according to whether the treatment was administered once or in several injections. But both researchers pointed out that the number of these multiple injections was still too small to conclude, calling for additional studies to confirm this point. Despite this short-term efficacy, the meta-analysis revealed a great variability of effect depending on patient profile, ranging from 40% efficacy on symptoms in some studies up to 70% in others. While these results seem rather conclusive in terms of efficacy, the authors acknowledged that another main conclusion of their work was the lack of data on the safety of ketamine in depressive patients.

Very recent work shows the interest of the association of glutamatergic modulators such as riluzole [35] or memantine [36] in the treatment of the resistant depression. However, it remains to refine the concept to make it generalizable.

Conclusion

Considerable progress has been made in the development of treatments for resistant depression. There are proposals of rodent models of treatment-resistant depression [37], or other biological paradigms [38]. The author believes, however, that the major problem is to distinguish more pertinently unipolar resistant depression from bipolar depression. Most developers in the pharmaceutical industry are not psychiatrists, and their concept of resistant depression is imprecise. The future in the development of such treatments is to revisit existing behavioral tests such as forced swimming test [39] with or without prior depletion [40]. Another avenue of investigation is to compare changes in brain neurotransmitters in two behavioral tests and to study how new treatments can restore or amplify them [41]. Finally opening the potassium channels facilitates the action of antidepressants [42, 43]; this could be a new avenue of research in the treatment of resistant depression [44].

References

1. Malhi GS, Byrow Y. Is treatment-resistant depression a useful concept? Evid Based Ment Health. 2016;19(1):1–3.
2. Souery D, Papakostas GI, Trivedi MH. Treatment-resistant depression. J Clin Psychiatry. 2006;67(Suppl 6):16–22.
3. David DJP, NicDhonnchadha BA, Jolliet P, Hascoët M, Bourin M. The use of animal models in defining antidepressant response. Brain Pharmacol. 2001;1:11–35.
4. Bourin M. New challenges for translational psychopharmacology. Front Psychol. 2010;1:1–2.
5. Tulogdi A, Biro L, Barsvari B, Stankovic M, Haller J, Toth M. Neural mechanisms of predatory aggression in rats-implications for abnormal intraspecific aggression. Behav Brain Res. 2015;283:108–15.
6. Willner P. The validity of animal models of depression. Psychopharmacology. 1984;83:1–16.
7. Willner P. Animal models as simulations of depression. Trends Pharmacol Sci. 1991;12:131–6.
8. Bourin M, Puech AJ, Chermat R, Doare L, Poncelet M, Simon P. The new versus the old antidepressant drugs: a comparative study of their psychopharmacological profiles. Encephale. 1981;7:235–42.
9. Bourin M. Is it possible to predict the activity of a new antidepressant in animals with simple psychopharmacological tests? Fundam Clin Pharmacol. 1990;4:49–64.
10. Bourin M, Poncelet M, Chermat R, Simon P. The value of the reserpine test in psychopharmacology. Arzneimittelforschung. 1983;33:1173–6.
11. Frances H, Chermat R, Simon P. Oxotremorine behavioural effects as a screening test in mice. Prog Neuropsychopharmacol. 1980;4:241–6.
12. Puech AJ, Chermat R, Poncelet M, Doaré L, Simon P. Antagonism of hypothermia and behavioral response to apomorphine: a simple, rapid and discriminating test for screening antidepressants and neuroleptics. Psychopharmacology. 1981;75:84–91.
13. Quinton RM, Halliwell G. Effects of alpha-Methyldopa and Dopa on the amphetamine excitatory response in reserpinezed rats. Nature. 1963;200:178–9.
14. Quinton RM. The increase in the toxicity of yohimbine induced by imipramine and other drugs in mice. Br J Pharmacol Chemother. 1963;21:51–66.
15. Petit-Demouliere B, Chenu F, Bourin M. Forced swimming test in mice: a review of antidepressant activity. Psychopharmacology. 2005;177:245–55.
16. Steru L, Chermat R, Thierry B, Simon P. The tail suspension test: a new method for screening antidepressants in mice. Psychopharmacology. 1985;85:367–70.
17. Willner P, Muscat R, Papp M. Chronic mild stress-induced anhedonia: a realistic animal model of depression. Neurosci Biobehav Rev. 1992;16:525–34.
18. van Riezen H, Schnieden H, Wren AF. Olfactory bulb ablation in the rat: behavioural changes and their reversal by antidepressant drugs. Br J Pharmacol. 1977;60:521–8.
19. Martinsson L, Wei Y, Xu D, Melas PA, Mathé AA, Schalling M, et al. Long-term lithium treatment in bipolar disorder is associated with longer leukocyte telomeres. Transl Psychiatry. 2013;3:e261.
20. Wei YB, Backlund L, Wegener G, Mathé AA, Lavebratt C. Telomerase dysregulation in the hippocampus of a rat model of depression: normalization by lithium. Int J Neuropsychopharmacol. 2015;18(7):pyv002.
21. Slattery ML, Herrick JS, Pellatt AJ, Wolff RK, Mullany LE. Telomere length, TERT, and miRNA expression. PLoS One. 2016;11(9):e0162077.
22. El Yacoubi M, Vaugeois JM. Genetic rodent models of depression. Curr Opin Pharmacol. 2007;7:3–7.
23. El Yacoubi M, Rappeneau V, Champion E, Malleret G, Vaugeois JM. The H/Rouen mouse model displays depression-like and anxiety-like behaviors. Behav Brain Res. 2013;256:43–50.
24. El Yacoubi M, Popa D, Martin B, Zimmer L, Hamon M, Adrien J, et al. Genetic association between helpless trait and depression-related phenotypes: evidence from crossbreeding studies with H/Rouen and NH/Rouen mice. Int J Neuropsychopharmacol. 2012;15:363–74.
25. Renard CE, Dailly E, Nic Dhonnchadha BA, Hascoet M, Bourin M. Is dopamine a limiting factor of the antidepressant-like effect in the mouse forced swimming test? Prog Neuro-Psychopharmacol Biol Psychiatry. 2004;28:1255–9.
26. Prica C, Hascoet M, Bourin M. Is co-administration of bupropion with SSRIs and SNRIs in forced swimming test in mice, predictive of efficacy in resistant depression? Behav Brain Res. 2008;194:92–9.
27. Bourin M, Chenu F, Prica C, Hascoët M. Augmentation effect of combination therapy of aripiprazole and antidepressants on forced swimming test in mice. Psychopharmacology. 2009;206:97–107.
28. Chenu F, Dailly E, Bourin M. Effect of antidepressant drugs on 6-OHDA-treated mice in the FST. Eur Neuropsychopharmacol. 2007;17:187–93.
29. Ripoll N, David DJ, Dailly E, Hascoët M, Bourin M. Antidepressant-like effects in various mice strains in the tail suspension test. Behav Brain Res. 2003;143:193–200.
30. Ikram H, Haleem DJ. Repeated treatment with reserpine as a progressive animal model of depression. Pak J Pharm Sci. 2017;30:897–902.
31. Zarate CA Jr, Brutsche NE, Ibrahim L, Franco-Chaves J, Diazgranados N, Cravchik A, et al. Replication of ketamine's antidepressant efficacy in bipolar depression: a randomized controlled add-on trial. Biol Psychiatry. 2012;71:939–46.
32. Salvadore G, Singh JB. Ketamine as a fast acting antidepressant: current knowledge and open questions. CNS Neurosci Ther. 2013;19:428–36.
33. Murrough JW, Perez AM, Pillemer S, Stern J, Parides MK, Aan Het Rot M, et al. Rapid and longer-term antidepressant effects of repeated ketamine infusions in

treatment-resistant major depression. Biol Psychiatry. 2013;74:250–6.
34. Coyle CM, Laws KR. The use of ketamine as an antidepressant: a systematic review and meta-analysis. Hum Psychopharmacol. 2015;30:152–63.
35. Mathew SJ, Gueorguieva R, Brandt C, Fava M, Sanacora G. A randomized, double-blind, placebo-controlled, sequential parallel comparison design trial of adjunctive riluzole for treatment-resistant major depressive disorder. Neuropsychopharmacology. 2017;42:2567–74.
36. Amidfar M, Réus GZ, Quevedo J, Kim YK, Arbabi M. Effect of co-administration of memantine and sertraline on the antidepressant-like activity and brain-derived neurotrophic factor (BDNF) levels in the rat brain. Brain Res Bull. 2017;128:29–33.
37. Caldarone BJ, Zachariou V, King SL. Rodent models of treatment-resistant depression. Eur J Pharmacol. 2015;753:51–65.
38. Samuels BA, Leonardo ED, Gadient R, Williams A, Zhou J, David DJ, et al. Modeling treatment-resistant depression. Neuropharmacology. 2011;61:408–13.
39. Kara NZ, Stukalin Y. Einat revisiting the validity of the mouse forced swim test: systematic review and meta-analysis of the effects of prototypic antidepressants. Neurosci Biobehav Rev. 2018;84:1–11.
40. Dailly E, Chenu F, Renard CE, Bourin M. Dopamine, depression and antidepressants. Fundam Clin Pharmacol. 2004;18:601–17.
41. Renard CE, Dailly E, David DJ, Hascoet M, Bourin M. Monoamine metabolism changes following the mouse forced swimming test but not the tail suspension test. Fundam Clin Pharmacol. 2003;17:449–55.
42. Redrobe JP, Pinot P, Bourin M. The effect of the potassium channel activator, cromakalim, on antidepressant drugs in the forced swimming test in mice. Fundam Clin Pharmacol. 1996;10:524–8.
43. Guo W, Todd K, Bourin M, Hascoet M, Kouadio F. Additive effects of glyburide and antidepressants in the forced swimming test: evidence for the involvement of potassium channel blockade. Pharmacol Biochem Behav. 1996;54:725–30.
44. Heurteaux C, Lucas G, Guy N, El Yacoubi M, Thümmler S, Peng XD, et al. Deletion of the background potassium channel TREK-1 results in a depression-resistant phenotype. Nat Neurosci. 2006;9:1134–41.

Integrated Approaches for Treatment-Resistant Psychiatric Disorders

6

Seon-Cheol Park and Yong-Ku Kim

6.1 Introduction

Conceptualizing treatment resistance of psychiatric disorders has been challenged by controversial issues, since its definition has generally been based not on causal risk factors but rather on post hoc analyses of clinical trials. Although the investigation of potential risk factors for treatment resistance in untreated patients with mental disorders is required for the identification of biological markers associated with treatment resistance, few such studies have been conducted [1]. Moreover, as the theoretical construct for psychiatric disorders has changed from "chemical imbalance" to "dysfunctional circuitry," a transition to "next-generation treatments" has been proposed [2]. Components of such "next-generation treatments" are as follows: molecular targets for new medications will transition from "monoamines, cholinergic pathways, and GABA receptors" to "glutamate receptors, neuropeptide receptors, neuroprotection, neurogenesis, synaptic plasticity, and epigenetic modifiers"; clinical targets will change from "psychosis, mood regulation, anxiety, and attention" to "a motivational states, attention bias, executive function, anhedonia, hopelessness, social deficits, and working memory"; and finally, clinical treatments will move from "medication, psychotherapy, and electroconvulsive therapy (ECT)" to "targeted medication, structured psychotherapy, somatic therapy, and combined treatments." Given the changes anticipated for "next-generation treatments," investigations of the clinical manifestations, underlying neurobiological correlates, and integrated approaches of pharmacological and non-pharmacological treatment options have been proposed as important components of conceptualizing treatment resistance in psychiatric disorders [3–5]. For example, treatment-resistant depression has been recently redefined through the identification of dysfunctional neural circuits and their gene expression correlates [6].

Interactions between genes and childhood trauma have been considered one of the most influential contributors to treatment resistance in psychiatric disorders. Interactions between genes and childhood trauma can effect gene expression, leading to structural and functional brain changes and affecting factors important to the development and prognosis of psychiatric disorders. Such mediating factors that might link exposure to childhood trauma with treatment resistance in psychiatric disorders include poor cognition, for psychotic disorder; severe symptoms, violent

S.-C. Park
Department of Psychiatry, Inje University College of Medicine and Haeundae Paik Hospital, Busan, Republic of Korea

Y.-K. Kim (✉)
Department of Psychiatry, College of Medicine, Korea University Ansan Hospital, Ansan, Republic of Korea
e-mail: yongku@korea.ac.kr

Y.-K. Kim (ed.), *Treatment Resistance in Psychiatry*, https://doi.org/10.1007/978-981-10-4358-1_6

suicide, and early onset, for bipolar disorder; severe symptoms and frequent recurrence, for depressive disorder; and severe symptoms and comorbidity, for post-traumatic stress disorder. Thus, understanding the influence of gene-childhood trauma interactions on the clinical manifestations of treatment-resistant psychiatric disorders can lead to improvements in therapeutic strategies [7, 8].

In addition, environmental factors can contribute to antidepressant effects in depressive and anxiety disorders, given that placebo response may account for 75–82% of the efficacy attributed to antidepressants in clinical trials [9, 10]. Strong responses to antidepressants and high remission rates have been shown to correlate with high socioeconomic status [11, 12]. Hence, interactions between the efficacy of antidepressants and environmental factors are thought to be an important variable in integrated therapeutic approaches for treatment-resistant psychiatric disorder. In addition, "plasticity-augmented psychotherapy" for treatment-resistant depressive and anxiety disorders has been proposed, in terms of the reconsolidation-updating paradigm and epigenetic modification. Evidence for the superiority of pharmacotherapy combined with psychotherapy, relative to pharmacotherapy alone, has been supported by neural plasticity data [13]. Thus, the corrective emotional experiences which are derived from psychodynamic psychotherapy can be supported by increased neuroplasticity with neurotransmitter regulators and epigenetic modifiers. For this reason, integrative therapeutic strategies for depressive and anxiety disorders have been recently proposed in the context of plasticity-augmented psychotherapy [13].

Moreover, a recent clinical study concluded that, with respect to inflammatory cytokines, depressed patients treated with combined ECT and pharmacotherapy show a decrease in interleukin-6 (IL-6) expression and an increase in tumor necrosis factor-α (TNF-α) expression, when compared to those treated with pharmacological therapy alone [14]. Plasma IL-6 and TNF-α have been consistently associated with the severity of depressive disorders and also with resistance to antidepressant treatment [15–17]. ECT combined with venlafaxine has been shown to be effective for treatment-resistant depressive patients, and the combination of repetitive transcranial magnetic stimulation (rTMS) with antidepressant therapy has also been effective in treating patients with resistant bipolar depression [18, 19]. Behavioral surgery has also been proposed as an option for managing treatment-resistant psychiatric disorders. For example, deep brain stimulation (DBS) may normalize decreased cerebral blood flow (CBF) in the prefrontal, premotor, dorsal anterior cingulate gyrus, and anterior insula and increased cerebral blood flow in the subgenual cingulate gyrus, in patients with major depressive disorder [20, 21]. Decreased volume and increased gray matter density of corticostriatal-thalamic circuits and increased baseline activity of orbitofrontal cortex, cingulate gyrus, and striatum have been identified as potential neurobiological correlates of obsessive-compulsive disorder [22, 23]. Given these research findings, one might speculate that brain stimulation techniques combined with pharmacotherapy may be a promising treatment option for treatment-resistant psychiatric disorders.

Integrated approaches to manage treatment-resistant psychiatric disorders are consistent with neuroplasticity hypotheses, including gene-environment interactions and epigenetic mechanisms. In terms of medication-only options, switching therapies, combination therapies, and augmentation strategies can be used to manage treatment-resistant psychiatric disorders [24, 25]. Furthermore, more comprehensive and integrated approaches for pharmacological and non-pharmacological treatment options may be required to manage treatment-resistant psychiatric disorders. With respect to such integrated approaches, psychotherapeutic approaches, brain stimulation techniques, and other non-pharmacological treatment options may be combined with pharmacotherapy to better treat treatment-resistant psychiatric disorders [4, 26, 27]. In this chapter, integrated approaches for treatment-resistant psychiatric disorders are summarized and discussed.

6.2 Treatment Resistance and Interaction Between Gene and Childhood Trauma

Evidence suggests that a synergistic interaction between certain genes and childhood trauma can increase the risk of poor outcomes for many psychiatric disorders. As genetic susceptibility can impact neurobiological responses to childhood trauma, thresholds for pathological responses associated with severe clinical presentations of psychiatric disorders may be reduced. Given such findings, childhood trauma and its interaction with specific genes have been thought to be an important factor affecting treatment resistance of psychiatric disorders [7, 28, 29]. The influence of gene-childhood trauma interactions on treatment resistance is described below, with respect to several different psychiatric disorders.

6.2.1 Schizophrenia

Despite the passing of the "golden age of psychopharmacology," a discrepancy exists between the beneficial effects of psychotropic agents and the limited improvements experienced by patients with schizophrenia [2, 8, 30]. In patients with schizophrenia, poor cognition is a key variable in terms of the influence of interactions between genes and childhood trauma on treatment resistance [7]. Early remission and social and occupational functioning in young adults with first-episode psychosis can be predicted by neurocognitive indicators [31]. In addition, among patients with schizophrenia, functional outcomes assessed after 1 year have been affected by specific neurocognitive deficits [32]. Several studies have reported that cognitive functions in patients with schizophrenia and other psychotic disorders may be influenced by childhood trauma interacting with single nucleotide polymorphisms (SNPs) in the brain-derived neurotrophic factor (BDNF) gene and length polymorphisms in the serotonin transporter (*SLC6A4/5-HTT*). Also, psychotic patients with the S/S version of the serotonin-transporter-linked polymorphic region (*5-HTTLPR*) and a high level of childhood trauma have lower cognitive function than those patients lacking childhood trauma and those with the L/L version of *5-HTTLPR* [33]. Moreover, psychotic patients with a history of childhood sexual abuse who also carry the BDNF methionine (*met*) allele have been characterized by decreased working memory, executive function and general cognition, enlarged lateral ventricles, and decreased hippocampal volume compared with patients who are homozygous for the valine (*val/val*) allele [34]. In summary, interactions between specific gene polymorphisms and a history of childhood trauma may contribute to poor prognosis and functioning in patients with schizophrenia [7].

6.2.2 Bipolar Disorder

While the influence of interactions between genes and childhood trauma on treatment resistance has not been well studied, a history of childhood trauma has been regarded as a primary correlate of severe symptoms in patients with bipolar disorder. In terms of a negative association between age at onset and childhood trauma, the modulating effects of specific genes have been described in patients with bipolar disorder. The combined effect of genetic variants in the Toll-like receptor 2 (*TLR 2*) gene together with childhood sexual abuse can influence the age of onset for bipolar disorder [35]. Also, interactions between the TLR2 *rs3804099* TT risk genotype and sexual abuse can affect the age at onset for bipolar disorder [36]. In addition, interactions between the BDNF *met* allele and childhood trauma can influence the risk of violent suicide [37, 38]. A negative association has also been described between early age of onset and poor treatment outcome in bipolar patients who are carriers of the BDNF *met* allele. This report also suggested that childhood sexual abuse may be a leading factor for early age at onset in bipolar patients who carry BDNF *met* alleles and also correlate with greater severity and persistence of symptoms in bipolar disorder [39].

6.2.3 Depressive Disorder

It has been reported that more influential effects on the relationship between childhood sexual abuse and adult depressive symptoms occur in depressed patients who are carriers of the S-allele of *5-HTTLPR*, compared to those with the L/L genotype for *5-HTTLPR*, and by depressed patients who are carriers of the met allele of the *BDNF val66met* polymorphism rather than those with carry the *val/val* genotype, respectively [40]. Another study has shown that the interaction between C677T methylenetetrahydrofolate reductase (*MTHFR*) variants and childhood trauma can influence the recurrence of major depressive disorder (MDD) and the interaction between the T allele version of C677T polymorphism (*rs1801133*) and childhood trauma can be associated with an increased risk for development of depressive symptoms and recurrence of MDD [41]. Moreover, an association between exposure to childhood trauma and reduced ability to bind glucocorticoid and mineralocorticoid receptors can contribute to changes in the stress response in adulthood of the hypothalamic-pituitary-adrenal (HPA) axis which can lead to an increased risk of depression [42, 43].

In terms of the interactions between gene and childhood trauma, differences in the activation of synapsin I, Erk 1/2, α-calcium-/calmodulin-dependent protein kinase (αCaM kinase II)/syntaxin-1, and αCaM kinase II/NMDA-receptor interactions in hippocampal synaptosomes have been seen in rats subjected to maternal separation in the first 2 weeks of life. Also, some (although not all) of the long-term effects of maternal separation were reversed with escitalopram treatment. These findings suggest that the interaction between early life stress and genes encoding synaptic proteins may influence life-long synaptic changes which are potentially associated with reduced treatment response to antidepressants [44].

6.2.4 Posttraumatic Stress Disorder (PTSD)

Several studies have identified an interaction between the FK506 binding protein 5 (*FKBP5*) gene and childhood trauma that can contribute to a greater vulnerability to PTSD in adulthood. More specifically, a "dose-dependent" genetic effect has been described, protecting against the severity of adult PTSD (in combination with childhood trauma) that arises from an additive interaction effect involving several SNPs within *FKBP5* (*rs9296158*, *rs3800373*, *rs1360780*, and *rs9470080*). Also, there has been a significant association between the severity of PTSD symptoms and *FKBP5* SNPs, which were associated with the total score on the Childhood Trauma Questionnaire. These findings have suggested that the greater symptom complexity of PTSD can be influenced by interactions between specific SNPs within the *FKBP5* gene and childhood abuse [45–47].

In addition, a study of male soldiers of European American ancestry has shown that interactions between the *rs2400707* SNP within the adrenoceptor beta 2 (*ADRB2*) gene and exposure to childhood adversity may be associated with the severity of PTSD symptoms. This finding, linking *rs2400707*, childhood trauma, and PTSD, has also been replicated in an independent, predominantly female African American cohort. However, a negative result for this interaction has also been reported [48]. In summary, these findings suggest that it is, in fact, not only adulthood trauma but also childhood trauma and its interaction with *ADRB2* gene variants that may contribute to the severity of adulthood PTSD. Thus, one might speculate that increased *ADRB2* gene expression, which has been associated with more efficient transcription, may lead to negative effects of adrenergic and noradrenergic activation in individuals with childhood trauma [7].

Interactions between the pituitary adenylate cyclase-activating polypeptide (PACAP) type I receptor (*ADCYAP1R1*) gene and childhood maltreatment have been associated with the severity of adulthood PTSD symptoms [49]. Also, in carriers of the C allele of the *ADCYP1R1* gene, the PTSD symptom severity can be predicted by the specific gene-childhood trauma interaction [50]. Consistent with these findings, the severity of PTSD symptoms and differential methylation of *ADCYP1R1* have been associated with levels of the PACAP protein in blood [51]. Moreover, the extent of epigenetic modifications in adulthood PTSD patients with childhood trauma has been estimated to be 12 times higher than those without childhood trauma. Hence, the differences in epigenetic modifications associated with exposure to childhood trauma can lead to different symptoms, courses, and treatment resistance in adulthood PTSD [52].

6.3 Combination of Pharmacotherapy and Psychotherapy for Treatment-Resistant Psychiatric Disorders

Despite the tendency to increasingly focus on pharmacotherapy for treating depressive and anxiety disorders, the effectiveness of psychotherapeutic options, including cognitive behavioral therapy (CBT) and interpersonal therapy (IPT), is equivalent to that of antidepressant medications of these disorders [53–56]. Moreover, in terms of treating depressive and/or anxiety disorders, it is well known that the effectiveness of psychotherapy combined with pharmacotherapy is greater than that of pharmacotherapy alone [4, 57–59]. Given the modest differences in the efficacies of the various antidepressant medications, the difference in the efficacy of combined pharmacotherapy and psychotherapy vs. pharmacotherapy alone is remarkable [60]. Similarly, with respect to treating panic disorder, efficacy for the combination of pharmacotherapy and CBT is greater than pharmacotherapy alone [61–63].

6.3.1 Interaction Between Antidepressant Effects and Environmental Factors

As mentioned previously, environmental factors can influence the effect of antidepressants [13]. A preclinical investigation using the chronic mild stress model in mice supports the state-dependent mood-elevating effects of antidepressants. The anhedonic symptoms assessed in mice randomly allocated to an enriched environment (EE)/EE, EE/stress, stress/EE, and stress/stress before and during the antidepressant treatments. Hence, the anhedonia improved only in the antidepressant treatment condition for the group with EE following exposure to stress. In contrast, anhedonia was aggravated in the antidepressant treatment condition for the group with exposure to stress following EE. Also, there were no significant changes in terms of the antidepressant effects for mice exposed to continuous stress or EE paradigms. These findings suggest that, by modulating the susceptibility to the effects of environmental factors, neural plasticity can be increased by the antidepressant treatment [64].

In terms of the state-dependent anxiolytic effects of antidepressants, consideration of fear conditioning may be necessary. With regard to fear conditioning, extinction can be described as suppressing learned fear, rather than manipulating the fear memory per se, which is followed by several phenomena including reinstatement (exposure to the same unconditional response), renewal (exposure in a shifted context), and spontaneous recovery (passage of time). "Fear erasure" refers to modification of the neural circuitry representing the fear memory without the occurrence of the three phenomena above (Choi and Kim 2016). A successful fear erasure associated with concurrent antidepressant treatment during extinction training has been demonstrated in an animal model. Also, attenuated fear in the vehicle/extinction group and its degree is comparable to that of the antidepressant/extinction group. Moreover, the vehicle/extinction group exhibited the reinstatement, renewal, and spontaneous recovery after the first week of extinction training, whereas the antidepressant/extinction group has not exhibited these phenomena. Remarkably, in terms of the interaction between antidepressant and environment, the antidepressant treatment without extinction training was not associated with the attenuation of learned fear. In addition, the antidepressant-induced *Bdnf* induction is a critical mechanism for the phenomena to occur based on the absence of the fear erasure effect in *Bdnf*$^{+/-}$ knockout mice [65]. In summary, the juvenile-like neuronal plasticity, which represents fear erasure, can be supported by fear erasure after extinction in juvenile mice and antidepressant-induced synaptic plasticity enhancement and immature neuronal marker increment [65–67].

6.3.2 Reconsolidation-Updating Mechanism

A behavioral paradigm known as "reconsolidation-updating mechanism" can erase a recently formed fear memory despite the resistance to extinction training of fear memory [68]. This finding may support the notion that extinction training can be enhanced by memory updating or modification during reconsolidation. The fear response has been persistently attenuated by extinction training 1 h after memory retention when applied 1 day after fear conditioning. For its full effectiveness, the extinction should occur within the reconsolidation window associated with the change from formed stable memory into transiently unstable memory, to be updated by new information [69]. Also, the attenuated fear response within the reconsolidation window has been applied to humans, and the persistence of attenuated fear effects has been shown to continue for at least a year [70–72].

The decreased activity in the hippocampus during memory retrieval in patients with PTSD was demonstrated in a functional magnetic resonance imaging (fMRI) study [73, 74]. The reactivation of the hippocampal memory trace activated during learning has been required by the reinstatement of a memory trace in the cortex during memory retrieval [75, 76]. In terms not only of extinction learning but also system reconsolidation after memory retrieval, the hippocampus is required [77, 78]. Consistent with these findings, it has also been reported that, after recent fear memory recall but not remote fear memory, increased levels of the c-fos and histone acetylation in the hippocampus have been observed (Graff et al. 2014). In one study, following memory retrieval and extinction training during the reconsolidation window, a systemic administration of histone acetylation 2 (HDAC2) inhibitor (Cl-994) was used to examine the causal relationship between hypoacetylation patterns, reduced reactivation of the hippocampus, and failure of reconsolidation-updating. Here, hypoacetylation was reversed, and neuronal reactivation occurred during remote memory retrieval. Also, a successful erasure of the remote contextual fear memory was demonstrated by the reconsolidation-updating mechanism [79]. Moreover, an HDAC2 inhibitor-induced release of constrained plasticity during remote recall was suggested by the exaggerated expression of neural plasticity-related genes during extinction training [79]. The epigenetic priming effects of HDAC2 inhibition have been supported by rodent study findings in which enhancement of both hippocampus- and amygdala-dependent memory formations was affected by genetic deletion of HDAC2 and use of an HDAC inhibitor [80, 81]. In addition, by reversing epigenetic constraints, the HDAC2 inhibitor valproic acid has been found to overcome refractoriness to anticancer treatments [82–84]. Moreover, epigenetic dysregulation has been associated with various psychiatric disorders, and HDAC inhibitors have been proposed as potential enhancers for treating Alzheimer's disease [79, 84–87].

6.3.3 HDAC Inhibitor-Augmented Psychotherapy to Modulate Dysfunctional Neural Circuits

Small hippocampal volumes in patients with PTSD have been associated with an overgeneralization of conditioned fear [88, 89]. In addition, in terms of a traumatic event, the degree of overgeneralization of conditioned fear has been positively associated with the intensity of the aversive experience [90]. The activity pattern of the hippocampal-amygdala network can be altered by excessive glucocorticoid levels which can lead to the failure of precise association between conditioned stimulus (CS) and unconditioned stimulus (US) in terms of learning and generalization of fear [91]. Moreover, the individual susceptibility of disease progression can be explained by hypofunctioning of the prefrontal cortex. In terms of the top-down regulation of medial prefrontal cortex (mPFC), recent studies showed that the overgeneralization of conditioned fear can be regulated by a neural circuit composed of the medial prefrontal cortex, nucleus reuniens, and hippocampus [92, 93]. In terms of the dysfunctional neural circuit associated with depressive symptom, the mPFC-dorsal raphe nucleus (DRN) projection has been highlighted. In the forced swim test, active coping behavior (reduced immobilization) has been facilitated by optogenetic stimulation of the mPFC-DRN projection, and serotonergic neuron in DRN and passive coping behavior (increased immobilization) has been increased by optogenetic stimulation of the mPFC-lateral habenula (LHb) projection [94]. In addition, in terms of social avoidance, low activity of the left mPFC is associated with high social avoidance, and normal activity of the left mPFC is associated with stress resilience [95]. Hence, in terms of the pathogenesis of depression, the mPFC has been significantly highlighted. Moreover, it has been reported that α-amino-3-hydroxy-5-methyl-4-isoxazolepropionic acid (AMPA) receptor blockade in mPFC or 5-HT deletion in DRN blocks the rapid antidepressant effect of ketamine [96].

Furthermore, the reconsolidation-updating paradigm supports the hypothesis that the HDAC inhibitor-augmented psychotherapy modulates dysfunctional neural circuits in depressive and anxiety disorders. In terms of the "plasticity-augmented psychotherapy," the integration of psychotherapy and pharmacotherapy might be conceptualized in the future to maximize the effectiveness of psychotherapy. In psychotherapy, the duration of each session should be extended to consider the reconsolidation window (10 min to 6 h). Also, in pharmacotherapy, the epigenetic constraints on the expression of neural plasticity-related genes should be removed by antidepressant and/or HDAC inhibitor (e.g., valproate). Hence, the treatment-resistant depressive and anxiety disorders may be treated by the integrated approach of psychotherapy and pharmacotherapy [13].

Conclusion

Based on the gene-childhood trauma interaction and epigenetic regulation, integrated approaches to treatment-resistant psychiatric disorders have been proposed consistent with the "next-generation treatments for psychiatric disorders." To conceptualize integrated approaches to treatment-resistant psychiatric disorders, modulating effects of the synergistic interaction between specific genes and childhood trauma on treatment-resistant psychiatric disorders should be regarded as significant clinical factors. Moreover, the "plasticity-augmented psychotherapy" to correct dysfunctional neural circuits can be hypothetically proposed as one of the integrated approaches to treatment-resistant psychiatric disorders.

References

1. Kim Y-K. Can we cope with treatment refractoriness in psychiatric disorders? Prog Neuro-Psychopharmcol Biol Psychiatry. 2016;70:101–2.
2. Insel TR. Next-generation treatments for mental disorders. Sci Transl Med. 2012;4:155psc19.
3. Park S-C, Choi J. Issues in the classification of psychotic depression. In: Kim Y-K, editor. Major depressive disorder: risk factors, characteristics and treatment options. New York: NOVA Science Publishers; 2017. p. 49–67.
4. Park S-C, Oh HS, Oh DH, Jung SA, Na KS, Lee HW, et al. Evidence-based, non-pharmacological treatment guideline for depression in Korea. J Korean Med Sci. 2014;29:12–22.
5. Won E, Park S-C, Han KM, Sung SH, Lee HY, Paik JW, et al. Evidence-based, pharmacological treatment guideline for depression in Korea, revised edition. J Korean Med Sci. 2014;29:468–84.
6. Akil H, Gordon J, Hen R, Javitch J, Mayberg H, McEwen B, et al. Treatment resistant depression: a multi-scale, systems biology approach. Neurosci Biobehav Rev. 2017;84:272–88. pii: S0149-7634(17)30368-8.
7. Kim JS, Lee S-H. Influence of interaction between genes and childhood trauma on refractoriness in psychiatric disorders. Prog Neuro-Psychopharmcol Biol Psychiatry. 2016;70:162–9.
8. Kim Y-K, Choi J, Park S-C. A novel bio-psychosocial-behavioral treatment model in schizophrenia. Int J Mol Sci. 2017;18:E734.
9. Kirsch I. Challenging received wisdom: antidepressants and placebo effect. Mcgill J Med. 2008;11:219–22.
10. Kirsch I, Deacon BJ, Huedo-Medina TB, Scoboria A, Moore TJ, Johnson BT. Initial severity and antidepressant benefits: a meta-analysis of data submit-

ted to the Food and Drug Administration. PLoS Med. 2008;5:e45.
11. Cohen A, Houck PR, Szanto K, Dew MA, Gliman SE, Reynolds CF. Social inequalities in response to antidepressant treatment in older adults. Arch Gen Psychiatry. 2006;63:50–6.
12. Trivedi ME, Rush AJ, Wisniewski SR, Nierenberg AA, Warden D, Ritz L, et al. Evaluation of outcomes with citalopram for depression using measurement-based care in STAR*D: implications for clinical practice. Am J Psychiatry. 2006;163:28–40.
13. Choi K-Y, Kim Y-K. Plasticity-augmented psychotherapy for refractory depressive and anxiety disorders. Prog Neuro-Psychopharmcol Biol Psychiatry. 2016;70:134–47.
14. Freire TFV, Rocha NSD, Fleck MPA. The association of electroconvulsive therapy to pharmacological treatment and its influence on cytokines. J Psychiatr Res. 2017;92:205–11.
15. Bay-Richter C, Linderholm KR, Lim CK, Samuelsson M, Traskman-Bendz L, Guillemin GJ, et al. A role for inflammatory metabolites as modulators of the glutamate N-methyl-D-aspartate receptor in depression and suicidality. Brain Behav Immun. 2015;43:110–7.
16. Dowlati Y, Herrmann N, Swardfager W, Liu H, Sham L, Reim EK, et al. A meta-analysis of cytokines in major depression. Biol Psychiatry. 2010;67:446–57.
17. Miller AH, Maletic V, Raison CL. Inflammation and its discontents: the role of cytokines in the pathophysiology of major depression. Biol Psychiatry. 2009;65:732–41.
18. Dell'Oso B, Mundo E, D'Urso N, Pozzoli S, Buoli M, Ciabatti MT, et al. Augmentative repetitive navigated transcranial magnetic stimulation (rTMS) in drug-resistant bipolar depression. Bipolar Disord. 2009;11:76–81.
19. Dibaz N, Sengul C, Okay T, Bayam G, Turkoglu A. The combined treatment of venlafaxine and ECT in treatment-resistant depressive patients. Int J Psychiatry Clin Pract. 2005;9:55–9.
20. Meyberg HS, Lozano AM, Voon V, McNeely HE, Seminowicz D, Hamani C, et al. Deep brain stimulation for treatment-resistant depression. Neuron. 2005;4:651–60.
21. Eljamel S. Strategies for the return of behavioral surgery. Surg Neurol Int. 2012;3:S4–9.
22. Hugo F, van Heerden BB, Zygo-Dirway N, Stein DJ. Functional brain imaging in obsessive-compulsive disorder secondary to neurological lesions. Depress Anxiety. 1999;10:129–36.
23. Rosenberg DR, Kehavan MD. Toward a neurodevelopmental model of obsessive-compulsive disorder. Biol Psychiatry. 1998;43:623–40.
24. Bares M, Novak T, Kopecek M, Stopkova P, Sos P. Is combined treatment more effective than switching to monotherapy in patients with resistant depression?: a retrospective study. Neuroendocrinol Lett. 2009;30:723–8.
25. Pridmore S, Tunier-Shea S. Medication options in the treatment of treatment-resistant depression. Aust N Z J Psychiatry. 2004;38:219–25.
26. Benedetti F, Riccaboni R, Locatelli C, Poletti S, Dallaspezia S, Colombo C. Rapid treatment response of suicidal symptoms to lithium, sleep deprivation, and light therapy (chronotherapeutics) in drug-resistant bipolar depression. J Clin Psychiatry. 2014;75:133–40.
27. Mura G, Moro MF, Patten SB, Carta MG. Exercise as an add-on strategy for the treatment of major depressive disorder: a systematic review. CNS Spectr. 2014;19:496–508.
28. Koek RJ, Schwartz HN, Scully S, Langevin J-P, Spangler S, Korotinsky A, et al. Treatment-refractory posttraumatic stress disorder (TRPTSD): a review and framework for the future. Prog Neuro-Psychopharmcol Biol Psychiatry. 2016;70:170–218.
29. Park S-C, Park YC, Lee MS, Chang HS. Plasma brain-derived neurotrophic factor level may contribute to the therapeutic response to eye movement desensitization and reprocessing in complex posttraumatic stress disorder: a pilot study. Acta Neuropsychiatr. 2012;24:384–6.
30. Kessler RC, Delmer O, Frank RG, Olfson M, Pincus HA, Walters EE, et al. Prevalence and treatment of mental disorders, 1990 to 2003. N Engl J Med. 2005;352:2515–23.
31. Torgalsboen AK, Suzuki H, Rabi K, Sheu YS, Polcari A, Teicher MH. Reduced prefrontal cortical gray matter volume in young adults exposed in the early course of first-episode schizophrenia. Psychiatry Res. 2014;216:1–5.
32. Fervaha G, Foussias G, Agid O, Remington G. Motivational and neurocognitive deficits are central to the prediction of longitudinal functional outcome in schizophrenia. Acta Psychiatr Scand. 2014;130:290–9.
33. Aas M, Djurovic S, Athanasiu L, Steen NE, Agartz I, Lorentzen S, et al. Serotonin transporter gene polymorphism, childhood trauma and cognition in patients with psychotic disorders. Schizophr Bull. 2012;38:15–22.
34. Aas M, Haukvik UK, Djurovic S, Bergmann O, Athanasiu L, Tesli MS, et al. BDNF val66met modulates the association between childhood trauma, cognitive and brain abnormalities in psychoses. Prog Neuro-Psychopharmacol Biol Psychiatry. 2013;46:181–8.
35. Oliveria J, Etain B, Lajnef M, Hamdani N, Bennabi M, Bengouga D, et al. Combined effects of TLR gene polymorphism and early life stress on the age at onset of bipolar disorders. PLoS One. 2015;10:e0119702.
36. Etain B, Henry C, Belliver F, Mathieu F, Leboyer M. Beyond genetics: childhood affective trauma in bipolar disorder. Bipolar Disord. 2008;10:867–76.
37. Perroud N, Courter P, Vincze I, Jausssent I, Jollant F, Belliveier F, et al. Interaction between BDNF Val66Met and childhood trauma on adult's violent suicide attempt. Genes Brain Behav. 2008;7:314–22.

38. Pregelj P, Nedic G, Paska AV, Zupanc Y, Nikolac M, Balazic J, et al. The association between brain-derived neurotrophic factor polymorphism (BDNF Val66Met) and suicide. J Affect Disord. 2011;128:287–90.
39. Miller S, Hallmayer J, Wang PW, Hill SJ, Johnson SL, Ketter TA. Brain-derived neurotrophic factor val66met genotype and early life stress effects upon bipolar course. J Psychiatr Res. 2013;44:511–20.
40. Aguilera M, Arias B, Wichers M, Barrantes-Vidal N, Moya J, Villa H, et al. Early adversity and 5-HTT/BDNF genes: new evidence of gene-environment interactions on depressive symptoms in a general population. Psychol Med. 2009;39:1425–32.
41. Lok A, Bockting CL, Koeter MW, Sneider H, Assies J, Mocking RJ, et al. Interaction between the MTHFR C677T polymorphism with traumatic childhood events predicts depression. Transl Psychiatry. 2013;3:e288.
42. Juruena MF. Early-life stress and HPA axis trigger recurrent adulthood depression. Epilepsy Behav. 2014;38:148–59.
43. Hardeveld F, Spijker J, Vreeburg SA, Graaf RD, Hendriks SM, Licht CM, et al. Increased cortisol awakening response was associated with time to recurrence of major depressive disorder. Psychoneuroendocrinology. 2014;50:62–71.
44. Musazzi L, Mallei A, Tardito D, Gruber SH, El Khourt A, Racagni G, et al. Early-life stress and antidepressant treatment involve synaptic signaling and Erk kinase in a gene-environment model of depression. J Psychiatr Res. 2010;44:511–20.
45. Bernstein DP, Stein JA, Newcomb MD, Walker E, Pogge D, Ahluvalia T, et al. Development and validation of a brief screening version of the Childhood Trauma Questionnaire. Child Abuse Negl. 2003;27:169–90.
46. Binder EB, Bradley RG, Liu W, Epstein MP, Deveau TC, Mercer KB, et al. Association of FKB5 polymorphisms and childhood abuse with risk of posttraumatic stress disorder symptoms in adults. JAMA. 2008;299:1291–305.
47. Cloitre M, Gavert DW, Brewin CR, Bryant RA, Maercker A. Evidence for proposed ICD-11 PTSD and complex PTSD: a latent profile analysis. Eur J Psychotraumato. 2013;4:20706.
48. Liberzon I, King AP, Ressler KJ, Almli LM, Zhang P, Ma ST, et al. Interaction of the ADRB2 gene polymorphism with childhood trauma in predicting adult symptoms of posttraumatic stress disorder. JAMA Psychiat. 2014;71:1174–82.
49. Uddin M, Chang SC, Zhang C, Ressler K, Mercer KB, Galea S, et al. Adcyap1r1 genotype, posttraumatic stress disorder, and depression among women exposed to childhood maltreatment. Depress Anxiety. 2013;30:251–8.
50. Almli LM, Mercer KB, Kerley K, Feng H, Bradley B, Conneely KN, et al. ADCYP1R1 genotype associates with post-traumatic stress symptoms in highly traumatized African-American female. Am J Genet B Neuropsychiatr Genet. 2013;162B:262–72.
51. Ressler KJ, Mercer KB, Bradley B, Jovanovic T, Mahan A, Kerley K, et al. Posttraumatic stress disorder is associated with PACAP and the PAC1 receptor. Nature. 2011;470:492–7.
52. Mehta D, Klengel T, Conneely KN, Smith AK, Altmann A, Pace TW, et al. Childhood maltreatment is associated with distinct genomic and epigenetic profiles in posttraumatic stress disorder. Proc Natl Acad Sci U S A. 2013;110:8302–7.
53. Elkin J, Shea MT, Watkins JT, Imber SD, Sotsky SM, Collins JF, et al. National institute of mental health treatment of depression collaborative research program. General effectiveness of treatment. Arch Gen Psychiatry. 1989;46:971–82.
54. Khan A, Faucett J, Lichtenberg P, Kirsch I, Brown WA. A systematic review of comparative treatments and controls for depression. PLoS One. 2012;7:e41778.
55. Marcus SC, Olfson M. National trends in the treatment for depression from 1998 to 2007. Arch Gen Psychiatry. 2010;67:1265–73.
56. Olfson M, Marcus SC, Druss B, Elinson L, Tanielian T, Pincus HA. National trends in the outpatient treatment of depression. JAMA. 2002;287:203–9.
57. Cuijepers P, Sijbrandij M, Koole SL, Andersson G, Beekman AT, Reynolds CF. Adding psychotherapy to antidepressant medication in depression and anxiety disorders: a meta-analysis. World Psychiatry. 2014;13:56–67.
58. Hollon SD, DeRubeis RJ, Fawcett J, Amsterdam JD, Shelton DC, Ziecka J, et al. Effect of cognitive therapy with antidepressant medication vs antidepressant alone on the rate of recovery in major depressive disorder: a randomized clinical trial. JAMA Psychiat. 2014;71:1157–64.
59. Schramm E, van Calker D, Dykierek P, Lieb K, Kech S, Zobel I, et al. An intensive treatment program of interpersonal psychotherapy plus pharmacotherapy for depressed inpatients: acute and long-term results. Am J Psychiatry. 2007;164:768–77.
60. Cipriani A, Furukawa TA, Salanti G, Geddes JR, Higgins JP, Churchill R, et al. Comparative efficacy and acceptability of 12 new-generation antidepressants: a multiple-treatments in meta-analysis. Lancet. 2009;373:746–58.
61. Barlow DH, Gorman JM, Shear MK, Woods SW. Cognitive-behavioral therapy, imipramine, or their combination for panic disorder: a randomized controlled trial. JAMA. 2000;283:2529–36.
62. Furukawa TA, Watanabe N, Churchill R. Combined psychotherapy plus antidepressant for panic disorder with or without agoraphobia. Cochrane Database Syst Rev. 2007:CD004364.
63. Otto MW, Smits JAJ, Reese HE. Cognitive-behavioral therapy for the treatment of anxiety disorders. J Clin Psychiatry. 2004;65:S34–41.
64. Branchi I, Santarelli S, Capoccia S, Poggini S, D'Andrea I, Cirulli F, et al. Antidepressant treatment outcome depends on the quality of the living environment: a pre-clinical investigation in mice. PLoS One. 2013;8:e62226.

65. Karpova NN, Pickenhagen A, Lindholm J, Tiraboschi E, Kulesskaya N, Agustsdottir A, et al. Fear erasure in mice requires synergy between antidepressant drugs and extinction training. Science. 2011;334:1731–4.
66. Castren E, Rantamaki T. The role of BDF and its receptors in depression and antidepressant action: reactivation of developmental plasticity. Dev Neurobiol. 2010;70:289–97.
67. Gorgolla N, Caroni P, Luthi A, Henry C. Perineuronal nets protect fear memories from erasure. Science. 2009;325:1258–61.
68. Mofils MS, Cowansage KK, Klann E, LeDoux JE. Extinction-reconsolidation boundaries: key to persistent attenuation of fear memories. Science. 2009;160:554–5.
69. Narder K, Hardt O. A single standard for memory: the case reconsolidation. Nat Rev Neurosci. 2009;10:224–34.
70. Agren T, Engman J, Frick A, Bjorkstrand J, Larsson E-M, Furmark T, et al. Disruption of reconsolidation erases a fear memory trace in the human amygdala. Science. 2012;337:1550–2.
71. Bjorkstrand J, Agren T, Frick A, Engman J, Larsson E-M, Furmark T, et al. Disruption of memory reconsolidation erases a fear memory trace in the human amygdala: an 18-month follow-up. PLoS Med. 2015;10:e100454.
72. Schiller D, Monfils MH, Raio CM, Johnson DC, LeDoux JE, Phelps EA. Preventing the return of fear in humans using reconsolidation update mechanisms. Nature. 2010;463:49–53.
73. Carrion VG, Haas BW, Garret A, Song S, Reiss AL. Reduced hippocampal activity in youth with posttraumatic stress symptoms: an fMRI study. J Pediatr Psychol. 2010;35:559–69.
74. Milad MR, Pitman RK, Ellis CB, Gold AL, Shin LM, Lasko NB, et al. Neurobiological basis of failure to recall extinction memory in posttraumatic stress disorder. Biol Psychiatry. 2009;66:1075–82.
75. Santoro A, Frankland PW. Chasing the engram: strategies to examine the memory trace. Mol Brain. 2014;5:32.
76. Tanaka KZ, Pevzner A, Hamidi AB, Nakazawa Y, Graham J, Wiltgen BJ. Cortical representations are reinstated by the hippocampus during memory retrieval. Neuron. 2014;84:347–54.
77. Bouton ME. Context and behavioral processes in extinction. Learn Mem. 2004;11:5–494.
78. Debiec J, LeDoux JE, Nader K. Cellular and systems reconsolidation in the hippocampus. Neuron. 2002;36:527–38.
79. Graff J, Kim D, Dobbin MM, Tsai LH. Epigenetic regulation of gene expression in physiological and pathological brain processes. Physiol Rev. 2011;91:603–49.
80. Fischer A, Sananbenesi F, Wang X, Dobbin M, Tsai L-H. Recovery of learning and memory is associated with chromatin remodeling. Nature. 2007;447:178–82.
81. Guan J-S, Haggarty SJ, Giacometti E, Dannenberg J-H, Joseph N, Gao J, et al. HDAC2 negatively regulates memory formation and synaptic plasticity. Nature. 2009;459:55–60.
82. Blagitko-Dorfs N, Jiang Y, Duque-Afonso J, Hiller J, Yalcin A, Greve G, et al. Epigenetic priming of AML blasts for all-trans retinoic acid-induced differentiation by the HDAC class-I selective inhibitor entinostat. PLoS One. 2013;8:e0129393.
83. Gu S, Tian Y, Chlenski A, Salwen HR, Lu Z, Rai JU, et al. Valproic acid shows a potent antitumor effect with alteration of DNA methylation in neuroblastoma. Anti-Cancer Drugs. 2012;23:1054–66.
84. Hubaux R, Vandermeers F, Cosse J-P, Crisanti C, Kapoor V, Albelda SM, et al. Valproic acid improves second-line regimen of small cell lung carcinoma in preclinical models. ERJ Open Res. 2015;1:00028.
85. Graff J, Tsai L-H. The potential of HDAC inhibitors as cognitive enhancers. Annu Rev Pharmacol Toxicol. 2013;53:311–30.
86. Noh H, Seo H. Age-dependent effects of valproic acid in Alzheimer's disease (AD) mice are associated with nerve growth factor (NGF) regulation. Neuroscience. 2014;266:255–65.
87. Xu K, Dai X-L, Huang H-C, Jiang Z-F. Targeting HDACs: a promising therapy for Alzheimer's disease. Oxidative Med Cell Longev. 2011;83:722–35.
88. Gilbertson MW, Shenton ME, Ciszewski A, Kasai K, Lasko NB, Orr SP, et al. Smaller hippocampal volume predicts pathologic vulnerability to psychological trauma. Nat Neurosci. 2002;5:1242–61.
89. Lindauer RJL, Vlieger E-J, Jalink M, Olff M, Carlier IVE, Majoie CBLM, et al. Smaller hippocampal volume in Dutch police officers with posttraumatic stress disorder. BPS. 2004;56:356–63.
90. Baldi E, Lorenzini CA, Bucherelli C. Footshock intensity and generalization in contextual and auditory-cued fear conditioning in the rat. Neurobiol Leran Mem. 2004;81:162–6.
91. Kaouane N, Porte Y, Vallee M, Brayda-Bruno L, Mons N, Calandreau L, et al. Glucocorticoids can induce PTSD-like memory impairments in mice. Science. 2012;334:1731–4.
92. Koenigs M, Grafman J. Posttraumatic stress disorder: the role of medial prefrontal cortex and amygdala. Neuroscientist. 2009;15:540–8.
93. Xu W, Sudhof TC. A neural circuit for memory specificity and generalization. Science. 2013;339:1290–5.
94. Warden MR, Selimbeyoglu A, Mirzabekov JJ, Lo M, Thompson KR, Kim S-Y, et al. A prefrontal cortex-brainstem neuronal projection that controls response to behavioural challenge. Nature. 2012;492:428–32.
95. Lee E, Hong J, Park Y-G, Chae S, Kim Y, Kim D. Left brain cortical activity modulates stress effects on social behavior. Sci Rep. 2015;5:13342.
96. Fukumoto J, Iijma M, Chaki S. The antidepressant effect of an mGlu2/3 receptor antagonist and ketamine require AMPA receptor stimulation in the mPFC and subsequent activation of the 5-HT neurons in the DRN. Neuropsychopharmacology. 2015;41:1046–56.

Part II

Treatment Resistance in Specific Disorders

7 Treatment-Resistant Depression: Understandings on the Neurobiological Etiology that Lead to Novel Pharmacological Treatment Options

Eunsoo Won, Byoung-Joo Ham, and Yong-Ku Kim

7.1 Introduction

The etiology of major depressive disorder (MDD) has mainly been attributed to the monoamine hypothesis of depression, which postulates deficits of certain neurotransmitters to be responsible for symptoms of depression [1]. The hypothesis was supported by the observation that the majority of antidepressant agents increased synaptic levels of neurotransmitters such as serotonin, norepinephrine, and dopamine. However, certain factors have led to the suggestion that the monoamine hypothesis is insufficient, such as the delayed therapeutic effects of antidepressants [2] and the insufficient response rates to pharmacological treatment [3]. The results of the STAR*D trial, which reported less than 70% of patients may improve in symptoms after four trials of antidepressants in 1 year [3], suggest a high rate of treatment resistance in patients with MDD. The term treatment-resistant depression (TRD) is used to describe depression that does not respond adequately to at least two antidepressant treatments [4]. High rates of treatment resistance cause a great burden, to not only the patients who are suffering from TRD but also the society as a whole, and effective treatment strategies for TRD are of great need. In order for novel treatment methods to emerge, a deep understanding of the neurobiological etiology of TRD is essential. In this chapter, we will discuss the recent findings on neurobiological mechanisms underlying TRD and corresponding novel pharmacological treatment strategies.

E. Won · B.-J. Ham
Department of Psychiatry, College of Medicine, Korea University, Seoul, Republic of Korea
e-mail: hambj@korea.ac.kr

Y.-K. Kim (✉)
Department of Psychiatry, College of Medicine, Korea University Ansan Hospital, Ansan City, Republic of Korea
e-mail: yongku@korea.ac.kr

7.2 Genetics

The contribution of genetic vulnerability to TRD has widely been investigated, and genes that influence monoaminergic neurotransmission have been implicated in TRD, such as the serotonin transporter gene (*SLC6A4*), tryptophan hydroxylase 2 gene (*TPH2*), norepinephrine transporter gene (*SLC6A2*), and catechol-O-methyltransferase gene (*COMT*). The possible influence of *SLC6A4* polymorphisms on the risk of TRD has been suggested, with lower serotonin transporter transcription alleles being correlated to a common resistant depression mechanism [5]. *TPH2* polymorphisms have been associated with

Y.-K. Kim (ed.), *Treatment Resistance in Psychiatry*, https://doi.org/10.1007/978-981-10-4358-1_7

the severity of TRD, with *TPH2* rs1386494 A/A genotype carrier patients showing significantly higher depression severity [6]. *SLC6A2* has been associated with the treatment outcome of TRD, with rs36024, an intronic single-nucleotide polymorphism (SNP) of *SLC6A2*, being associated with response to olanzapine-fluoxetine combination treatment in patients with TRD [7]. Regarding *COMT*, the G allele of *COMT* was correlated to the occurrence of TRD, and homozygous G allele carrier patients were evidenced to be more sensitive to modified electroconvulsive therapy than heterozygous G allele carriers [8]. However, such studies focusing on functional variants of risk genes in TRD are considered to have several limitations. The majority of findings could not be generalized, due to factors such as ethnic variability, with the frequency of genes varying substantially across ethnicities. Also, the etiology of depression is complex, with multiple interactions of various factors underlying its etiology, and the sole influence of genetic vulnerability cannot lead to TRD. Stress has been suggested to interact with genetic susceptibility and contribute to the development of the disorder [9]. As a result, epigenetics is recently receiving much attention, with early-life stress considered to influence changes in DNA methylation and histone modification, altering how genes are expressed without changing the underlying DNA sequence [10]. The recurrence of depression is being associated with epigenetic changes of genes such as the brain-derived neurotrophic factor (BDNF) promoter gene in recent studies [11]. Further studies on the association between epigenetics and TRD are needed.

7.3 Neural Substrates

Alterations in brain structure in TRD have been implicated by previous imaging studies. Studies on brain structure have reported decreased volume of brain regions, such as the superior temporal gyrus, lateral inferior frontal gyrus, prefrontal cortex [12], hippocampus [13], and entorhinal cortex (in females) [14]. On the other hand, increased volume of the cuneus and precuneus [12] and no difference in entorhinal cortex volume (in males) [14], cortical thickness, or hippocampal volume [15] have also been reported. Such inconsistencies of the study results may be in part due to differences in confounding factors such as medication status, early-life stress, and gender.

Alterations in brain function in TRD have also been implicated by functional magnetic resonance imaging (fMRI) studies. The default mode network (DMN) has been of particular interest in TRD, which consists of brain regions such as the medial prefrontal cortex, anterior/posterior cingulate, cuneus, and precuneus. Not only is the DMN hyperactive in patients with MDD compared to healthy controls, this hyperactivity is even more prominent in TRD [16, 17]. Furthermore, alterations in functional connectivity of specific brain regions, such as decreased cerebellum–cerebellar functional connectivity [17], and increased connectivity from the temporal gyrus to the frontal and angular gyrus, precuneus, and rectus [18] have been reported. Patients with TRD have shown increased regional homogeneity in regions such as the temporal gyrus and insula and decreased regional homogeneity in regions including the precuneus and inferior frontal gyrus [19]. Patients with TRD have also shown increased metabolism in the amygdala and uncus in positron emission tomography studies [20]. The underlying mechanisms of such alterations in neural substrates may be attributed to the following etiological factors.

7.4 Neuroinflammation, Neurogenesis, and Neurodegeneration

Increased inflammation has been widely implicated in depression, with elevated pro-inflammatory cytokine levels, such as interleukin (IL)-6 and tumor necrosis factor alpha (TNF-α), being observed in MDD [21]. Decreased levels of anti-inflammatory cytokines have also been suggested to contribute to the development of depression [22]. The role of inflammation has also been emphasized in TRD, as previous studies have reported TNF-α antagonists, such as infliximab, to be effective in patients with TRD with elevated inflammatory markers at baseline [23]. The major intermediate target of pro-inflammatory cytokines in the brain is microglia, with insufficient microglial function leading to reduced neuroprotection and excess microglia activity leading to neuronal cell damage [24]. Increased levels of pro-inflammatory cytokines and microglia are suggested to underlie the pathophysiology of MDD, with both being synergistic to each other's activity [25]. Pro-inflammatory cytokines promote the activation of microglia, and activated microglia, in turn, release pro-inflammatory cytokines. Furthermore, activated microglia can also increase glutamatergic neurotransmission which may result in excitotoxicity and apoptosis. Glutamate and microglia are also interactive, and disruption in glutamatergic neurotransmission may in turn lead to the activation of microglia [26]. Recent studies have reported pro-inflammatory mediators to be associated with treatment response in patients with MDD, such as alterations in IL-6 levels being associated with response to treatment [27].

Neurogenesis is the process by which nervous system cells, also known as neurons, are produced by neural stem cells [28]. Neurogenesis occurs not only prenatally but also continuously in specific regions in the adult brain [29], including the subgranular zone which is part of the dentate gyrus of the hippocampus [30]. Adult neurogenesis in the hippocampus has been associated with learning and memory, conditioning, and investigative behaviors [31]. Numerous studies have implicated an association between adult hippocampal neurogenesis and MDD [32], with decreased neurogenesis being observed in animal models of MDD [33], and treatments with antidepressant effects, such as medication and electroconvulsive therapy, increasing neurogenesis. Therefore, neurogenesis is considered to be a fundamental process in the development and progression of the disorder.

Both neurogenesis and neurodegeneration are greatly influenced by neuroinflammation. For neurogenesis, pro-inflammatory cytokine receptors which are highly expressed in the hippocampus [34], may inhibit the process of neurogenesis [35]. The most widely reported cytokine is IL-1β, with its inhibition leading to a protective effect against stress-induced reductions in neurogenesis [36]. Accordingly, a continuous expression of IL-1β in the hippocampus has been shown to have negative influence on adult neurogenesis [37]. IL-1β also has influence on other pro-inflammatory cytokine-induced reduction of neurogenesis, such as interferon-gamma (IFN-γ) [38]. Another cytokine which has been implicated in neurogenesis is leukemia inhibitory factor (LIF), which shares glycoprotein 130 (gp130) with other IL-6 cytokine family members [39]. In relation to its effects on neurogenesis, LIF has been shown to have influence on neuroinflammation, glial cell activation, and various transcription pathways [40]. Neuronal functioning acquires adequate levels of LIF, with LIF knockout mice exhibiting abnormal cell activities of microglia and astrocytes and CNS insults leading to excessive LIF, which have been associated with schizophrenia-like symptoms [41]. TNF-α also has been numerously implicated in neurogenesis and neurodegeneration [42], with CNS insults leading to activation of TNF-α by glial cells [43]. There are two receptors of TNF-α, TNF receptor (TNFR)-1 and TNFR-2, with TNFR-1 mainly taking part in processes such as neurodegeneration and apoptosis and TNFR-2 mainly associated with processes of neurogenesis [44, 45]. Accordingly, previous studies have reported TNFR-1 to have detrimental effects on adult neurogenesis in the hippocampus [46, 47] and TNFR-2 to enhance neurogenesis [48, 49]. Furthermore, the relation of TNF-α with α-amino-3-hydroxy-5-methyl-4-isoxazolepropionic acid (AMPA) receptors is also known to greatly contribute to synaptic plasticity, as AMPA receptors control glutamatergic neurotransmission [50].

7.5 Glutamatergic Neurotransmission

Glutamatergic neurotransmission is now considered to play an essential role in the etiology of TRD [51]. Being the major and primary excitatory neurotransmitter, glutamate has been the center of attention when discussing calcium influx-associated neurotoxicity [52], but recently its role in synaptic plasticity is being emphasized through N-methyl-D-aspartate receptor (NMDAR) neurotransmission [53]. Glutamate receptors can be categorized as ionotropic or metabotropic depending on which signal transduction mechanism the receptor relies on [54]. NMDARs, AMPARs, and kainate receptors are all ionotropic receptors, and the antagonism of extrasynaptic NMDARs and AMPARs is considered to play an essential role in the etiology and treatment of TRD [55].

Although glutamate's activity had been once considered dependent on the intensity of neurotransmission accompanied by calcium influx [56], the location of NMDARs is considered nowadays to be essential in the process of excitotoxicity and related apoptosis and neurodegeneration [57]. Extrasynaptic NMDAR-mediated glutamatergic neurotransmission has been shown to have detrimental effects such as excitotoxicity, but synaptic neurotransmission has been shown to have positive effects on synaptic plasticity [58]. Synaptic glutamate is transported into glial cells via excitatory amino acid transporters (EAATs) and, once converted to glutamine, is then again transported to presynaptic neurons, where glutamine is converted back to glutamate and then released to the synapse [59]. Inappropriate uptake of the glial cells resulting in excess glutamate leads to the diffusion and uptake of glutamate by extrasynaptic NMDARs; hence insufficient activity of EAATs may lead to extrasynaptic neurotransmission, contributing to excitotoxicity [60]. Therefore, enhanced synaptic NMDAR neurotransmission along with diminished extrasynaptic neurotransmission is considered to play a pivotal role in neuronal survival [58]. The detrimental effects of extrasynaptic NMDAR neurotransmission have been numerously reported, such as the inhibition of extracellular signal-regulated kinases (ERK) [61], cyclic adenosine monophosphate response element-binding protein (CREB) activation [62], and the increase in beta-induced nitric oxide production [63], all of which exert opposing effects on neuronal plasticity and survival. Accordingly, synaptic NMDAR neurotransmission has been shown to have opposite effects and activate ERK and CREB [61, 62].

Metabotropic glutamate receptors (mGlus) can be divided into three groups, with group I including mGlu1 and mGlu5, which are situated alongside NMDARs. Antagonism of mGlu5 has been shown to lead to NMDAR inhibition, and agonism of mGlu5 has been shown to lead to NMDAR enhancement [64, 65]; hence mGlu5 has been widely studied in relation to TRD [66]. Groups II and III include mGlu2 and mGlu3 and mGlu4, mGlu6, mGlu7, and mGlu8, respectively [67]. The majority of group II receptors are present in the hippocampus and prefrontal cortex and inhibit glutamatergic release via negative feedback [68]; hence the activation of these receptors decreases glutamatergic release and may enhance neuroprotection [69].

7.6 Glial Cells

Glial cells are the most abundant nonneuronal cells in the brain and include microglia, astrocytes, and oligodendrocytes [70]. Contrary to the belief that glial cells only functioned as structural support to neurons, glial cells are now considered to play a central role in the etiology of MDD. Astrocytes mainly express synaptic EAATs, and neuronal activity is greatly influenced by astrocyte-released glutamate [71]. Hence, astrocyte dysfunction can lead to a decline in synaptic neurotransmission and an increase in the direct binding of glutamate to extrasynaptic NMDARs [72].

Microglia cells are essential in neuroinflammatory processes and react promptly to changes in the environment; hence CNS insults directly lead to activation of microglia [73]. Although inadequate microglia activation can lead to inadequate defense against insults, excess activation may also lead to neurotoxicity due to excess amounts of inflammatory mediators being released [25]. The increase in pro-inflammatory cytokines due to abnormal microglia activation is considered a fundamental factor in the etiology of MDD. Previous studies have reported peripheral inflammation to induce microglia-dependent alterations of glutamatergic synaptic transmission and hippocampal plasticity [74] and to induce loss of EAAT1 expression in astrocytes, resulting in decreased reuptake of synaptic glutamate [75]. Microglia are also related to presynaptic mGlus, through dipeptide gliotransmitter N-acetylaspartylglutamate (NAAG), which exist in all glial cells [76]. When glial cells are activated, microglial NAAG increases, which may lead to excess glutamatergic release that induces excitotoxicity [77]. As all receptors of glutamate are present in microglia, glutamate has substantial influence on microglial function and is controlled normally through AMPARs with adenosine triphosphate-mediated signals [78]. However, in inflammatory conditions, GluA2 is shown to have more control over microglial activation; hence deficiencies in GluA2 that lead to abnormal glutamate neurotransmission may have a key role in inducing microglia and pro-inflammatory cytokine-mediated chronic inflammation [26]. Inflammatory pathways are also influenced by microglia via p38 mitogen-activated protein kinase (MAPK), which suppresses glucocorticoid receptor function and in turn influences susceptibility to stressors [79].

7.7 Novel Treatment Options: Anti-inflammatory Medications and Ketamine

Based on the understandings on the neurobiological etiology of TRD, novel pharmacological treatment options have been recommended for TRD, such as anti-inflammatory medications and NMDAR antagonists such as ketamine.

Antidepressant treatment agents are now considered to exert its treatment effects by not only modulating monoamines [80] but also by mediating inflammatory processes [81] and promoting neuroplasticity [82]. Therefore, other agents that prevent or restore the neurotoxic effects caused by excess inflammation may be beneficial in treating depression. Previous studies have reported adjunctive cyclooxygenase-2 selective nonsteroidal anti-inflammatory medications and TNF inhibiting agents to exert antidepressant efficacies [83–88]. Furthermore, acetylsalicylic acid and tetracycline antibiotics have also been reported as potential adjunctive antidepressant agents [89, 90]. Furthermore, anti-inflammatory agents have been shown to reinforce neuro-regenerative processes [91, 92]. Based on the existing evidence, anti-inflammatory agents may be considered as strong candidates when treating TRD.

Currently available antidepressants are considered to have major limitations as stated above. The delay in treatment effects and the high rate of treatment resistance are suggested to be most problematic [93, 94]. Ketamine, a NMDAR antagonist, has been suggested as a potential treatment agent that may overcome such shortcoming of conventional antidepressants. The rapid antidepressant effects of ketamine have been numerously reported by previous studies, along with its efficacy in TRD [95], and suicidality, although the therapeutic effects are generally known not to exceed 2 weeks [96]. Ketamine's treatment effects on TRD are suggested to be mediated by NMDAR antagonism, AMPAR potentiation, and enhanced BDNF-initiated intracellular signaling [97]. Although the long-term treatment effects and safety of ketamine have not yet been adequately studied, it is evident that ketamine has great potential as a candidate antidepressant of TRD.

Conclusion

In this chapter, we discussed the neurobiological etiology and novel pharmacological treatment options in TRD. Genetics, along with interactions with environmental factors, and alterations in neural substrates have been deeply implicated in TRD. Furthermore, changes in neuroinflammatory conditions, glutamatergic neurotransmission, and glial cell pathology, which in turn influence neurogenesis and neurodegeneration, are all considered to play key roles in the pathophysiology of TRD. Based on the speculated etiological factors, novel treatment agents that have substantially different mechanisms of action from conventional treatment agents, such as anti-inflammatory drugs and ketamine, are suggested as potent candidates that will aid us to treat TRD. Future studies are needed to investigate the long-term efficacies and safety of such treatment options.

References

1. Nutt DJ. Relationship of neurotransmitters to the symptoms of major depressive disorder. J Clin Psychiatry. 2008;69(Suppl E1):4–7.
2. Garfield S, Francis SA, Smith FJ. Building concordant relationships with patients starting antidepressant medication. Patient Educ Couns. 2004;55(2):241–6.
3. Gaynes BN, Rush AJ, Trivedi MH, Wisniewski SR, Spencer D, Fava M. The STAR*D study: treating depression in the real world. Cleve Clin J Med. 2008;75(1):57–66.
4. Wijeratne C, Sachdev P. Treatment-resistant depression: critique of current approaches. Aust N Z J Psychiatry. 2008;42(9):751–62.
5. Bonvicini C, Minelli A, Scassellati C, Bortolomasi M, Segala M, Sartori R, et al. Serotonin transporter gene polymorphisms and treatment-resistant depression. Prog Neuro-Psychopharmacol Biol Psychiatry. 2010;34(6):934–9.
6. Anttila S, Viikki M, Huuhka K, Huuhka M, Huhtala H, Rontu R, et al. TPH2 polymorphisms may modify clinical picture in treatment-resistant depression. Neurosci Lett. 2009;464(1):43–6.
7. Houston JP, Lau K, Aris V, Liu W, Fijal BA, Heinloth AN, et al. Association of common variations in the norepinephrine transporter gene with response to olanzapine-fluoxetine combination versus continued-fluoxetine treatment in patients with treatment-resistant depression: a candidate gene analysis. J Clin Psychiatry. 2012;73(6):878–85.
8. Lin Z, He H, Zhang C, Wang Z, Jiang M, Li Q, et al. Influence of Val108/158Met COMT gene polymorphism on the efficacy of modified electroconvulsive therapy in patients with treatment resistant depression. Cell Biochem Biophys. 2015;71(3):1387–93.
9. Liu RT, Alloy LB. Stress generation in depression: a systematic review of the empirical literature and recommendations for future study. Clin Psychol Rev. 2010;30(5):582–93.
10. Heim C, Binder EB. Current research trends in early life stress and depression: review of human studies on sensitive periods, gene-environment interactions, and epigenetics. Exp Neurol. 2012;233(1):102–11.
11. Na KS, Won E, Kang J, Chang HS, Yoon HK, Tae WS, et al. Brain-derived neurotrophic factor promoter methylation and cortical thickness in recurrent major depressive disorder. Sci Rep. 2016;6:21089.
12. Shah PJ, Ebmeier KP, Glabus MF, Goodwin GM. Cortical grey matter reductions associated with treatment-resistant chronic unipolar depression. Controlled magnetic resonance imaging study. Br J Psychiatry J Ment Sci. 1998;172:527–32.
13. Maller JJ, Daskalakis ZJ, Thomson RH, Daigle M, Barr MS, Fitzgerald PB. Hippocampal volumetrics in treatment-resistant depression and schizophrenia: the devil's in de-tail. Hippocampus. 2012;22(1):9–16.
14. Furtado CP, Maller JJ, Fitzgerald PB. A magnetic resonance imaging study of the entorhinal cortex in treatment-resistant depression. Psychiatry Res. 2008;163(2):133–42.
15. Phillips JL, Batten LA, Tremblay P, Aldosary F, Blier P. A prospective, longitudinal study of the effect of remission on cortical thickness and hippocampal volume in patients with treatment-resistant depression. Int J Neuropsychopharmacol. 2015;18(8):1–9.
16. de Kwaasteniet BP, Rive MM, Ruhe HG, Schene AH, Veltman DJ, Fellinger L, et al. Decreased resting-state connectivity between neurocognitive networks in treatment resistant depression. Front Psych. 2015;6:28.
17. Guo W, Liu F, Xue Z, Gao K, Liu Z, Xiao C, et al. Abnormal resting-state cerebellar-cerebral functional connectivity in treatment-resistant depression and treatment sensitive depression. Prog Neuro-Psychopharmacol Biol Psychiatry. 2013;44:51–7.
18. Ma C, Ding J, Li J, Guo W, Long Z, Liu F, et al. Resting-state functional connectivity bias of middle temporal gyrus and caudate with altered gray matter volume in major depression. PLoS One. 2012;7(9):e45263.
19. Wu QZ, Li DM, Kuang WH, Zhang TJ, Lui S, Huang XQ, et al. Abnormal regional spontaneous neural activity in treatment-refractory depression revealed by resting-state fMRI. Hum Brain Mapp. 2011;32(8):1290–9.
20. Paillere Martinot ML, Martinot JL, Ringuenet D, Galinowski A, Gallarda T, Bellivier F, et al. Baseline brain metabolism in resistant depression and response to transcranial magnetic stimulation. Neuropsychopharmacology. 2011;36(13):2710–9.
21. Dowlati Y, Herrmann N, Swardfager W, Liu H, Sham L, Reim EK, et al. A meta-analysis of cytokines in major depression. Biol Psychiatry. 2010;67(5):446–57.
22. Kim YK, Na KS, Myint AM, Leonard BE. The role of pro-inflammatory cytokines in neuroinflammation, neurogenesis and the neuroendocrine system in major depression. Prog Neuro-Psychopharmacol Biol Psychiatry. 2016;64:277–84.
23. Raison CL, Rutherford RE, Woolwine BJ, Shuo C, Schettler P, Drake DF, et al. A randomized controlled trial of the tumor necrosis factor antagonist infliximab for treatment-resistant depression: the role of baseline inflammatory biomarkers. JAMA Psychiatry. 2013;70(1):31–41.
24. Nelson LH, Lenz KM. Microglia depletion in early life programs persistent changes in social, mood-related,

and locomotor behavior in male and female rats. Behav Brain Res. 2017;316:279–93.
25. Fenn AM, Gensel JC, Huang Y, Popovich PG, Lifshitz J, Godbout JP. Immune activation promotes depression 1 month after diffuse brain injury: a role for primed microglia. Biol Psychiatry. 2014;76(7):575–84.
26. Noda M. Dysfunction of glutamate receptors in microglia may cause neurodegeneration. Curr Alzheimer Res. 2016;13(4):381–6.
27. Lindqvist D, Dhabhar FS, James SJ, Hough CM, Jain FA, Bersani FS, et al. Oxidative stress, inflammation and treatment response in major depression. Psychoneuroendocrinology. 2017;76:197–205.
28. Emsley JG, Mitchell BD, Kempermann G, Macklis JD. Adult neurogenesis and repair of the adult CNS with neural progenitors, precursors, and stem cells. Prog Neurobiol. 2005;75(5):321–41.
29. Ernst A, Frisen J. Adult neurogenesis in humans-common and unique traits in mammals. PLoS Biol. 2015;13(1):e1002045.
30. Vadodaria KC, Gage FH. SnapShot: adult hippocampal neurogenesis. Cell. 2014;156(5):1114–e1.
31. Cameron HA, Glover LR. Adult neurogenesis: beyond learning and memory. Annu Rev Psychol. 2015;66:53–81.
32. Odaka H, Adachi N, Numakawa T. Impact of glucocorticoid on neurogenesis. Neural Regen Res. 2017;12(7):1028–35.
33. Vollmayr B, Mahlstedt MM, Henn FA. Neurogenesis and depression: what animal models tell us about the link. Eur Arch Psychiatry Clin Neurosci. 2007;257(5):300–3.
34. Parnet P, Kelley KW, Bluthe RM, Dantzer R. Expression and regulation of interleukin-1 receptors in the brain. Role in cytokines-induced sickness behavior. J Neuroimmunol. 2002;125(1–2):5–14.
35. Arai K, Matsuki N, Ikegaya Y, Nishiyama N. Deterioration of spatial learning performances in lipopolysaccharide-treated mice. Jpn J Pharmacol. 2001;87(3):195–201.
36. Koo JW, Duman RS. IL-1beta is an essential mediator of the antineurogenic and anhedonic effects of stress. Proc Natl Acad Sci U S A. 2008;105(2):751–6.
37. Wu MD, Hein AM, Moravan MJ, Shaftel SS, Olschowka JA, O'Banion MK. Adult murine hippocampal neurogenesis is inhibited by sustained IL-1beta and not rescued by voluntary running. Brain Behav Immun. 2012;26(2):292–300.
38. Kaneko N, Kudo K, Mabuchi T, Takemoto K, Fujimaki K, Wati H, et al. Suppression of cell proliferation by interferon-alpha through interleukin-1 production in adult rat dentate gyrus. Neuropsychopharmacology. 2006;31(12):2619–26.
39. Taga T, Kishimoto T. Gp130 and the interleukin-6 family of cytokines. Annu Rev Immunol. 1997;15:797–819.
40. Holmberg KH, Patterson PH. Leukemia inhibitory factor is a key regulator of astrocytic, microglial and neuronal responses in a low-dose pilocarpine injury model. Brain Res. 2006;1075(1):26–35.
41. Watanabe Y, Hashimoto S, Kakita A, Takahashi H, Ko J, Mizuno M, et al. Neonatal impact of leukemia inhibitory factor on neurobehavioral development in rats. Neurosci Res. 2004;48(3):345–53.
42. Aharoni R, Arnon R, Eilam R. Neurogenesis and neuroprotection induced by peripheral immunomodulatory treatment of experimental autoimmune encephalomyelitis. J Neurosci Off J Soc Neurosci. 2005;25(36):8217–28.
43. Sheng W, Zong Y, Mohammad A, Ajit D, Cui J, Han D, et al. Pro-inflammatory cytokines and lipopolysaccharide induce changes in cell morphology, and upregulation of ERK1/2, iNOS and sPLA(2)-IIA expression in astrocytes and microglia. J Neuroinflammation. 2011;8:121.
44. Yang L, Lindholm K, Konishi Y, Li R, Shen Y. Target depletion of distinct tumor necrosis factor receptor subtypes reveals hippocampal neuron death and survival through different signal transduction pathways. J Neurosci Off J Soc Neurosci. 2002;22(8):3025–32.
45. Marchetti L, Klein M, Schlett K, Pfizenmaier K, Eisel UL. Tumor necrosis factor (TNF)-mediated neuroprotection against glutamate-induced excitotoxicity is enhanced by N-methyl-D-aspartate receptor activation. Essential role of a TNF receptor 2-mediated phosphatidylinositol 3-kinase-dependent NF-kappa B pathway. J Biol Chem. 2004;279(31):32869–81.
46. Dybedal I, Bryder D, Fossum A, Rusten LS, Jacobsen SE. Tumor necrosis factor (TNF)-mediated activation of the p55 TNF receptor negatively regulates maintenance of cycling reconstituting human hematopoietic stem cells. Blood. 2001;98(6):1782–91.
47. Iosif RE, Ekdahl CT, Ahlenius H, Pronk CJ, Bonde S, Kokaia Z, et al. Tumor necrosis factor receptor 1 is a negative regulator of progenitor proliferation in adult hippocampal neurogenesis. J Neurosci Off J Soc Neurosci. 2006;26(38):9703–12.
48. Chen J, Jacobs-Helber SM, Barber DL, Sawyer ST. Erythropoietin-dependent autocrine secretion of tumor necrosis factor-alpha in hematopoietic cells modulates proliferation via MAP kinase--ERK-1/2 and does not require tyrosine docking sites in the EPO receptor. Exp Cell Res. 2004;298(1):155–66.
49. Arnett HA, Mason J, Marino M, Suzuki K, Matsushima GK, Ting JP. TNF alpha promotes proliferation of oligodendrocyte progenitors and remyelination. Nat Neurosci. 2001;4(11):1116–22.
50. Beattie EC, Stellwagen D, Morishita W, Bresnahan JC, Ha BK, Von Zastrow M, et al. Control of synaptic strength by glial TNFalpha. Science. 2002;295(5563):2282–5.
51. Serafini G, Howland RH, Rovedi F, Girardi P, Amore M. The role of ketamine in treatment-resistant depression: a systematic review. Curr Neuropharmacol. 2014;12(5):444–61.
52. Choi DW. Glutamate neurotoxicity in cortical cell culture is calcium dependent. Neurosci Lett. 1985;58(3):293–7.
53. Balazs R. Trophic effect of glutamate. Curr Top Med Chem. 2006;6(10):961–8.

54. Nakanishi S. Molecular diversity of glutamate receptors and implications for brain function. Science. 1992;258(5082):597–603.
55. Lapidus KA, Soleimani L, Murrough JW. Novel glutamatergic drugs for the treatment of mood disorders. Neuropsychiatr Dis Treat. 2013;9:1101–12.
56. Lipton SA, Kater SB. Neurotransmitter regulation of neuronal outgrowth, plasticity and survival. Trends Neurosci. 1989;12(7):265–70.
57. Zhou X, Chen Z, Yun W, Ren J, Li C, Wang H. Extrasynaptic NMDA receptor in excitotoxicity: function revisited. Neuroscientist: Rev J Bringing Neurobiol Neurol Psychiatry. 2015;21(4):337–44.
58. Hardingham GE, Bading H. Synaptic versus extrasynaptic NMDA receptor signalling: implications for neurodegenerative disorders. Nat Rev Neurosci. 2010;11(10):682–96.
59. Popoli M, Yan Z, McEwen BS, Sanacora G. The stressed synapse: the impact of stress and glucocorticoids on glutamate transmission. Nat Rev Neurosci. 2011;13(1):22–37.
60. Zheng K, Scimemi A, Rusakov DA. Receptor actions of synaptically released glutamate: the role of transporters on the scale from nanometers to microns. Biophys J. 2008;95(10):4584–96.
61. Ivanov A, Pellegrino C, Rama S, Dumalska I, Salyha Y, Ben-Ari Y, et al. Opposing role of synaptic and extrasynaptic NMDA receptors in regulation of the extracellular signal-regulated kinases (ERK) activity in cultured rat hippocampal neurons. J Physiol. 2006;572(Pt 3):789–98.
62. Kaufman AM, Milnerwood AJ, Sepers MD, Coquinco A, She K, Wang L, et al. Opposing roles of synaptic and extrasynaptic NMDA receptor signaling in cocultured striatal and cortical neurons. J Neurosci Off J Soc Neurosci. 2012;32(12):3992–4003.
63. Molokanova E, Akhtar MW, Sanz-Blasco S, Tu S, Pina-Crespo JC, McKercher SR, et al. Differential effects of synaptic and extrasynaptic NMDA receptors on Abeta-induced nitric oxide production in cerebrocortical neurons. J Neurosci Off J Soc Neurosci. 2014;34(14):5023–8.
64. Doherty AJ, Palmer MJ, Bortolotto ZA, Hargreaves A, Kingston AE, Ornstein PL, et al. A novel, competitive mGlu(5) receptor antagonist (LY344545) blocks DHPG-induced potentiation of NMDA responses but not the induction of LTP in rat hippocampal slices. Br J Pharmacol. 2000;131(2):239–44.
65. Awad H, Hubert GW, Smith Y, Levey AI, Conn PJ. Activation of metabotropic glutamate receptor 5 has direct excitatory effects and potentiates NMDA receptor currents in neurons of the subthalamic nucleus. J Neurosci Off J Soc Neurosci. 2000;20(21):7871–9.
66. Palucha-Poniewiera A, Wieronska JM, Branski P, Burnat G, Chruscicka B, Pilc A. Is the mGlu5 receptor a possible target for new antidepressant drugs? Pharmacol Rep : PR. 2013;65(6):1506–11.
67. Anwyl R. Metabotropic glutamate receptors: electrophysiological properties and role in plasticity. Rev Neurosci. 1992;3(3):217–31.
68. Wright RA, Johnson BG, Zhang C, Salhoff C, Kingston AE, Calligaro DO, et al. CNS distribution of metabotropic glutamate 2 and 3 receptors: transgenic mice and [(3)H]LY459477 autoradiography. Neuropharmacology. 2013;66:89–98.
69. Williams CJ, Dexter DT. Neuroprotective and symptomatic effects of targeting group III mGlu receptors in neurodegenerative disease. J Neurochem. 2014;129(1):4–20.
70. Kettenmann H, Verkhratsky A. Neuroglia: the 150 years after. Trends Neurosci. 2008;31(12):653–9.
71. Parpura V, Basarsky TA, Liu F, Jeftinija K, Jeftinija S, Haydon PG. Glutamate-mediated astrocyte-neuron signalling. Nature. 1994;369(6483):744–7.
72. Krystal JH, Sanacora G, Duman RS. Rapid-acting glutamatergic antidepressants: the path to ketamine and beyond. Biol Psychiatry. 2013;73(12):1133–41.
73. Davalos D, Grutzendler J, Yang G, Kim JV, Zuo Y, Jung S, et al. ATP mediates rapid microglial response to local brain injury in vivo. Nat Neurosci. 2005;8(6):752–8.
74. Riazi K, Galic MA, Kentner AC, Reid AY, Sharkey KA, Pittman QJ. Microglia-dependent alteration of glutamatergic synaptic transmission and plasticity in the hippocampus during peripheral inflammation. J Neurosci Off J Soc Neurosci. 2015;35(12):4942–52.
75. Blakely PK, BK K-DM, Tyler KL, Irani DN. Disrupted glutamate transporter expression in the spinal cord with acute flaccid paralysis caused by West Nile virus infection. J Neuropathol Exp Neurol. 2009;68(10):1061–72.
76. Zhong C, Luo Q, Jiang J. Blockade of N-acetylaspartylglutamate peptidases: a novel protective strategy for brain injuries and neurological disorders. Int J Neurosci. 2014;124(12):867–73.
77. Passani L, Elkabes S, Coyle JT. Evidence for the presence of N-acetylaspartylglutamate in cultured oligodendrocytes and LPS activated microglia. Brain Res. 1998;794(1):143–5.
78. Fontainhas AM, Wang M, Liang KJ, Chen S, Mettu P, Damani M, et al. Microglial morphology and dynamic behavior is regulated by ionotropic glutamatergic and GABAergic neurotransmission. PLoS One. 2011;6(1):e15973.
79. Wang X, Wu H, Miller AH. Interleukin 1alpha (IL-1alpha) induced activation of p38 mitogen-activated protein kinase inhibits glucocorticoid receptor function. Mol Psychiatry. 2004;9(1):65–75.
80. Heninger GR, Delgado PL, Charney DS. The revised monoamine theory of depression: a modulatory role for monoamines, based on new findings from monoamine depletion experiments in humans. Pharmacopsychiatry. 1996;29(1):2–11.
81. Hashioka S, McGeer PL, Monji A, Kanba S. Anti-inflammatory effects of antidepressants: possibili-

ties for preventives against Alzheimer's disease. Cent Nerv Syst Agents Med Chem. 2009;9(1):12–9.
82. Pittenger C, Duman RS. Stress, depression, and neuroplasticity: a convergence of mechanisms. Neuropsychopharmacology. 2008;33(1):88–109.
83. Muller N, Schwarz MJ, Dehning S, Douhe A, Cerovecki A, Goldstein-Muller B, et al. The cyclooxygenase-2 inhibitor celecoxib has therapeutic effects in major depression: results of a double-blind, randomized, placebo controlled, add-on pilot study to reboxetine. Mol Psychiatry. 2006;11(7):680–4.
84. Abbasi SH, Hosseini F, Modabbernia A, Ashrafi M, Akhondzadeh S. Effect of celecoxib add-on treatment on symptoms and serum IL-6 concentrations in patients with major depressive disorder: randomized double-blind placebo-controlled study. J Affect Disord. 2012;141(2–3):308–14.
85. Akhondzadeh S, Jafari S, Raisi F, Nasehi AA, Ghoreishi A, Salehi B, et al. Clinical trial of adjunctive celecoxib treatment in patients with major depression: a double blind and placebo controlled trial. Depress Anxiety. 2009;26(7):607–11.
86. Tyring S, Gottlieb A, Papp K, Gordon K, Leonardi C, Wang A, et al. Etanercept and clinical outcomes, fatigue, and depression in psoriasis: double-blind placebo-controlled randomised phase III trial. Lancet. 2006;367(9504):29–35.
87. Menter A, Augustin M, Signorovitch J, Yu AP, Wu EQ, Gupta SR, et al. The effect of adalimumab on reducing depression symptoms in patients with moderate to severe psoriasis: a randomized clinical trial. J Am Acad Dermatol. 2010;62(5):812–8.
88. Ertenli I, Ozer S, Kiraz S, Apras SB, Akdogan A, Karadag O, et al. Infliximab, a TNF-alpha antagonist treatment in patients with ankylosing spondylitis: the impact on depression, anxiety and quality of life level. Rheumatol Int. 2012;32(2):323–30.
89. Mendlewicz J, Kriwin P, Oswald P, Souery D, Alboni S, Brunello N. Shortened onset of action of antidepressants in major depression using acetylsalicylic acid augmentation: a pilot open-label study. Int Clin Psychopharmacol. 2006;21(4):227–31.
90. Miyaoka T, Wake R, Furuya M, Liaury K, Ieda M, Kawakami K, et al. Minocycline as adjunctive therapy for patients with unipolar psychotic depression: an open-label study. Prog Neuro-Psychopharmacol Biol Psychiatry. 2012;37(2):222–6.
91. Ajmone-Cat MA, Cacci E, Minghetti L. Non steroidal anti-inflammatory drugs and neurogenesis in the adult mammalian brain. Curr Pharm Des. 2008;14(14):1435–42.
92. Monje ML, Toda H, Palmer TD. Inflammatory blockade restores adult hippocampal neurogenesis. Science. 2003;302(5651):1760–5.
93. Uppal A, Singh A, Gahtori P, Ghosh SK, Ahmad MZ. Antidepressants: current strategies and future opportunities. Curr Pharm Des. 2010;16(38):4243–53.
94. Huynh NN, McIntyre RS. What are the implications of the STAR*D trial for primary care? A review and synthesis. Prim Care Companion J Clin Psychiatry. 2008;10(2):91–6.
95. Dutta A, McKie S, Deakin JF. Ketamine and other potential glutamate antidepressants. Psychiatry Res. 2015;225(1–2):1–13.
96. McGirr A, Berlim MT, Bond DJ, Fleck MP, Yatham LN. Lam RW. A systematic review and meta-analysis of randomized, double-blind, placebo-controlled trials of ketamine in the rapid treatment of major depressive episodes. Psychol Med. 2015;45(4):693–704.
97. Autry AE, Adachi M, Nosyreva E, Na ES, Los MF, Cheng PF, et al. NMDA receptor blockade at rest triggers rapid behavioural antidepressant responses. Nature. 2011;475(7354):91–5.

Treatment-Resistant Schizophrenia: Assessment and Management

8

Sandeep Grover, Harsh Garekar, and Anisha Agarwal

8.1 Introduction

Schizophrenia is a chronic debilitating disorder, which affects 1% of the world population, with no differences across countries or cultures [1]. With the discovery of chlorpromazine in the 1950s, pharmacological treatment became the mainstay of treatment. This was soon followed by introduction of thioridazine, haloperidol, fluphenazine, and several other antipsychotics [2]. Clozapine was the first "atypical" antipsychotic, discovered in Switzerland in 1958. It is a dibenzodiazepine derivative, with ten times greater affinity for D4 receptors than D2 receptors; in addition it has high affinity for 5-HT receptors. Due to its effectiveness and lack of extrapyramidal effects, it was approved for use in Europe in 1972 and was used extensively in patients with psychosis. But in 1975, significant hematological side effects associated with clozapine were recognized, and about 50 patients around the world had died due to granulocytopenia [3]. Clozapine was subsequently withdrawn from the market and was forgotten till 1988, when John Kane and others, after approval from the US Food and Drug Administration (FDA), conducted a multicenter trial on its effectiveness in treatment-refractory psychosis. Comparing the effects of clozapine with chlorpromazine in patients with TRS, the study showed a 30% response rate for clozapine as compared to 4% for chlorpromazine, with significantly greater improvements on Brief Psychiatric Rating Scale (BPRS), Clinical Global Impression (CGI) Scale, and Nurses' Observation Scale for Inpatient Evaluation (NOSIE). The improvement was seen in both positive and negative symptoms [4]. This led to the emergence of concept of treatment-resistant schizophrenia (TRS), which was considered as an indication for use of clozapine. The concept of TRS has evolved over the last three decades, and various definitions of TRS have emerged, based on past evidence and clinical applicability.

The 1990s also saw the introduction of the second-generation antipsychotic drugs (SGAs) such as risperidone, olanzapine, quetiapine, ziprasidone, aripiprazole, and paliperidone. The SGAs not only reduced the burden of extrapyramidal symptoms but also improved outcomes in patients not responding to the first generation of antipsychotics (FGAs). Despite such expansion in the range of available drugs, a significant number of patients still fail to achieve full remission, and another subgroup of patients remains severely ill with persistent psychotic symptoms. Due to this, the concept of TRS is still relevant in the clinical practice, and clozapine has its role in the management of schizophrenia. The chapter focuses on the

S. Grover (✉) · H. Garekar · A. Agarwal
Department of Psychiatry, Postgraduate Institute of Medical Education and Research, Chandigarh, India

Y.-K. Kim (ed.), *Treatment Resistance in Psychiatry*, https://doi.org/10.1007/978-981-10-4358-1_8

evolution of the concept of treatment resistance and the treatment strategies developed so far to manage it.

8.2 Definitions of Treatment-Resistant Schizophrenia

During the 1970s, chronic hospitalization (hospitalization for more than 2 years) was considered one of the most important indicators of treatment resistance in schizophrenia. This approach was of little help in ascertaining treatment responsiveness as reasons for chronic hospitalization varied from poor treatment adherence to inadequate psychosocial rehabilitation. However, deinstitutionalization and the emergence of a host of antipsychotics led to the transfer of some of symptomatic patients, who were not violent and aggressive, from custodial care to the community care. Some of these patients were symptomatic but still could be managed at the community level. Accordingly, the focus for treatment resistance shifted to symptoms, rather than the duration of hospitalization. Subsequent revisions of diagnostic systems (Diagnostic and Statistical Manual of Mental Disorders [DSM] and International Classification of Diseases [ICD]) also led to a more narrow definition of schizophrenia. Positive symptoms were given more importance in diagnosis and consequently became the focus of management. Accordingly, when Kane et al. (1988) defined the criteria for TRS, persistent positive symptoms despite adequate drug therapy were the essential criterion for treatment resistance in schizophrenia. They considered a patient to have TRS if [5–7]:

1. Historically: Treatment with at least two different classes of antipsychotics at doses equal to 1000 mg/day of chlorpromazine for at least three periods of 6 weeks in the last 5 years without significant clinical improvement
2. Actual: BPRS score of at least 45. Score of at least ≥4 on two of the following BPRS items of conceptual disorganization, unusual thoughts, hallucinatory behavior, and suspiciousness and Clinical Global Impression (CGI) score of ≥4 (moderately ill)
3. Prospective: No improvement after 6 weeks of treatment with haloperidol (up to 60 mg/day or higher); improvement defined as reduction of at least 20% on BPRS as compared with the level of severity defined by the actual criteria and/or a posttreatment CGI of ≤3 or BPRS ≤35

This definition paved the way for use of clozapine in a subset of patients with remarkable results. Further, proper monitoring for agranulocytosis showed that the incidence of agranulocytosis was lower than that reported earlier. This led to an expansion of clinician experience with the use of clozapine, and gradually the molecule emerged as the gold standard for management of TRS. Since the beginning, the concept of TRS as defined by Kane et al. has been questioned by contemporary researchers, and this has led to the proliferation of multiple definitions of TRS (Table 8.1). Brenner et al. (1990) proposed a dimensional approach to TRS and described seven levels of response ranging from full clinical remission to severely refractory. This definition implies that some patient's levels of response may worsen over time and also takes into account patients' functional, social, and personal levels and not just the existence of active symptoms [8]. Meltzer in 1992 proposed to assess treatment resistance in schizophrenia according to different parameters, i.e., psychopathology, cognitive function, extrapyramidal functions, social functioning, independence and work functioning, quality of life, reinstatement, dependences, cost of the illness, as well as treatment [9]. His criteria are considered to be less strict and more useful in clinical practice. But the disadvantage of this approach is that all partial responders are considered equal and not to differ qualitatively from patients who are completely refractory. The original criteria proposed by Kane et al. also underwent modification driven by pharmacological evidence that doses of more than 400 mg/day of chlorpromazine led to blockade of 80–90% of dopaminergic receptors [10]. Accordingly, the criteria were modified as [6]:

1. Historical: at least three treatments with typical antipsychotic from two different chemical

Table 8.1 Various definitions of TRS

Year	Author	Definition of TRS			
1988	Kane et al. [5]	Persistent positive symptoms (PPS) despite adequate drug therapy to be the essential criterion			
		1. Historical: Treatment with at least two different classes of antipsychotics at doses equal to 1000 mg/day of chlorpromazine for at least three periods of 6 weeks in the last 5 years without significant clinical improvement			
		2. Actual: BPRS score of at least 45. Score of at least ≥4 on two of the following BPRS items of conceptual disorganization, unusual thoughts, hallucinatory behavior, and suspiciousness and CGI score ≥4 (moderately ill)			
		3. Prospective: No improvement after 6 weeks of treatment with haloperidol (up to 60 mg/day or higher); improvement is defined as reduction of at least 20% on BPRS as compared with the level of severity defined by the actual criteria and/or a posttreatment CGI of ≤3 or BPRS ≤35			
1988–1990	Brenner et al. [10]	Level 1	Clinical remission	No need for a formal rehabilitation program	Rapid response to antipsychotics at recommended doses. Patient may show anhedonia or another negative symptom. CGI normal and score <2 on BPRS. Good functional level without supervision
		Level 2	Partial remission	No need for a formal rehabilitation program	Rapid reduction of psychotic symptoms. Mild signs of residual psychotic symptoms. CGI score of 2. None of the BPRS scale items are ≥3
		Level 3	Light resistance	Need for a rehabilitation program	Slight or incomplete reduction of symptoms with positive and negative residual symptoms. Alteration of social or personal functioning in at least two areas and requiring occasional supervision. No more than one item with a score ≥4 on the BPRS
		Level 4	Moderate resistance	Need for a rehabilitation program	Reduction of symptoms but with a clear persistence of them, affecting six or more areas of social and personal functioning and requiring frequent supervision. CGI 4. A score of 4 or 2 BPRS items. A BPRS score ≥45 on the 18-item version and 60 on the 24-item version
		Level 5	Severe resistance	Need for a continuous strategy, individual and oriented toward attempts with atypical antipsychotics and adjuvant treatment	Reduction of symptoms but with a clear persistence of them, affecting six or more areas of social and personal functioning and requiring frequent supervision. CGI 5. A score of 5 on 1 BPRS item or ≥4 on 3 items. A total BPRS >50 on the 18-item version and 67 on the 24-item version
		Level 6	Refractoriness	Longer-term hospitalization with pharmacological and psychosocial attempts	Reduction of mild or non-demonstrable symptoms and persistence of positive and negative symptoms with marked alteration in all areas of social and personal functioning. CGI 6. A score of 6 on 1 BPRS item or of ≥5 on 2 items. Total BPRS score of ≥5 per level
		Level 7	Severe refractoriness	Longer-term hospitalization with pharmacological and psychosocial attempts	No reduction of symptoms with many positive and negative symptoms associated with behavioral alterations. All areas of social and personal functioning have deteriorated, requiring constant supervision. CGI 7. A score of 7 on 1 BPRS item. Total score of ≥5 per level
1989	Wilson et al. [11]	Persistence of symptoms after 2.5 years of treatment with three different classes of neuroleptics (dosage of 1000 mg of chlorpromazine equivalents) for 8 weeks in the last 5 years			
1989	Schüssler et al. [12]	Insufficient improvement after administering neuroleptic treatment for 4 weeks			
1991	Keefe et al. [13]	There is no sufficient improvement after their neuroleptic treatment (40 mg haloperidol/day) during 6 weeks			

classes at doses equivalent to 400–600 mg/day of chlorpromazine for a period of at least 6 weeks, without significant relief. No period of good functioning within the preceding 5 years.
2. Actual: A score of at least 45 in the BPRS with score of ≥4 in two of the following: conceptual disorganization, unusual thought content, hallucinatory behavior, and suspiciousness and CGI score ≥4 (moderately ill).
3. Prospective: No improvement after 6 weeks of treatment with haloperidol (up to 60 mg/day or higher); improvement is defined as reduction of at least 20% on the Brief Psychiatric Rating Scale (BPRS) as compared with the level of severity defined by the actual criteria; and BPRS ≤35 points on the BPRS and CGI score ≤3.

Over the last decade, with more experience in the use of clozapine and reduction in the dread of using clozapine, more and more authors rely on using modified Kane's criteria for defining TRS. Various treatment guidelines have also adopted similar definitions and diluted the same further (Table 8.2). In general these guidelines suggest that if a patient has a lack of satisfactory clinical improvement despite sequential use of the recommended doses of at least two antipsychotics for 6–8 weeks, at least one of which should be an atypical, and then the patient should be considered as having TRS.

Table 8.2 Definition of TRS as per various treatment guidelines

Author	Criterion of treatment resistance
APA 2004 [14]	Insufficient response to two clinical trials of 4- or 6-week duration using monotherapy with two different SGAs or two trials with FGAs, if SGAs are not available. It is considered that the patient is treatment-resistant and is a candidate for clozapine
Maudsley 2015 [15]	Failure to respond to at least two antipsychotics (either SGA/FGA), each given for at least for 2–3 weeks. If some response detected, continue for a total of at least 4 weeks before abandoning treatment
NICE 2014 [16]	Lack of satisfactory clinical improvement despite sequential use of the recommended doses for 6–8 weeks of at least two antipsychotics, at least one of which should be SGA
IPAP 2006 [17]	No period of good functioning in the previous 5 years
	Prior nonresponse to at least two antipsychotics of two different chemical classes for at least 4–6 weeks each at doses ≥400 mg equivalents of CPZ or 5 mg/day of risperidone
	Moderate to severe psychopathology, especially positive symptoms: conceptual disorganization, hallucinatory behavior, suspiciousness, or delusions

APA American Psychiatric Association, *NICE* National Institute of Clinical Excellence, *IPAP* International Psychopharmacology Algorithm Project

8.3 Current Perspective of TRS

Treatment resistance in schizophrenia is a concept that still holds different positions in clinical settings and research areas. Categorical and criteria-based approach with more emphasis on positive symptoms is preferred for research, while individualized and holistic view for treatment resistance seems appropriate for day-to-day clinical situations. Regarding pharmacological treatment of TRS, till now only clozapine has demonstrated conclusive favorable evidence. The management of TRS is a persistent public health problem, because patients with TRS experience the worst outcomes, such as suicide and homelessness. TRS can manifest as failure to achieve remission from the initial episode of psychosis, failure to maintain remission, or gradual deterioration in the patient's status.

8.4 Factors Associated with TRS

Some of the studies have attempted to identify the risk factors for TRS. Studies which have evaluated neurodevelopment predictors of poor response to treatment among patients of schizophrenia have shown a link of poor treatment response to lower level of premorbid functioning, presence of deficit state, male gender, cavum septum pellucidum, higher prevalence of obstetrical complications, lateral and third ventricular enlargement, and vulnerability to tardive dyskinesia [18–20]. Other factors which have been linked to some degree of treatment refractoriness among patients of schizophrenia include male gender, early onset of illness, positive family history of schizophrenia, absence of affective symptoms, severe and lengthy premorbid manifestations, longer duration of untreated psychosis, severe negative and cognitive symptoms, presence of soft neurological signs, early onset of abnormal involuntary movements, and low level of social functioning [20–36]. A recent Danish register-based study included 8044 patients of which 1703 (21%) patients fulfilled the main proxy definition of TRS (earliest instance of either clozapine initiation or hospital admission for schizophrenia after having had two periods of different antipsychotic monotherapy) with a median follow-up period of 9.1 years. The factors which were found to be significantly associated with TRS included younger age, living in a less urban area, primary education level, more than 30 bed-days in psychiatric hospital in the year before first schizophrenia diagnosis, inpatient at first schizophrenia diagnosis, paranoid subtype, comorbid personality disorder, psychotropic drug use, use of benzodiazepines, and previous suicide attempt [37].

A recent systematic review evaluated the neuroimaging findings among patients with TRS. Computerized tomography (CT)-based studies have shown smaller prefrontal sulcal prominence reflecting prefrontal atrophy in patients with TRS. Magnetic resonance imaging (MRI) studies show that, compared to healthy controls, patients with TRS have more widespread reduction in cortical thickness (frontal, parietal, temporal, and occipital regions) than patients with non-TRS (frontal regions). When compared to patients with non-TRS, MRI studies suggested a greater reduction in left dorsolateral prefrontal cortex (DLPFC) volume in patients with TRS [38].

8.5 Pharmacotherapy of Treatment-Resistant Schizophrenia

Treatment resistance can occur in approximately 20–30% of all patients with schizophrenia [39]. It is vital that before classifying a patient as treatment-resistant, the possibility of pseudo-resistance be ruled out. The clinician should consider the following steps to rule out pseudo-resistance [40]:

- Upward titration of antipsychotic medications till effective dose range is reached. Checking serum levels if required. Assessing pharmacokinetic interactions with other drugs and smoking.
- Optimizing the duration of antipsychotic therapy, typically a 4- to 6-week trial, with optimal dosing.
- Side effects of psychiatric drugs and other medications may mimic worsening positive (akathisia, delirium) or negative (hypokinesia) symptoms. In such a scenario, reduction in doses may be beneficial.
- Reevaluating the diagnosis of schizophrenia, along with ruling out other general medical or neurologic condition that may be presenting with psychotic symptoms.
- Evaluation for comorbid conditions such as substance use disorders, personality disorders, mania or depression with psychotic symptoms, and obsessive-compulsive disorder (OCD).
- Ensuring drug compliance through pill count, measuring serum levels, checking pharmacy refill dates, and using depot antipsychotic injections [41].

Once the clinicians have ensured that these factors have been taken care of, the patients need to be considered as having true TRS and managed accordingly.

8.6 Management of TRS

Treatment-resistant schizophrenia can often generate feeling of nihilism in the clinician, due to the unrelenting nature of symptoms. Various guidelines therefore warn against such an outlook and advise clinicians to be hopeful of more positive outcomes and continue to treat using the best available evidence. There is no "lost cause," and clinicians should focus on identifying the target symptoms and building an individually tailored treatment program, rather than an algorithm driven.

8.7 Clozapine in TRS

Since the resurgence of clozapine, with Kane et al. showing its superiority over clozapine, its effectiveness in patients with schizophrenia, i.e., those with TRS, has never been questioned much. Many studies after the initial evaluation by Kane et al. have evaluated the effectiveness of clozapine. Lieberman et al. reported that 50% of patients with treatment-refractory illness and 76% of the treatment-intolerant patients respond to clozapine, with treatment continued up to 52 weeks [23]. The safety and efficacy of clozapine were also studied in the UK by the Clozapine Study Group, which found marked improvements in psychopathology in 20 of the 26 inpatients, who completed the 26-week study [42]. The superior effectiveness of clozapine has been supported by two large independently funded studies: Clinical Antipsychotic Trial of Intervention Effectiveness (CATIE) and Cost Utility of the Latest Antipsychotic Drugs in Schizophrenia Study (CUtLASS). In phase 2 of the CATIE trial, the time to all-cause medication discontinuation and the primary outcome measure were significantly better for clozapine compared with all the other antipsychotics (quetiapine, risperidone, ziprasidone, and perphenazine) under evaluation except for olanzapine. Clozapine was significantly superior to olanzapine, quetiapine and risperidone in terms of time to discontinuation due to inadequate therapeutic effect [43]. In CUtLASS study, clozapine was found to be significantly superior to non-clozapine SGAs with regard to symptom reduction and the quality of life [44].

Over the years, understanding about the symptom dimension of schizophrenia broadened and the five-factor model, i.e., positive, negative, cognitive, disorganized, and affective symptoms, is considered as the dimension which represents the clinical picture of schizophrenia. Further, the understanding about the outcome measures has expanded beyond symptom reduction or remission. Accordingly, studies have evaluated the effectiveness of clozapine on various treatment outcomes and symptom dimensions of schizophrenia. Clozapine has also been evaluated in special population like children, adolescents, and elderly, and there is some data on its safety in pregnancy and lactation. Besides its benefit in management of schizophrenia, clozapine has also been shown to have beneficial effect on tardive syndromes.

8.7.1 Positive and Negative Symptoms

Using data from published systematic reviews and meta-analysis, clozapine response rates among people with TRS have been found to be around 40%, with a mean reduction of 22 points on PANSS [45]. Another meta-analysis of two decades of data from 30 randomized clinical trials, which evaluated the short-term outcome of 2530 patients assigned to different treatments, showed that patients treated with clozapine had better clinical improvement and had significantly lower number of relapses during treatment. This meta-analysis also showed that the risk for blood dyscrasias with long-term use of clozapine was as high as 7% [46]. A subsequent meta-analysis which included studies comparing clozapine with other antipsychotics and took into account the heterogeneity and duration of the studies, the initial psychopathology of patients, the year of publication, and sponsorship in the selected clinical trials still found an effect size of 0.44 in favor of clozapine [47]. Another recent systematic review and meta-analysis included the data from 21 RCTs evaluating the efficacy of clozapine against other antipsychotics. It included data of 1131 patients enrolled in the clozapine arm and 1233 patients in the control medication arm. Of these patients, final follow-up data was available for 801 and 799 patients in the clozapine and other antipsychotic arms, respectively. This meta-analysis showed that clozapine was superior in reducing positive psychotic symptoms in both the short (less than 3 months) and long term (more than 3 months). For negative symptoms, clozapine was superior in the short term but not in the long term. When compared to specific antipsychotics, clozapine was found to be superior to olanzapine, haloperidol, and chlorpromazine in the short term, while these differences were not significant when compared with olanzapine and risperidone in the long term. A lack of efficacy for negative symptoms may explain this lack of difference in the long term [48].

8.7.2 Cognitive Symptoms

Several studies over the past decades have tried to assess the impact of atypical antipsychotics on cognitive function in patients with schizophrenia, based on their effects on cholinergic and 5-HT2a-mediated neurotransmission. While all atypical antipsychotics have shown variable levels of improvement, clozapine has been consistently found to improve verbal fluency, attention, and motor speed in patients with TRS [49, 50].

8.7.3 Suicidality and Aggression

There is emerging evidence to suggest that clozapine can be particularly effective in reducing specific behavioral problems of violence, aggression, and suicidality in patients with schizophrenia. Clozapine is the only FDA-recommended treatment for reducing suicidal risk in schizophrenia. This was demonstrated in the International Suicide Prevention Trial (Inter SePT), a 2-year, multicenter, randomized study comparing clozapine and olanzapine in 980 people with schizophrenia, at a high risk for suicide. During the study period, compared to patients receiving olanzapine, lower number of patients on clozapine attempted suicide (34 vs. 55%) and required hospitalizations (82 vs. 107%) and rescue interventions (118 vs. 155%) to prevent suicide [51]. A population-based cohort study of 2370 individuals with TRS from 1996 to 2013, extracting information from the Danish National Prescription Registry, found that non-clozapine antipsychotic treatment was associated with an increased rate of self-harm, with hazard ratio of 1.36 compared to clozapine. The results also demonstrated a nearly twofold higher mortality rate among those not treated with clozapine [52].

However, a recent systematic review, which evaluated the data published during 2005–2014, showed that, with the strengthening of the restriction in access to lethal means and school-based awareness programs, the anti-suicidal effect of clozapine is substantiated, but it might be less specific than thought earlier [53]. Clozapine can reduce violence and persistent impulsive aggression in patients with schizophrenia and other psychiatric disorders, independent of their effects on core psychopathology. The anti-aggressive effect is particularly marked in those with TRS [54–56].

8.7.4 Depressive Symptoms

Clozapine has also been shown to have better antidepressant effect in patients with schizophrenia compared to other antipsychotic medications. A reanalysis of the CATIE trial data showed that clozapine was as effective as olanzapine and risperidone but was more effective than quetiapine [57].

8.7.5 Catatonic Symptoms

Although systematic studies are lacking, data in the form of case reports suggest that clozapine can be beneficial in patients with persistent catatonia and recurrent catatonia [58].

8.7.6 Quality of Life

The effect of clozapine on the quality of life of patients with TRS has been evaluated extensively. Meltzer et al. in 1990, using the quality-of-life scale, provided an objective measure of changes in patients' psychosocial functioning, who had been on clozapine for 6 months. Significant improvements were reported in all factors of quality of life, namely, material and physical well-being, relationships, social activities, and personal development [59]. Another study reported improvement in quality of life only in patients who continued to take clozapine for 2 years [60]. Subsequent studies including RCTs have shown that, compared to haloperidol and other atypical antipsychotics, clozapine has a significant positive impact on quality of life at 1 year [61, 62]. However, occasional studies do not support the beneficial effect of clozapine in terms of quality of life [63]. Multiple surveys of patients highlight the positive regard and high subjective satisfaction with clozapine as compared to other neuroleptics [64, 65].

8.7.7 Children and Adolescents

The use of clozapine in children and adolescents for childhood-onset schizophrenia (COS) has followed the same pattern as in adults. Despite not being currently approved for treatment in pediatric population, clozapine has been used in patients not responding to first- or second-line medications. There are a number of case series and open trials, which have shown the efficacy of clozapine in children and adolescents who have not responded to conventional neuroleptics [66, 67]. However only a handful of small randomized controlled trials have been conducted to test its effectiveness in treatment-refractory COS. In a 6-week double-blind comparison, with haloperidol in 21 patients, with onset before the age of 12 years, who had been unresponsive to conventional neuroleptics, clozapine was superior on all measures of psychosis [68]. In another 8-week randomized, double-blind trial, with a 2-year open-label follow-up, clozapine when compared with olanzapine showed a significant reduction in both positive and negative symptoms. However, clozapine was associated with more overall adverse events, such as lipid abnormalities and seizures [69]. In a meta-analysis of current evidence of use of antipsychotics in childhood-onset schizophrenia, when clozapine was compared with other antipsychotics, clozapine was more efficacious than other antipsychotics with effect size of 0.848 (based upon 85 participants; CI 0.748–0.948) [70]. So in conclusion, it can be stated that, despite the burden of side effects, clozapine remains the most effective medication for treatment-refractory COS.

8.7.8 Clozapine in Pregnancy and Postpartum

Pregnancy and the immediate postpartum period are being increasingly recognized as a high-risk period for psychotic exacerbations; however studies on clozapine use during this period are limited. The effectiveness of clozapine in treatment-refractory cases during pregnancy has been stated only in case reports and small case series [71, 72]. Clozapine is currently included in category B by the US FDA, implying no evidence of risk in humans and under the L3 category (moderately safe) for lactation. This is in contrast to other atypical and typical antipsychotics, which are category C drugs and are associated with potential risks. A recent review of 21 studies which included case series and case reports did not find an increased risk of congenital malformations in fetuses exposed to clozapine but possibly contributed to increased rates of floppy baby syndrome, decreased heart rate variability, and seizures in infancy [73]. Clozapine use has also been associated with increased risk of gestational diabetes, in women who have pre-existing risk factors such as diabetes, obesity or a family history of diabetes. The developmental effects of clozapine, in comparison with other atypical antipsychotics, were investigated in a 12-month study of 63 infants. The study showed that clozapine-exposed infants showed no difference in cognitive, language, motor, social, and emotional development at all time points, but adaptive behavior was delayed at 2 and 6 months of age [74]. In terms of pharmacokinetics, the plasma concentration of clozapine can decrease during pregnancy due to increased hepatic metabolism and volume of distribution. A review of case reports and pharmacovigilance data of nearly 200 patients has recommended that clozapine dose should be increased during psychotic symptom exacerbation and a typical antipsychotic like perphenazine, trifluoperazine or haloperidol can be added to clozapine [75]. Substitution of clozapine is not recommended as it can lead to psychotic exacerbation during pregnancy. The dual goal of reducing infant exposure and controlling symptoms can only be achieved by an individualized risk-benefit analysis in partnership with the patient. Each case must be evaluated on an individual basis by taking into account the number and severity of previous episodes.

8.7.9 Elderly

The use of clozapine in the elderly is particularly fraught with danger due to a high susceptibility for not just the serious adverse effects like agranulocytosis, myocarditis, seizures, and metabolic syndrome but also for the commoner side effects like sedation, constipation, urinary incontinence, and hypersalivation [76]. Despite the potential pitfalls, clozapine has been found to be an effective drug for resistant cases in studies carried out in the geriatric population. In a retrospective chart review of 527 elderly patients, with chronic resistant schizophrenia, rehospitalization rates were found to be significantly lower for clozapine, and mortality was equal to that of other antipsychotics [77]. In another review of 133 elderly patients, clozapine showed marked to moderate improvements in psychotic symptoms at a relatively low mean dose of 134 mg/day, which was well tolerated [78]. Although clozapine efficacy in treatment-resistant cases in the elderly is similar to that in the younger age group, the burden of side effects is higher. The risk of agranulocytosis has been estimated to be five to ten times higher than the quoted 1% risk for general population [79]. Fatal myocarditis has also been reported in the elderly [80]. While other common side effects of clozapine are often manageable, clozapine use in the elderly must be done with caution after a careful assessment of the risk to benefit ratio.

8.7.10 Clozapine in Patients with Tardive Syndromes

Tardive syndromes are delayed-onset syndromes, which include tardive dyskinesia, tardive dystonia, tardive akathisia, tardive stereotypy, tardive tourettism, tardive myoclonus, tardive tremor, and tardive parkinsonism. They are associated with both atypical and typical antipsychotic exposure, with possible pathogenic mechanism involving hypersensitivity of dopamine receptors. Clozapine is associated with the lowest risk of extrapyramidal side effects, and current evidence suggests that clozapine can significantly diminish dyskinetic movements in patients with tardive syndromes. However some reports have also suggested conflicting findings of development/worsening of tardive syndromes [81]. In an 18-week study of clozapine in patients with TRS, with coexisting tardive dyskinesia, chronic akathisia, and parkinsonism, the use of low-dose clozapine led to improvement rates of 74% for tardive dyskinesia, 69% for parkinsonism, and 78% for chronic akathisia [82]. In a case series including patients with affective psychosis with tardive syndromes, low-dose clozapine showed response rates varying from 50% to 100% [83]. A systematic review of 15 trials and 28 case series/reports supported the beneficial effects of clozapine, taking in to account reports which suggested emergence of tardive syndromes with clozapine [84].

8.8 Clozapine: Prescription Practices and Barrier in Use

While clozapine has maintained its place as the treatment of choice in TRS and endorsed as the gold standard of therapy in all practice guidelines, its use has been found to be lower than recommended [85]. It has been found that clozapine accounts for <5% of the antipsychotics prescribed, and an estimated five to ten times more patients could benefit from clozapine than who are now receiving it [86, 87]. Despite the available evidence in favor of clozapine in treatment of TRS, it is often seen that in many patients starting of clozapine is delayed. Studies across the world show that starting of clozapine is often delayed, by 1.6–4.5 years in patients of schizophrenia, despite patients fulfilling the criteria of TRS [88, 89]. A survey of psychiatrists from India showed that, in about 28% of patients, clozapine was not prescribed though indicated [90]. Clinicians resort to use of polypharmacy prior to starting clozapine. Clinicians are reluctant to start clozapine because of fear of agranulocytosis and associated blood monitoring. Other factors, which have been shown to be associated with lower prescription of clozapine, include history of poor medication compliance, lower awareness among prescribers, and fear of side effects [91, 92]. In a study assessing attitude toward clozapine, in patients who are eligible for clozapine, but not yet prescribed so, it was found that the necessity for hospital admission was seen as the greatest barrier to starting clozapine (49% of respondents). In addition, concerns about side effects were another reason for clozapine refusal in 43% of respondents. Around 24% of the respondents felt that clozapine would be a useful option for them. So overall, it is apparent that the overall acceptability of clozapine can be increased by enhanced education about clozapine's benefits, improving management of its side effects and initiating clozapine on an outdoor clinic basis [93].

8.9 Predictors of Response to Clozapine

A number of studies have tried to evaluate the factors associated with good clinical outcomes with the use of clozapine. Some of the demographic and clinical factors which have been shown to be associated with favorable clinical response to clozapine include female gender, presence of extrapyramidal side effects, paranoid subtype, and presence of 22q11.2 deletion [94, 95]. The clinical features which are associated with poor response include early age of onset, catatonia and deficit syndromes [23, 96–99]. Among the biological measures, low pretreatment CSF homovanillic (HVA)/5-hydroxyindoleaceticacid (HIAA) acid levels predict a superior clozapine response, consistent with the dopaminergic and serotonergic components of its mechanism of action [100]. Clinical improvement with clozapine has also been related with the anatomy and metabolic activity of specific brain areas. Improvement in positive symptoms with clozapine was directly related to temporal gray matter volume, whereas improvement of negative symptoms is seen in patients with high baseline DLPF cortical volume and metabolic activity [101, 102]. The effects of clozapine have also been attributed to changes in regional blood flow. Responders to clozapine show a higher thalamic, left basal ganglia and right prefrontal perfusion prior to starting of clozapine, while clozapine treatment increases bilateral frontal/caudate perfusion ratio; hence across studies it seems that subcortical perfusion of the responders decreases when they received clozapine [103–106]. Despite a growing list of laboratory-based findings, which could function as a predictor of response to clozapine, unequivocal evidence of reproducibility, specificity, and clinical feasibility is absent.

Oral dosage and pharmacokinetic factors also play a pivotal part in determining response. A number of studies have related blood levels with clinical response, recommending a concentration of more than 350 ng/ml for clinical response [107]. The plasma clozapine concentration is influenced by a number of patient factors such as altered cytochrome P450 1A4 activity, age, gender, and smoking. While pivotal studies have used clozapine in the dose range of 100–900 mg, it is suggested that for clinical response, doses above 400 mg must be used [108]. Furthermore, one study has indicated a dose-response relationship, better clinical response with doses of 600 mg/day group than 300 mg/day and least benefit with a dose 100 mg/day [109]. Another important point to note regarding the pharmacokinetics of clozapine is the wide interindividual variability at a given dose. In a Chinese sample of inpatients with schizophrenia, eightfold variability at a given dose was reported [110]. Due to these pharmacokinetic and pharmacodynamic properties of clozapine, an adequate trial with clozapine should last for 4–6 months, with plasma trough levels maintained at 350–400 ng/L for at least 8 weeks [111, 112].

8.10 How to Use Clozapine

In view of side effects (both serious and nonserious), different guidelines have been recommended for starting and maintaining hematological monitoring while using clozapine (Table 8.3). However, occasional reports from resource poor countries have questioned very frequent monitoring and suggest that monitoring at a frequency of 3 months after stabilization of the dose of clozapine may be considered [113]. However, there is lack of systematic data for the same. Besides hematological monitoring, another issue, which has received significant attention, is the development of metabolic disturbances like diabetes mellitus, obesity/weight gain and metabolic syndrome. In fact, as per the American Diabetes Association (ADA) and the American Psychiatric Association (APA) consensus statement on antipsychotic drugs, clozapine along with olanzapine has the highest potential to cause metabolic syndrome [114]. Studies, which have evaluated the prevalence of metabolic syndrome among patients receiving clozapine, have reported it to range from 44% to 64% [115–117]. However, few authors have questioned this high prevalence rate on the basis of the fact that many patients would have fulfilled metabolic syndrome prior to starting of clozapine. Few longitudinal studies, which have evaluated the prevalence of metabolic syndrome, prior to starting clozapine and subsequently, and reevaluated the same after 3–6 months of clozapine, suggest that only about half of the prevalence of metabolic syndrome in patients with clozapine may be attributed to it and the rest of the patients fulfill the criteria of metabolic syndrome prior to starting of clozapine [118, 119]. However, in view of the risk of metabolic syndrome, close monitoring of metabolic parameters is recommended by the APA/ADA consensus statement (Table 8.4).

Table 8.3 Pretreatment assessment and monitoring for clozapine

Baseline evaluation	Complete blood count that includes an absolute neutrophil count (ANC)
	Weight and height (body mass index), waist circumference, fasting blood sugar (or HbA1c), fasting lipids
	Physical examination and vital signs
	ECG
	Liver function tests (LFTs)
	Consider troponin, CRP, beta natriuretic peptide, ESR monitoring (if persisting tachycardia or fever; suspected myocarditis) [120]. Not mandatory but recommended in some guidelines
	Pregnancy test in women of childbearing age
Required blood monitoring	Before initiating therapy – complete blood count that includes an absolute neutrophil count (ANC); WBC >3500/mm^3 and ANC >2000/mm^3
	Mandatory blood monitoring (country specific) [121]
	USA – weekly for the first 26 weeks, then biweekly for 26 weeks, and then monthly
	UK – weekly for the first 18 weeks, then biweekly from 19 to 52 weeks, and then monthly
	Japan – weekly for the first 26 weeks and then biweekly thereafter

ANC absolute neutrophil count, *ECG* electrocardiogram, *CRP* C-reactive protein, *WBC* white blood cell count

Table 8.4 Monitoring of metabolic parameters while using clozapine

Recommended monitoring	Weight/BMI/waist – baseline and then at 1, 3, 6, and 12 months
	Plasma glucose and lipids – at month 1, 6, and 12 months
	Liver function tests – baseline and at 6 months

8.11 Side Effects of Clozapine and Its Management

Clozapine is associated with a wide range of adverse effects, some of which can be potentially life-threatening. Clozapine also has poorer tolerability compared to other antipsychotics. The common side effects of clozapine include sedation, constipation, sialorrhea, weight gain, metabolic disturbances, sinus tachycardia, fever, seizures, and nocturnal enuresis (Table 8.5). The serious side effects of clozapine are agranulocytosis, seizures and myocarditis. These usually require discontinuation of clozapine even before target plasma levels are reached [122, 123]. Therefore, anticipating and addressing these adverse side effects are vital for a clinician to improve adherence. Among the life-threatening adverse effects, agranulocytosis and myocarditis require careful monitoring during the first 3–6 months of clozapine treatment (Table 8.6). Clozapine-induced agranulocytosis can occur in 1% of treated individuals and can be fatal if not detected early. The US Food and Drug Administration (FDA) requires a neutrophil count >1500/microL, to start clozapine, and treatment should be stopped if absolute neutrophil count (ANC) falls below 1000/microL [124].

Table 8.5 Common adverse effects of clozapine and their management

Adverse effect	Frequency/time course	Management
Sedation	Incidence: 10–60% Diminishes over 4–6 weeks	Decreasing dose Slower titration Higher doses at night
Hypersalivation	Incidence: 30–80% Worse at night May persist	Chewing gum, to increase swallowing Using towel over pillow at night Glycopyrrolate, hyoscine, atropine Amisulpride (100–400 mg/day) Amitriptyline Modafinil
Constipation	Incidence: 15–60% Can occur in acute and maintenance phase Can be life-threatening due to necrosis and perforation	High-fiber diet Adequate fluid intake Exercise Stool softeners, osmotic laxatives, enemas
Tachycardia	Incidence: 25% Within first 4 weeks Can persist	Persistent tachycardia can be treated with atenolol, metoprolol, and ivabradine If associated with hypotension, chest pain, fever; may indicate myocarditis
Weight gain	4.45 kg over 10 weeks Can continue over 5 years	Exercise-based weight management program Lifestyle modifications Dietary intervention
Hypotension	Incidence: 10% Tolerance after 4–6 weeks	Reduce dose/slower titration Increase fluid and salt intake Rise slowly from sitting/lying position If severe, consider fludrocortisones
Fever	First 2–3 weeks Lasts for few days Usually benign	Paracetamol Check blood counts Rule out myocarditis and neuroleptic malignant syndrome
Seizures	Incidence: ~6% Related to dose Increased risk at >600 mg/day, rapid escalation of dose and pre-existing seizure disorder	Consider prophylactic valproate, lamotrigine, or gabapentin at high dose (>500 mg/day) Restart at half the previous dose after a seizure
Nocturnal enuresis	Incidence:0.23–41% May occur anytime Spontaneous remission can occur	Behavioral techniques, using an alarm clock Desmopressin nasal spray Anticholinergic agents

Table 8.6 Serious adverse effects with clozapine and their management

Adverse event	Risk/time course	Management
Neutropenia and agranulocytosis	Neutropenia Incidence: 2.7% during first year Incidence: 0.69% during second year Agranulocytosis Incidence: 0.73% during first year Incidence: 0. 07% during second year 80% of cases are seen within 18 weeks of treatment	Mild neutropenia (100–1500/microL) Monitor absolute neutrophil count (ANC) three times weekly till>1500/microL Moderate neutropenia (500–1000/microL) Stop clozapine Monitor ANC daily till>1000 Then monitor three times/week till>1500 Then weekly for 4 weeks Severe neutropenia (<500/microL) Discontinue clozapine Daily ANC till>1000/microL Then three times weekly till ANC>1500 Use granulocyte colony-stimulating factor as a rescue treatment after consultation with hematologist Generally reexposure should not be attempted
Myocarditis and cardiomyopathy	Incidence: 1% 80% of the cases occur during the first 6 weeks	Careful monitoring is essential Baseline – pulse, blood pressure, temperature, respiratory rate, blood counts, ECG Daily – pulse, blood pressure, temperature, respiratory rate; ask about chest pain, fever, cough, shortness of breath, exercise capacity Weekly till 4 weeks – CRP, troponin, complete blood counts, ECG, and echocardiography if possible If CRP > 100 mg/L or troponin > twice upper limit of normal – stop clozapine; repeat echo Rechallenge with clozapine associated with high mortality rates
Neuroleptic malignant syndrome	Few case reports Low risk when compared to other neuroleptics	Early recognition Cessation of clozapine Supportive care Dopamine agonists/dantrolene

ANC absolute neutrophil count, *ECG* electrocardiogram, *CRP* C-reactive protein

Clozapine-treated patients are also at a higher risk to develop both transient and persistent anemia, neutrophilia, and eosinophilia, but these generally do not require treatment interruption. Male patients have been found to be at a higher risk for persistent neutrophilia and eosinophilia, while concomitant treatments with mood stabilizers (or benzodiazepines) and antidepressants have been associated with transient anemia and eosinophilia, respectively [125]. A number of case reports have suggested elevated clozapine levels during infections. A systematic review of these reports (40 cases) has demonstrated elevated clozapine levels associated with infections particularly of respiratory origin and hence advised consideration of reduction of dose to minimize side effects [126].

A summary of the suggested pretreatment assessment and monitoring schedule is given in Table 8.3. Before starting clozapine, it is important that patients and family/caregivers are given full information about the risks and benefits of clozapine treatment, the need for blood regular blood testing and the need for lifestyle changes. There should be a discussion about the common side effects and potential medical complications, and arrangements should be made to ensure availability of the medical help, apart from the usual clinic hours, in case of emergency.

8.11.1 Treatment Strategies Other than Clozapine for TRS

As some of the clinicians are reluctant to use clozapine, available data also suggest use of treatment strategies other than clozapine in the management of TRS. These include the use of combination of antipsychotics other than clozapine, use of combination of antipsychotics other than clozapine and ECT, and use of suprathreshold doses of other antipsychotics.

8.11.1.1 Combined Use of Non-clozapine Antipsychotics and Electroconvulsive Therapy

Some of the studies have evaluated the effectiveness of combination of non-clozapine antipsychotic and ECT against the same antipsychotic medications among patients with TRS. A recent meta-analysis included data from 11 RCTs involving 818 patients who were treated with a combination of an antipsychotic medication (chlorpromazine, flupenthixol, olanzapine, quetiapine, risperidone, and ziprasidone) and ECT or the same antipsychotic being used alone. In these trials, TRS was defined as failure to respond to two or more adequate antipsychotic trials (one study), three or more adequate trials (nine studies), and four or more antipsychotic trials (one study). Findings of this meta-analysis suggest that the use of adjunctive ECT was superior to use of antipsychotic alone in terms of improvement in symptoms, with difference seen between the two groups as early as 1–2 weeks. Response and remission rates as defined by various studies were superior with the combined treatment when compared to antipsychotic monotherapy. The number needed to treat for response and remission with the combined treatment was 6 and 8, respectively. However the combined treatment was more often associated with headache with number needed for harm (NNH) to be 6, and for memory impairment, NNH was 3 [127]. Accordingly, it can be said that augmentation with ECT may be an important treatment option for management of patients with TRS, in case there is contraindication for use of clozapine.

8.11.1.2 Combinations of Two Antipsychotics

There is limited data on the use of combination of two antipsychotics other than clozapine for patients with TRS. The combinations include the use of two oral antipsychotics, an oral antipsychotic combined with a depot preparation, and use of combination of two depot preparations.

8.11.1.3 Non-clozapine Antipsychotic Combination Therapy (NCCAT)

A recent review documented 19 studies on SGA + SGA, 4 studies on FGA + FGA, 3 studies on SGA + FGA, and 2 studies on FGA + SGA. Among the SGAs, ten studies evaluated the use antipsychotic augmentation with non-clozapine antipsychotics. Combination therapy was found to be superior to monotherapy in terms of symptom reduction, but superiority was only apparent in open-label and low-quality trials and not in double-blind and high-quality trials. Findings regarding symptom reduction were similar in augmentation studies of clozapine with a SGA or a FGA ($n = 514$), clozapine with a SGA ($n = 512$), and non-clozapine with a SGA ($n = 52$) and studies augmenting with a partial D2 agonist ($n = 54$) and those augmenting with D2 antagonists ($n = 512$). Results persisted independent of the nonresponse definition (strict, two adequate trial failures vs. lenient, one adequate trial failure). Again, differences were non-significant when analyzing only high-quality studies. Commonly used SGA + SGA were aripiprazole plus risperidone and sulpiride plus olanzapine. In addition, no double-blind evidence for additional adverse effect burden was associated with antipsychotic combination. Augmentation with a partial D2 agonist can also be considered to lessen metabolic adverse effects in patients where switching to a low-risk agent is not an option [128].

8.11.1.4 Use of Long-Acting Injectable (LAI) Antipsychotics

A prospectively gathered nationwide database study (29,823 patients) has recently shown that the use of LAI antipsychotics in patients with schizophrenia is associated with a substantially lower risk of relapse and rehospitalization [129]. The use of LAI antipsychotics in TRS has been evaluated in a few studies. In a 12-month, multicenter, prospective, observational study that included unstable and severe TRS patients with and without dopamine supersensitivity psychosis (judged on the basis of the clinical courses and neurological examinations), 115 patients with TRS were administered risperidone LAI (RLAI) adjunctively once every 2 weeks along with oral antipsychotics. BPRS total scores and Clinical Global Impression-Severity of Illness (CGI-S) scores were significantly reduced in both groups [130]. Data on beneficial effect of two depots has been reported in a few case reports. One case report used two long-acting antipsychotics (haloperidol and olanzapine) simultaneously to target psychotic symptoms in treatment-resistant schizophrenia, safely and effectively when alternative therapies such as clozapine were not effective [131].

8.11.1.5 High-Dose/Suprathreshold Antipsychotic Therapy

High-dose antipsychotic use involves prescribing a dose higher than that stated by regulatory authorities and the summary of product characteristics. High-dose antipsychotics have been used in clinical practice when patients fail to respond to standard doses and in patients who display persistent aggression. The decision to prescribe high doses should involve an individual risk-benefit analysis in consultation with the patient and the family. A baseline and regular monitoring of ECG should be carried out during the therapy to rule out prolonged QTc interval. A QTc > 440 ms in men and > 470 ms in women should prompt the clinician to stop therapy and seek cardiology consultation. The evidence for efficacy, based on published controlled trials, provides little support for the use of high-dose strategy. In a systematic review, eight RCTs were identified which compared high-dose non-clozapine antipsychotics with standard-dose clozapine therapy. Pooled analysis failed to show any difference between the two groups, while one trial reported significant improvement in BPRS scores in the standard-dose clozapine arm compared with high-dose risperidone [132]. Patients on high-dose non-clozapine antipsychotics had a higher incidence of extrapyramidal symptoms as compared to the clozapine group [133].

8.11.2 Post-clozapine Augmentation Strategies

Unfortunately, a significant proportion of patients (30%) do not respond to clozapine. This group of patients is known to have 'ultra-treatment resistance' or 'clozapine-resistant schizophrenia'. In view of this, many studies have attempted to augment clozapine with various other treatment strategies. The various treatments, which have been evaluated, include ECT, other SGAs, FGAs (haloperidol, trifluoperazine, depot), mood stabilizers, antidepressants, and other agents such as memantine and omega-3 fatty acids. However, it is important to remember that the use of additional drugs can increase the side effect burden for the patient and can even potentiate complex drug interactions; therefore all augmentation strategies must be carefully carried out and should be abandoned after 3–6 months.

8.11.2.1 Electroconvulsive Therapy

Out of the various modalities evaluated, ECT has been shown to have the maximum beneficial effect among patients not responding to clozapine. The data for use of ECT is available in the form of case reports, case series, and open-label studies. In recent times, an RCT has found that augmentation of clozapine with ECT can be an effective and safe treatment option. The study randomized 39 individuals with clozapine-resistant schizophrenia, to ECT plus clozapine or treatment as usual (clozapine) group, and found that after 8 weeks, 50% of the treatment group met the response criteria of 40% reduction in symptoms. In addition, during the crossover phase, nonresponders from the clozapine-only group showed a response rate of 47% after ECT [134]. A systematic review of current evidence reported the efficacy range from 37.5% to 100% in the short term, while sustained long-term (3 weeks to 24 months) improvement was seen in only a few studies. Of the 208 patients identified in the review, only 9 patients experienced side effects such as delirium, tachycardia and prolonged seizures. Some of the available data on the use of maintenance ECT in patients not responding adequately to clozapine also suggest that this combination strategy may be of use in long run too [135]. The combination of antipsychotics and ECT has been effectively used to achieve rapid alleviation of symptoms in acutely psychotic patients with TRS in a recent case report [136]. A meta-analysis of clinical trials, retrospective chart reviews, case series, and case reports from 1980 to 2015 demonstrated an overall response rate of 66%, while adverse events were reported in 14% of cases. The data also suggested that a higher number of ECT treatments (mean, 11.2) might be required, as compared to other clinical conditions. In addition, 32% of cases relapsed after the end of ECT treatment [137]. A recent single-blinded sham-controlled pilot study has failed to show any beneficial effect of ECT when used for augmentation of clozapine [138]; hence, further placebo-controlled trials with larger samples are warranted. However, based on the majority of ECT studies, combination of ECT with antipsychotic medications seems to be superior to either modality alone and should be considered as an important treatment option in clozapine-resistant schizophrenia.

8.12 Augmentation with Other Antipsychotics

Treatment resistance has been attributed to a number of biological changes such as reduced presynaptic striatal dopamine synthesis, dopamine super sensitivity, and abnormalities in glutaminergic system. The clinical utility of these proposed mechanisms are continually being investigated. From the perspective of pharmacology, clozapine with its low D2 receptor binding properties can be combined with drugs with a strong D2 receptor affinity, such as risperidone, amisulpride, or haloperidol, to increase response.

8.12.1 Risperidone

The combination of risperidone with clozapine has been widely studied in partial responders to clozapine, with mixed results. In a randomized, double-blind placebo-controlled trial of 8 weeks, involving 68 patients, no statistically significant difference in symptomatic benefit was found between augmentation with risperidone and placebo [139]. In another 6-week double-blind, placebo-controlled study involving 30 patients, adjunctive risperidone therapy did not significantly improve psychopathology or quality of life compared to placebo [140]. When compared with active treatments such as sulpiride and ziprasidone in combination with clozapine, risperidone did not show any difference for a clinically significant response [141]. One RCT has reported the efficacy of risperidone augmentation compared to placebo. In a 12-week trial of 40 patients, with risperidone given up to 6 mg, there was an improvement in both positive and negative symptoms. The combination was also safe and tolerated well [142]. The use of risperidone long-acting injection along with clozapine has also shown some beneficial effects such as markedly reduced duration and frequencies of hospitalizations. The use of risperidone LAI has also been reported in a case series for patients poorly adherent to oral clozapine. In all the four cases, the durations and frequencies of hospitalizations markedly declined after LAI augmentation [143].

8.12.2 Amisulpride

Amisulpride binds preferentially to D2/D3 receptors in the limbic region and also has a high affinity for HT2B antagonism. Amisulpride augmentation has been used mainly for persistent negative symptoms in clinical practice, but its efficacy in combination with clozapine continues to be analyzed in robust RCTs. In a placebo-controlled trial of 16 patients, partially responsive to clozapine, augmentation with amisulpride (dose, 600 mg) led to improvements in subscores of "activity" on BPRS and in secondary outcome measures of global improvement, as assessed by GAF (Global Assessment of Functioning), CGI (Clinical Global Impression), and MADRS (Montgomery-Åsberg Depression Rating Scale) score [144]. In an open nonrandomized study, augmentation with amisulpride, over a 6-month period, led to improvements in positive and negative symptoms, without worsening the side effect burden [145]. In another study, comparing amisulpride augmentation to quetiapine, over an 8-week period, improvements associated with amisulpride were significantly greater for both positive and negative symptoms [146]. The beneficial effect of amisulpride augmentation is also supplemented by its amelioration of clozapine-induced hypersalivation.

8.12.3 Aripiprazole

Aripiprazole is a partial dopaminergic agonist, whose effectiveness as an augmentation agent has been reported in various case reports and studied in few randomized clinical trials. In a 24-week, double-blind, randomized, placebo-controlled trial, at a dose of 15 mg/day, aripiprazole was significantly more efficacious than placebo. Aripiprazole was more efficacious in reducing positive symptoms such as delusions and bizarre behavior and in the negative symptom of alogia [147]. In another randomized, double-blind, placebo-controlled, 8-week study of 62 patients, although no improvement was seen in total symptom severity, a favorable change was observed in the negative symptom domain [148]. In a direct head-to-head comparison with haloperidol as an augmenting agent, aripiprazole did not offer any additional benefit with regard to symptoms over the course of 3 months [149]. Additionally in a naturalistic 12-month follow-up study comparing aripiprazole to haloperidol, the change in BPRS scores was similar in both groups, but aripiprazole was perceived to be more tolerable than haloperidol [150]. In addition to its effects on psychotic symptoms, add-on aripiprazole therapy has shown favorable results on body weight, fasting glucose, total cholesterol, and obsessive-compulsive symptoms [151–153].

Various other antipsychotic agents have been used to augment clozapine including ziprasidone, haloperidol, olanzapine and pimozide [154–156]. Ziprasidone has been found to be equally efficacious as risperidone in a controlled trial [157]. The evidence base for these strategies remains weak due to absence of controlled trials. Furthermore, head-to-head trials need to be carried out in order to compare the efficacy and tolerability of the mentioned augmentation approaches. Several meta-analyses of antipsychotic combinations in treatment-resistant schizophrenia have been performed which suggest only a marginal therapeutic benefit of combined treatment, based on a weak evidence base and only a modest or absent effect [157, 158]. A Cochrane review of all currently available studies of combinations of clozapine with other antipsychotics also did not find any evidence for differential recommendations [159]. A summary of the above findings is given in Table 8.7.

8.13 Augmentation with Mood Stabilizers

The use of mood stabilizers such as valproic acid, lamotrigine, lithium, and topiramate is a common augmentation strategy in TRS, despite a lack of conclusive evidence.

8.13.1 Valproate

Valproate is one of the most commonly prescribed mood stabilizers for this population. Early reports of valproate augmentation on treatment-resistant psychosis suggested reduction of positive symptoms and more specifically hostile/disruptive behavior [160]. However larger trials have failed to replicate these initial findings [161]. A retrospective study examined the use of adjunctive divalproex compared to clozapine monotherapy in patients with TRS

Table 8.7 Clozapine augmentation with other antipsychotics

Authors	Design	Sample	Duration	Outcome
Risperidone				
Yagcioglu et al. [140]	DB placebo-controlled RCT	30	6 weeks	No significant improvement in psychopathology or quality of life
Josiassen et al. [142]	DB placebo-controlled RCT	40	12 weeks	Significant reduction in BPRS total and positive subscale scores and reduction in SANS score
Honer et al. [139]	DB placebo-controlled RCT	68	8 weeks	No significant improvements on PANSS
Amisulpride				
Assion et al. [144]	DB placebo-controlled RCT	16	6 weeks	No improvement in BPRS Improvements in secondary outcome measures GAF, CGI, MADRS
Munro et al. [145]	Open nonrandomized study	28	6 months	Significant improvement in the mean scores for PANSS, SANS, and GAF
Genc et al. [146]	Single-blind RCT amisulpride versus quetiapine	56	8 weeks	Significantly greater improvement with amisulpride on BPRS, SAPS, SANS
Aripiprazole				
Muscatello et al. [147]	DB placebo-controlled RCT	31	24 weeks	Significantly more efficacious than placebo in reducing positive symptoms and overall psychopathology (SAPS, BPRS)
Chang et al. [148]	DB placebo-controlled RCT	62	8 weeks	No significant difference in the primary outcome measures of BPRS Secondary analyses showed significant improvements in negative symptoms
Barbui et al. [149]	RCT Aripiprazole versus haloperidol	106	3 months	No difference in symptom scores (BPRS) Aripiprazole better in terms of side effects
Ziprasidone				
Zink et al. [157]	RCT Ziprasidone versus risperidone	24	6 weeks	No significant difference, but both groups showed significant reductions of positive and negative symptoms
Muscatello et al. [147]	DB placebo-controlled RCT	40	16 weeks	Ziprasidone added to clozapine was effective on negative and cognitive symptoms

DB double blind, *RCT* randomized controlled trial, *SANS* Scale for the Assessment of Negative Symptoms, *BPRS* Brief Psychiatric Rating Scale, *CGI* Clinical Global Impression Scale, *GAF* Global Assessment of Functioning, *MADRS* Montgomery-Åsberg Depression Rating Scale, *PANSS* Positive and Negative Syndrome Scale, *SAPS* Scale for the Assessment of Positive Symptoms

and found a trend toward greater reduction of global symptoms, driven by hostility and anxiety, in the first month of adjunct treatment as compared to clozapine monotherapy [162]. Meta-analytical studies have since showed that while valproate augmentation is beneficial for a faster response and those with sever hostility and aggression, its impact on core psychotic features is unconvincing [163, 164]. However, a recent meta-analysis of RCTs on the use of adjunctive sodium valproate in TRS (6 RCTs, $n = 430$) has shown significant improvements in positive and general symptom severity compared to clozapine monotherapy, with no significant differences in adverse drug reactions [165].

8.13.2 Lithium

Lithium has been used effectively as an augmenting agent along with clozapine in patients with schizoaffective disorder, where improvements have occurred in both negative symptoms and cognitive domain. However, these results have not been seen in those with schizophrenia [166–168]. The use of lithium with clozapine is well tolerated, and the usefulness of this combination has been highlighted in cases of clozapine-induced neutropenia. Lithium can be used to increase neutrophil blood counts and prevent neutropenia recurrence after clozapine rechallenge [169].

8.13.3 Lamotrigine

Like other anticonvulsants, lamotrigine is a voltage-gated sodium channel inhibitor, but it has also been shown to inhibit glutamate. Glutamate is an excitatory neurotransmitter, which has been implicated in the pathophysiology of schizophrenia. Based on this probable mechanism of action, as a stabilizer of glutamate neurotransmission, lamotrigine has been studied as an augmentation agent with positive results. A meta-analysis and systematic review of five randomized placebo-controlled trials, of 10–24-week duration, involving 161 patients, evaluated the effectiveness of lamotrigine augmentation in clozapine-resistant patients. It was found that lamotrigine augmentation was effective for both positive and negative symptoms [170–172]. However, subsequent placebo-controlled studies have failed to show benefits, and the need for further investigation is evident [173]. In addition, current evidence also does not support the use of lamotrigine in patients on antipsychotics other than clozapine. Lamotrigine is generally well tolerated in combination with clozapine, with a small but important risk of Steven-Johnson syndrome, which necessitates a slow titration of dose.

8.13.4 Topiramate

Augmentation studies based on topiramate have shown varied results. A 17-week, double-blind, placebo-controlled study on 80 patients failed to show significant benefits in psychotic symptoms [174], while a12-week naturalistic, open study led to a 14% reduction in BPRS scores and a 2.5% decrease in body weight [175]. In another 24-week double-blind, randomized, placebo-controlled trial of 43 patients with TRS on clozapine, add-on topiramate was scarcely effective in reducing clinical symptomatology and also led to cognitive complaints confirmed by impairments on certain cognitive tasks [176]. Based on current evidence, the benefits of augmentation with topiramate appear meager; however it can be particularly useful in offsetting the weight loss induced by clozapine (Table 8.8).

8.14 Augmentation with Antidepressants

Antidepressants can be effectively used to treat depressive symptoms in schizophrenia. In addition, augmentation with antidepressants is being increasingly done to treat negative symptoms, comorbid obsessive-compulsive symptoms, and even some psychotic symptoms and treatment resistance.

8.14.1 Fluvoxamine

Fluvoxamine is an inhibitor of cytochrome P450 1A2 and increases clozapine plasma levels. The increase in dose can increase response in patients in whom adequate clozapine levels have not been reached. Addition of 50 mg/day of fluvoxamine to low-dose clozapine (100 mg/day) can increase clozapine levels to over 400 ng/ml [177, 178]. Several trials have demonstrated that adjunctive use of fluvoxamine can also increase clozapine efficacy by reducing plasma norclozapine-clozapine ratios [179, 180]. A systematic review of adjunctive fluvoxamine with clozapine based on 24 case reports/series, 7 cohort studies, and 2 randomized controlled trials showed that the combination can increase the probability of response and reduce metabolic side effects of clozapine, but further studies are needed to explore clinical implication [181, 182].

Table 8.8 Clozapine augmentation with other agents

Augmenting agent	Authors	Design	Sample	Duration	Outcome
Valproate	Kelly et al. [163]	Non-randomized, retrospective study	15	6 months	Significantly more effective in reducing global symptoms (BPRS) mainly in hostility and anxiety
Lithium	Small et al. [168]	Placebo-controlled trial	Ten patients with schizophrenia and ten patients with schizoaffective disorder	4 weeks	Improvements in schizoaffective patients on CGI and PANSS and cognitive measures, but no improvements in schizophrenic patients
Lamotrigine	Tiihonen et al. [171]	Placebo-controlled crossover RCT	34	14 weeks	Lamotrigine more effective in reducing positive and general psychopathological symptoms (PANSS), no improvement in negative symptoms
	Zoccali et al. [172]	DB placebo-controlled RCT	60	24 weeks	Beneficial effect mainly on the negative and general psychopathological symptomatology
Topiramate	Muscatello et al. [176]	DB placebo-controlled RCT	43	24 weeks	Ineffective for reducing clinical symptomatology
	Hahn et al. [175]	Open-label, naturalistic	20	12 weeks	14% reduction in BPRS scores, 2.5% reduction in weight
Fluvoxamine	Silver et al. [180]	Open-label pilot study	11	6 weeks	4/11 (36.4%) had improvement of >20% in BPRS scores
					2/11 (18.2%) had improvement of >20% in SANS scores
	Lammers et al. [182]	Case series	18	5 weeks	Five patients were treatment responders (BPRS reduction >50%)
					Significant improvement in measures of cognitive speed
	Lu et al. [178]	Prospective open study	18	4 weeks	Addition of fluvoxamine (50 mg/day) to low-dose clozapine (100 mg/day) can raise plasma clozapine levels to at least 300 ng/mL
Fluoxetine	Buchanan et al. [184]	DB placebo-controlled RCT	33	8 weeks	No significant differences in positive, negative, and depressive symptoms
Mirtazapine	Zoccali et al. [185]	DB placebo-controlled RCT	24	8 weeks	Significant reduction on SANS total scores and subscales of avolition/apathy and anhedonia/asociality
Memantine	Veerman et al. [187]	DB placebo-controlled RCT, crossover	26	12 weeks	Significant improvement in verbal recognition memory and paired associate learning task scores and PANSS negative subscale scores
	De Lucena et al. [189]	DB placebo-controlled study	21	12 weeks	Significant improvement on the total BPRS score, its subscales of positive and negative symptoms, the CGI score, and the MMSE score

DB double blind, *RCT* randomized controlled trial, *SANS* Scale for the Assessment of Negative Symptoms, *BPRS* Brief Psychiatric Rating Scale, *CGI* Clinical Global Impression Scale, *GAF* Global Assessment of Functioning, *PANSS* Positive and Negative Syndrome Scale, *SAPS* Scale for the Assessment of Positive Symptoms, *MMSE* Mini-Mental Status Examination

8.14.2 Fluoxetine

Fluoxetine, like fluvoxamine, can increase clozapine levels through enzyme inhibition, but the effects are not as marked as fluvoxamine. When added at a dose of 20 mg/day to clozapine (150–200 mg/day), mean plasma concentrations of clozapine, norclozapine, and clozapine N-oxide increased significantly by 58%, 36%, and 38%, respectively [183]. Few studies have been carried out to assess the effects on psychotic symptoms, but a double-blind, placebo-controlled trial failed to show any difference in positive or negative symptoms [184].

8.14.3 Mirtazapine

Mirtazapine is a noradrenergic and specific serotonergic antidepressant (NaSSAs), and because of their specific mechanism of action, they do not produce many of the side effects associated with SSRIs. An 8-week double-blind, randomized, placebo-controlled trial of 30 mg adjunctive mirtazapine to clozapine therapy conducted in 24 patients showed a significant reduction on the SANS and BPRS scores [185]. In addition to their effects on psychopathology, mirtazapine has also been found to improve akathisia and extrapyramidal symptoms [186]. However more studies are needed to confirm these results.

8.14.4 Memantine

N-methyl-d-aspartate (NMDA) neurotransmission in the prefrontal cortex has been suggested as a probable cause of negative, positive and cognitive symptoms in schizophrenia. Hence, clozapine augmentation with memantine, an NMDA antagonist used for moderate Alzheimer's disease, has shown promise. In a 12-week placebo-controlled study, add-on memantine group showed improvements in verbal and visual memory and negative symptoms without serious side effects [187]. In the 1-year open-label extension of the study, the favorable effects were sustained, and further improvements were seen in both positive and negative symptoms [188]. Similar results were also obtained in another double-blind, placebo-controlled study, with memantine at 20 mg/day dose associated with improvements in both positive and negative symptoms [189]. While adjunctive memantine has shown positive results with clozapine, its addition to other atypical antipsychotics has failed to show improvements in psychopathology [190].

8.14.5 NMDA/Glycine Modulators

NMDA/glycine site modulators include full and partial glycine agonists such as glycine, D-serine, and D-cycloserine. These agents have been found to be helpful in ameliorating negative and cognitive symptoms in schizophrenia in several trials [191, 192]. Hence their use in treatment-resistant schizophrenia, as an augmenting agent, is being studied, with mixed results. Low-dose D-cycloserine (DCS) is a partial agonist at the glycine site of the NMDA-associated receptor complex, and its effectiveness as an augmenting agent was evaluated in one preliminary randomized, double-blind, placebo-controlled trial of 17 patients. The results suggested worsening of negative symptoms compared to placebo with no effect on the positive symptoms [193]. Other RCTs evaluating the effects of glycine and D-serine to clozapine augmentation have failed to exhibit symptom improvement, with no worsening of symptoms [194–196]. These results have suggested that glycine site agonists may be less effective when combined with clozapine than they are when combined with conventional antipsychotics.

8.15 Conclusion and Future Directions

The concept of TRS was given about three decades ago, and over the years, it has been widely accepted by the clinicians and researchers. Over the last three decades, the concept has evolved from a very strict definition to a more flexible and relaxed criteria. Initially the definition was kept very strict as the concept evolved around clozapine, a molecule that was banned due to a history of serious side effects and consequent deaths. Accordingly, the definition was kept such that clozapine was not used indiscriminately. Over the years, with a slow but gradual increase in its use, there is increased confidence among clinicians that this molecule can be safely used, if the monitoring is kept proper. The regular monitoring while using clozapine has not only established the safety of clozapine, but it has somehow also brought psychiatry as a discipline close to medicine and has made mental health professionals to focus on the physical health of mentally ill patients too. The current concept of TRS allows the use of clozapine at a much earlier stage than the past.

Clozapine has been the mainstay of therapy for treatment-resistant schizophrenia over the last three decades, which has been consistently reflected in nearly all clinical practice guidelines. In addition to psychotic symptoms, clozapine has been found to be useful in those at risk for suicide and aggression and in those with tardive syndromes. Patient and clinician's concern over clozapine side effects and the need for continuous laboratory monitoring have restricted its use in clinical practice. Hence, optimizing the use of clozapine and increasing the knowledge base among prescribers need to be addressed effectively. While research on physician and patient's attitude to clozapine is forthcoming, future research should focus on identifying mechanisms used to deliver and monitor clozapine.

The evidence for clozapine augmentation strategies is currently weak with low to moderate effects. Of the various augmentation strategies, the combination of clozapine and ECT has been found to be of maximum benefit among patients not responding to clozapine. Trials involving other augmenting agents ranging from other antipsychotics, mood stabilizers, or antidepressants have shown equivocal results. However the use of these augmenting strategies can be undertaken based on symptom profile and side effect profile of the patient. Future studies on treatment resistance should focus on robust double-blind RCT methodology with a larger sample size.

References

1. Bhugra D. The global prevalence of schizophrenia. PLoS Med. 2005;2(5):e151.
2. Shen WW. A history of antipsychotic drug development. Compr Psychiatry. 1999;40:407–14.
3. Idänpään-Heikkilä J, Alhava E, Olkinuora M, Palva I. Clozapine and agranulocytosis. Lancet. 1975;306:611.
4. Kane J, Honigfeld G, Singer J, Meltzer H. Clozapine for the treatment-resistant schizophrenic. A double-blind comparison with chlorpromazine. Arch Gen Psychiatry. 1988;45:789–96.
5. Kane JM. Schizophrenia. New Eng J Med. 1996;334:34–41.
6. Kane JM, Honigfeld G, Singer J, Meltzer HY, and the Clozaril Collaborative Study Group. Clozapine for the treatment-resistant schizophrenic. Arch Gen Psychiatry. 1988;45:789–96.
7. Kane JM, d Marder SR. Psychopharmacologic treatment of schizophrenia. Schizophr Bull. 1993;19:113–28.
8. Meltzer HY. Treatment of the neuroleptic-nonresponsive schizophrenic patient. Schizophr Bull. 1992;18:515–42.
9. Fabre LF, Nordström AL, Wiesel FA, Pauli S, Halldin C, Sedvall G. Positron emission tomographic analysis of central D1 and D2 dopamine receptors occupancy in patient treated with classical neuroleptic and clozapine: relation to extrapyramidal side effects. Arch Gen Psychiatry. 1992;49:538e44.
10. Brenner HD. Defining treatment refractoriness in schizophrenia. Schizophr Bull. 1990;16:551.
11. Wilson WH. Clinical review of clozapine treatment in a state hospital. Hosp Commun Psychiatry. 1992;43:700–3.
12. López-Ibor MI, López-Ibor JJ. The evolving concept of treatment-resistant schizophrenia. Actas Esp Psiquiatr. 2011;39:236–50.
13. Keefe RS, Lobel DS, Mohs RC, Silverman JM, Harvey PD, Davidson M, et al. Diagnostic issues in chronic schizophrenia: kraepelinian schizophrenia, undifferentiated schizophrenia, and state-independent negative symptoms. Schizophr Res. 1991;4:71–9.
14. American Psychiatric Association. Practice guidelines for the treatment of schizophrenia. Washington, DC: American Psychiatric Association; 1997.
15. Taylor D, Paton C, Kapur S. The Maudsley prescribing guidelines in psychiatry. 12th ed. Oxford: Wiley-Blackwell; 2015.
16. National Institute of Clinical Excellence. Psychosis and schizophrenia in adults. 2014. Retrieved from: https://www.nice.org.uk/guidance/cg178.
17. International Psychopharmacology Algorithm Project. Treatment resistant schizophrenia. The international psychopharmacology algorithm project. 2006. Retrieved from: http://www.ipap.org/pdf/schiz/IPAP_Schiz_treatment_resistant.pdf.

18. Murray RM, O'Callaghan E, Castle DJ, Lewis SW. A neurodevelopmental approach to the classification of schizophrenia. Schizophr Bull. 1992;18:319–32.
19. Weinberger DR. From neuropathology to neurodevelopment. Lancet. 1995;346:552–7.
20. Lieberman J, Jody D, Geisler S. Time course and biologic correlates of treatment response in first-episode schizophrenia. Arch Gen Psychiatry. 1993;50:369–76.
21. Chakos M, Lieberman J, Hoffman E, Bradford D, Sheitman B. Effectiveness of second-generation antipsychotics in patients with treatment-resistant schizophrenia: a review and meta-analysis of randomized trials. Am J Psychiatry. 2001;158:518–26.
22. Robinson DG. Predictors of treatment response from a first episode of schizophrenia or schizoaffective disorder. Am J Psychiatry. 1999;156:544–9.
23. Lieberman JA, Safferman AZ, Pollack S, Szymanski S, Johns C, Howard A, et al. Clinical effects of clozapine in chronic schizophrenia: response to treatment and predictors of outcome. Am J Psychiatry. 1994;151:1744–52.
24. Meltzer HY. Age at onset and gender of schizophrenic patients in relation to neuroleptic resistance. Am J Psychiatry. 1997;154:475–82.
25. Malaspina D. Relation of familial schizophrenia to negative symptoms but not to the deficit syndrome. Am J Psychiatry. 2000;157:994–1003.
26. Alvir JMJ, Woerner MG, Gundduz H, Degreef G, Lieberman JA. Obstetric complications predict treatment response in first-episode schizophrenia. Psychol Med. 1999;29:621–7.
27. Lieberman JA. Psychobiologic correlates of treatment response in schizophrenia. Neuropsychopharmacology. 1996;14:13S–21S.
28. Bartkó G, Frecska E, Horváth S, Zádor G, Arató M. Predicting neuroleptic response from a combination of multilevel variables in acute schizophrenic patients. Acta Psychiatr Scand. 1990;82:408–12.
29. Bailer J, Bräuer W, Rey ER. Premorbid adjustment as predictor of outcome in schizophrenia: results of a prospective study. Acta Psychiatr Scand. 1996;93:368–77.
30. Wieselgren IM, Lindström LH. A prospective 1–5 year outcome study in first-admitted and readmitted schizophrenic patients; relationship to heredity, premorbid adjustment, duration of disease and education level at index admission and neuroleptic treatment. Acta Psychiatr Scand. 1996;93:9–19.
31. Lieberman JA. Prospective study of psychobiology in first-episode Schizophrenia at Hillside Hospital. Schizophr Bull. 1992;18:351–71.
32. Edwards J, Maude D, McGorry PD, Harrigan SM, Cocks JT. Prolonged recovery in first-episode psychosis. Br J Psychiatry. 1998;172:107–16.
33. Kinon BJ, Kane JM, Chakos M, Munne R. Possible predictors of neuroleptic-resistant schizophrenic relapse: influence of negative symptoms and acute extrapyramidal side effects. Psychopharmacol Bull. 1993;29:365–9.
34. Kolakowska T, Williams A, Jambor K, Ardern M. Schizophrenia with good and poor outcome. III: Neurological'soft'signs, cognitive impairment and their clinical significance. Br J Psychiatry. 1985;146:348–57.
35. Schultz SC, Conley RR, Kahn EM, Alexander J. Nonresponders to neuroleptics: a distinct subtype. In: Schultz C, Taminga CA, editors. Schizophrenia: scientific progress. New York, Oxford: Oxford University Press; 1989. p. 341–50.
36. Wiersma D. Social disability in schizophrenia: its development and prediction over 15 years in incidence cohorts in six European centres. Psychol Med. 2000;30:1155–67.
37. Wimberley T. Predictors of treatment resistance in patients with schizophrenia: a population-based cohort study. Lancet Psychiatry. 2016;3:358–66.
38. Nakajima S. Neuroimaging findings in treatment-resistant schizophrenia: a systematic review. Schizophr Res. 2015;164:164–75.
39. Sadock BJ, Sadock VA, Kaplan HI. Kaplan & Sadock's comprehensive textbook of psychiatry. Philadelphia: Lippincott Williams & Wilkins; 2005.
40. Dold M, Leucht S. Pharmacotherapy of treatment-resistant schizophrenia: a clinical perspective. Evid Based Ment Health. 2014;17:33–7.
41. Velligan DI, Weiden PJ, Sajatovic M, Scott J, Carpenter D, Ross R, et al. The expert consensus guideline series: adherence problems in patients with serious and persistent mental illness. J Clin Psychiatry. 2009;70(Suppl 4):1–46.
42. Clozapine Study Group. The safety and efficacy of clozapine in severe treatment-resistant schizophrenic patients in the UK. Br J Psychiatry. 1993;163:150–4.
43. McEvoy JP, Lieberman JA, Stroup TS, Davis SM, Meltzer HY, Rosenheck RA, et al. Effectiveness of clozapine versus olanzapine, quetiapine, and risperidone in patients with chronic schizophrenia who did not respond to prior atypical antipsychotic treatment. Am J Psychiatry. 2006;163:600–10.
44. Lewis SW, Barnes TR, Davies L, Murray RM, Dunn G, Hayhurst KP, et al. Randomized controlled trial of effect of prescription of clozapine versus other second-generation antipsychotic drugs in resistant schizophrenia. Schizophr Bull. 2006;32:715–23.
45. Siskind D, Siskind V, Kisely S. Clozapine response rates among people with treatment-resistant schizophrenia: data from a systematic review and meta-analysis. Can J Psychiatr. 2017;62:772. https://doi.org/10.1177/0706743717718167.
46. Wahlbeck K, Cheine M, Essali A, Adams C. Evidence of clozapine's effectiveness in schizophrenia: a systematic review and meta-analysis of randomized trials. Am J Psychiatry. 1999;156:990–9.
47. Moncrieff J. Clozapine v. conventional antipsychotic drugs for treatment-resistant schizophrenia: a re-examination. Br J Psychiatry. 2003;183:161–6.
48. Siskind D, McCartney L, Goldschlager R, Kisely S. Clozapine v. first- and second-generation antipsychotics in treatment-refractory schizophrenia: systematic review and meta-analysis. Br J Psychiatry. 2016;209:385–92.

49. Meltzer HY, McGurk SR. The effects of clozapine, risperidone, and olanzapine on cognitive function in schizophrenia. Schizophr Bull. 1999;25:233–55.
50. McGurk SR. The effects of clozapine on cognitive functioning in schizophrenia. J Clin Psychiatry. 1999;60(Suppl 12):24–9.
51. Meltzer HY, Alphs L, Green AI, Altamura AC, Anand R, Bertoldi A, et al. Clozapine treatment for suicidality in schizophrenia: international suicide prevention trial (InterSePT). Arch Gen Psychiatry. 2003;60:82–91.
52. Wimberley T, MacCabe JH, Laursen TM, Sorensen HJ, Astrup A, Horsdal HT, et al. Mortality and self-harm in association with clozapine in treatment-resistant schizophrenia. T Am J Psychiatry. 2017;174:990. https://doi.org/10.1176/appi.ajp.2017.16091097.
53. Zalsman G, Hawton K, Wasserman D, van Heeringen K, Arensman E, Sarchiapone M, et al. Suicide prevention strategies revisited: 10-year systematic review. Lancet Psychiatry. 2016;3:646–59.
54. Frogley C, Taylor D, Dickens G, Picchioni M. A systematic review of the evidence of clozapine's anti-aggressive effects. Neuropsychopharmacology. 2012;15:1351–71.
55. Glazer WM, Dickson RA. Clozapine reduces violence and persistent aggression in schizophrenia. J Clin Psychiatry. 1998;59(Suppl 3):8–14.
56. Spivak B, Mester R, Wittenberg N, Maman Z, Weizman A. Reduction of aggressiveness and impulsiveness during clozapine treatment in chronic neuroleptic-resistant schizophrenic patients. Clin Neuropharmacol. 1997;20(5):442–6.
57. Nakajima S, Takeuchi H, Fervaha G, Plitman E, Chung JK, Caravaggio F, et al. Comparative efficacy between clozapine and other atypical antipsychotics on depressive symptoms in patients with schizophrenia: analysis of the CATIE phase 2E data. Schizophr Res. 2015;161:429–33.
58. Hung YY, Yang PS, Huang TL. Clozapine in schizophrenia patients with recurrent catatonia: report of two cases. Psychiatry Clin Neurosci. 2006;60:256–8.
59. Meltzer HY, Burnett S, Bastani B, Ramirez LF. Effects of six months of clozapine treatment on the quality of life of chronic schizophrenic patients. Hosp Comm Psychiatry. 1990;41:892–7.
60. Meltzer HY, Cola P, Way L, Thompson PA, Bastani B, Davies MA, et al. Cost effectiveness of clozapine in neuroleptic-resistant schizophrenia. Am J Psychiatry. 1993;150:1630–8.
61. Lewis SW, Davies L, Jones PB, Barnes TR, Murray RM, Kerwin R, et al. Randomised controlled trials of conventional antipsychotic versus new atypical drugs, and new atypical drugs versus clozapine, in people with schizophrenia responding poorly to, or intolerant of, current drug treatment. Health Technol Assess. 2006;10(17):iii–v, ix–xi, 1–165
62. Raoul Y, Manesse P, Delage M. Quality of life of schizophrenic patients and clozapine. L'Encephale. 1997;23(4):12–6.
63. RE MC. Clozapine improves symptoms but not quality of life compared with other second-generation antipsychotics in people with treatment resistant schizophrenia. Evid Based Ment Health. 2007;10:57.
64. Waserman J, Criollo M. Subjective experiences of clozapine treatment by patients with chronic schizophrenia. Psychiatr Serv. 2000;51:666–8.
65. Taylor D, Shapland L, Laverick G, Bond J, Munro J. Clozapine – a survey of patient perceptions. Psychiatr Bull. 2000;24:450–2.
66. Turetz M, Mozes T, Toren P, Chernauzan N, Yoran-Hegesh R, Mester R, et al. An open trial of clozapine in neuroleptic-resistant childhood-onset schizophrenia. Br J Psychiatry. 1997;170:507–10.
67. Mozes T, Toren P, Chernauzan N, Mester R, Yoran-Hegesh R, Blumensohn R, et al. Clozapine treatment in very early onset schizophrenia. J Am Acad Child Adolesc. 1994;33:65–70.
68. Kumra S, Frazier JA, Jacobsen LK, McKenna K, Gordon CT, Lenane MC, et al. Childhood-onset schizophrenia. A double-blind clozapine-haloperidol comparison. Arch Gen Psychiatry. 1996;53:1090–7.
69. Shaw P, Sporn A, Gogtay N, Overman GP, Greenstein D, Gochman P, et al. Childhood-onset schizophrenia: a double-blind, randomized clozapine-olanzapine comparison. Arch Gen Psychiatry. 2006;63:721–30.
70. Sarkar S, Grover S. Antipsychotics in children and adolescents with schizophrenia: a systematic review and meta-analysis. Indian J Pharmacol. 2013;45:439–46.
71. Sethi S. Clozapine in pregnancy. Indian J Psychiatry. 2006;48:196–7.
72. Duran A, Ugur MM, Turan S, Emul M. Clozapine use in two women with schizophrenia during pregnancy. J Psychopharmacol (OxfordEngland). 2008;22:111–3.
73. Mehta TM, Van Lieshout RJ. A review of the safety of clozapine during pregnancy and lactation. Arch Womens Ment Health. 2017;20:1–9.
74. Shao P, Ou J, Peng M, Zhao J, Chen J, Wu R. Effects of clozapine and other atypical antipsychotics on infants development who were exposed to as fetus: a post-hoc analysis. PLoS One. 2015;10:e0123373.
75. Nguyen HN, Lalonde P. Clozapine and pregnancy. L'Encephale. 2003;29:119–24.
76. Bishara D, Taylor D. Adverse effects of clozapine in older patients: epidemiology, prevention and management. Drugs Aging. 2014;31:11–20.
77. Pridan S, Swartz M, Baruch Y, Tadger S, Plopski I, Barak Y. Effectiveness and safety of clozapine in elderly patients with chronic resistant schizophrenia. Int Psychogeriatr. 2015;27:131–4.
78. Barak Y, Wittenberg N, Naor S, Kutzuk D, Weizman A. Clozapine in elderly psychiatric patients: tolerability, safety, and efficacy. Compr Psychiatry. 1999;40:320–5.
79. Herst L, Powell G. Is clozapine safe in the elderly? Aust N Z J Psychiatry. 1997;31:411–7.

80. Thomas K, Susan S, Jayaprakash K. Clozapine-induced cardiac failure. Indian J Psychiatry. 2006;48:128–9.
81. Casey DE. Clozapine: neuroleptic-induced EPS and tardive dyskinesia. Psychopharmacology. 1989;99(Suppl):S47–53.
82. Spivak B, Mester R, Abesgaus J, Wittenberg N, Adlersberg S, Gonen N, et al. Clozapine treatment for neuroleptic-induced tardive dyskinesia, parkinsonism, and chronic akathisia in schizophrenic patients. J Clin Psychiatry. 1997;58:318–22.
83. Grover S, Hazari N, Kate N, Chakraborty K, Sharma A, Singh D, et al. Management of tardive syndromes with clozapine: a case series. Asian J Psychiatry. 2014;8:111–4.
84. Hazari N, Kate N, Grover S. Clozapine and tardive movement disorders: a review. Asian J Psychiatry. 2013;6:439–51.
85. Warnez S, Alessi-Severini S. Clozapine: a review of clinical practice guidelines and prescribing trends. BMC Psychiatry. 2014;14:102.
86. Stahl SM. Clozapine: is now the time for more clinicians to adopt this orphan? CNS Spectr. 2014;19:279–81.
87. Cohen D. Prescribers fear as a major side-effect of clozapine. Acta Psychiatr Scand. 2014;130:154–5.
88. Grover S, Hazari N, Chakrabarti S, Avasthi A. Delay in initiation of clozapine: a retrospective study from a tertiary care hospital in North India. Psychiatry Res. 2015;226:181–5.
89. Grover S, Balachander S, Chakarabarti S, Avasthi A. Prescription practices and attitude of psychiatrists towards clozapine: a survey of psychiatrists from India. Asian J Psychiatry. 2015;18:57–65.
90. Ucok A, Cikrikcili U, Karabulut S, Salaj A, Ozturk M, Tabak O, et al. Delayed initiation of clozapine may be related to poor response in treatment-resistant schizophrenia. Int Clin Psychopharmacol. 2015;30:290–5.
91. Nielsen J, Dahm M, Lublin H, Taylor D. Psychiatrists' attitude towards and knowledge of clozapine treatment. J Psychopharmacol (Oxford, England). 2010;24:965–71.
92. Gee S, Vergunst F, Howes O, Taylor D. Practitioner attitudes to clozapine initiation. Acta Psychiatr Scand. 2014;130:16–24.
93. Gee SH, Shergill SS, Taylor DM. Patient attitudes to clozapine initiation. Int Clin Psychopharmacol. 2017;32:337–42.
94. Ciapparelli A, Ducci F, Carmassi C, Carlini M, Paggini R, Catena M, et al. Predictors of response in a sample of treatment-resistant psychotic patients on clozapine. Eur Arch Psychiatry Clin Neurosci. 2004;254:343–6.
95. Usall J, Suarez D, Haro JM. Gender differences in response to antipsychotic treatment in outpatients with schizophrenia. Psychiatry Res. 2007;153:225–31.
96. Pickar D, Owen RR Jr, Litman RE, Hsiao JK, Su TP. Predictors of clozapine response in schizophrenia. J Clin Psychiatry. 1994;55(Suppl B):129–32.
97. Butcher NJ, Fung WL, Fitzpatrick L, Guna A, Andrade DM, Lang AE, et al. Response to clozapine in a clinically identifiable subtype of schizophrenia. Br J Psychiatry. 2015;206:484–91.
98. Rajkumar AP, Chitra C, Bhuvaneshwari S, Poonkuzhali B, Kuruvilla A, Jacob KS. Clinical predictors of response to clozapine in patients with treatment resistant schizophrenia. Psychopharmacol Bull. 2011;44:51–65.
99. Fenton WS, Lee B. Can clozapine response be predicted? A naturalistic pilot study. J Nerv Ment Dis. 1993;181:62–4.
100. Pickar D, Owen RR, Litman RE, Konicki E, Gutierrez R, Rapaport MH. Clinical and biologic response to clozapine in patients with schizophrenia. Crossover comparison with fluphenazine. Arch Gen Psychiatry. 1992;49:345–53.
101. Mauri MC, Volonteri LS, Colasanti A, Fiorentini A, De Gaspari IF, Bareggi SR. Clinical pharmacokinetics of atypical antipsychotics: a critical review of the relationship between plasma concentrations and clinical response. Clin Pharmacokinet. 2007;46:359–88.
102. Molina V, Reig S, Sarramea F, Sanz J, Francisco Artaloytia J, Luque R, et al. Anatomical and functional brain variables associated with clozapine response in treatment-resistant schizophrenia. Psychiatry Res. 2003;124:153–61.
103. Lauriello J, Mathalon DH, Rosenbloom M, Sullivan EV, Faustman WO, Ringo DL, et al. Association between regional brain volumes and clozapine response in schizophrenia. Biol Psychiatry. 1998;43:879–86.
104. Ertugrul A, Volkan-Salanci B, Basar K, KarliOguz K, Demir B, Ergun EL, et al. The effect of clozapine on regional cerebral blood flow and brain metabolite ratios in schizophrenia: relationship with treatment response. Psychiatry Res. 2009;174:121–9.
105. Rodriguez VM, Andree RM, Castejon MJ, Zamora ML, Alvaro PC, Delgado JL, et al. Fronto-striato-thalamic perfusion and clozapine response in treatment-refractory schizophrenic patients. A 99mTc-HMPAO study. Psychiatry Res. 1997;76:51–61.
106. Molina Rodriguez V, Montz Andree R, Perez Castejon MJ, Capdevila Garcia E, Carreras Delgado JL, Rubia Vila FJ. SPECT study of regional cerebral perfusion in neuroleptic-resistant schizophrenic patients who responded or did not respond to clozapine. Am J Psychiatry. 1996;153:1343–6.
107. Perry PJ, Miller DD, Arndt SV, Cadoret RJ. Clozapine and norclozapine plasma concentrations and clinical response of treatment-refractory schizophrenic patients. Am J Psychiatry. 1991;148:231–5.
108. Davis JM, Chen N. Dose response and dose equivalence of antipsychotics. J Clin Psychopharmacol. 2004;24:192–208.
109. Simpson GM, Josiassen RC, Stanilla JK, de Leon J, Nair C, Abraham G, et al. Double-blind study of clozapine dose response in chronic schizophrenia. Am J Psychiatry. 1999;156:1744–50.

110. Tang YL, Mao P, Li FM, Li W, Chen Q, Jiang F, et al. Gender, age, smoking behaviour and plasma clozapine concentrations in 193 Chinese inpatients with schizophrenia. Br J Clin Pharmacol. 2007;64:49–56.
111. Schulte P. What is an adequate trial with clozapine?: therapeutic drug monitoring and time to response in treatment-refractory schizophrenia. Clin Pharmacokinet. 2003;42:607–18.
112. Meltzer HY, Bastani B, Kwon KY, Ramirez LF, Burnett S, Sharpe J. A prospective study of clozapine in treatment-resistant schizophrenic patients. I. Preliminary report. Psychopharmacology. 1989;99(Suppl):S68–72.
113. Tharyan P. Haematological monitoring with clozapine therapy in India. Br J Psychiatry. 1998;172:540.
114. American Diabetes Association; American Psychiatric Association; American Association of Clinical Endocrinologists; North American Association for the Study of Obesity. Consensus development conference on antipsychotic drugs and obesity and diabetes. Diabetes Care. 2004;27:596–601.
115. Grover S, Nebhinani N, Chakrabarti S, Avasthi A, Kulhara P. Metabolic syndrome among patients receiving clozapine: a preliminary estimate. Indian J Pharmacol. 2011;43:591–5.
116. Lee JS, Kwon JS, Kim D, Kim SW, Kim JJ, Kim JH, et al. Prevalence of metabolic syndrome in patients with schizophrenia in Korea: a multicenter Nationwide cross-sectional study. Psychiatry Investig. 2017;14:44–50.
117. Richard J, Dawn F, Jessica C, Rita S, Adlai J, Ronald P, et al. An archival, follow-forward exploration of the metabolic syndrome in randomly selected, clozapine-treated patients. Clin Schizophr Relat Psychoses. 2009;3:87–96.
118. Grover S, Nebhinani N, Padmavati R, Chadda RK, Tirupati S, Pallava A. Metabolic syndrome in antipsychotic naive patients with schizophrenia: pooled analysis of data from three Indian studies. Early Interv Psychiatry. 2015;9:357–62.
119. Lamberti JS, Olson D, Crilly JF, Olivares T, Williams GC, Tu X, et al. Prevalence of the metabolic syndrome among patients receiving clozapine. Am J Psychiatry. 2006;163:1273–6.
120. Fehily SR, Forlano R, Fitzgerald PB. C-reactive protein: an early critical sign of clozapine-related myocarditis. Australas Psychiatry. 2016;24:181–4.
121. Nielsen J, Young C, Ifteni P, Kishimoto T, Xiang YT, Schulte PF, et al. Worldwide differences in regulations of clozapine use. CNS Drugs. 2016;30:149–61.
122. Legge SE, Hamshere M, Hayes RD, Downs J, O'Donovan MC, Owen MJ, et al. Reasons for discontinuing clozapine: a cohort study of patients commencing treatment. Schizophr Res. 2016;174:113–9.
123. Fabrazzo M, Prisco V, Sampogna G, Perris F, Catapano F, Monteleone AM, et al. Clozapine versus other antipsychotics during the first 18 weeks of treatment: a retrospective study on risk factor increase of blood dyscrasias. Psychiatry Res. 2017;256:275–82.
124. Clark SR, Warren NS, Kim G, Jankowiak D, Schubert KO, Kisely S, et al. Elevated clozapine levels associated with infection: a systematic review. Schizophr Res. 2017;192:50.
125. Davis MC, Fuller MA, Strauss ME, Konicki PE, Jaskiw GE. Discontinuation of clozapine: a 15-year naturalistic retrospective study of 320 patients. Acta Psychiatr Scand. 2014;130:30–9.
126. Mohapatra S. New food and drug administration recommendations for clozapine prescribing and monitoring requirements. Indian J Psychol Med. 2016;38:488–9.
127. Zheng W, Cao XL, Ungvari GS, Xiang YQ, Guo T, Liu ZR, et al. Electroconvulsive therapy added to non-clozapine antipsychotic medication for treatment resistant schizophrenia: Meta-analysis of randomized controlled trials. PLoS One. 2016;11:e0156510.
128. Galling B, Roldan A, Hagi K, Rietschel L, Walyzada F, Zheng W, et al. Antipsychotic augmentation vs. monotherapy in schizophrenia: systematic review, meta-analysis and meta-regression analysis. World Psychiatry. 2017;16:77–89.
129. Tiihonen J, Mittendorfer-Rutz E, Majak M, Mehtala J, Hoti F, Jedenius E, et al. Real-world effectiveness of antipsychotic treatments in a nationwide cohort of 29823 patients with schizophrenia. JAMA Psychiat. 2017;74:686–93.
130. Kimura H, Kanahara N, Komatsu N, Ishige M, Muneoka K, Yoshimura M, et al. A prospective comparative study of risperidone long-acting injectable for treatment-resistant schizophrenia with dopamine supersensitivity psychosis. Schizophr Res. 2014;155:52–8.
131. Scangos KW, Caton M, Newman WJ. Multiple long-acting injectable antipsychotics for treatment-resistant schizophrenia: case report. J Clin Psychopharmacol. 2016;36:283–5.
132. Rayikanti R, Lentowicz I, Birur B, Li L. Combined antipsychotics and electroconvulsive therapy in an acutely psychotic patient with treatment-resistant schizophrenia. Psychopharmacol Bull. 2017;47:57–62.
133. Azorin JM, Spiegel R, Remington G, Vanelle JM, Pere JJ, Giguere M, et al. A double-blind comparative study of clozapine and risperidone in the management of severe chronic schizophrenia. Am J Psychiatry. 2001;158:1305–13.
134. Combination and high-dose atypical antipsychotic therapy in patients with schizophrenia: systematic review. CADTH Technol Overv. 2012;2:e2301.
135. Petrides G, Malur C, Braga RJ, Bailine SH, Schooler NR, Malhotra AK, et al. Electroconvulsive therapy augmentation in clozapine-resistant schizophrenia: a prospective, randomized study. Am J Psychiatry. 2015;172:52–8.
136. Grover S, Hazari N, Kate N. Combined use of clozapine and ECT: a review. Acta Neuropsychiatr. 2015;27:131–42.

137. Lally J, Tully J, Robertson D, Stubbs B, Gaughran F, MacCabe JH. Augmentation of clozapine with electroconvulsive therapy in treatment resistant schizophrenia: a systematic review and meta-analysis. Schizophr Res. 2016;171:215–24.
138. Melzer-Ribeiro DL, Rigonatti SP, Kayo M, Avrichir BS, Ribeiro RB, Santos BD, et al. Efficacy of electroconvulsive therapy augmentation for partial response to clozapine: a pilot randomized ECT sham controlled trial. Arch Clin Psychiatry (São Paulo). 2017;44:45–50.
139. Honer WG, Thornton AE, Chen EY, Chan RC, Wong JO, Bergmann A, et al. Clozapine alone versus clozapine and risperidone with refractory schizophrenia. N Engl J Med. 2006;354:472–82.
140. Anil Yagcioglu AE, Kivircik Akdede BB, Turgut TI, Tumuklu M, Yazici MK, Alptekin K, et al. A double-blind controlled study of adjunctive treatment with risperidone in schizophrenic patients partially responsive to clozapine: efficacy and safety. J Clin Psychiatry. 2005;66:63–72.
141. Barber S, Olotu U, Corsi M, Cipriani A. Clozapine combined with different antipsychotic drugs for treatment-resistant schizophrenia. Cochrane Database Syst Rev. 2017;3:Cd006324.
142. Josiassen RC, Joseph A, Kohegyi E, Stokes S, Dadvand M, Paing WW, et al. Clozapine augmented with risperidone in the treatment of schizophrenia: a randomized, double-blind, placebo-controlled trial. Am J Psychiatry. 2005;162:130–6.
143. Se Hyun K, Dong Chung J, Yong Min A, Yong Sik K. The combined use of risperidone long-acting injection and clozapine in patients with schizophrenia non-adherent to clozapine: a case series. J Psychopharmacol. 2010;24:981–6.
144. Assion HJ, Reinbold H, Lemanski S, Basilowski M, Juckel G. Amisulpride augmentation in patients with schizophrenia partially responsive or unresponsive to clozapine. A randomized, double-blind, placebo-controlled trial. Pharmacopsychiatry. 2008;41:24–8.
145. Munro J, Matthiasson P, Osborne S, Travis M, Purcell S, Cobb AM, et al. Amisulpride augmentation of clozapine: an open non-randomized study in patients with schizophrenia partially responsive to clozapine. Acta Psychiatr Scand. 2004;110:292–8.
146. Genc Y, Taner E, Candansayar S. Comparison of clozapine-amisulpride and clozapine-quetiapine combinations for patients with schizophrenia who are partially responsive to clozapine: a single-blind randomized study. Adv Ther. 2007;24:1–13.
147. Muscatello MR, Bruno A, Pandolfo G, Mico U, Scimeca G, Di Nardo F, et al. Effect of aripiprazole augmentation of clozapine in schizophrenia: a double-blind, placebo-controlled study. Schizophr Res. 2011;127:93–9.
148. Chang JS, Ahn YM, Park HJ, Lee KY, Kim SH, Kang UG, et al. Aripiprazole augmentation in clozapine-treated patients with refractory schizophrenia: an 8-week, randomized, double-blind, placebo-controlled trial. J Clin Psychiatry. 2008;69:720–31.
149. Barbui C, Accordini S, Nose M, Stroup S, Purgato M, Girlanda F, et al. Aripiprazole versus haloperidol in combination with clozapine for treatment-resistant schizophrenia in routine clinical care: a randomized, controlled trial. J Clin Psychopharmacol. 2011;31:266–73.
150. Cipriani A, Accordini S, Nose M, Purgato M, Girlanda F, Tansella M, et al. Aripiprazole versus haloperidol in combination with clozapine for treatment-resistant schizophrenia: a 12-month, randomized, naturalistic trial. J Clin Psychopharmacol. 2013;33:533–7.
151. Srisurapanont M, Suttajit S, Maneeton N, Maneeton B. Efficacy and safety of aripiprazole augmentation of clozapine in schizophrenia: a systematic review and meta-analysis of randomized-controlled trials. J Psychiatr Res. 2015;62:38–47.
152. Englisch S, Esslinger C, Inta D, Weinbrenner A, Peus V, Gutschalk A, et al. Clozapine-induced obsessive-compulsive syndromes improve in combination with aripiprazole. Clin Neuropharmacol. 2009;32:227–9.
153. Schonfelder S, Schirmbeck F, Waltereit R, Englisch S, Zink M. Aripiprazole improves olanzapine-associated obsessive compulsive symptoms in schizophrenia. Clin Neuropharmacol. 2011;34:256–7.
154. Rajarethinam R, Gilani S, Tancer M, DeQuardo J. Augmentation of clozapine partial responders with conventional antipsychotics. Schizophr Res. 2003;60:97–8.
155. Gupta S, Sonnenberg SJ, Frank B. Olanzapine augmentation of clozapine. Ann Clin Psychiatry. 1998;10:113–5.
156. Gunduz-Bruce H, Oliver S, Gueorguieva R, Forselius-Bielen K, D'Souza DC, Zimolo Z, et al. Efficacy of pimozide augmentation for clozapine partial responders with schizophrenia. Schizophr Res. 2013;143:344–7.
157. Zink M, Kuwilsky A, Krumm B, Dressing H. Efficacy and tolerability of ziprasidone versus risperidone as augmentation in patients partially responsive to clozapine: a randomised controlled clinical trial. J Psychopharmacol. 2009;23:305–14.
158. Paton C, Whittington C, Barnes TR. Augmentation with a second antipsychotic in patients with schizophrenia who partially respond to clozapine: a meta-analysis. J Clin Psychopharmacol. 2007;27:198–204.
159. Taylor DM, Smith L. Augmentation of clozapine with a second antipsychotic – a meta-analysis of randomized, placebo-controlled studies. Acta Psychiatr Scand. 2009;119:419–25.
160. Morinigo A, Martin J, Gonzalez S, Mateo I. Treatment of resistant schizophrenia with valproate and neuroleptic drugs. Hillside J Clin Psychiatry. 1989;11:199–207.
161. Basan A, Kissling W, Leucht S. Valproate as an adjunct to antipsychotics for schizophrenia: a systematic review of randomized trials. Schizophr Res. 2004;70:33–7.
162. Glick ID, Bosch J, Casey DE. A double-blind randomized trial of mood stabilizer augmentation using

lamotrigine and valproate for patients with schizophrenia who are stabilized and partially responsive. J Clin Psychopharmacol. 2009;29:267–71.
163. Kelly DL, Conley RR, Feldman S, Yu Y, McMahon RP, Richardson CM. Adjunct divalproex or lithium to clozapine in treatment-resistant schizophrenia. Psychiatric Q. 2006;77(1):81–95.
164. Tseng PT, Chen YW, Chung W, Tu KY, Wang HY, Wu CK, et al. Significant effect of valproate augmentation therapy in patients with schizophrenia: a meta-analysis study. Medicine. 2016;95:e2475.
165. Zheng W, Xiang YT, Yang XH, Xiang YQ, de Leon J. Clozapine augmentation with antiepileptic drugs for treatment-resistant schizophrenia: a meta-analysis of randomized controlled trials. J Clin Psychiatry. 2017;78(5):e498–505.
166. Lally J, Tully J, MacCabe JH. Clozapine augmentation for treatment-resistant schizoaffective disorder. Cochrane Database Syst Rev. 2016;3:CD012104.
167. Kontaxakis VP, Ferentinos PP, Havaki-Kontaxaki BJ, Roukas DK. Randomized controlled augmentation trials in clozapine-resistant schizophrenic patients: a critical review. Eur Psychiatry. 2005;20:409–15.
168. Small JG, Klapper MH, Malloy FW, Steadman TM. Tolerability and efficacy of clozapine combined with lithium in schizophrenia and schizoaffective disorder. J Clin Psychopharmacol. 2003;23:223–8.
169. Simon L, Cazard F. Clozapine rechallenge after neutropenia in resistant schizophrenia: a review. L'Encephale. 2016;42:346–53.
170. Tiihonen J, Wahlbeck K, Kiviniemi V. The efficacy of lamotrigine in clozapine-resistant schizophrenia: a systematic review and meta-analysis. Schizophr Res. 2009;109:10–4.
171. Tiihonen J, Hallikainen T, Ryynanen OP, Repo-Tiihonen E, Kotilainen I, Eronen M, et al. Lamotrigine in treatment-resistant schizophrenia: a randomized placebo-controlled crossover trial. Biol Psychiatry. 2003;54(11):1241–8.
172. Zoccali R, Muscatello MR, Bruno A, Cambria R, Micò U, Spina E, et al. The effect of lamotrigine augmentation of clozapine in a sample of treatment-resistant schizophrenic patients: a double-blind, placebo-controlled study. Schizophr Res. 93(1):109–16.
173. Vayisoglu S, Anil Yagcioglu AE, Yagcioglu S, Karahan S, Karci O, Gurel SC, et al. Lamotrigine augmentation in patients with schizophrenia who show partial response to clozapine treatment. Schizophr Res. 2013;143:207–14.
174. Behdani F, Hebrani P, RezaeiArdani A, Rafee E. Effect of topiramate augmentation in chronic schizophrenia: a placebo-controlled trial. Arch Iranian Med. 2011;14:270–5.
175. Hahn MK, Remington G, Bois D, Cohn T. Topiramate augmentation in clozapine-treated patients with schizophrenia: clinical and metabolic effects. J Clin Psychopharmacol. 2010;30:706–10.
176. Muscatello MR, Bruno A, Pandolfo G, Mico U, Bellinghieri PM, Scimeca G, et al. Topiramate augmentation of clozapine in schizophrenia: a double-blind, placebo-controlled study. J Psychopharmacol. 2011;25(5):667–74.
177. Olesen OV, Linnet K. Fluvoxamine-clozapine drug interaction: inhibition in vitro of five cytochrome P450 isoforms involved in clozapine metabolism. J Clin Psychopharmacol. 2000;20:35–42.
178. Lu ML, Lane HY, Chen KP, Jann MW, Su MH, Chang WH. Fluvoxamine reduces the clozapine dosage needed in refractory schizophrenic patients. J Clin Psychiatry. 2000;61(8):594–9.
179. Wetzel H, Anghelescu I, Szegedi A, Wiesner J, Weigmann H, Harter S, et al. Pharmacokinetic interactions of clozapine with selective serotonin reuptake inhibitors: differential effects of fluvoxamine and paroxetine in a prospective study. J Clin Psychopharmacol. 1998;18:2–9.
180. Silver H, Kushnir M, Kaplan A. Fluvoxamine augmentation in clozapine-resistant schizophrenia: an open pilot study. Biol Psychiatry. 40:671–4.
181. Polcwiartek C, Nielsen J. The clinical potentials of adjunctive fluvoxamine to clozapine treatment: a systematic review. Psychopharmacology. 2016;233:741–50.
182. Lammers CH, Deuschle M, Weigmann H, Hartter S, Hiemke C, Heese C, et al. Coadministration of clozapine and fluvoxamine in psychotic patients – clinical experience. Pharmacopsychiatry. 1999;32:76–7.
183. Spina E, Avenoso A, Facciola G, Fabrazzo M, Monteleone P, Maj M, et al. Effect of fluoxetine on the plasma concentrations of clozapine and its major metabolites in patients with schizophrenia. Int Clin Psychopharmacol. 1998;13:141–5.
184. Buchanan RW, Kirkpatrick B, Bryant N, Ball P, Breier A. Fluoxetine augmentation of clozapine treatment in patients with schizophrenia. Am J Psychiatry. 1996;153:1625–7.
185. Zoccali R, Muscatello MR, Cedro C, Neri P, La Torre D, Spina E, et al. The effect of mirtazapine augmentation of clozapine in the treatment of negative symptoms of schizophrenia: a double-blind, placebo-controlled study. Int Clin Psychopharmacol. 2004;19:71–6.
186. Kishi T, Iwata N. Meta-analysis of noradrenergic and specific serotonergic antidepressant use in schizophrenia. Int J Neuropsychopharmacol. 2014;17:343–54.
187. Veerman SR, Schulte PF, Smith JD, de Haan L. Memantine augmentation in clozapine-refractory schizophrenia: a randomized, double-blind, placebo-controlled crossover study. Psychol Med. 2016;46:1909–21.
188. Veerman SR, Schulte PF, Deijen JB, de Haan L. Adjunctive memantine in clozapine-treated refractory schizophrenia: an open-label 1-year extension study. Psychol Med. 2017;47:363–75.
189. de Lucena D, Fernandes BS, Berk M, Dodd S, Medeiros DW, Pedrini M, et al. Improvement of negative and positive symptoms in treatment-refractory

schizophrenia: a double-blind, randomized, placebo-controlled trial with memantine as add-on therapy to clozapine. J Clin Psychiatry. 2009;70:1416–23.
190. Lieberman JA, Papadakis K, Csernansky J, Litman R, Volavka J, Jia XD, et al. A randomized, placebo-controlled study of memantine as adjunctive treatment in patients with schizophrenia. Neuropsychopharmacology. 2009;34:1322–9.
191. Javitt DC. Glycine modulators in schizophrenia. Curr Opin Investig Drugs. 2002;3:1067–72.
192. Goff DC, Tsai G, Manoach DS, Flood J, Darby DG, Coyle JT. D-cycloserine added to clozapine for patients with schizophrenia. Am J Psychiatry. 1996;153:1628–30.
193. Goff DC, Henderson DC, Evins AE, Amico E. A placebo-controlled crossover trial of D-cycloserine added to clozapine in patients with schizophrenia. Biol Psychiatry. 1999;45:512–4.
194. Guochuan ET, Pinchen Y, Li-Chen C, Tsai IC, Chung-Wen Tsai A, Joseph TC. d-Serine added to clozapine for the treatment of schizophrenia. Am J Psychiatry. 1999;156:1822–5.
195. Evins AE, Fitzgerald SM, Wine L, Rosselli R, Goff DC. Placebo-controlled trial of glycine added to clozapine in schizophrenia. Am J Psychiatry. 2000;157:826–8.
196. Potkin SG, Jin Y, Bunney BG, Costa J, Gulasekaram B. Effect of clozapine and adjunctive high-dose glycine in treatment-resistant schizophrenia. Am J Psychiatry. 1999;156:145–7.

9 Treatment Resistance in Bipolar Disorders

Marsal Sanches, João Quevedo, and Jair C. Soares

9.1 Introduction

Bipolar disorder (BD) is among the most prevalent severe mental illnesses in the general population. Epidemiological findings from the World Mental Health Survey point to a prevalence of bipolar spectrum disorders as high as 4.4% in the United States [1]. Over the last two decades, considerable advances have been made in regard to a better understanding of BD, not only from a pathophysiological but also from a clinical perspective. Nevertheless, BD remains a leading cause of disability worldwide and is associated with elevated rates of suicide [2, 3].

Even though there is no consensus about the rates of resistance to treatment in BD, evidence indicates that lack of response (or only limited response) to treatment is extremely common among bipolar patients. Data from the STEP-BD study indicate a rate of recovery of less than 60% among bipolar patients, with almost 50% of the participants having displayed recurrence in symptoms during the 2-year follow-up period [4]. These numbers highlight the magnitude of the problem represented by lack of response or partial response to the current available therapeutic approaches.

The current chapter aims at performing a critical evaluation of the current status of resistance

M. Sanches (✉)
Center of Excellence on Mood Disorders, Department of Psychiatry and Behavioral Sciences, McGovern Medical School, The University of Texas Health Science Center at Houston (UTHealth), Houston, TX, USA

Department of Psychiatry and Behavioral Sciences, University of North Dakota School of Medicine, Grand Forks, ND, USA

J. Quevedo
Center of Excellence on Mood Disorders, Department of Psychiatry and Behavioral Sciences, McGovern Medical School, The University of Texas Health Science Center at Houston (UTHealth), Houston, TX, USA

Translational Psychiatry Program, Department of Psychiatry and Behavioral Sciences, McGovern Medical School, The University of Texas Health Science Center at Houston (UTHealth), Houston, TX, USA

Neuroscience Graduate Program, The University of Texas MD Anderson Cancer Center UTHealth Graduate School of Biomedical Sciences, Houston, TX, USA

Laboratory of Neurosciences, Graduate Program in Health Sciences, Health Sciences Unit, University of Southern Santa Catarina (UNESC), Criciúma, SC, Brazil
e-mail: Joao.L.DeQuevedo@uth.tmc.edu

J. C. Soares
Center of Excellence on Mood Disorders, Department of Psychiatry and Behavioral Sciences, McGovern Medical School, The University of Texas Health Science Center at Houston (UTHealth), Houston, TX, USA
e-mail: Jair.C.Soares@uth.tmc.edu

Y.-K. Kim (ed.), *Treatment Resistance in Psychiatry*, https://doi.org/10.1007/978-981-10-4358-1_9

to treatment in BD, in light of available evidence. It begins with general aspects of treatment-resistant BD from a clinical standpoint, followed by a discussion of some of the pathophysiological factors possibly involved in the pathophysiology of this condition. Finally, an evaluation of the current status of the possible therapeutic approaches aiming at improving response to treatment in BD is performed, with a subsequent analysis of some future perspectives in the understanding and clinical management of this condition.

9.2 Concept of Treatment Resistance in Bipolar Disorder

There is no consensus as for the concept of treatment resistance in BD. Factors such as the cyclic nature of that condition and its heterogeneity in terms of clinical presentation and progression make the description of objective parameters to characterize resistance to treatment particularly challenging [5]. The different attempts to establish criteria for resistance in BD have mostly focused on lack of improvement in core symptoms during specific mood states (mania and depression), although longitudinal factors, including frequency of episodes, residual symptoms between episodes, and functional status, should possibly be taken into account as well. Moreover, from a clinical standpoint, factors that can negatively impact response to treatment, such as lack of compliance or tolerability to therapeutic agents, comorbid conditions, and diagnostic accuracy, need to be ruled out or at least considered before a case can be labeled as treatment-resistant [5].

The International Society for Bipolar Disorders (ISBD) conceptualizes refractoriness to treatment in BD as follows [6]:

1. Mania: no significant decreases in the YMRS or MRS scores or significant increase in the MADRS or HDRS scores, or MADRS or HDRS higher than 6, over a treatment period of 8–10 weeks
2. Depression: no significant decrease in the MADRS or HDRS scores, or increase in the YMRS or MRS scores, or YMRS or MRS scores higher than 5, over a treatment period of 10–12 weeks
3. Maintenance: No change in episode frequency, or MADRS/HDRS scores >6 or YMRS/MRS scores >7 in the inter-episode period, over a 1-year treatment period

Although the ISBD criteria above likely represent the most comprehensive and operational concept of treatment resistance in BD (specially for research purposes), it still faces limitations. Comorbidities such as substance use disorder and features such as anxiety, irritability, and cognitive impairment are not contemplated by the ISBD concept of treatment-resistant BD [6].

Furthermore, differently from schizophrenia and unipolar depression, the class effect regarding pharmacological agents in the treatment of BD (especially bipolar depression) is very modest. As the different available guidelines for the treatment of BD indicate, off-label use of medications (supported by different levels of evidence) tends to be the rule rather than the exception in the management of BD. Antidepressants, often cited as ineffective in the treatment of bipolar depression, are listed among the treatment options in the ISBD guidelines for BD, as long as they are associated with mood stabilizers [7]. If a stricter approach were adopted and only FDA-approved agents were adopted as acceptable treatment strategies to characterize resistance, the prevalence of treatment-resistant BD would likely be overestimated and not well-correlated with observations coming from clinical practice. The same possibly applies to the time frames established to characterize resistance, since the different times for the onset of the expected therapeutic effect vary from agent to agent and some medications seem to have bimodal curves of treatment response over time.

It is also important to notice that the vast majority of literature data available on treatment-resistant bipolar disorder focus on resistant bipolar depression. That is likely a result of the paradigm change observed over the last two decades, based on literature findings indicating that depressive symptoms, rather than manic or hypomanic ones, tend to be more pervasive and associated with a higher degree of morbidity, mortality, and functional impairment [8]. In addition to the at times limited treatment response observed during index episodes of bipolar depression, subsyndromal depressive symptoms are common among BD patients in partial remission. Furthermore, patients with bipolar depression are often more accessible for inclusion in controlled studies from a practical standpoint. On the other hand, most of the literature on resistant mania comes from anecdotal reports and case series, usually describing innovative therapeutic interventions, which will be discussed in the next sections of the present chapter.

Finally, some authors attempted to identify clinical features that seem to be associated with treatment-resistant bipolar disorder. These studies usually utilize a retrospective approach, with different definitions of resistance. In a recently published naturalistic study [9], treatment resistance was established based on the number of psychiatric medications and mood stabilizers received. Resistance was found to be associated with female gender, older age, later onset of illness, strong family history of depression, personality traits such as irritability and interpersonal sensitivity, employment status, benzodiazepine use, and comorbid anxiety disorders and medical conditions. Similarly, mixed states are often cited as indicators of poor response to treatment in BD [10]. The relationship between poor treatment response and several of these factors is likely bidirectional, with some of them possibly representing risk factors for poor response while others are probably consequences of the functional and psychopathological impact of the limited response to treatment. On the other hand, there is a certain consensus in the literature indicating that rapid cycling (the presence of four or more mood episodes over the course of 1 year) is an indicator of poor response to treatment and worse prognosis [10]. Similarly, the number of mood episodes has been described as associated with higher severity and worse prognosis among bipolar patients [11].

In conclusion, the concept of treatment-resistant BD is not well established, and there is not enough evidence to support it as a single construct. The ISBD-proposed criteria are probably the most appropriate for research purposes, while from a clinical standpoint, a more global concept, taking into consideration a number of therapeutic agents necessary to achieve remission, degree of response to treatment, functional impact of the condition, and residual symptoms, is likely more realistic and closely correlated with clinician's observations. The different definitions of resistance as well as the multitude of therapeutic regimens potentially considered adequate for the treatment of BD across its different phases make the comparison of different literature findings on the topic particularly challenging.

9.3 Pathophysiological Factors and Resistance

Literature data on the pathophysiological basis of treatment resistance in bipolar disorder is notoriously scant. Yet, it is possible to make some inferences from biological research addressing factors of poor prognosis among bipolar patients, as well as from studies assessing the possible role of degenerative processes in the pathophysiology of bipolar disorder. Further, some studies have analyzed biological predictors of response to certain therapeutic interventions.

For instance, the fact that patients with a stronger family history of depression are more likely to display resistance to treatment [10] indicates that the degree of genetic load for bipolar disorder may impact response to treatment in bipolar disorder. The heterogeneity of the concept of treatment-resistant BD is likely behind the lack of studies addressing genetic factors associated with treatment resistance. Pharmacogenetic studies have identified several candidate genes associated with good response to lithium therapy among bipolar patients [12], although the evidence is less strong when it comes to other mood stabilizers. Some of these findings may conversely be seen as possible indicators of treatment resistance.

Similarly, the finding that the number of episodes is a factor of poor response to treatment in bipolar disorder suggests that, over the course of the illness, the bipolar brain suffers some degree of desensitization and possibly neurodegeneration. The *kindling* theory hypothesizes that, while in early phases of the disease, environmental factors play a major role in triggering mood episodes among bipolar patients, as the disease progresses, the threshold for triggering of a mood episode decreases, with sometimes minor stressors being associated with relapses and recurrence in mood symptoms [13]. It has been recently hypothesized that, in early phases of the disease, putative endogenous compensatory mechanisms are able to counterbalance the negative impact that mood episodes seem to have on the brain of bipolar patients. However, as the disease progresses, the compensatory mechanisms become overwhelmed, resulting in neuroprogression and, likely, in resistance to treatment [13]. Evidence suggests that, among bipolar patients, intensity and chronicity of illness are associated cognitive impairment in the inter-episode period, and neuroimaging studies point to correlations between illness progression and the volume of several brain structures [14]. These findings support the possible involvement of neurodegenerative processes among bipolar patients. At a biochemical level, evidence suggests that factors such as inflammatory process, mitochondrial dysfunctions, and abnormalities in the gene expression on brain-derived neurotrophic factors are involved in these neurodegenerative changes [13].

9.4 Therapeutic Approaches for Treatment Resistance in BD

9.4.1 Pharmacological Agents

While certain agents have been identified as of particular interest for the treatment of resistant patients, no particular medications have received specific FDA approval for that purpose. Several currently available guidelines offer evidence-based options for the treatment of bipolar disorder in a stepwise fashion, therefore indirectly targeting some of the resistant-to-treatment cases. Yet, no specific guideline focusing on those cases is currently available.

9.4.1.1 Resistant Bipolar Depression

According to the ISBD guidelines, published in 2009 and updated in 2013 [7], lithium, lamotrigine, quetiapine, and quetiapine ER should be considered as first-line monotherapy medications for the treatment of bipolar depression. Based on available evidence, divalproex and lurasidone are listed as second-line agents, while carbamazepine and olanzapine appear as third-line monotherapy agents. A large number of combinations are listed as alternative treatments as first-, second-, and third-line agents. Despite the controversy regarding use of antidepressants in patients with bipolar depression (due to concerns about the risk of manic-induced switch, rapid cycling, and possible lack of efficacy), they are listed among the recommendations, although not recommended as monotherapy. The guidelines state that SSRIs (except for paroxetine) and bupropion may be used in the acute treatment of bipolar depression, in combination with a mood stabilizer, with an ultimate goal of having the antidepressants tapered off 6–8 weeks after remission of the depressive episode [7]. Venlafaxine and tricyclic antidepressants should be avoided, although they (as well as MAOI inhibitors) do appear as third-line option in combination with mood stabilizers. Current evidence does not support the use of ziprasidone in the treatment of bipolar depression. Similarly, randomized clinical trials failed to demonstrate a significant effect of aripiprazole in the treatment of depression in BD, although some open-label trials did suggest possible improvement among depressed bipolar patients treated with that medication. Finally, augmentation with modafinil, as well as pramipexole (the latter, in combination with lithium), is listed as second- and third-line option for the treatment of bipolar depression [7].

On the other hand, the International College of Neuro-Psychopharmacology (CINP) recently published its own guidelines for the clinical management of BD, including bipolar depression [15]. It adopted a stepwise process similar to the proposed by the ISBD, including however a broader range of agents and a higher number of steps. According to the CINP guidelines, quetiapine and lurasidone should be considered as first-line agents in the treatment of bipolar depression, and monotherapy with aripiprazole does appear as a treatment option for the treatment of bipolar depression, as a step 3 strategy. Curiously, monotherapy with some antidepressants (including imipramine, phenelzine, and tranylcypromine) is listed as a viable option for the treatment of bipolar depression, although the authors do state that, at the therapist's discretion, an antimanic agent may be added as a prophylactic measure against manic switching [15]. The CINP recommendations include several alternative agents as possible augmentation strategies, including pioglitazone (second step), lithium in combination with oxcarbazepine or sulpiride (third step), and mood stabilizers in combination with levothyroxine, armodafinil, or ketamine (fourth step).

Very few trials addressed the treatment of resistant bipolar depression. As part of the STEP-BD study, a randomized, open-label study analyzed the effects of add-on inositol (compared to lamotrigine and risperidone) in the treatment of resistant bipolar depression [16]. Participants were receiving an optimized mood stabilizer regimen (lithium, valproic acid, carbamazepine, or lithium plus valproic acid) in addition to either one or two antidepressants. The overall recovery rate was low, and no differences were observed across the three treatment groups.

Among the alternative agents mentioned above, ketamine is considered a promising agent for the treatment of bipolar depression, although the strength of the evidence is not as high as it is in regard to the treatment of unipolar patients. Nevertheless, at least four randomized clinical trials have analyzed the efficacy of ketamine infusions in patents with bipolar depression [17]. Evidence suggests that the antidepressant response associated with that medicine in bipolar patients is similar to the one observed among unipolar patients, with improvements observed from 40 min to several hours following the infusion. Yet, the studies in question largely differ as for several methodological issues (e.g., patient profile, use of saline versus midazolam in the control group).

In the only study to specifically address treatment-resistant, depressed bipolar patients, ketamine infusions were found to produce a rapid and significant improvement in anhedonia, even when controlling for the total antidepressant effect, suggesting that the medication had an specific anti-anhedonic effect in resistant bipolar depression [18]. Also of notice, improvement in anhedonia was more pronounced among patients who were receiving lithium than among those receiving valproic acid, and there was a direct correlation between the anti-anhedonic effect and increase in glucose metabolism (as observed through PET) in the dorsal anterior cingulate cortex and in the putamen, following the ketamine infusion. Given the mechanism of action of ketamine (an NMDA receptor partial agonist), the finding above suggests that dysfunctions in the glutamatergic system are likely involved in the pathophysiology of anhedonia among resistant, depressed bipolar patients. In a small, open-label study, patients with treatment-resistant bipolar depression were treated for 8 weeks with D-cycloserine, an antibiotic with NMDA antagonism properties, following a single ketamine infusion [19]. Acute improvement was a predictor of response at 8 weeks, with five patients having completed the study and four (out of a total of seven participants) achieved remission at 8 weeks.

The potential role of other alternative agents in the treatment of resistant bipolar depression is less clear, although several novel agents seem to be promising. Scopolamine, a muscarinic receptor antagonist, seems to produce rapid improvement in depressive symptoms, not only in unipolar patients but also in BD [20]. Similarly, riluzole, a glutamatergic modulator, has been found to produce improvements when utilized as an augmentation to lithium in depressed bipolar patients unresponsive to lithium as monotherapy [20]. Omega-3 fatty acids have been extensively studied in regard to their role in the treatment of mood disorder, including bipolar disorder.

Evidence suggests that they may be effective in the treatment of bipolar depression, in contrast with their role in the treatment of manic symptoms, which is not clear at this point [21].

Furthermore, given the large amount of research pointing to the possible role of inflammation in the pathophysiology of BD, the efficacy of agents with anti-inflammatory properties in the treatment of BD (particularly bipolar depression) is of high interest. These agents include nonsteroidal anti-inflammatory drugs (especially cox-2 inhibitors such as celecoxib, cimicoxib, and rofecoxib), N-acetylcysteine (which also seems to have antioxidant and anti-glutamatergic effects), and minocycline, an antibiotic with important anti-inflammatory properties, which seem to be independent of its antimicrobial effects [22, 23]. Pioglitazone, an antidiabetic medication, has also recently been tested in the treatment of bipolar depression, with positive results [24].

Nevertheless, in a recent meta-analysis, the possible role of different agents (including anti-inflammatory drugs, N-acetylcysteine, omega-3 fatty acids, and pioglitazone) in the treatment of bipolar depression was addressed [25]. When findings regarding all agents with anti-inflammatory properties were pooled and compared to conventional treatments, a moderate antidepressant effect was observed. However, when considered separately, the effect sizes of omega-3 fatty acids, pioglitazone, and nonsteroidal anti-inflammatory drugs were not considered to be statistically significant. N-acetylcysteine was the only agent that seemed to have independent positive effects as an adjunctive treatment for bipolar depression, although the effect size resulted from one single study. The authors concluded that, despite their promising role, it is not yet possible to recommend the use of any specific agents in question for the treatment of bipolar depression, in light of the available evidence.

Finally, despite its popularity in the treatment of unipolar depression as an augmentation strategy, the efficacy of thyroid hormones as augmentation agents in the treatment of bipolar depression is not clear at this point [26]. To date, studies seem to have elicited conflicting results, and the role of these agents in the treatment of depressed patients with bipolar disorder still demands further investigation.

9.4.1.2 Resistant Mania

The management of treatment-resistant mania/hypomania has been a neglected area of study. The ISBD guidelines for the treatment of BD list monotherapy with lithium, valproic acid, and several atypical antipsychotics (risperidone, quetiapine, quetiapine XR, aripiprazole, ziprasidone, asenapine, and paliperidone) as first-line option for the treatment of mania [7]. Monotherapy with carbamazepine, carbamazepine ER, or haloperidol appears as second option, while third option includes chlorpromazine, clozapine, oxcarbazepine, tamoxifen, and cariprazine as monotherapy. Several medication combinations are presented as alternatives to monotherapy, usually involving a mood stabilizer and an antipsychotic.

In contrast, in the CINP guidelines (which combine recommendations for manic and mixed states), monotherapy with lithium appears as a second-step strategy, while valproic acid or an atypical antipsychotic (aripiprazole, quetiapine, cariprazine, paliperidone, quetiapine, risperidone, or asenapine) should be considered as first-line therapy [15]. The recommendations emphasize that past history of psychotic symptoms should be taken into consideration. Adjunctive treatment with allopurinol, medroxyprogesterone, and celecoxib, which are not included in the ISBD guidelines for mania, is listed as second-step option, while tamoxifen, either as monotherapy or an adjunct to lithium or valproic acid, is listed as a fourth-step strategy.

The strength of the evidence supporting the use of some of the alternative agents mentioned above varies. The role of clozapine in the management of resistant mania has been well established by several studies and was addressed in a recent systematic review [27]. A case series described the potential benefits of clozapine rapid titration in patients with resistant mania [28]. To our knowledge, however, no randomized clinical trials have analyzed the usefulness and safety of clozapine under those conditions.

Similarly, a recent meta-analysis supports the use of tamoxifen, a protein-kinase C inhibitor, in the treatment of patients with manic symptoms [29]. Allopurinol has been found to be effective as an adjunctive agent in the treatment of acute mania in at least four randomized clinical trials, but its side-effect profile limits the use of that medication [30]. In the ISBD guidelines, allopurinol is mentioned only as an alternative treatment for patients that are "refractory to other first-, second-, and third-line treatments." Celecoxib, a Cox-2 inhibitor previously assessed in regard to its possible role in the treatment of bipolar depression, also seems to have potential benefits in the treatment of mania. In a recent randomized clinical trial, celecoxib was found to be superior to placebo when combined with valproic acid in the treatment of nonpsychotic mania [31].

9.4.1.3 Resistance During Maintenance Treatment

There is limited evidence on the pharmacological treatment of resistant bipolar disorder during the maintenance phase, likely due to the difficulties in characterizing refractoriness during that period. The ISBD guideline recommendations for maintenance include a large number of agents as first-, second-, and third-line options, emphasizing that antidepressants should not be used as maintenance agents as monotherapy [7]. Of notice, omega-3-fatty acids are mentioned as adjunctive agents, as a third-line medication. The CINP guidelines emphasize the need to take into consideration the predominant polarity of each patient (based on number of previous depressive versus manic or hypomanic episodes) when deciding what medication regimen to be utilized during maintenance [15]. It also recommends that the medications utilized during the index episode should be kept for at least 2 months following remission, before changes are made to the medication regimen.

As mentioned above, the use of omega-3 fatty acids in bipolar disorder remains a controversial issue. In addition to its apparent positive effects on the treatment of bipolar depression, there is also evidence suggesting that dietary supplementation with omega-3 fatty acids may be useful in reducing subsyndromal mood symptoms of bipolar disorder in children [32]. Given the benign side-effect profile of these agents and their apparent safety as a long-term maintenance medication, further research should assess their usefulness as a maintenance agent among BD patients, especially those with partial remission and residual symptoms.

Similarly, the role of cognitive impairment in euthymic bipolar disorder patients has been the object of several studies, although limited evidence supports the use of medications in the management of those symptoms [33]. Cholinesterase inhibitors seem to have limited value in the management of cognitive deficits in bipolar disorder. Anecdotic reports suggest memantine may have some role in the treatment of acute mania, but there is no evidence supporting its role in the treatment of cognitive impairment during the maintenance phase. In one study, mifepristone, a glucocorticoid receptor antagonist, seemed to produce some improvements in the cognitive performance of depressed bipolar patients, but to our knowledge, no study has addressed its efficacy during the maintenance phase of BD [33]. Another study showed improvements in executive functioning associated with the use of intranasal insulin among bipolar patients, possibly due to neuroplastic effects of that agent on the dorsolateral prefrontal cortex [34].

Finally, given the growing evidence supporting the conceptualization of BD as a chronic and potentially disabling condition, psychosocial interventions seem to play a prominent role in its management during the maintenance phase. This issue will be addressed in the section "psychosocial approaches" of this chapter (see below).

9.4.2 Neurostimulation

Although electroconvulsive therapy (ECT) is generally considered an effective option in the management of treatment-resistant mood disorders, the efficacy of ECT in the treatment of refractory bipolar disorder comes mostly from anecdotic or open-label studies. Yet, the ISBD guidelines list ECT as a third-line option in the treatment of bipolar depression and a second-line option for the treatment of mania [7]. Among depressed patients, the guidelines emphasize that early consideration should be given to ECT among patients with psychotic symptoms, at high suicide risk, and in those with ongoing medical complications due to poor ingestion of fluids and food. ECT is also mentioned as a third-line option for the maintenance treatment of BD, as an adjunctive agent. On the other hand, in the CINP guidelines, ECT is mentioned as a fifth step option in the management of mania, bipolar depression, and also in the maintenance phase [15].

In a recent naturalistic, observational study with 522 patients, ECT was found to be effective in approximately two-thirds of the patients with depressed manic or mixed features and 80% of those with catatonic features [35]. Predictors of nonresponse included length of the index mood episode and global severity of the illness. Despite the promising results displayed above, the several methodological issues inherent to the nature of the study limit the generalization of its conclusions. In a meta-analysis, the rates of response to ECT were found to be similar among patients with bipolar and unipolar depression. In a randomized study, ECT was compared to an evidence-based pharmacological algorithm for the treatment of resistant bipolar depression [36]. Results indicated a higher response rate in the ECT group than in the algorithm-based pharmacological treatment group, but no statistically significant differences between groups were found with respect to the remission rate. Concerns regarding the use of ECT in BD are related to the risk of manic switch (among patients with bipolar depression) and worsening cognitive impairment. In one of the studies mentioned above, though, the risk of manic switch was found to be "almost nonexistent," and, in another study, ECT was found as not being associated with worsening in the cognitive function when utilized in the treatment of resistant bipolar disorder patients [37].

Transcranial magnetic stimulation (TMS) is a different modality of neurostimulation technique that allows the electrical stimulation of the brain through magnetic fields produced by a coil [38]. It is considered a noninvasive technique, and its efficacy in the treatment of unipolar depression has been widely demonstrated. Yet, few studies have specifically addressed its role in the management of bipolar disorder. Most of the evidence available comes from case reports or small, open-label studies, often without a sham group. Nevertheless, these results point to possible benefits from excitatory TMS targeting the prefrontal cortex in patients with bipolar depression [38]. Two other studies analyzed the efficacy of inhibitory TMS targeting the right dorsolateral prefrontal cortex in bipolar depression, with positive results, although the conclusions were limited by the small sample size in one of the studies [39] and lack of a sham group in the other [40]. Similarly, the efficacy of TMS in mania has been addressed in a small number of studies, and evidence points to possible benefits of right prefrontal cortex excitatory TMS in the treatment of mania [41]. Last, there is not clear evidence regarding the possible role of traditional TMS in the maintenance treatment of BD, although a recent study pointed to decreases in the rates of depressive relapses among unipolar and bipolar patients treated with deep TMS, a novel modality of TMS [42]. TMS is not mentioned in the ISBD guidelines for the treatment of BD and is listed by the CINP guidelines as not recommended for the treatment of mania or acute bipolar depression [15].

Similar to TMS, vagus nerve stimulation (VNS) is a well-studied therapeutic modality, widely accepted for the treatment of resistant unipolar depressive disorder. It consists of an implanted stimulator that transmits electrical pulses to the left vagus nerve [43]. Evidence regarding the efficacy of VNS in bipolar patients is scant and usually comes from studies that pooled unipolar and bipolar depressed patients under the label "resistant depressive disorder." A small, open-label study assessing the efficacy of VNS in the treatment of rapid cycling bipolar patients pointed to benefits over a period of 12 months [44].

Finally, there is very limited efficacy regarding the efficacy of other neurostimulation techniques in BD. A noninvasive technique, transcranial direct current stimulation (TDCS), involves the application of a weak direct electric current through two scalp electrodes [38]. Literature findings suggest it may be promising in the treatment of bipolar depression, although very few studies, usually with small sample sizes, specifically analyzed its role in the management of depression in bipolar disorder, and there are concerns about the possible risk of manic switching associated with the treatment [45]. Moreover, deep brain stimulation (DBS), another technique, has been used in the treatment of severe, resistant unipolar depression. In DBS, an electric stimulator sends pulses to specific brain areas through implanted wires [38]. Due to concerns about possible DBS-induced manic or hypomanic symptoms, patients with bipolar depression are usually excluded from these studies, although a case report of a bipolar patient treated with DBS suggested that the risk of a manic switch can be minimized by concomitant use of mood stabilizer and decreases in the intensity of the stimulation [38]. Magnetic seizure therapy (MST), an experimental therapeutic intervention, combines aspects of ECT and TMS, aiming at producing improvement in mood symptoms by inducing seizure activity, with a lower risk of cognitive impairment when compared with ECT [46]. Very few studies with MST included bipolar patients, and the actual advantages and disadvantages of that therapeutic modality when compared to ECT in the management of treatment-resistant bipolar disorder are still not clear.

Last, a prospective study analyzed the longitudinal effects of a psychosurgical intervention (subcaudate tractotomy and cingulotomy) in the treatment of patients with severe, refractory bipolar disorder [47]. Results over a 7-year period of follow-up pointed to significant reductions in the depressive symptomatology, while no apparent effects were observed in regard to manic symptoms.

9.4.3 Psychosocial Interventions

There is a consensus as for the recommendation for long-term pharmacological treatment for patients with bipolar disorder. Yet, psychosocial interventions may be of benefit in the management of treatment-resistant bipolar disorder, specially in the maintenance phase. These interventions may include psychoeducational approaches aiming at improving adherence to treatment, as well as other interventions focusing on improving coping strategies and eventually decreasing the risk of a mood relapse associated with stressors. Studies support the role of psychoeducation, cognitive-behavioral therapy (CBT), mindfulness-based interventions, family therapy, and interpersonal and social rhythm therapy (IPSRT) in BD [48].

Yet, systematic reviews and meta-analysis focusing on the effects of psychosocial interventions in the treatment of bipolar patients have reached inconsistent conclusions. For example, the efficacy of CBT as an adjunctive treatment in BD has been questioned in regard to its impact on relapse prevention [49]. In a recent meta-analysis, CBT was associated with mild-to-moderate effect sizes in regard to improvement not only in depressive symptoms but also in mania severity and psychosocial functioning [50]. Group psychoeducation has been found to produce positive effects in terms of reducing frequency and number of relapses, as well as duration of acute episodes and length of hospitalizations.

On the other hand, in a recent systematic review focusing on the impact of different psychosocial treatments in BD, psychoeducation seemed to be effective only on a very specific subgroup of bipolar patients, with optimized mood stabilization and full (or "very good") remission [51]. The same review presented a rather guarded scenario when it comes to the efficacy of other psychosocial interventions in the management of BD, with family interventions displaying possible benefits primarily for caregivers and unclear effects in regard to patient's outcomes. Studies focusing on interventions aiming at improving the cognitive performance of bipolar patients, such as cognitive remediation and functional remediation, were found to display basically negative results. In the review in question, mindfulness-based interventions seem to be effective only in reducing anxiety symptoms, while in another recent review/meta-analysis, mindfulness-based interventions were found to be effective in reducing depressive and anxious symptoms (but not manic symptoms) among bipolar patients in the within-group analysis, but not when compared to the control groups [52].

Finally, in a recently published network meta-analysis, the relative effectiveness of several different psychosocial interventions in the treatment of BD was compared, with a focus on relapse rates, mood symptoms, functioning, and medication adherence [53]. Results indicated that therapeutic interventions targeting family members seem to be the only ones effective in reducing rates of relapse. CBT did not seem to decrease risk of relapse, although it did seem to improve adherence and functional status, as well as decreasing manic symptoms, when associated with psychosocial interventions.

In summary, given the mixed results involving the efficacy of psychosocial therapies in BD, their role in the management of treatment-resistant cases seems to be even more unclear. While common sense would suggest that patients with treatment-resistant bipolar disorder should be offered nonpharmacological treatments as adjunct interventions aiming at having their management optimized, some of the results mentioned above suggest that specific subgroups of patients likely benefit from some nonpharmacological interventions and not from others. Additional research is necessary in order to better clarify the individual role and potential benefit of the different psychosocial interventions according to specific patient profiles.

Conclusions

Treatment-resistant bipolar disorder is an important yet neglected area of study. While research on the factors associated with the development of resistance to treatment are not totally clear, some alternative pharmacological strategies (including not only novel agents but also different combinations of traditional agents) are currently available.

Yet, the strength of the evidence supporting the use of these strategies is rather heterogeneous, and clinicians may often rely on their personal clinical experience, as well as on expert reports, when making a decision regarding the management of a treatment-resistant patient. There is considerable inconsistence across the different available guidelines for the treatment of BD, and that seems to contribute to the lack of consensus as for the management of resistant cases. As our understanding of the pathophysiology of BD continues to improve, more novel therapeutic strategies will likely be identified, and controlled studies will be necessary to characterize their role in the treatment of this condition.

With respect to nonpharmacological biological treatments, ECT seems to display good efficacy in the treatment of resistant case, despite the shortage of controlled studies in treatment-resistant bipolar disorder. Other neurostimulation techniques still seem to be in a preliminary phase regarding their role in the treatment of refractory BD, and it is expected that future studies will address their efficacy and safety.

Finally, adjunct psychosocial interventions will continue to have a role in the treatment of BD, including resistant cases. However, considering the large variation in the different study findings and the different factors that seem to affect the impact these interventions seem to have on the acute symptomatology and on the course of illness in BD, future research should likely focus on strategies aiming at identifying predictors of response to certain interventions, with the ultimate goal of optimizing the recommendation process of the different modalities of psychosocial interventions, therefore maximizing their potential benefits.

References

1. Merikangas KR, Jin R, He J-P, Kessler RC, Lee S, Sampson NA, et al. Prevalence and correlates of bipolar spectrum disorder in the world mental health survey initiative. Arch Gen Psychiatry. 2011;68(3):241.
2. Rosa AR, Reinares M, Michalak EE, Bonnin CM, Sole B, Franco C, et al. Functional impairment and

disability across mood states in bipolar disorder. Value Health. 2010;13(8):984–8.
3. Schaffer A, Isometsä ET, Tondo L, Moreno DH, Sinyor M, Kessing LV, et al. Epidemiology, neurobiology and pharmacological interventions related to suicide deaths and suicide attempts in bipolar disorder: part I of a report of the International Society for Bipolar Disorders Task Force on suicide in bipolar disorder. Aust N Z J Psychiatry. 2015;49(9):785–802.
4. Perlis RH, Ostacher MJ, Patel JK, Marangell LB, Zhang H, Wisniewski SR, et al. Predictors of recurrence in bipolar disorder: primary outcomes from the systematic treatment enhancement program for bipolar disorder (STEP-BD). Am J Psychiatry. 2006;163(2):217–24.
5. Fountoulakis KN. Refractoriness in bipolar disorder: definitions and evidence-based treatment: refractoriness in bipolar disorder. CNS Neurosci Ther. 2012;18(3):227–37.
6. Tohen M, Frank E, Bowden CL, Colom F, Ghaemi SN, Yatham LN, et al. The International Society for Bipolar Disorders (ISBD) Task Force report on the nomenclature of course and outcome in bipolar disorders. Bipolar Disord. 2009;11(5):453–73.
7. Yatham LN, Kennedy SH, Parikh SV, Schaffer A, Beaulieu S, Alda M, et al. Canadian Network for Mood and Anxiety Treatments (CANMAT) and International Society for Bipolar Disorders (ISBD) collaborative update of CANMAT guidelines for the management of patients with bipolar disorder: update 2013: CANMAT guidelines for bipolar disorder. Bipolar Disord. 2013;15(1):1–44.
8. Pacchiarotti I, Mazzarini L, Colom F, Sanchez-Moreno J, Girardi P, Kotzalidis GD, et al. Treatment-resistant bipolar depression: towards a new definition. Acta Psychiatr Scand. 2009;120(6):429–40.
9. Parker GB, Graham RK. Clinical characteristics associated with treatment-resistant bipolar disorder. J Nerv Ment Dis. 2017;205(3):188–91.
10. Cole AJ, Scott J, Ferrier IN, Eccleston D. Patterns of treatment resistance in bipolar affective disorder. Acta Psychiatr Scand. 1993;88(2):121–3.
11. Magalhães PV, Dodd S, Nierenberg AA, Berk M. Cumulative morbidity and prognostic staging of illness in the systematic treatment enhancement program for bipolar disorder (STEP-BD). Aust N Z J Psychiatry. 2012;46(11):1058–67.
12. Rybakowski JK. Genetic influences on response to mood stabilizers in bipolar disorder: current status of knowledge. CNS Drugs. 2013;27(3):165–73.
13. da Costa SC, Passos IC, Lowri C, Soares JC, Kapczinski F. Refractory bipolar disorder and neuroprogression. Prog Neuro-Psychopharmacol Biol Psychiatry. 2016;70:103–10.
14. Goodwin GM, Martinez-Aran A, Glahn DC, Vieta E. Cognitive impairment in bipolar disorder: neurodevelopment or neurodegeneration? An ECNP expert meeting report. Eur Neuropsychopharmacol. 2008;18(11):787–93.
15. Fountoulakis KN, Grunze H, Vieta E, Young A, Yatham L, Blier P, et al. The International College of Neuro-Psychopharmacology (CINP) treatment guidelines for Bipolar disorder in adults (CINP-BD-2017), part 3: the clinical guidelines. Int J Neuropsychopharmacol. 2017;20(2):180–195.
16. Nierenberg AA, Ostacher MJ, Calabrese JR, Ketter TA, Marangell LB, Miklowitz DJ, et al. Treatment-resistant bipolar depression: a STEP-BD equipoise randomized effectiveness trial of antidepressant augmentation with lamotrigine, inositol, or risperidone. Am J Psychiatry. 2006;163(2):210–6.
17. Grunebaum MF, Ellis SP, Keilp JG, Moitra VK, Cooper TB, Marver JE, et al. Ketamine versus midazolam in bipolar depression with suicidal thoughts: a pilot midazolam-controlled randomized clinical trial. Bipolar Disord. 2017;19(3):176–83.
18. Lally N, Nugent AC, Luckenbaugh DA, Ameli R, Roiser JP, Zarate CA. Anti-anhedonic effect of ketamine and its neural correlates in treatment-resistant bipolar depression. Transl Psychiatry. 2014;4(10):e469.
19. Kantrowitz JT, Halberstam B, Gangwisch J. Single-dose ketamine followed by daily D-Cycloserine in treatment-resistant bipolar depression. J Clin Psychiatry. 2015;76(6):737–8.
20. Sanches M, Newberg AR, Soares JC. Emerging drugs for bipolar disorder. Expert Opin Emerg Drugs. 2010;15(3):453–66.
21. Sarris J, Mischoulon D, Schweitzer I. Omega-3 for bipolar disorder: meta-analyses of use in mania and bipolar depression. J Clin Psychiatry. 2012;73(1):81–6.
22. Dodd S, Fernandes BS, Dean OM. Future directions for pharmacotherapies for treatment-resistant bipolar disorder. Curr Neuropharmacol. 2015;13(5):656–62.
23. Soczynska JK, Kennedy SH, Alsuwaidan M, Mansur RB, Li M, McAndrews MP, et al. A pilot, open-label, 8-week study evaluating the efficacy, safety and tolerability of adjunctive minocycline for the treatment of bipolar I/II depression. Bipolar Disord. 2017;19(3):198–213.
24. Zeinoddini A, Sorayani M, Hassanzadeh E, Arbabi M, Farokhnia M, Salimi S, et al. Pioglitazone adjunctive therapy for depressive episode of bipolar disorder: a randomized, double-blind, placebo-controlled trial. Depress Anxiety. 2015;32(3):167–73.
25. Rosenblat JD, Kakar R, Berk M, Kessing LV, Vinberg M, Baune BT, et al. Anti-inflammatory agents in the treatment of bipolar depression: a systematic review and meta-analysis. Bipolar Disord. 2016;18(2):89–101.
26. Chakrabarti S. Thyroid functions and bipolar affective disorder. J Thyroid Res. 2011;2011:1–13.
27. Li X-B, Tang Y-L, Wang C-Y, de Leon J. Clozapine for treatment-resistant bipolar disorder: a systematic review. Bipolar Disord. 2015;17(3):235–47.
28. Aksoy Poyraz C, Turan Ş, Demirel ÖF, Usta Sağlam NG, Yıldız N, Duran A. Effectiveness of ultra-rapid dose titration of clozapine for treatment-resistant bipolar mania: case series. Ther Adv Psychopharmacol. 2015;5(4):237–42.
29. Armani F, Andersen ML, Galduróz JCF. Tamoxifen use for the management of mania: a review of current

preclinical evidence. Psychopharmacology (Berl). 2014;231(4):639–49.
30. Chen AT, Malmstrom T, Nasrallah HA. Allopurinol augmentation in acute mania: a meta-analysis of placebo-controlled trials. J Affect Disord. 2018;226:245–50.
31. Arabzadeh S, Ameli N, Zeinoddini A, Rezaei F, Farokhnia M, Mohammadinejad P, et al. Celecoxib adjunctive therapy for acute bipolar mania: a randomized, double-blind, placebo-controlled trial. Bipolar Disord. 2015;17(6):606–14.
32. Fristad MA, Young AS, Vesco AT, Nader ES, Healy KZ, Gardner W, et al. A randomized controlled trial of individual family psychoeducational psychotherapy and omega-3 fatty acids in youth with subsyndromal bipolar disorder. J Child Adolesc Psychopharmacol. 2015;25(10):764–74.
33. Sanches M, Bauer IE, Galvez JF, Zunta-Soares GB, Soares JC. The management of cognitive impairment in bipolar disorder: current status and perspectives. Am J Ther. 2015;22(6):477–86.
34. McIntyre RS, Soczynska JK, Woldeyohannes HO, Miranda A, Vaccarino A, MacQueen G, et al. A randomized, double-blind, controlled trial evaluating the effect of intranasal insulin on neurocognitive function in euthymic patients with bipolar disorder: intranasal insulin in bipolar disorder. Bipolar Disord. 2012;14(7):697–706.
35. Perugi G, Medda P, Toni C, Mariani MG, Socci C, Mauri M. The role of electroconvulsive therapy (ECT) in bipolar disorder: effectiveness in 522 patients with bipolar depression, mixed-state, mania and catatonic features. Curr Neuropharmacol. 2017;15(3):359–71.
36. Schoeyen HK, Kessler U, Andreassen OA, Auestad BH, Bergsholm P, Malt UF, et al. Treatment-resistant bipolar depression: a randomized controlled trial of electroconvulsive therapy versus algorithm-based pharmacological treatment. Am J Psychiatry. 2015;172(1):41–51.
37. Kessler U, Schoeyen HK, Andreassen OA, Eide GE, Malt UF, Oedegaard KJ, et al. The effect of electroconvulsive therapy on neurocognitive function in treatment-resistant bipolar disorder depression. J Clin Psychiatry. 2014;75(11):e1306–13.
38. Loo C, Katalinic N, Mitchell PB, Greenberg B. Physical treatments for bipolar disorder: a review of electroconvulsive therapy, stereotactic surgery and other brain stimulation techniques. J Affect Disord. 2011;132(1–2):1–13.
39. Tamas RL, Menkes D, El-Mallakh RS. Stimulating research: a prospective, randomized, double-blind, sham-controlled study of slow transcranial magnetic stimulation in depressed bipolar patients. J Neuropsychiatr Clin Neurosci. 2007;19(2):198–9.
40. Dell'Osso B, Mundo E, D'Urso N, Pozzoli S, Buoli M, Ciabatti M, et al. Augmentative repetitive navigated transcranial magnetic stimulation (rTMS) in drug-resistant bipolar depression. Bipolar Disord. 2009;11(1):76–81.
41. Praharaj SK, Ram D, Arora M. Efficacy of high frequency (rapid) suprathreshold repetitive transcranial magnetic stimulation of right prefrontal cortex in bipolar mania: a randomized sham controlled study. J Affect Disord. 2009;117(3):146–50.
42. Rapinesi C, Bersani FS, Kotzalidis GD, Imperatori C, Del Casale A, Di Pietro S, et al. Maintenance Deep Transcranial Magnetic Stimulation Sessions are Associated with Reduced Depressive Relapses in Patients with Unipolar or Bipolar Depression. Front Neurol [Internet]. 2015;6. Available from: http://journal.frontiersin.org/Article/10.3389/fneur.2015.00016/abstract.
43. Cimpianu C-L, Strube W, Falkai P, Palm U, Hasan A. Vagus nerve stimulation in psychiatry: a systematic review of the available evidence. J Neural Transm. 2017;124(1):145–58.
44. Marangell LB, Suppes T, Zboyan HA, Prashad SJ, Fischer G, Snow D, et al. A 1-year pilot study of vagus nerve stimulation in treatment-resistant rapid-cycling bipolar disorder. J Clin Psychiatry. 2008;69(2):183–9.
45. Dondé C, Amad A, Nieto I, Brunoni AR, Neufeld NH, Bellivier F, et al. Transcranial direct-current stimulation (tDCS) for bipolar depression: a systematic review and meta-analysis. Prog Neuro-Psychopharmacol Biol Psychiatry. 2017;78:123–31.
46. Cretaz E, Brunoni AR, Lafer B. Magnetic seizure therapy for unipolar and bipolar depression: a systematic review. Neural Plast. 2015;2015:1–9.
47. Cho D-Y, Lee W-Y, Chen C-C. Limbic leukotomy for intractable major affective disorders: a 7-year follow-up study using nine comprehensive psychiatric test evaluations. J Clin Neurosci. 2008;15(2):138–42.
48. McMahon K, Herr NR, Zerubavel N, Hoertel N, Neacsiu AD. Psychotherapeutic treatment of bipolar depression. Psychiatr Clin North Am. 2016;39(1):35–56.
49. Lynch D, Laws KR, McKenna PJ. Cognitive behavioural therapy for major psychiatric disorder: does it really work? A meta-analytical review of well-controlled trials. Psychol Med. 2010;40(1):9–24.
50. Chiang K-J, Tsai J-C, Liu D, Lin C-H, Chiu H-L, Chou K-R. Efficacy of cognitive-behavioral therapy in patients with bipolar disorder: a meta-analysis of randomized controlled trials. Mazza M, editor. PLOS ONE. 2017;12(5):e0176849.
51. Miziou S, Tsitsipa E, Moysidou S, Karavelas V, Dimelis D, Polyzoidou V, et al. Psychosocial treatment and interventions for bipolar disorder: a systematic review. Ann Gen Psychiatry [Internet]. 2015;14(1). Available from: http://www.annals-general-psychiatry.com/content/14/1/19.
52. Chu C-S, Stubbs B, Chen T-Y, Tang C-H, Li D-J, Yang W-C, et al. The effectiveness of adjunct mindfulness-based intervention in treatment of bipolar disorder: a systematic review and meta-analysis. J Affect Disord. 2018;225:234–45.
53. Chatterton ML, Stockings E, Berk M, Barendregt JJ, Carter R, Mihalopoulos C. Psychosocial therapies for the adjunctive treatment of bipolar disorder in adults: network meta-analysis. Br J Psychiatry. 2017;210(5):333–41.

Treatment Resistance in Post-traumatic Stress Disorder

10

Alexander Cowell McFarlane

10.1 Background

There has been a long-standing suggestion that patients with post-traumatic stress disorder (PTSD) after multiple trauma exposures such as veterans have a worse outcome with both psychological and pharmacological treatments than single incident traumatic events [1, 2]. Despite this harbinger of less than adequate treatment outcomes, there has been little systematic exploration of the question of treatment resistance in the traumatic stress field [3–7]. Rather, PTSD has been treated as a unitary disorder by most treatment guidelines, suggesting that there is a uniform set of interventions that can be broadly applied independent of the initiating traumatic event or the duration of illness [1, 8]. The issue of treatment resistance in PTSD is remarkably underdeveloped in contrast to other disorders such as major depression and anxiety disorders including generalised anxiety disorder and obsessive-compulsive disorder [9–15].

This is somewhat surprising, given over two decades of evidence about the fact that approximately 50% people who develop PTSD go on to have a chronic course as was demonstrated in the first US national comorbidity study, despite many receiving treatment [16]. Using a lifetime disorder approach, this analysis suggested the treatment decreased the duration of illness but did not significantly improve the numbers going into remission. Furthermore, the seminal Vietnam Veterans' Readjustment Study that was conducted in 1988 found that there was a lifetime prevalence of 18.7% of PTSD with 9.1% continuing to suffer from the disorder at the time of the study [17]. These results highlighted that even 15 years or more after their service, substantial morbidity remained. Subsequently major steps were put in place to improve the quality of treatment for Vietnam veterans in the light of an increasingly developed treatment literature. Despite this, when this cohort was assessed 25 years later, 16% of theatre veterans reported an increase, and 7.6% reported a decrease of PTSD symptoms. This highlights the continued morbidity despite the services provided to this cohort [18].

One of the reasons why the issue of treatment resistance has not gained more attention in the PTSD field is because of the advocacy of therapists for their particular interventions, many who have been leaders in the field. In particular, there has been a significant conflict between CBT therapists and those practising EMDR [19]. When reviews have been published that are critical of the effect sizes that have been calculated, using wait list controls rather than an active alternative therapy, these have been met with strong rebuttals in the light of minimal differences in

A. C. McFarlane
The Centre for Traumatic Stress Studies, The University of Adelaide, Adelaide, SA, Australia
e-mail: alexander.mcfarlane@adelaide.edu.au

Y.-K. Kim (ed.), *Treatment Resistance in Psychiatry*, https://doi.org/10.1007/978-981-10-4358-1_10

outcomes. For example, when a meta-analysis by Benish et al. [20] concluded that CBT was no more effective than other active non-trauma-focused therapies, this evoked strong counterclaim by a group of senior therapists from the cognitive behavioural school [21, 22]. This type of dialectic has not encouraged a questioning of the effectiveness of trauma-focused therapies as should have occurred.

More recent research has confirmed the lack of differences between trauma-focused therapies and a present-centred approach [23]. Furthermore, a meta-analysis by Steenkamp et al. [24], founded approximately two thirds of veterans continue to retain their PTSD diagnosis following treatment with cognitive processing therapy and prolonged exposure. Trauma-focused therapy is the only marginally superior compared with non-trauma-focused approaches. These findings highlight the need to have more effective interventions, the extent of treatment resistance and the predictors of treatment response.

10.2 Conceptual Issues About Treatment Resistance and PTSD

In addressing the issue of treatment resistance and PTSD, there are several bodies of literature that have been relevant to this discussion. Critical issues are the existence of a series of phenotypes and the progression of the disorder. These are underpinned by the increasing body of evidence about the role of delayed onset in post-traumatic stress disorder. Longitudinal studies that have been highlighted are significantly more prevalent than had previously been anticipated [25].

10.2.1 The Utility of a Staging Model of PTSD

Advances in improving treatment resistance in PTSD requires a more sophisticated classification of PTSD that takes account of the heterogeneity of this condition and the progressions which occur with chronicity that impact on treatment responsiveness.

A clinical staging strategy utilises on the substantial body of research on the longitudinal course of PTSD and the progressive sequential shifts in its neurobiology following traumatic stress exposure [25]. This methodology has been advocated as a valuable framework to better define the unpredictable treatment response and course of disorders, such as bipolar disorder and schizophrenia [26, 27]. The staging approach is thought to permit the identification of clear and detectible inflexion points in the course of a disease process that inform severity, prognosis and treatment [28]. Staging moves away from a reliance on cross-sectional descriptions and highlights the importance of studying illnesses longitudinally. The advantage of a longitudinal approach is that it offers the potential for the early prediction of a range of later outcomes that reflect different trajectories and phenotypes. The increasing recognition of the prevalence of comorbidity with PTSD and the lack of specificity of most intervention strategies across psychiatry highlight the need for more sophisticated diagnostic reasoning.

PTSD is no different. The lack of utilisation of a longitudinal perspective is reflected in the study of the way the biology of PTSD is lumped together without consideration of the differences due to duration of illness and earlier treatment interventions. In this regarded, PTSD tends to be seen as a unitary entity without consideration that it may reflect a series of stages in the progression of the disorder, and this is necessary to better characterise treatment nonresponse. The literature about delayed-onset disorder highlights the imperative of this approach.

10.2.2 The Issue of Delayed Onset: M/L Paper Trajectory ADF

The importance of the impact of the longitudinal course on the responses to traumatic events is highlighted by the increasing recognition that delayed-onset PTSD is much more common than previously thought. Delayed-onset PTSD was initially recognised in the DSM-III formulation published in 1980 [29]. DSM-IV specifically defines that delayed-onset PTSD should be diagnosed if "…the onset of symptoms is at least 6 months after the stressor" [30, Page 468]. A historical review about the delayed-onset PTSD emphasised how much of the confusion about this construct has arisen from different definitions of delayed-onset PTSD [31]. For example, different interpretations of the construct included whether or not an individual who has had subsyndromal symptoms who has subsequently crossed a threshold of clinical severity has a delayed onset or whether the term should be preserved for individuals who have been asymptomatic and then at some later point developed a disorder.

The existence of the delayed form of PTSD emphasises how a traumatic experience can apparently lie relatively symptomatically dormant within an individual only to become manifest at some future point. This raises important questions about the mechanism of how a subclinical state is triggered into a full-blown syndrome and how these switches may impact on treatment responsiveness. There is a broad body of scientific literature available that can assist in answering these questions.

There is substantial literature highlighting the risk of subsyndromal symptoms and the later emergence of full-blown disorder in the form of delayed-onset PTSD [32–35]. One of the difficulties summarising this literature is the variable periods of follow-up. One meta-analysis [36] indicated that most studies have followed populations for less than 2 years, which provides little information about the longer-term cumulative risk. Specifically, Smid et al. [36] found that the mean duration of longitudinal studies was 25 months and the maximum range of 60 months. In the combined study population, 24.8% (95% CI = 22.6–27.2%) had delayed-onset PTSD. A regression analysis of this data showed that the proportion of individuals with delayed-onset PTSD was larger when the duration of follow-up was longer. They also found that traumatic exposures in military populations were associated with a greater proportion of delayed-onset PTSD and when the cumulative incidence was lower.

One important limitation of the literature is that the probability of symptoms increasing across much longer time periods has only limited examination literature. For example, a 20-year follow-up of a group of veterans with combat stress reactions and a group of veterans without stress reactions indicated that in the latter group, the total number of symptoms was greater 20 years after combat than at any of the previous assessment points. This study was of Israeli veterans of the 1982 Lebanon War and found that the rates of delayed-onset PTSD emerged relatively soon in the aftermath of the war but again 17 years after the period of military service [35]. In fact, 23% of the Israeli veterans who did not develop an immediate acute stress disorder subsequently went on to develop a delayed-onset PTSD. Furthermore, in the Australian Vietnam Veterans Study, rates of lifetime PTSD were found to increase over a decade, going from 20% in the 1990s to 28% in the 2000s [37]. These studies highlight the long-term and continual increase in PTSD morbidity following trauma. In other words, the degree of symptomatic distress even in those without PTSD does not seem to decrease with time. In those without combat stress reactions, 14% of individuals had PTSD in the 1st year in contrast to 26% at the 20th year assessment [35].

These studies have been of populations who have access to treatment services. If treatment was effective, there would be an expectation that with the passage of time, the rates of disorder would decrease. The findings suggest the opposite, namely, that the combination of age and time, despite the effects of treatment, leads to increasing rates for disorder highlighting the importance of considering the issue of treatment resistance. Given the interest in the longitudinal course of PTSD, it is surprising that there has not been a more systematic examination of this critically important clinical issue. Hence the literature suggests that PTSD passes through a series of stages as well as different subtypes where treatment response should not be assumed to be unitary.

10.2.3 The Impact of Cumulative Stress Exposure

A further related issue that has not been systematically addressed in the treatment literature for

PTSD is the risk of developing PTSD following exposure to an event and how this changes with multiple exposures. A change in the probability of developing the disorder would also suggest a change in the probability of treatment response with multiple exposures.

The importance of this issue is supported by evidence from a variety of research that indicates that the cumulative impact of trauma exposure increases the risk of PTSD [38]. Population studies show that the number of trauma exposures is a significant risk for post-traumatic stress disorder and other adverse health outcomes [39]. In particular, it is not simply exposure to a single traumatic event but repeated trauma exposure that results in the further sensitisation and neurobiological dysregulation which ultimately lead to the onset of clinical disorder. Thus, it is important to consider lifetime trauma history accumulated as a determinant of treatment response and treatment resistance.

Similarly, studies of veterans have illustrated that lifetime trauma exposure is an important predictor of both PTSD and depressive symptoms, over and above the effects of combat experiences [40, 41]. Equally, the cumulative exposures to traumatic events predict the risk of PTSD, depression and alcohol abuse [42, 43].

In summary, studies have shown that the effect of trauma is cumulative, in that previous exposure to trauma signals a greater risk of mental disorder from subsequent trauma [44]. The impact of 'cumulative trauma' has also demonstrated that the number of trauma types experienced is associated with significantly greater probability of disorder [45]. The effects have also been demonstrated in police officers where the cumulative burden of stress exposure has been identified as leading to increasing neurobiological dysregulation [46]. This highlights how cumulative stress exposure has an enduring neurobiological effect which in turn is likely to impact on treatment responsiveness. However, this is not addressed in the treatment literature. There are several mechanisms that may account for this cumulative impact and, in turn, the effects on treatment responsiveness.

10.2.4 Sensitisation, Kindling and Onset of Disorder

Firstly, sensitisation provides a theoretical perspective for examining the risk of consequences of repeated exposure to major traumatic stresses prior to the onset of any disorder. This mechanism is likely to underpin how repeated exposure to traumatic stresses increases the probability that those individuals will suffer from PTSD with a further exposure [47–49]. Heim et al. [50] have highlighted how this process of sensitisation to symptoms arising from trauma exposure has been supported at a biological level. In a number of studies, a link between childhood trauma and sensitisation of their neuroendocrine stress response modified by immune activation, glucocorticoid resistance and reduced hippocampal volume has been identified. Hence, there is a significant body of evidence demonstrating that repeated stress exposures prior to the onset of the first episode of a disorder increased the risk of PTSD and a range of other conditions, particularly depression.

An important question arises as to which individuals are vulnerable to the impact of further triggering and activation of their traumatic memories. One study of accident victims showed that those who went on to develop delayed-onset PTSD symptoms had significantly more symptoms 8 days after the trauma than those who did not develop PTSD. Importantly, the majority of the injury survivors in this study had low levels of symptoms in the acute setting, and these persisted over time. The initial symptoms which were particularly indicative of risk were intensity and frequency of the arousal and re-experiencing symptoms [51]. These data demonstrate how subsyndromal PTSD can increase in severity due the process of sensitisation, particularly in the first year after a major traumatic incident.

The literature about sensitisation and kindling in the onset of depression is an important model for PTSD, particularly in the light of the regular comorbidity of these disorders. For a long time, it has been recognised that major depression has a complex aetiology that involves both the role of stressful life events and genetic risk factors as is now increasingly the case with PTSD. One meta-analysis [52] concluded that the first onset of major depression was more likely to be preceded by severe life stress than were recurrent episodes of depression. In other words, milder events can trigger the onset of depressive episodes as the number of episodes of depression increases. Ultimately this process can reach a point where the illness becomes relatively autonomous of stress in situations where the stressors are not required to trigger the onset or what to an outside observer would be regarded as a stressor is absent [53]. It is important to examine whether a similar process is occurring with PTSD and leading to increasing treatment resistance.

Kendler et al. [54] have concluded that kindling is particularly important in people who do not have a major genetic predisposition to depression, and this is a model likely to be applicable to PTSD. Furthermore, this kindling effect has been shown to disappear after approximately nine episodes when the process becomes increasingly autonomous and may provide a model for emerging treatment resistance in PTSD. This is in keeping with the kindling hypothesis that suggests that there is a threshold beyond which there can be no additional sensitisation to the depressive state as maybe the case with PTSD. This implies a transitioning to a pattern of increasingly autonomous illness, where an increasing number of episodes have been correlated with relative treatment refractiveness [47].

In the case of PTSD, once the disorder has developed, triggers play a particularly important role in reinforcing the intrusive memories and the associated psychophysiological activity. These memories increasingly become more and more spontaneous as a consequence of a kindling-like progression. The support for the commonality of this mechanism also comes from the role of serotonin in the rate of development of amygdala kindling and the role of serotonin reuptake inhibitors in the treatment of all of these conditions.

Sensitisation is also likely to play an important role via kindling-like mechanisms in the somatic symptoms associated with PTSD such as pain. Given the significant interrelationship between PTSD and somatic symptoms, these shared mechanisms are of particular relevance in assessing the importance and contribution of stress exposure to conditions such as chronic back pain and fatigue-like syndromes and their role in treatment refractoriness [55, 56]. The role of these somatic symptoms in the treatment responsiveness in PTSD has received remarkably little attention in the literature.

10.2.5 The Model of Allostatic Load

A further body of evidence highlights the underlying mechanisms by which stress exposure can modify subsequent reactivity to challenge, with exposure to stress leading to modification of a range of biological systems. This results in increasing allostatic load due to the up-regulation of the inhibitory systems [57–59]. The allostatic load model has been used to refocus the stress disease literature, emphasising that their multiple biological systems are vulnerable to a temporal cascade of dysregulation [55]. These progressive dysregulations lead to the emergence of a range of disease trajectories as well as treatment resistance. This approach provides a broader construct than traditional models used in biomedical practice for understanding how repeated challenges from the environment lead to increasingly maladaptive disruptions of homeostatic mechanisms. The essence of the allostatic load model is that the body is subject to wear and tear with repeated activation during stressful situations [60].

At a neurobiological level, these inhibitory systems are reflected in the prefrontal/amygdala circuitry [60, 61]. Similarly, the HPA axis and other neurohormonal systems are vulnerable to these mechanisms of sensitisation [57, 58]. Hence, when individuals who has suffered a major trauma exposure and then attempts to adapt to day-to-day life including the normal stressors that occur within the community, the dysregulation of these underlying regulatory systems modifies their adaptability. Progressively, they react to the presence of stressors with greater amplitude or intensity and ultimately develop an overgeneralised reactivity to a range of stimuli that remind them of the traumatic event [62]. This cycle of increasing reactivity to a widening range of cues serves to further reinforce the distress response. This may, however, only become manifest as frank disorder after the passage of time and also logically lead to decreased treatment responsiveness as the disorder becomes more chronic. Again, the lack of examination of this question in the treatment literature is surprising.

10.2.6 Shared Neural Circuitry

The models of sensitisation, kindling and allostatic load in PTSD highlight the importance of the biological mechanisms of the onset and chronicity of this disorder. The underlying circuitry neural regions which have been identified as being relevant to the aetiology of PTSD are equally those involved in depression and the emergence of treatment resistance. For example, amygdala reactivity has been identified as a primary area of interest in PTSD, and this nucleus plays a central role in determining fear reactivity [63, 64]. The amygdala has also been extensively involved in the investigation of depression [65].

For example, Ramel et al. [66] highlighted how amygdala reactivity is an important issue in people with a history of depression in contrast to those without such a history. These results indicate how the amygdala plays a central role in modulating mood congruent memory, particularly during the induction of sad states of mind in individuals who are vulnerable to depression. Hence, a known risk for individuals with PTSD is further exposure to environments that have traumatic triggers because the obvious risks of activation of fear-related circuitry are similar to the risks for individuals with depression to activate the neural systems associated with the vulnerability to negative emotion and the onset of depressive episodes [67, 68]. Further evidence suggested the underlying biological mechanisms of how the duration of depression impacts on cognitive functioning and disability. Against this background, the lack of investigation of this domain in the PTSD is surprising as it is highly probable that similar observations would be made.

This effect is related to the sensitivity of the hippocampus to stress, a critical issue in PTSD. In depression, it has been found that the length of past depression impairs memory performance and that there is a significant toxic link between the burden of depression and cognition [9]. The role of the hippocampus in the aetiology of post-traumatic stress disorder has been similarly extensively researched with several meta-analyses concluding that individuals with post-traumatic stress disorder have a smaller hippocampal volume than individuals without this condition who are trauma exposed and that this difference cannot be solely attributed to a pre-existing vulnerability as suggested by the study of [69].

There is now a range of literature which suggests that the hippocampus is one structure that is vulnerable to morphological damage caused by untreated illness such as in depression and schizophrenia. This issue has been investigated in PTSD. It has been found that the longer the duration of illness, the greater degree of hippocampal atrophy in post-traumatic stress disorder. Importantly, the hippocampus is part of a neural network associated with the dorsolateral prefrontal cortex and the anterior cingulate whose activation is critical to the outcomes of cognitive behavioural therapy. Hence the damage to this network diminishes the probability of an adequate treatment response in cognitive behavioural therapy. Logically, the longer the illness goes untreated and the greater the degree of the disruption of these networks, the less the probability that the individual will have an adequate treatment response. Furthermore, changes in the hippocampus have been associated with insomnia severity in PTSD. The importance of this finding is that the structural abnormalities and the progressive disruption of hippocampal function at the time of post-traumatic stress disorder have also been specifically tied to the phenomenological outcomes that are of clinical relevance [70].

These findings have been studied in the aftermath of a number of different types of traumas [71]. In this sample, the severity of the re-experiencing symptoms was greater in those officers with smaller total and left hippocampal volume. They highlighted how the chronic stress of having PTSD symptoms can contribute to smaller hippocampal volume [72]. In this study, the PTSD subjects had had their symptoms for approximately 3 years highlighting the possibility that these changes had occurred.

Finally, further neuroimaging studies have demonstrated increased activation of these regions of interest in patients who have successful outcomes from cognitive behavioural therapy. Therefore, factors that lessen the probability that these neural networks can be recruited in the course of treatment are likely to lessen the probability of effective treatment outcomes. This literature highlights the characteristics of these predictors of treatment outcome that have been examined in PTSD but have not led to more general consideration of the issue of treatment resistance in PTSD.

10.3 The Relevance of Other Issues from the General Literature

10.3.1 Duration of Illness

There is no direct research that has examined the impact of duration of illness on treatment outcome in PTSD, despite the extensive research into this question with other disorders. However, the majority of the naturalistic studies concluded that it did not impact on the effectiveness of interventions, but these were substantially flawed from a methodological perspective. The studies that have considered this question of the impact of a delay in implementation of treatment in PTSD [2, 73–75] have done this by re-examining existing treatment studies. None were specifically designed to answer this question; rather, this is being addressed in secondary analyses.

The Resick et al. [73] study compares CBT and cognitive reprocessing treatment and found that the duration of disorder did not influence the effectiveness, i.e. the time that had elapsed since the traumatic exposure. However, people who present late for treatment cannot be presumed to have a disorder that has the same severity or course as those presenting to closer proximity to the trauma. The Gillespie et al. study [75] was an effectiveness study following the Omagh bombing, and the outcomes of those who presented early for care were compared with those presenting in the latter period of the treatment service. Again those presenting in the immediate aftermath of bombing cannot be presumed to be the same as those presenting later. In particular, those presenting later may have a delayed-onset PTSD where the high levels of acute distress in those without a delayed onset may be indicative of differential risk factors. A study of sertraline [2] in combat veterans where the mean duration of treatment was 17 years found no effect of the duration of treatment, but this is not surprising, given that sertraline was not demonstrated to be an effective intervention in this population.

In contrast, the study of Duffy et al. [74] of patients with PTSD in the context of terrorism in Northern Ireland did find that the longer the delay for presenting for treatment, the worse the outcome.

Hence, these studies do not provide an adequate scientific investigation of this question, and the lack of investigation of this issue in PTSD in contrast to major depression, bipolar disorder and GAD is in fact surprising. Furthermore, there is a general consensus reflected in the general psychiatric literature about the gains that are obtained from the early intervention of psychiatric disorder [76–78].

Given the commonality of the underpinnings of the aetiology in depression and PTSD, it is reasonable to extrapolate from the factors that have been identified as influencing treatment response. Kravitz et al. [79] reviewed the evidence and in a study of a further sample identified that recovery from a major depressive episode was most strongly correlated with the length of the current episode. Similar findings have been identified in a number of other studies where the longer the illness length, the greater the delay in the remission onset [10–12]. It is improbable that the duration of illness is not a substantial determinant of treatment responsive of PTSD.

10.4 Partial Remission to Treatment as a Protector of Relapse

There is a substantial body of research that has examined the impact of partial remission following treatment in the course of a major depressive disorder on longitudinal course and recurrence. This perspective is of equal relevance to PTSD but has received virtually no systematic examination. Pintor et al. [13] followed up a population suffering from unipolar depression and identified that the relapse rate in patients with partial remission was 67%. This study emphasised the importance of complete remission as an issue required to decrease the rates of short-term relapse. This is an important finding in the context of the fact that in the order of 80% of individuals have second episodes. These findings about major depressive episodes are pertinent particularly to individuals who have a comorbid major depressive disorder and PTSD but are also likely to be applicable to those without the secondary comorbidity.

10.5 The Utility of a Staging Approach to Addressing Treatment Resistance in PTSD

A staging approach to PTSD as with other disorders would provide a framework for addressing the changing patterns of treatment response if it was systematically applied in treatment studies. It requires an acknowledgement of the inadequate outcomes that current treatments, psychotherapeutic and pharmacological alike provide for a significant percentage of those with PTSD. The staging approach highlights the need to characterise the biological progression of the disease and how this impacts on treatment response. This has been characterised in major depressive disorder, with particular emphasis on the early treatment of preclinical stages as described above [27]. Similarly in PTSD, it is necessary to identify which early symptoms are the likely markers of the risk to chronic illness. Clinically and theoretically, there has been a propensity to normalise the early symptoms of distress following traumatic stress exposure [80, 81], thereby depriving the field of important prognostic indicators for those who may be en route to a chronic course of illness. Fortunately, biological studies of the acute stress response in those who develop PTSD at a later time have shown that there are important predictors that differentiate these individuals from those who demonstrate minimal reactivity [82, 83].

The question becomes, if trauma survivors have different biological alterations at early stages of illness that appear to predict symptoms later on, even if they do not seem to have particularly different symptomatic presentations in the early aftermath of trauma, should the biological information be used to determine further treatment? Staging may be of considerable benefit if it is able to differentiate patients who are likely to have good treatment outcomes with early intervention from those who are less likely to benefit. The probable adverse effect of duration of illness is one important predictor of prognosis. In PTSD, like other psychiatric disorders, the need to document the continually evolving dysregulation that has a substantial probability of impacting on treatment outcome is highlighted [84]. This worsening treatment outcome with increasing duration of untreated illness is a further argument for a staging model. There needs to be more attention to defining the phenotypes and neurobiology of those who are treatment resistance to allow a systematic examination of second-order treatments.

Specifically, if the course of PTSD rests on the fact that post-trauma neurobiological alterations reach a point that results in persistent or progressive illness [4], then staging would have considerable clinical utility. To test this hypothesis, disease markers that have a direct clinicopathological correlation to the underlying pathophysiology need to be characterised, and these need to reflect the emerging increasing severity of the disorder [5, 85–90]. The research strategy has to involve longitudinal investigation of the relationship between the biological characteristics of PTSD and its stages. This approach also needs to consider the related somatic comorbidities that have a shared biology. The aim of the staging approach is to identify biomarkers that have an adequate degree of specificity for PTSD and to differentiate those that act as disease markers from indicators of risk and vulnerability across the different stages, markers of disease progression and epiphenomena [26].

The staging model further allows a framework for examining different biological models for PTSD and how they overlap [25]. This requires a long window of observation to investigate models such as stress-induced sensitisation and increasing inflammatory reactivity [91]. The neurobiology of the secondary adaptations of chronic hyperreactivity and associated numbing in the context of emerging mood disorder is likely to be of particular importance in understanding chronicity and treatment resistance. In essence, time is a critical dimension in dissecting the interplay of the matrix of biological phenomena that has been examined in PTSD and treatment responsiveness [92, 93]. The development of a model of clinical stages of PTSD has much to recommend itself to inform future possible novel treatments.

10.6 Candidate Strategies

The substantial body of the treatment studies in PTSD has trialled interventions as a primary intervention for PTSD. The literature has very few studies that consider the issues of augmentation or second-line interventions that address treatment resistance.

10.6.1 Medication Approaches

A recent consensus statement about psychopharmacological approaches for PTSD statement highlighted the paucity of treatment alternatives. It concluded that there was no visible horizon for advancements in PTSD treatment [94]. The SSRIs remain the only FDA-approved treatments for PTSD [8]. In clinical practice, a variety of off-label usages underpin the polypharmacy that is frequent. Hence most prescribing has little empirical guidance regarding risks and benefits. A number of potential strategies such as the atypical antipsychotics [95], anticonvulsants [96], ketamine [97, 98] and prazosin [99, 100] have not met up to their initial promise in the outcomes from clinical trials. MDMA-assisted psychotherapy is currently receiving considerable attention [101]. However, other agents that have been trialled to assist cognitive behavioural interventions such as propranolol [102] and d-cycloserine [103] have not provided substantial evidence of benefits.

Perhaps the strategies that should be utilised to further the knowledge about treatment resistance should be adapted from the depression literature. There is an increasingly sophisticated literature about the role of inflammation in PTSD, and this may be a target for intervention [25]. Trials that investigate the potential augmentation benefits of minocycline and aspirin that have been shown to have benefit in major depressive disorder should be considered [104]. Equally raised C reactive protein has been found to be a predictor of improved response in depression to different types of antidepressants [105]. When the C reactive protein is greater than one, targeting both noradrenergic and serotoninergic neurotransmission leads to better treatment response [105]. In contrast, medications targetting serotoninergic neurotransmission alone showed better treatment response when C reactive protein levels were less than one. Hence inflammation is another domain worthy of examining in determining treatment response to medications in PTSD.

Also, the cognitive deficits in PTSD are an important cause of impairment and disability in PTSD [106]. The use of medications such as dexamphetamine, donepezil and rivastigmine has some promising findings but has not been subject to large systematic trials [107].

The lack of interest of the pharmaceutical industry in funding such trials highlights the importance of treatment resistance needing to be addressed by organisations such as the Departments of Veterans Affairs and organising registries that assist in improving treatment outcomes. The personalised medicine approach where interventions are trialled in settings where there is a substantial neurobiological database collected on patients prior to the commencement of treatment has much to recommend itself.

10.6.2 Psychotherapeutic Strategies

While some trials have examined the combination of medications and psychotherapy, these have not demonstrated any consistent gains in treatment effect sizes [8]. Most psychotherapy studies are head-to-head studies and do not consider the possibility that different approaches may have an additive effect. For example, anger has been shown to be a predictor of poorer outcomes in CBT, and interventions aimed to address anger as an initial step in treatment may improve the later use of CBT [108].

Similarly, the impact of PTSD on interpersonal relationships has led to the demonstrated benefits of interpersonal psychotherapy [109 to get]. However, there is no evidence of whether this approach can be combined with trauma-focused psychotherapy to improve treatment gains.

10.6.3 Physical Interventions

While trials have been conducted using transcranial magnetic stimulation in PTSD, the results have been equivocal [110]. Similarly, the role of direct current stimulations remains unclear. Neurofeedback is another approach that has promise [111]. Again, a personalised approach is likely to be required to demonstrate the clinical utility of these approaches [112]. The literature suggests that there are a series of different patterns of network abnormalities and functional connectivity in PTSD. It is only when these treatments are targeted to abnormalities that have been characterised prior to treatment that their role in addressing treatment resistant PTSD will be properly identified [112].

10.6.4 Others

There are frequent media stories about novel approaches to the treatment of PTSD, particularly in the veterans' community that evoke considerable interest and advocacy. These include studies of yoga [113], exercise [114, 115] and meditation [116]. There is an emerging literature about their benefits. However, where this sits in the therapeutic armamentarium is far from clear. These are likely to be nonspecific approaches that should optimally be trialled in conjunction with more symptom-focused approaches such as CBT. These interventions are likely to be of particular use to address areas such as social inclusion and engagement. Equally assistance dogs and equine therapy are unlikely to be treatments for PTSD but rather provide methods to address the social withdrawal and hypervigilance that are important causes of disability.

Conclusion

Treatment resistance in PTSD has been subject to surprisingly little systematic consideration despite the substantial evidence of the limited effectiveness of first-line evidence-based treatments in a substantial percentage of cases. If this situation is to be improved, there needs to be a systematic approach to addressing treatment resistance in PTSD. The utilisation of a personalised medicine approach that characterises the phenomenological and neurobiological underpinnings of treatment response is likely to be a high-yield strategy. There is a need to address the neurobiology, the meaning and context of the traumatic events and the disabilities and related social impairments. It is probable that a multi-tiered approach simultaneously addresses these dimensions of morbidity. However, this requires a coordinated initiative of interested parties such as insurers dealing with accident victims, emergency service organisations and government departments dealing with veterans.

References

1. Foa EB, Keane TM, Friedman MJ, Cohen JA, editors. Effective treatments for PTSD: practice guidelines from the International Society for Traumatic Stress Studies. New York: Guilford Press; 2008.
2. Friedman MJ, Marmar CR, Baker DG, Sikes CR, Farfel GM. Randomized, double-blind comparison of sertraline and placebo for posttraumatic stress dis-

order in a Department of Veterans Affairs setting. J Clin Psychiatry. 2007;68:711–20.
3. Boulos D, Zamorski MA. Do shorter delays to care and mental health system renewal translate into better occupational outcome after mental disorder diagnosis in a cohort of Canadian military personnel who returned from an Afghanistan deployment? BMJ Open. 2015;5(12):e008591.
4. Koek RJ, Schwartz HN, Scully S, Langevin JP, Spangler S, Korotinsky A, et al. Treatment-refractory posttraumatic stress disorder (TRPTSD): a review and framework for the future. Prog Neuro-Psychopharmacol Biol Psychiatry. 2016;70:170–218.
5. Hamner MB, Robert S, Frueh BC. Treatment-resistant posttraumatic stress disorder: strategies for intervention. CNS Spectr. 2004;9(10):740–52.
6. Dunlop BW, Kaye JL, Youngner C, Rothbaum B. Assessing treatment-resistant posttraumatic stress disorder: the Emory treatment resistance interview for PTSD (E-TRIP). Behav Sci. 2014;4(4):511–27.
7. Simon NM, Connor KM, Lang AJ, Rauch S, Krulewicz S, LeBeau RT, et al. Paroxetine CR augmentation for posttraumatic stress disorder refractory to prolonged exposure therapy. J Clin Psychiatry. 2008;69:400–5.
8. Australian Centre for Posttraumatic Mental Health 2013. Australian guidelines for the treatment of acute stress disorder and posttraumatic stress disorder. Melbourne: ACPMH; 2013.
9. Gorwood P, Corruble E, Falissard B, Goodwin GM. Toxic effects of depression on brain function: impairment of delayed recall and the cumulative length of depressive disorder in a large sample of depressed outpatients. Am J Psychiatr. 2008;165(6):731–9.
10. O'Leary D, Costello F, Gormley N, Webb M. Remission onset and relapse in depression: an 18-month prospective study of course for 100 first admission patients. J Affect Disord. 2000;57(1):159–71.
11. Gormley N, O'Leary D, Costello F. First admissions for depression: is the 'no-treatment interval' a critical predictor of time to remission? J Affect Disord. 1999;54(1):49–54.
12. Scott J, Eccleston D, Boys R. Can we predict the persistence of depression? Br J Psychiatry. 1992;161(5):633–7.
13. Pintor L, Gastó C, Navarro V, Torres X, Fañanas L. Relapse of major depression after complete and partial remission during a 2-year follow-up. J Affect Disord. 2003;73(3):237–44.
14. Roy-Byrne P. Treatment-refractory anxiety; definition, risk factors, and treatment challenges. Dialogues Clin Neurosci. 2015;17(2):191.
15. Fava M. Diagnosis and definition of treatment-resistant depression. Biol Psychiatry. 2003;53(8):649–59.
16. Kessler RC, Sonnega A, Bromet E, Hughes M, Nelson CB. Posttraumatic stress disorder in the National Comorbidity Survey. Arch Gen Psychiatry. 1995;52(12):1048–60.
17. Marshall RD, Turner JB, Lewis-Fernandez R, Koenan K, Neria Y, Dohrenwend BP. Symptom patterns associated with chronic PTSD in male veterans: new findings from the National Vietnam Veterans Readjustment Study. J Nerv Ment Dis. 2006;194(4):275–8.
18. Marmar CR, Schlenger W, Henn-Haase C, Qian M, Purchia E, Li M, et al. Course of posttraumatic stress disorder 40 years after the Vietnam War: findings from the National Vietnam Veterans Longitudinal Study. JAMA Psychiat. 2015;72(9):875–81.
19. Russell MC. Scientific resistance to research, training and utilization of eye movement desensitization and reprocessing (EMDR) therapy in treating post-war disorders. Soc Sci Med. 2008;67(11):1737–46.
20. Benish SG, Imel ZE, Wampold BE. The relative efficacy of bona fide psychotherapies for treating posttraumatic stress disorder: a meta-analysis of direct comparisons. Clin Psychol Rev. 2008;28(5):746–58.
21. Ehlers A, Bisson J, Clark DM, Creamer M, Pilling S, Richards D, et al. Do all psychological treatments really work the same in posttraumatic stress disorder? Clin Psychol Rev. 2010;30(2):269–76.
22. Wampold BE, Imel ZE, Laska KM, Benish S, Miller SD, Flűckiger C, et al. Determining what works in the treatment of PTSD. Clin Psychol Rev. 2010;30(8):923–33.
23. Hoge CW, Chard KM. A window into the evolution of trauma-focused psychotherapies for posttraumatic stress disorder. JAMA. 2018;319(4):343–5.
24. Steenkamp MM, Litz BT, Hoge CW, Marmar CR. Psychotherapy for military-related PTSD: a review of randomized clinical trials. JAMA. 2015;314(5):489.
25. McFarlane AC, Lawrence-Wood E, Van Hooff M, Malhi GS, Yehuda R. The need to take a staging approach to the biological mechanisms of PTSD and its treatment. Curr Psychiatry Rep. 2017;19(2):10.
26. McGorry P, Keshavan M, Goldstone S, Amminger P, Allott K, Berk M, et al. Biomarkers and clinical staging in psychiatry. World Psychiatry. 2014;13(3):211–23.
27. Verduijn J, Milaneschi Y, Schoevers RA, Hickie IB, Penninx BW, Beekman AT. Clinical staging of major depressive disorder: an empirical exploration. J Clin Psychiatry. 2015;76(9):1200–8.
28. Gonnella JS, Hornbrook MC, Louis DZ. Staging of disease. A case-mix measurement. JAMA. 1984;251(5):637–44.
29. American Psychiatric Association. Diagnostic and statistical manual of mental disorders. 3rd ed. Washington, DC: American Psychiatric Association; 1980.
30. American Psychiatric Association. Diagnostic and statistical manual of mental disorders, Text revision. 4th ed. Washington, DC: American Psychiatric Association; 2000.

31. Andrews B, Brewin CR, Philpott R, Stewart L. Delayed-onset posttraumatic stress disorder: a systematic review of the evidence. Am J Psychiatr. 2007;164(9):1319–26.
32. Carty J, O'Donnell ML, Creamer M. Delayed-onset PTSD: a prospective study of injury survivors. J Affect Disord. 2006;90(2):257–61.
33. Grieger TA, Cozza SJ, Ursano RJ, Hoge C, Martinez PE, Engel CC, et al. Posttraumatic stress disorder and depression in battle-injured soldiers. Am J Psychiatr. 2006;163(10):1777–83.
34. Orcutt HK, Erickson DJ, Wolfe J. The course of PTSD symptoms among Gulf War veterans: a growth mixture modeling approach. J Trauma Stress. 2004;17(3):195–202.
35. Solomon Z, Mikulincer M. Trajectories of PTSD: a 20-year longitudinal study. Am J Psychiatr. 2006;163(4):659–66.
36. Smid GE, Mooren TT, van der Mast RC, Gersons BP, Kleber RJ. Delayed posttraumatic stress disorder: systematic review, meta-analysis, and meta-regression analysis of prospective studies. J Clin Psychiatry. 2009;70(11):1572.
37. O'Toole BI, Catts SV, Outram S, Pierse KR, Cockburn J. The physical and mental health of Australian Vietnam veterans 3 decades after the war and its relation to military service, combat, and post-traumatic stress disorder. Am J Epidemiol. 2009;170(3):318–30.
38. Karam EG, Friedman MJ, Hill ED, Kessler RC, McLaughlin KA, Petukhova M, et al. Cumulative traumas and risk thresholds: 12-month PTSD in the World Mental Health (WMH) surveys. Depress Anxiety. 2014;31(2):130–42.
39. Del Gaizo AL, Elhai JD, Weaver TL. Posttraumatic stress disorder, poor physical health and substance use behaviors in a national trauma-exposed sample. Psychiatry Res. 2011;188(3):390–5.
40. Dedert EA, Green KT, Calhoun PS, Yoash-Gantz R, Taber KH, Mumford MM, et al. Association of trauma exposure with psychiatric morbidity in military veterans who have served since September 11, 2001. J Psychiatr Res. 2009;43(9):830–6.
41. Iversen AC, Fear NT, Ehlers A, Hughes JH, Hull L, Earnshaw M, et al. Risk factors for post-traumatic stress disorder among UK Armed Forces personnel. Psychol Med. 2008;38(4):511–22.
42. Harvey SB, Milligan-Saville JS, Paterson HM, Harkness EL, Marsh AM, Dobson M, et al. The mental health of fire-fighters: an examination of the impact of repeated trauma exposure. Aust N Z J Psychiatry. 2016;50(7):649–58.
43. Jahnke SA, Poston WS, Haddock CK, Murphy B. Firefighting and mental health: experiences of repeated exposure to trauma. Work. 2016;53(4):737–44.
44. Breslau N, Chilcoat HD, Kessler RC, Davis GC. Previous exposure to trauma and PTSD effects of subsequent trauma: results from the Detroit Area Survey of Trauma. Am J Psychiatr. 1999;156(6):902–7.
45. Cabrera OA, Hoge CW, Bliese PD, Castro CA, Messer SC. Childhood adversity and combat as predictors of depression and post-traumatic stress in deployed troops. Am J Prev Med. 2007;33(2):77–82.
46. Regehr C, LeBlanc V, Jelley RB, Barath I, Daciuk J. Previous trauma exposure and PTSD symptoms as predictors of subjective and biological response to stress. Can J Psychiatry. 2007;52(10):675–83.
47. Post RM, Weiss SR. Sensitization and kindling phenomena in mood, anxiety, and obsessive–compulsive disorders: the role of serotonergic mechanisms in illness progression. Biol Psychiatry. 1998;44(3):193–206.
48. Bremner JD, Southwick SM, Johnson DR, Yehuda R, Charney DS. Childhood physical abuse and combat-related posttraumatic stress disorder in Vietnam veterans. Am J Psychiatry. 1993;150(2):235.
49. Yehuda R, Kahana B, Schmeidler J, Southwick SM. Impact of cumulative lifetime trauma and recent stress on current posttraumatic stress disorder symptoms in Holocaust survivors. Am J Psychiatry. 1995;152(12):1815.
50. Heim C, Nemeroff CB. Neurobiology of posttraumatic stress disorder. CNS Spectr. 2009;14(1 Suppl 1):13–24.
51. O'Donnell ML, Elliott P, Lau W, Creamer M. PTSD symptom trajectories: from early to chronic response. Behav Res Ther. 2007;45(3):601–6.
52. Stroud CB, Davila J, Moyer A. The relationship between stress and depression in first onsets versus recurrences: a meta-analytic review. J Abnorm Psychol. 2008;117(1):206.
53. Patten SB. Sensitization: the sine qua non of the depressive disorders? Med Hypotheses. 2008;71(6):872–5.
54. Kendler KS, Thornton LM, Gardner CO. Genetic risk, number of previous depressive episodes, and stressful life events in predicting onset of major depression. Am J Psychiatr. 2001;158(4):582–6.
55. McFarlane AC. Stress-related musculoskeletal pain. Best Pract Res Clin Rheumatol. 2007;21(3):549–65.
56. Post RM. Do the epilepsies, pain syndromes, and affective disorders share common kindling-like mechanisms? Epilepsy Res. 2002;50(1–2):203–19.
57. Marshall RD, Garakani A. Psychobiology of the acute stress response and its relationship to the psychobiology of post-traumatic stress disorder. Psychiatr Clin N Am. 2002;25(2):385–95.
58. McFarlane AC. The long-term costs of traumatic stress: intertwined physical and psychological consequences. World Psychiatry. 2010;9(1):3–10.
59. Post RM, Weiss SR, Smith M, Li H, McCann U. Kindling versus quenching. Ann N Y Acad Sci. 1997;821(1):285–95.
60. McEwen BS, Wingfield JC. The concept of allostasis in biology and biomedicine. Horm Behav. 2003;43(1):2–15.
61. Rauch SL, Shin LM, Phelps EA. Neurocircuitry models of posttraumatic stress disorder and extinction: human neuroimaging research—past, present, and future. Biol Psychiatry. 2006;60(4):376–82.

62. McEwen BS. Physiology and neurobiology of stress and adaptation: central role of the brain. Physiol Rev. 2007;87(3):873–904.
63. Etkin A, Wager TD. Functional neuroimaging of anxiety: a meta-analysis of emotional processing in PTSD, social anxiety disorder, and specific phobia. Am J Psychiatr. 2007;164(10):1476–88.
64. Shin LM, Liberzon I. The neurocircuitry of fear, stress, and anxiety disorders. Neuropsychopharmacology. 2010;35(1):169.
65. Drevets WC, Price JL, Furey ML. Brain structural and functional abnormalities in mood disorders: implications for neurocircuitry models of depression. Brain Struct Funct. 2008;213(1–2):93–118.
66. Ramel W, Goldin PR, Eyler LT, Brown GG, Gotlib IH, McQuaid JR. Amygdala reactivity and mood-congruent memory in individuals at risk for depressive relapse. Biol Psychiatry. 2007;61(2):231–9.
67. Leppänen JM. Emotional information processing in mood disorders: a review of behavioral and neuroimaging findings. Curr Opin Psychiatry. 2006;19(1):34–9.
68. Hamilton JP, Gotlib IH. Neural substrates of increased memory sensitivity for negative stimuli in major depression. Biol Psychiatry. 2008;63(12):1155–62.
69. Gilbertson MW, Shenton ME, Ciszewski A, Kasai K, Lasko NB, Orr SP, et al. Smaller hippocampal volume predicts pathologic vulnerability to psychological trauma. Nat Neurosci. 2002;5(11):1242.
70. Neylan TC, Mueller SG, Wang Z, Metzler TJ, Lenoci M, Truran D, et al. Insomnia severity is associated with a decreased volume of the CA3/dentate gyrus hippocampal subfield. Biol Psychiatry. 2010;68(5):494–6.
71. Lindauer RJ, Vlieger EJ, Jalink M, Olff M, Carlier IV, Majoie CB, et al. Smaller hippocampal volume in Dutch police officers with posttraumatic stress disorder. Biol Psychiatry. 2004;56(5):356–63.
72. Pitman RK. Hippocampal diminution in PTSD: more (or less?) than meets the eye. Hippocampus. 2001;11(2):73–4.
73. Resick PA, Nishith P, Weaver TL, Astin MC, Feuer CA. A comparison of cognitive-processing therapy with prolonged exposure and a waiting condition for the treatment of chronic posttraumatic stress disorder in female rape victims. J Consult Clin Psychol. 2002;70(4):867.
74. Duffy M, Gillespie K, Clark DM. Post-traumatic stress disorder in the context of terrorism and other civil conflict in Northern Ireland: randomised controlled trial. BMJ. 2007;334(7604):1147.
75. Gillespie K, Duffy M, Hackmann A, Clark DM. Community based cognitive therapy in the treatment of post-traumatic stress disorder following the Omagh bomb. Behav Res Ther. 2002;40(4):345–57.
76. Beddington J, Cooper CL, Field J, Goswami U, Huppert FA, Jenkins R, et al. The mental wealth of nations. Nature. 2008;455(7216):1057.
77. McGorry PD, Hickie IB, Yung AR, Pantelis C, Jackson HJ. Clinical staging of psychiatric disorders: a heuristic framework for choosing earlier, safer and more effective interventions. Aust N Z J Psychiatry. 2006;40(8):616–22.
78. Herrman H, Chopra P. Quality of life and neurotic disorders in general healthcare. Curr Opin Psychiatry. 2009;22(1):61–8.
79. Kravitz HM, Bloom RW, Fawcett J. Recovery from a recurrent major depressive episode. Depress Anxiety. 2000;12(1):40–3.
80. Jones E, Wessely S. A paradigm shift in the conceptualization of psychological trauma in the 20th century. J Anxiety Disord. 2007;21(2):164–75.
81. Maercker A, Brewin CR, Bryant RA, Cloitre M, Reed GM, van Ommeren M, et al. Proposals for mental disorders specifically associated with stress in the International Classification of Diseases-11. Lancet. 2013;381(9878):1683–5.
82. Yehuda R, McFarlane A, Shalev A. Predicting the development of posttraumatic stress disorder from the acute response to a traumatic event. Biol Psychiatry. 1998;44(12):1305–13.
83. Galatzer-Levy IR, Karstoft KI, Statnikov A, Shalev AY. Quantitative forecasting of PTSD from early trauma responses: a machine learning application. J Psychiatr Res. 2014;59:68–76.
84. Maguen S, Madden E, Neylan TC, Cohen BE, Bertenthal D, Seal KH. Timing of mental health treatment and PTSD symptom improvement among Iraq and Afghanistan veterans. Psychiatr Serv. 2014;65(12):1414–9.
85. Van Rooij SJ, Kennis M, Vink M, Geuze E. Predicting treatment outcome in PTSD: a longitudinal functional MRI study on trauma-unrelated emotional processing. Neuropsychopharmacology. 2016;41(4):1156.
86. Lobo I, Portugal LC, Figueira I, Volchan E, David I, Pereira MG, et al. EEG correlates of the severity of posttraumatic stress symptoms: a systematic review of the dimensional PTSD literature. J Affect Disord. 2015;183:210–20.
87. Kaczkurkin AN, Burton PC, Chazin SM, Manbeck AB, Espensen-Sturges T, Cooper SE, et al. Neural substrates of overgeneralized conditioned fear in PTSD. Am J Psychiatr. 2016;174(2):125–34.
88. Shin LM, Davis FC, VanElzakker MB, Dahlgren MK, Dubois SJ. Neuroimaging predictors of treatment response in anxiety disorders. Biol Mood Anxiety Disord. 2013;3(1):15.
89. Karatzias A, Power K, McGoldrick T, Brown K, Buchanan R, Sharp D, et al. Predicting treatment outcome on three measures for post-traumatic stress disorder. Eur Arch Psychiatry Clin Neurosci. 2007;257(1):40–6.
90. Bryant RA, Felmingham K, Whitford TJ, Kemp A, Hughes G, Peduto A, et al. Rostral anterior cingulate volume predicts treatment response to cognitive-behavioural therapy for posttraumatic stress disorder. J Psychiatry Neurosci: JPN. 2008;33(2):142.
91. Michopoulos V, Jovanovic T. Chronic inflammation: a new therapeutic target for post-traumatic stress disorder? Lancet Psychiatry. 2015;2(11):954–5.
92. Lindqvist D, Dhabhar FS, James SJ, Hough CM, Jain FA, Bersani FS, et al. Oxidative stress, inflam-

mation and treatment response in major depression. Psychoneuroendocrinology. 2017;76:197–205.
93. Miller AH, Maletic V, Raison CL. Inflammation and its discontents: the role of cytokines in the pathophysiology of major depression. Biol Psychiatry. 2009;65(9):732–41.
94. Krystal JH, Davis LL, Neylan TC, Raskind MA, Schnurr PP, Stein MB, et al. It is time to address the crisis in the pharmacotherapy of posttraumatic stress disorder: a consensus statement of the PTSD Psychopharmacology Working Group. Biol Psychiatry. 2017;82(7):e51–9.
95. Liu XH, Xie XH, Wang KY, Cui H. Efficacy and acceptability of atypical antipsychotics for the treatment of post-traumatic stress disorder: a meta-analysis of randomized, double-blind, placebo-controlled clinical trials. Psychiatry Res. 2014;219(3):543–9.
96. Kozaric-Kovacic D, Eterovic M. Lamotrigine abolished aggression in a patient with treatment-resistant posttraumatic stress disorder. Clin Neuropharmacol. 2013;36(3):94–5.
97. D'Andrea D, Sewell RA. Transient resolution of treatment-resistant posttraumatic stress disorder following ketamine infusion. Biol Psychiatry. 2013;74(9):e13–4.
98. Hartberg J, Garrett-Walcott S, De Gioannis A. Impact of oral ketamine augmentation on hospital admissions in treatment-resistant depression and PTSD: a retrospective study. Psychopharmacology. 2018;235(2):393–8.
99. Berardis DD, Marini S, Serroni N, Iasevoli F, Tomasetti C, de Bartolomeis A, et al. Targeting the noradrenergic system in posttraumatic stress disorder: a systematic review and meta-analysis of prazosin trials. Curr Drug Targets. 2015;16(10):1094–106.
100. Green B. Prazosin in the treatment of PTSD. J Psychiatr Pract. 2014;20(4):253–9.
101. Sessa B. MDMA and PTSD treatment: PTSD: from novel pathophysiology to innovative therapeutics. Neurosci Lett. 2017;649:176–80.
102. Giustino TF, Fitzgerald PJ, Maren S. Revisiting propranolol and PTSD: memory erasure or extinction enhancement? Neurobiol Learn Mem. 2016;130:26–33.
103. de Kleine RA, Hendriks GJ, Kusters WJ, Broekman TG, van Minnen A. A randomized placebo-controlled trial of D-cycloserine to enhance exposure therapy for posttraumatic stress disorder. Biol Psychiatry. 2012;71(11):962–8.
104. Savitz JB, Teague TK, Misaki M, Macaluso M, Wurfel BE, Meyer M, et al. Treatment of bipolar depression with minocycline and/or aspirin: an adaptive, 2×2 double-blind, randomized, placebo-controlled, phase IIA clinical trial. Transl Psychiatry. 2018;8(1):27.
105. Jha MK, Minhajuddin A, Gadad BS, Greer T, Grannemann B, Soyombo A, et al. Can C-reactive protein inform antidepressant medication selection in depressed outpatients? Findings from the CO-MED trial. Psychoneuroendocrinology. 2017;78:105–13.
106. Qureshi SU, Long ME, Bradshaw MR, Pyne JM, Magruder KM, Kimbrell T, et al. Does PTSD impair cognition beyond the effect of trauma? J Neuropsychiatry Clin Neurosci. 2011;23(1):16–28.
107. Friedman MJ, Donnelly CL, Mellman TA. Pharmacotherapy for PTSD. Psychiatr Ann. 2003;33(1):57–62.
108. Van Minnen A, Arntz A, Keijsers GP. Prolonged exposure in patients with chronic PTSD: predictors of treatment outcome and dropout. Behav Res Ther. 2002;40(4):439–57.
109. Bleiberg KL, Markowitz JC. A pilot study of interpersonal psychotherapy for posttraumatic stress disorder. Am J Psychiatr. 2005;162(1):181–3.
110. Karsen EF, Watts BV, Holtzheimer PE. Review of the effectiveness of transcranial magnetic stimulation for post-traumatic stress disorder. Brain Stimul (Basic, Translational, and Clinical Research in Neuromodulation). 2014;7(2):151–7.
111. Kluetsch RC, Ros T, Théberge J, Frewen PA, Calhoun VD, Schmahl C, et al. Plastic modulation of PTSD resting-state networks and subjective wellbeing by EEG neurofeedback. Acta Psychiatr Scand. 2014;130(2):123–36.
112. Lanius RA, Frewen PA, Tursich M, Jetly R, McKinnon MC. Restoring large-scale brain networks in PTSD and related disorders: a proposal for neuroscientifically-informed treatment interventions. Eur J Psychotraumatol. 2015;6(1):27313.
113. van der Kolk BA, Stone L, West J, Rhodes A, Emerson D, Suvak M, et al. Original research yoga as an adjunctive treatment for posttraumatic stress disorder: a randomized controlled trial. J Clin Psychiatry. 2014;75(6):e559–65.
114. Banks K, Newman E, Saleem J. An overview of the research on mindfulness-based interventions for treating symptoms of posttraumatic stress disorder: a systematic review. J Clin Psychol. 2015;71(10):935–63.
115. Goldstein LA, Mehling WE, Metzler TJ, Cohen BE, Barnes DE, Choucroun GJ, et al. Veterans Group Exercise: a randomized pilot trial of an integrative exercise program for veterans with posttraumatic stress. J Affect Disord. 2018;227:345–52.
116. Vancampfort D, Stubbs B, Richards J, Ward PB, Firth J, Schuch FB, et al. Physical fitness in people with posttraumatic stress disorder: a systematic review. Disabil Rehabil. 2017;39(24):2461–7.

Treatment Resistance in Obsessive-Compulsive Disorder

11

Rachel Middleton, Michael G. Wheaton, Reilly Kayser, and H. Blair Simpson

11.1 Introduction

Obsessive-compulsive disorder (OCD) is characterized by obsessions (recurrent thoughts, images, or urges that typically provoke anxiety and distress) and compulsions (repetitive behaviors that the individual feels driven to perform, often to alleviate distress or prevent feared consequences). To warrant a diagnosis of OCD, obsessions and/or compulsions must be time-consuming (e.g., present for more than 1 hour per day) and cause significant distress or impairment in an individual's daily functioning [1]. The severity of symptoms can be assessed using the Yale-Brown Obsessive Compulsive Scale (YBOCS) [2].

OCD has an estimated lifetime prevalence rate of 2–3% in the population, making it more than twice as common as schizophrenia. OCD typically starts in childhood or adolescence (with a median onset of 19 years old) and persists throughout a person's life, with symptoms typically following a chronic waxing and waning course. OCD produces substantial impairment in functioning due to the severe and chronic nature of the illness. Earlier age of onset can disrupt normal developmental trajectories and thus lead to greater impairment. Males often have an earlier OCD onset age, but by adulthood, OCD is estimated to affect equal numbers of men and women [3].

Practice guidelines from the American Psychiatric Association (APA) [4] recommend beginning treatment with either pharmacotherapy with serotonin reuptake inhibitors (SRIs), cognitive-behavioral therapy (CBT), or their combination. SRIs include the selective serotonin reuptake inhibitors (SSRIs, i.e., fluoxetine, fluvoxamine, sertraline, paroxetine, citalopram) as well as the nonselective SRI clomipramine; which have been shown in large, multisite, randomized controlled trials (RTCs) to outperform placebos in reducing OCD symptoms [5]. The recommended form of CBT is that consisting of Exposure and Ritual (Response) Prevention (ERP), a structured psychotherapy that involves two major components: systematic confrontation with feared situations and stimuli (i.e., exposures) and voluntary restriction from engaging in compulsive rituals (i.e., ritual prevention component). SRIs and ERP, either on their own, or used together, will help

R. Middleton · R. Kayser · H. B. Simpson (✉)
New York State Psychiatric Institute/Columbia Psychiatry, Columbia University Medical Center, New York, NY, USA
e-mail: Rachel.Middleton@nyspi.columbia.edu; Reilly.Kayser@nyspi.columbia.edu; Blair.Simpson@nyspi.columbia.edu

M. G. Wheaton
New York State Psychiatric Institute/Columbia Psychiatry, Columbia University Medical Center, New York, NY, USA

Barnard College, Columbia University, New York, NY, USA
e-mail: Michael.Wheaton@nyspi.columbia.edu

Y.-K. Kim (ed.), *Treatment Resistance in Psychiatry*, https://doi.org/10.1007/978-981-10-4358-1_11

many patients reduce their OCD symptoms and about half achieve minimal symptoms [6–9].

However promising, these results indicate that these treatment options are not universally effective, as up to 40–60% of individuals fail to respond to these first-line treatments [10, 11]. A "treatment response" in OCD clinical trials has historically been operationalized as a decrease of 25–35% in OCD symptoms, typically assessed with the YBOCS, and often combined with a rating of "improved" or "very much improved" on the Clinical Global Impressions-Improvement Scale (CGI-I) [12]. Individuals who fail to achieve a sufficient response, and those who continue to experience clinically significant symptoms despite a 25–35% decrease, are often referred to as "treatment-resistant" [13]. When a first-line treatment is not enough, several alternatives are available, depending on the type and degree of treatment resistance (i.e., resistance to SSRIs, ERP, or both), as discussed below.

11.2 Treatment Resistance with Pharmacotherapy

11.2.1 Predictors of SRI Response

In the Cochrane review [14] meta-analysis of 17 RCTs (comprising more than 3000 participants), researchers found SRIs to be associated with significant reductions in OCD symptoms, with an average YBOCS reduction for patients who respond to SRIs to be 30–60% from baseline. In this analysis, no individual medication emerged as more efficacious. However, because the side effects associated with clomipramine can be more severe [5, 14, 15], treating clinicians typically begin with an SSRI.

Ineffective dosages or insufficient duration may be responsible for poor response to SRI treatment, the so-called technical failure. Studies show that higher doses yield, on average, higher rates of improvement in symptoms [16]. Similarly, data suggest that doses should be maintained for at least 8–12 weeks for maximum therapeutic effects [17]. However, higher doses of SSRIs produce more side effects, leading some patient to prematurely discontinue the medication [18]. Therefore, it is recommended that patients begin at low doses and increase their dose to the maximum tolerated. The maximally tolerated dose should be maintained for a minimum of 6 weeks to be considered an adequate therapeutic trial [3, 16].

Several clinical factors can also predict poor response to SRIs. Higher levels of symptoms at baseline have been associated with lower levels of SRI response in multiple trials [12, 19, 20]. Comorbid tic disorders, such as Tourette's, have also been linked to poorer SRI outcomes. For example, in a study of 33 OCD patients on fluvoxamine, 52% of OCD patients without a history of tic disorders achieved a significant decrease in symptoms (assessed by the YBOCS), compared to only 21% of OCD patients in the comorbid tic group [21]. These findings have been replicated in children and adolescents with the SSRIs sertraline and paroxetine [22, 23]. However, in a small pilot study, comorbid tics did not appear to adversely impact response to clomipramine [21]. One issue complicating the interpretation of these data is that higher rates of comorbid tic disorders have been linked to earlier OCD onset [24]. Early age of OCD onset has also been linked to treatment nonresponse across several SRIs [25–29], including fluvoxamine, paroxetine, citalopram, and clomipramine [28, 29].

Patients with OCD often present with comorbid psychiatric conditions, most frequently anxiety disorders (e.g., panic disorder, social anxiety disorder, generalized anxiety disorder, specific phobias), which appear in about 75% of OCD patients [30]. However, the impact of comorbid anxiety disorders on SRI response remains unclear. Most OCD studies have not found comorbid anxiety disorders to interfere with SRI response [17, 31], though an earlier review of this literature came to a different conclusion [32]. Unexpectedly, some reports have found that comorbid PTSD predicts better responses in individuals with certain OCD symptoms (hoarding, contamination fears, illness concerns, mental rituals, and/or superstition) [33]. A "post-traumatic" OCD subtype has been proposed as a potential explanation for these findings, though further research on this area is warranted [34]. Although panic disorder has not been shown to impact SSRI response in OCD, higher doses of SSRIs in these individuals have been linked to increases in panic attacks in multiple studies [17].

Medication adherence has also been linked to the likelihood of responding to SRI treatment, with nonadherent patients at risk for treatment failure [28]. Unwanted medication effects are a barrier to adherence for many patients. Common side effects with SRIs include gastrointestinal problems (nausea, constipation, and diarrhea), weight gain, tremors, apathy, sleep disturbances (insomnia and/or vivid dreams), fatigue and somnolence, dry mouth, and sexual dysfunction (decreased libido, trouble ejaculating, anorgasmia) [16, 35], the latter three of which have been found to be the most predictive of medication discontinuation for patients beginning pharmacotherapy [35]. Other patients may have difficulty with adherence to medication due to particular aspects of their presentation of OCD (e.g., those with contamination fears may be concerned about what they ingest, making them more hesitant to take medicine [36]).

A patient's degree of insight may also impact his or her adherence to medication. Insight can be defined as the degree to which an individual recognizes the maladaptive nature of their symptoms. Several studies have reported poor insight as a significant predictor of poor SRI response [37, 38].

11.2.2 Management of Resistance with SRIs

Patients who do not experience an adequate response to SSRIs may explore several different options. If they do not have dose-limiting side effects, a practical first step is to increase their dose. The FDA has approved the following SSRI dose ranges for OCD: fluoxetine 20–60 mg/day, fluvoxamine 100–300 mg/day, paroxetine 40–60 mg/day, sertraline 50–200 mg/day, citalopram up to 40 mg/day (20 mg/day in patients older than 60), and escitalopram 10–20 mg/day [39]. However, higher doses are recommended in practice guidelines and are commonly used in clinical practice (e.g., fluoxetine up to 120 mg/day, fluvoxamine up to 450 mg/day, paroxetine up to 100 mg/day, sertraline up to 400 mg/day, citalopram up to 120 mg/day, and escitalopram up to 60 mg/day) [17]. As noted above, since higher SRI doses may increase the risk for side effects in some patients, dosing should begin on the lower end after which dosages can be increased every 1–2 weeks to determine the maximally tolerated dose. Only following 6 weeks at this dose should a patient be considered treatment-resistant [16].

Switching SSRIs or exploring monotherapy with clomipramine are both alternatives for patients who have experienced little to no response to an initial SSRI trial. It has been estimated that less than half of patients will benefit from switching from one SSRI to another, and the likelihood of response diminishes as the number of failed adequate trials increases [16, 25]. Switching to clomipramine, a tricyclic antidepressant that inhibits the reuptake of both serotonin and norepinephrine, is often tried after two different SSRIs have not produced a significant relief from symptoms. Although not typically a first-line agent due to its side effect profile (e.g., sedation, dry mouth, constipation, urinary delay, orthostatic hypotension, and cardiac conduction delay), some meta-analyses find that clomipramine can lead to larger effects than SSRIs [39].

When patients experience a partial response to serotonergic medication but continue to have clinically impairing symptoms, SRI augmentation is often considered. In general, augmentation strategies involve the addition of either psychotherapy (ERP) or an antipsychotic medication such as risperidone. In our recent trial, we found ERP augmentation to be more efficacious than risperidone, even among patients who preferred medication over ERP [7, 40]. Given this result, as well as the side effect profile of antipsychotics, augmentation with ERP is the best to try first [41, 42].

However, ERP is not available to all patients, and not all are willing to try it. Therefore, antipsychotic augmentation remains a viable strategy for some patients. Haloperidol, risperidone, quetiapine, olanzapine, and aripiprazole have all been shown in RCTs to enhance response to

SRIs, though not all trials with these agents have had positive results [41–43]. It is unclear if mixed responses found across antipsychotic trials reflect true differences in efficacy between these agents or methodological issues with specific trials. Meta-analyses across all of these trials [42, 44, 45] suggest that around one third of OCD patients on an SRI will have a treatment response when an antipsychotic medication is added. Some data suggest that OCD patients with comorbid tics are more likely to respond, particularly, to risperidone and haloperidol [44]. Although effective for some, antipsychotics are associated with weight gain, metabolic syndrome, and a variety of extrapyramidal side effects including acute dyskinesias and dystonic reactions, tardive dyskinesia, parkinsonism, akinesia, akathisia, and neuroleptic malignant syndrome [44]. Patients starting an antipsychotic should be monitored closely for side effects, and the medication should be discontinued if no benefits are observed after an adequate therapeutic trial of 1 month [16].

There is some evidence from case studies to support augmentation with other pharmacological agents such as lithium, buspirone, and clonazepam. However, none were found to outperform placebo in small clinical trials, which may suggest that these drugs are only effective for a subset of patients [46].

Monotherapy with other medications has also been explored, including venlafaxine and mirtazapine. Venlafaxine had robust effects on OCD symptoms in both open-label and double-blind comparator studies. However, these effects were not replicated in a placebo-controlled trial [47]. In one small study, mirtazapine was shown to be effective in patients who have had no more than one failed SSRI trial [48].

11.3 Treatment Resistance with ERP

11.3.1 Predictors of Treatment Resistance

Although the evidence supporting ERP is substantial [17], not all patients benefit. Some patients discontinue treatment prematurely, and of those who complete, a subset does not respond [8]. Substantial effort has been made to describe predictors of ERP outcomes in order to identify patients at risk for poor outcomes. Both patient factors (e.g., patient adherence, comorbidity, degree of insight) and treatment factors (e.g., treatment intensity and duration) can influence outcome [49].

Patient adherence is the strongest predictor of ERP outcome. ERP requires patients to confront fears and refrain from compulsive rituals, both in therapy sessions (under therapist supervision) and between therapy sessions (as homework assignments). Several studies have shown that the degree to which patients adhere to ERP assignments robustly predicts acute outcomes [50], and also outcomes 6 months later [51]. Monitoring patient adherence, particularly adherence to ritual prevention instructions, has also been shown to prospectively forecast who will benefit from treatment, allowing treating clinicians to make individualized treatment predictions [40].

Some studies have found that higher initial OCD symptom severity and severe comorbid depression can also predict poor ERP outcomes [52]. However, other studies have not replicated these findings, and a recent meta-analysis found no relationship between either baseline OCD severity or depression severity and ERP effect size [53]. One potential explanation for these mixed results is that it may only be severe depression that predicts ERP response, which has been excluded in many ERP trials. Severe depression can also impact patient adherence to treatment, which may mediate the link with poor outcomes. Similarly, other common comorbid disorders found in OCD populations (e.g., obsessive-compulsive personality disorder and comorbid anxiety disorders) warrant clinical attention when they impact a patient's ability to adhere to treatment [17].

Some studies have reported that patients with poor insight are less likely to experience an ERP treatment response compared to patients with good or fair insight [30, 54]. However, other studies have found no association between insight and treatment response [17, 50, 55]. One possible explanation for these different outcomes is restriction in range of insight, as few patients with the poorest insight present for treatment. The link between insight and outcome may also be via patient adherence. For example, early studies found that approximately 25–30% of patients who begin ERP drop out due to the nature of ERP (i.e., ERP requires the patient to confront their anxiety [56]). Thus, the APA recommends that clinicians gauge patient insight as a preliminary step to the establishment of a treatment plan [17]. Assessing insight before treatment selection can inform the clinician of their patient's motivation and willingness to adhere; this information can in turn be factored into the patient's treatment plan.

Therapist fidelity to ERP is another factor that may play a role in treatment outcomes. If ERP is not administered effectively, patients may not respond [57]. Effective ERP administration involves exposing patients to distress-provoking stimuli and then persisting in the exposure for a sufficient amount of time in order for the patient to learn that the situation can be managed without giving into compulsive rituals [52]. Therapist failure to follow these treatment procedures during sessions may interfere with patients' ability to benefit from ERP. Some data also suggest that the frequency of sessions also can affect treatment outcomes, as reviewed below.

Finally, other factors have also been identified in individual studies to affect ERP outcomes, including gender, marital status, and baseline quality of life/functioning. For example, some studies have reported that females have poorer ERP response as compared to males [58], while others have found that married/partnered patients fare better than single patients [59]. Similarly, Maher et al. reported that individuals with worse quality of life at baseline had poorer ERP responses [58], while Wheaton et al. found that greater problems in functioning at baseline predicted poorer ERP response [60]. However, for each of these variables, multiple other studies have reported null results [61]. It may be that many factors each play a small role in ERP outcomes which can vary from sample to sample in terms of strength, with patient adherence to the ERP playing a major role and showing a consistent relationship with ERP outcomes [58]. Given how effective ERP is for individuals with OCD, further study is warranted and should include both therapist and patient factors as well as biological, psychological, behavioral, and sociocultural variables.

11.3.2 Management of Treatment Resistance with ERP

When a trial of ERP does not yield a sufficient treatment response, therapists should consider increasing exposure intensity (i.e., utilize stimuli that induce higher levels of anxiety) and/or increasing the duration and frequency of sessions before considering a different type of therapy or exploring pharmacological options. There is some evidence that ERP sessions are more effective when administered intensively (at least twice weekly); however, this benefit may plateau at five sessions per week in outpatient treatment [10, 17]. Increasing dose and intensity may be particularly helpful for patients who need extra support in adherence outside of session ERP assignments, including those with poor insight [10, 62].

Residential treatment is another option when outpatient ERP does not succeed. In the United States, several specialty residential programs have been established focusing on OCD, including programs at Rogers Memorial Hospital and the McLean Institute at Massachusetts General Hospital. Even though these programs tend to enroll patients with high illness severity, who often also have multiple comorbidities, both programs have reported positive results in terms of reducing OCD and depressive symptoms [63–65]. Residential programs allow patients to receive multiple hours per day of ERP work, delivered in both group and individual formats.

When ERP does not succeed as a monotherapy, it can be combined with either medications or other techniques from other forms of psychotherapy. For example, psychotherapy incorporating cognitive therapy may offer an alternative or an augmentation strategy to standard ERP [66]. Cognitive therapy involves identification and modification of distorted or dysfunctional beliefs, and some trials have found it to be effective at reducing OCD symptoms, although these trials have not been as extensive those for ERP [46, 67].

11.4 Treatment Resistance to Both SRIs and ERP

SRIs and ERP alone, or in combination, can help up to 50% of OCD patients become well [7, 9]. However, any of the aforementioned factors can interfere with achieving wellness, and thus many continue to suffer. After thoroughly exploring the treatment options outlined above, the use of more experimental therapies may be warranted. These include neuromodulatory treatments and even neurosurgery.

Transcranial magnetic stimulation (TMS) is a noninvasive method for either stimulating or inhibiting neural transmission. Greenberg et al. (1997) found that a single session of stimulation of the right lateral prefrontal cortex (PFC) led to a decrease in compulsive urges that lasted for 8 hours. Since then, there have been several trials of repetitive TMS (rTMS) targeting different brain regions [46]. Meta-analyses of existing trials of rTMS studies suggest that rTMS of prefrontal regions (specifically the dorsolateral PFC) may not be effective in OCD, but low-frequency rTMS targeting the supplemental motor area appears to be promising [68–70].

Patients deemed treatment refractory (i.e., failed at least three adequate SRI trials, several augmentation trials (e.g., with an antipsychotic or clonazepam), and at least one adequate CBT trial) are potential candidates for neurosurgical interventions. These interventions include either making targeted lesions in cortico-striatal-thalamic-cortical (CTSC) circuits or altering activity within these circuits using deep brain stimulation (DBS).

DBS involves delivering electrical impulses to various areas of the brain via surgically implanted electrodes. Recent literature has focused on the CSTC circuit as a target for this treatment modality [71], with a double-blind trial and several case reports/series focusing on the anterior limbs of the internal capsules (ALIC) and the subthalamic nucleus. A case series investigation in which the ALIC was targeted using DBS found a greater than 25% decrease in YBOCS scores in 73% of participants. Studies using the subthalamic nucleus as a target have not reported significant decreases in YBOCS scores [72, 73]. While DBS is reversible (in the sense that the stimulation can be turned off and the electrodes removed from the brain), risks include brain hemorrhage, infection, and new onset of seizures. For these reasons, DBS is only used in treatment-refractory populations [17].

Neurosurgical lesions can be produced either surgically or using radiosurgical ("Gamma Knife") techniques. Different lesions have been tried: subcaudate tractotomy, capsulotomy, cingulotomy, and limbic leucotomy [74, 75]. Case series find that 30–70% of patients have at least minimal improvement symptoms following these procedures [10, 76]. The first RTC of gamma knife capsulotomy was conducted in 2014. The final report found that two of the eight patients who received the procedure responded at the 12-month follow-up and an additional two responded at the 54-month follow-up [77]. A second report during an open phase of the same study found significant improvement in two out of four patients who were elected to undergo the procedure after initial randomization to the sham condition. No patients in the sham condition of either phase reported an improvement in symptoms [78]. Ablative procedures are irreversible and can lead to serious adverse events (SAEs) including seizures, increased executive dysfunction, apathy, disinhibition, suicide, weight gain, brain hemorrhage, stroke, edema, hydrocephalus, and personality change [75, 79]. Thus, ablation is only used in treatment-refractory populations.

11.5 Biological Predictors of Treatment-Resistant OCD: Current Research

Current research continues to examine the mechanisms underlying obsessions and compulsions as well as how our current treatments work. These data may help explain why some individuals respond to current treatments and others do not, and may lead to novel targets for treatment development and markers of disease that can guide treatment choice.

One approach has been to study the basic neural processes that may lead to obsessions and compulsions. For example, some have investigated whether dysfunction in the learning or extinction of fear contributes to OCD [80], and impairment in fear extinction has been demonstrated in laboratory studies in patients with OCD [81]. Others have examined whether abnormalities in goal-directed versus habitual behavior explain the compulsions seen in OCD. For example, Gillan et al. (2011) found evidence of disruption in goal-directed action control among OCD patients [82], and these findings have been replicated in other samples [80, 83]. However, whether any of these abnormalities predict treatment response remains to be tested.

Another approach has been to identify brain signatures of obsessions and compulsions using neuroimaging [84]. While abnormalities have been identified in CSTC circuits as well as in other areas [80] linked to compulsivity [85], it is not clear whether these brain abnormalities cause OCD or result from it. In addition, it remains unclear the extent to which neural functioning can be used to predict treatment outcome. A recent study by Fullana et al. (2017) found a significant association between decreased connectivity in the basolateral amygdala–ventromedial prefrontal cortex and better ERP treatment outcomes [86]. However, these findings yielded a relatively small effect size, similar to many other imaging studies conducted with the OCD population [87].

Neuroinflammatory markers are a third area of interest. One theory holds that neuroinflammation may cause obsessions and compulsions in a subset of OCD patients, and research on pediatric autoimmune neuropsychiatric disease (PANS/PANDAS) has highlighted this connection [36]. In addition, a recent paper found evidence for neuroinflammation in CSTC circuits in unmedicated OCD patients [88]. Thus, neuroinflammatory markers might identify a subset of individuals that are potentially resistant to existing treatments. The role of neuroinflammation in OCD deserves further study as it opens up a new pathway for treatment development.

Finally, researchers are interested in using genetic studies to identify which treatments will work best for individual patients. Genome-wide association studies (GWAS) offer one approach to identifying common genetic risk factors, but the studies in OCD are still underpowered, and no findings with genome-wide significance have yet been identified [89, 90]. An alternative is to search for rare or de novo (DN) mutations using whole-genome or exome sequencing in select samples. This approach has been applied in two studies [91, 92] utilizing parent-child trios (i.e., children with OCD and their parents). In one of these studies, researchers identified two risk genes, SCUBEI and CHD8, in the children. Both of these genes contained significant clusters of damaging DN variants [91]. The long-term goal of this line of research is to identify gene variants that might explain why certain individuals developed OCD and might guide more precise treatment selection.

11.6 Alternative Treatment Modalities: Current Research

Given that first-line treatments fail in up to half of OCD patients (as reviewed above), new and alternative treatments are needed. In terms of alternative psychotherapies, recent work has investigated acceptance and commitment therapy (ACT), which integrates mindfulness and acceptance-based processes with values-connected behaviors [93]. Initial data supports the use of ACT as an OCD treatment, but further research on this method is warranted [94]. Similarly, mindfulness therapy is currently being explored in the literature. This approach focuses on creating awareness and subsequent detachment between an individual and their symptoms. A recent review of this approach has suggested that it may be useful for some OCD patients [95, 96].

With regards to medications, glutamatergic agents have garnered much attention because of data from genetic and neuroimaging studies implicating the glutamate system in OCD. Many different glutamatergic agents have been investigated in the last 5 years, including N-acetylcysteine, memantine, and riluzole [78–81]. These medications have been shown to benefit some OCD patients in both open-label and placebo-controlled trials, although there have also been failed trials [97–101]. In a proof-of-concept crossover study, a single dose of IV ketamine (an antagonist at the N-methyl-D-aspartate receptor [NMDA] receptor) led to the rapid resolution of obsessions in unmedicated adults with OCD [82], introducing the exciting possibility of developing rapidly acting medications for OCD.

The potential role of the endocannabinoid (eCB) system in the treatment of OCD has attracted new interest. Studies in mice have linked activity within the eCB system to altered functionality within frontal-striatal circuits that regulate the balance between goal-directed and habitual action strategies [102]. Exogenously delivered cannabinoids can reduce marble-burying, a repetitive behavior thought to be a proxy for compulsions in OCD [103–107]. Both mouse models and human studies suggest that cannabidiol (CBD, a non-psychoactive constituent of the marijuana plant) can enhance fear extinction, suggesting that agents targeting the eCB system may be beneficial when combined with exposure-based treatments [99]. However, to date, human studies involving cannabinoid agents in OCD populations are limited to two case reports. Both describe patients with treatment-resistant OCD who experienced an improvement in symptoms after dronabinol was added to ongoing treatment with an SRI [108].

The potential role of neuroinflammation in OCD has led some to reconsider the effects of drugs like N-acetylcysteine (NAC) and celecoxib. The efficacy of NAC, a glutamate-modulator with anti-inflammatory properties, has been supported in an RTC, with further evidence from prior case studies [109]. Similarly, celecoxib has found support as an adjunctive treatment to fluvoxamine and fluoxetine in two RTCs [110].

Finally, studies are investigating how to combine different types of noninvasive neuromodulation (i.e., rTMS and tDCS) with pharmacotherapy [111, 112] or with ERP [80, 113]. In addition, new targets for interventions are being examined. For example, several case studies have found positive results targeting the inferior thalamic peduncle in treatment-resistant OCD patients, and results were maintained at a 1-year follow-up [63].

Conclusion

While there is substantial evidence for effective first-line treatments for OCD, many individuals fail to sufficiently respond. These individuals are considered treatment-resistant. Many factors have been shown to predict treatment resistance. Suboptimal response has been linked to "technical failures." These include insufficient dose, duration, and/or type of treatment, as well as clinical factors such as symptom severity, comorbidities, age of onset, insight, and patient adherence. To avoid these issues, treatment guidelines recommend thorough evaluation and treatment planning to ensure appropriate progression of treatment types.

Management options for treatment-resistant OCD should be evaluated based on the level of response the individual demonstrates. Management of partial response to initial first-line treatments can include increasing dose and duration, or augmentation of SRIs with ERP, or vice versa. For patients with minimal to no response, options include switching medications or augmenting with an antipsychotic. Patients who continue to see an inadequate response to these treatments can explore novel treatment strategies including new glutamate medications. Only in the most severe cases should neurosurgical approaches (e.g., DBS or ablation) be considered.

Recent advances in genetic, neuroimaging, and neurobehavioral studies may allow future research to uncover what causes OCD while also aiding in the development of new treatment options. Ideally, treatment will one day be tailored to each individual, and as a result, treatment outcomes and quality of life will improve for these individuals, and for the patients of the future.

References

1. American Psychiatric Association. Diagnostic and statistical manual of mental disorders. Arlington; 2013.
2. Goodman Wayne K, Price Lawrence H, Rasmussen SA, Mazure C, Fleischmann RL, Hill CL, et al. Yale-Brown obsessive compulsive scale: development, use, and reliability. Arch Gen Psychiatry. 1989;46:1006–11.
3. Pittenger C, Kelmendi B, Bloch M, Krystal JH, Coric V. Clinical treatment of obsessive compulsive disorder. Psychiatry. 2005;2:34–43.
4. Foa E, Yadin E, Lichner T. Exposure and response (ritual) prevention for obsessive-compulsive disorder: therapist guide (treatments that work). 2nd ed. New York: Oxford University Press; 2012.
5. Simpson HB. Pharmacotherapy for obsessive-compulsive disorder in adults. Up to date. 2015.
6. Foa EB, Liebowitz MR, Kozak MJ, et al. Randomized, placebo-controlled trial of exposure and ritual prevention, clomipramine, and their combination in the treatment of obsessive-compulsive disorder. Am J Psychiatry. 2005;162:151–61.
7. Simpson HB, Foa EB, Liebowitz MR, et al. Cognitive-behavioral therapy vs risperidone for augmenting serotonin reuptake inhibitors in obsessive-compulsive disorder. JAMA Psychiat. 2013;70:1190.
8. Simpson HB, Huppert JD, Petkova E, Foa EB, Liebowitz MR. Response versus remission in obsessive-compulsive disorder. J Clin Psychiatry. 2006;67:269–76.
9. Simpson HB, Foa EB, Liebowitz MR, Ledley R, Huppert JD, Cahill S, et al. A randomized, controlled trial of cognitive-behavioral therapy for augmenting pharmacotherapy in obsessive-compulsive disorder. Am J Psychiatry. 2008;165:621–30.
10. Gershkovich M, Wheaton M, Simpson H. Management of treatment-resistant obsessive-compulsive disorder. Curr Treat Options Psychiatry. 2017;4:357–70.
11. Haverkampf J. Treatment-resistant OCD. J Psychiatry Psychother Commun. 2014;3:91–4.
12. Mataix-Cols D, Rauch SL, Manzo PA, Jenike MA, Baer L. Use of factor-analyzed symptom dimensions to predict outcome with serotonin reuptake inhibitors and placebo in the treatment of obsessive-compulsive disorder. Am J Psychiatry. 1999;156:1409–16.
13. Farris SG. NIH Public Access. 2014;74:685–90.
14. Soomro GM, Altman DG, Rajagopal S, Oakley Browne M. Selective serotonin re-uptake inhibitors (SSRIs) versus placebo for obsessive compulsive disorder (OCD). Cochrane Database Syst Rev. 2008; https://doi.org/10.1002/14651858.CD001765.pub3.
15. R a H, Saxena S, Rauch SL, Hoehn-Saric R, Taber KH. Predicting treatment response in obsessive-compulsive disorder. J Neuropsychiatr Clin Neurosci. 2002;14:249–53.
16. Blair Simpson H. Pharmacotherapy for obsessive-compulsive disorder in adults. Uptodate. 2015.
17. Koran LM, Hollander E, Nestadt G, Simpson HB. Practice guideline for the treatment of patients with obsessive-compulsive disorder. Am J Psychiatry. 2007;64:5–53.
18. Bloch M, McGuire J, Landeros-Weisenberger A, Leckman JF, Pittenger C. Meta-analysis of the dose-response relationship of SSRI in obsessive-compulsive disorder. Mol Psychiatry. 2010;15:850–5.
19. Tukel R, Bozkurt O, Polat A, Genc A, Atli H. Clinical predictors of response to pharmacotherapy with selective serotonin reuptake inhibitors in obsessive-compulsive disorder. Psychiatry Clin Neurosci. 2006;60:404–9.
20. Stein D, Montgomery S, Kasper S, Tanghoi P. Predictors of response to pharmacotherapy with citalopram in obsessive-compulsive disorder. Int Clin Psychopharmacol. 2001;16:357–61.
21. Miguel EC, Shavitt RG, Ferrão YA, Brotto SA, Diniz JB. How to treat OCD in patients with Tourette syndrome. J Psychosom Res. 2003;55:49–57.
22. March JS, Franklin ME, Leonard H, Garcia A, Moore P, Freeman J, et al. Tics moderate treatment outcome with sertraline but not cognitive-behavior therapy in pediatric obsessive-compulsive disorder. Biol Psychiatry. 2007;61:344–7.
23. Geller D, Biederman J, Stewart S, Mullin B, Farrell C, Wagner K, et al. Impact of comorbidity on treatment response to paroxetine in pediatric obsessive-compulsive disorder: is the use of exclusion criteria empirically supported in randomized clinical trials? J Child Adolesc Psychopharmacol. 2003;13:S19–29.
24. Arumugham SS, Reddy JY. Augmentation strategies in obsessive-compulsive disorder. Expert Rev Neurother. 2013;13:187–203.
25. Kellner M. Drug treatment of obsessive-compulsive disorder. Dialogues Clin Neurosci. 2010;12:187–97.
26. Shetti C, Reddy Y, Kandavel T, Kashyap K, Singisetti S, Hiremath A, et al. Clinical predictors of drug nonresponse in obsessive-compulsive disorder. J Clin Psychiatry. 2005;66:1517–23.

27. Ravizza L, Barzega G, Bellino S, Bogetto F, Maina G. Predictors of drug treatment response in obsessive-compulsive disorder. J Clin Psychiatry. 1995;56:368–73.
28. Erzegovesi S, Cavallini M, Cavallini M, Diaferia G, Locatelli M, Bellodi L. Clinical predictors of drug response in obsessive-compulsive disorder. J Clin Psychiatry. 2001;21:488–92.
29. Rosario-Campos M, Leckman J, Mercadante M, Shavitt R, Prado H, Sada P, et al. Adults with early-onset obsessive-compulsive disorder. Am J Psychiatry. 2001;158:1899–903.
30. Fenske JN, Petersen K. Obsessive-compulsive disorder: diagnosis and Management. Am Fam Physician. 2015;92(10):896–903.
31. Koran LM, Simpson HB. Guideline watch (March 2013): practice guideline for the treatment of patients with obsessive-compulsive disorder. Arlington: American Psychiatric Association; 2013.
32. Carrasco J, Hollander E, Schneier F, Leibowitz M. Treatment outcome of obsessive compulsive disorder with comorbid social phobia. J Clin Psychiatry. 1992;53:387–91.
33. Shavitt RG, Valério C, Fossaluza V, Da Silva EM, Cordeiro Q, Diniz JB, et al. The impact of trauma and post-traumatic stress disorder on the treatment response of patients with obsessive-compulsive disorder. Eur Arch Psychiatry Clin Neurosci. 2010;260:91–9.
34. Fontenelle LF, Cocchi L, et al. Towards a post-traumatic subtype of obsessive–compulsive disorder. J Anxiety Disord. 2012;26:377–83.
35. Kelly K, Posternak M, Alpert JE. Toward achieving optimal response: understanding and managing antidepressant side effects. Dialogues Clin Neurosci. 2008;10:409–18.
36. Pallanti S, Grassi G, Sarrecchia ED, Cantisani A, Pellegrini M. Obsessive-compulsive disorder comorbidity: clinical assessment and therapeutic implications. Front Psychol. 2011;2:1–11.
37. Erzegovesi S, Cavallini M, Cavedini P, Diaferia G, Locatelli M, Bellodi L. Clinical predictors of drug response in obsessive-compulsive disorder. J Clin Psychopharmacol. 2001;21:488–92.
38. Catapano F, Perris F, Fabrazzo M, Cioffi V, Giacco D, De Santis V, et al. Obsessive-compulsive disorder with poor insight: a three-year prospective study. Prog Neuro-Psychopharmacology Biol Psychiatry. 2010;34:323–30.
39. Reid J, Reghunandanan S, Roberts A, Fineberg NA. Standard evidence-based pharmacological treatment for OCD. In: Pittenger C, editor. Obsessive-compulsive disorder: Phenomenology, pathophysiology, and treatment. 1st ed. New York: Oxford University Press; 2017. p. 443–61.
40. Wheaton MG, Galfalvy H, Steinman SA, Wall MM, Foa EB, Simpson HB. Patient adherence and treatment outcome with exposure and response prevention for OCD: which components of adherence matter and who becomes well? Behav Res Ther. 2016;85:6–12.
41. Dold M, Aigner M, Lanzenberger R, Kasper S. Antipsychotic augmentation of serotonin reuptake inhibitors in treatment-resistant obsessive-compulsive disorder: a meta-analysis of double-blind, randomized, placebo-controlled trials. Int J Neuropsychopharmacol. 2013;16:557–74.
42. Veale D, Miles S, Smallcombe N, Ghezai H, Goldacre B, Hodsoll J. Atypical antipsychotic augmentation in SSRI treatment refractory obsessive-compulsive disorder: a systematic review and meta-analysis. BMC Psychiatry. 2014;14:317.
43. Komossa K, Depping AM, Meyer M, Kissling W, Leucht S. Second-generation antipsychotics for obsessive compulsive disorder. Cochrane Database Syst Rev. 2010; https://doi.org/10.1002/14651858.CD008141.pub2.
44. Bloch MH, Landeros-Weisenberger A, Kelmendi B, Coric V, Bracken MB, Leckman JF. A systematic review: antipsychotic augmentation with treatment refractory obsessive-compulsive disorder. Mol Psychiatry. 2006;11:622–32.
45. Dold M, Aigner M, Lanzenberger R, Kasper S. Antipsychotic augmentation of serotonin reuptake inhibitors in treatment-resistant obsessive-compulsive disorder: an update meta-analysis of double-blind, randomized, placebo-controlled trials. Int J Neuropsychopharmacol. 2015;18:1–11.
46. Simpson HB. Overview of the treatment of obsessive-compulsive disorder. 1st ed. New York: Oxford University Press; 2017.
47. Fineberg NA, Gale TM. Evidence-based pharmacotherapy of obsessive – compulsive disorder. Int J Neuropsychopharmacol. 2005;8:107–29.
48. Koran LM, Gamel NN, Choung HW, Smith EH, Aboujaoude EN. Mirtazapine for obsessive-compulsive disorder: an open trial followed by double-blind discontinuation. J Clin Psychiatry. 2005;66:515–20.
49. McKay D, Sookman D, Neziroglu F, Wilhelm S, Stein DJ, Kyrios M, et al. Efficacy of cognitive-behavioral therapy for obsessive-compulsive disorder. Psychiatry Res. 2015;227:104–13.
50. Simpson HB, Maher MJ, Wang Y, Bao Y, Foa EB, Franklin M. Patient adherence predicts outcome from cognitive behavioral therapy in obsessive-compulsive disorder. J Consult Clin Psychol. 2011;79:247–52.
51. Albert U, Aguglia A, Bogetto F, Cieri L, Daniele M, Maina G, et al. Effectiveness of cognitive-behavioral therapy addition to pharmacotherapy in resistant obsessive-compulsive disorder: a multicenter study. Psychother Psychosom. 2012;81:383–5.
52. Zitterl W, Demal U, Aigner M, Lenz G, Urban C, Zapotoczky H-G, et al. Naturalistic course of obsessive compulsive disorder and comorbid depression. Psychopathology. 2000;33:75–80.
53. Olatunji BO, Davis ML, Powers MB, Smits JAJ. Cognitive-behavioral therapy for obsessive-compulsive disorder: a meta-analysis of treatment outcome and moderators. J Psychiatr Res. 2013;47:33–41.

54. Foa EB, Abramowitz JS, Franklin ME, Kozak MJ. Feared consequences, fixity of belief, and treatment outcome in patients with obsessive-compulsive disorder. Behav Ther. 1999;30:717–24.
55. Eisen JL, Rasmussen SA, Phillips KA, Price LH, Davidson J, Lydiard RB, et al. Insight and treatment outcome in obsessive-compulsive disorder. Compr Psychiatry. 2001;42:494–7.
56. Abramowitz J. The psychological treatment of obsessive compulsive disorder. Can J Psychiatr. 2006;51:407–16.
57. Gillihan SJ, Williams MT, Malcoun E, Yadin E, Foa EB. Journal of obsessive-compulsive and related disorders common pitfalls in exposure and response prevention (EX/RP) for OCD. J Obsessive Compuls Relat Disord. 2012;1:251–7.
58. Maher M, Ph D, Huppert JD, Chen H, Foa EB, Liebowitz MR, et al. Compulsive Disord. 2014;40:2013–23.
59. Marks IM, Lelliott P, Basoglu M, Noshirvani H, Monteiro W, Cohen D, et al. Clomipramine, self-exposure and therapist-aided exposure for obsessive-compulsive rituals. Br J Psychiatry. 1988;152:522. LP-534
60. Wheaton MG, Rosenfield D, Foa EB, Simpson HB. Augmenting serotonin reuptake inhibitors in obsessive-compulsive disorder: what moderates improvement? J Consult Clin Psychol. 2015;83: 926–37.
61. Knopp J, Knowles S, Bee P, Lovell K, Bower P. A systematic review of predictors and moderators of response to psychological therapies in OCD: do we have enough empirical evidence to target treatment? Clin Psychol Rev. 2013;33:1067–81.
62. Abramowitz J, Foa E, Franklin M. Exposure and ritual prevention for obsessive-compulsive disorder: effects of intensive versus twice-weekly sessions. J Consult Clin Psychol. 2003;71:394–8.
63. Leonard RC, Franklin ME, Wetterneck CT, Riemann BC, Simpson HB, Kinnear K, et al. Residential treatment outcomes for adolescents with obsessive-compulsive disorder. Psychother Res. 2016;26:727–36.
64. Stewart SE, Stack DE, Farrell C, Pauls DL, Jenike MA. Effectiveness of intensive residential treatment (IRT) for severe, refractory obsessive-compulsive disorder. J Psychiatr Res. 2005;39:603–9.
65. Stewart E. Obsessive-compulsive disorder. In: Camprodon J, Rauch S, Greenberg B, Dougherty D, editors. Psychiatric neurotherapeutics. New York: Humana Press; 2016. p. 23–50.
66. Whittal M. Cognitive Therapy for OCD. In: Pittenger C, editor. Obsessive-compulsive disorder: Phenomenology, pathophysiology, and treatment. 1st ed. New York: Oxford University Press; 2017. p. 421–9.
67. Wilhelm S, Berman N, Keshaviah A, Schwartz R, Steketee G. Mechanisms of change in cognitive therapy for obsessive compulsive disorder: role of maladaptive beliefs and schemas. Behav Res Ther. 2015;65:5–10.
68. Jaafari N, Rachid F, Rotge JY, Polosan M, El-Hage W, Belin D, et al. Safety and efficacy of repetitive transcranial magnetic stimulation in the treatment of obsessive-compulsive disorder: a review. World J Biol Psychiatry. 2012;13:164–77.
69. Berlim MT, Van Den Eynde F, Daskalakis ZJ. Efficacy and acceptability of high frequency repetitive transcranial magnetic stimulation (RTMS) versus electroconvulsive therapy (ECT) for major depression: a systematic review and meta-analysis of randomized trials. Depress Anxiety. 2013;30:614–23.
70. Lapidus KAB, Stern ER, Berlin HA, Goodman WK. Neuromodulation for obsessive-compulsive disorder. Neurotherapeutics. 2014;11:485–95.
71. Bourne SK, Eckhardt CA, Sheth SA, Eskandar EN. Mechanisms of deep brain stimulation for obsessive compulsive disorder: effects upon cells and circuits. Front Integr Neurosci. 2012;6:1–14.
72. Cleary DR, Ozpinar A, Raslan AM, Ko AL. Deep brain stimulation for psychiatric disorders: where we are now. Neurosurg Focus. 2015;38:E2.
73. Alonso P, Cuadras D, Gabriëls L, et al. Deep brain stimulation for obsessive-compulsive disorder: a meta-analysis of treatment outcome and predictors of response. PLoS One. 2015;10:1–16.
74. Greenberg BD, Price LH, Rauch SL, Friehs G, Noren G, Malone D, et al. Neurosurgery for intractable obsessive-compulsive disorder and depression: critical issues. Neurosurg Clin N Am. 2003;14:199–212.
75. Brown LT, Mikell CB, Youngerman BE, Zhang Y, Ii GMM, Sheth SA. System Rev Observational Stud. 2015;124:77–89.
76. Sheth SA, Neal J, Tangherlini F, Mian MK, Gentil A, Rees Cosgrove G, et al. Limbic system surgery for treatment-refractory obsessive-compulsive disorder: a prospective long-term follow-up of 64 patients. J Neurosurg. 2013;118:491–7.
77. Lopes AC, Greenberg BD, Canteras MM, et al. Gamma ventral capsulotomy for obsessive-compulsive disorder: a randomized clinical trial. JAMA Psychiat. 2014;71:1066–76.
78. Keen E, Widge A, Dougherty DD. Functional neurosurgery in severe and treatment-refractory OCD. In: Pittenger C, editor. Obsessive-compulsive disorder: Phenomenology, pathophysiology, and treatment. 1st ed. New York: Oxford University Press; 2017. p. 507–16.
79. Rück C, Karlsson A, Steele J, et al. Capsulotomy for obsessive-compulsive disorder: long-term follow-up of 25 patients. Arch Gen Psychiatry. 2008;65:914–21.
80. Milad MR, Rauch SL. Obsessive-compulsive disorder: beyond segregated cortico-striatal pathways. Trends Cogn Sci. 2012;16:43–51.
81. Milad MR, Rosenbaum BL, Simon NM. Neuroscience of fear extinction: implications for assessment and treatment of fear-based and anxiety related disorders. Behav Res Ther. 2014;62:17–23.
82. Gillan CM, Papmeyer M, Morein-Zamir S, Sahakian BJ, Fineberg NA, Robbins TW, et al. Disruption in the balance between goal-directed behavior and

habit learning in obsessive-compulsive disorder. Am J Psychiatry. 2011;168:718–26.
83. Gillan CM, Robbins TW. Goal-directed learning and obsessive – compulsive disorder. Philos Trans R Soc Lond Ser B Biol Sci. 2014;369:20130475.
84. Stern ER, Taylor SF. Cognitive neuroscience of obsessive-compulsive disorder. Psychiatr Clin NA. 2014;37:337–52.
85. Van Den Heuvel OA, Van Wingen G, Soriano-Mas C, Alonso P, Chamberlain SR, Nakamae T, et al. Brain circuitry of compulsivity. Eur Neuropsychopharmacol. 2016;26:810–27.
86. Fullana MA, Zhu X, Alonso P, et al. Basolateral amygdala-ventromedial prefrontal cortex connectivity predicts cognitive behavioural therapy outcome in adults with obsessive-compulsive disorder. J Psychiatry Neurosci. 2017;42:378–85.
87. Boedhoe PSW, Schmaal L, Mataix-Cols D, et al. Association and causation in brain imaging in the case of OCD: response to McKay et al. Am J Psychiatry. 2017;174:597–9.
88. Attwells S, Setiawan E, AA W, et al. Inflammation in the neurocircuitry of obsessive-compulsive disorder. JAMA Psychiat. 2017;74:833–40.
89. (OCGAS) IOCDFGC (IOCDF-G and OCDCGAS). Revealing the complex genetic architecture of obsessive-compulsive disorder using meta-analysis. Mol Psychiatry. 2017;5:1181–8.
90. Taylor S. Molecular genetics of obsessive–compulsive disorder: a comprehensive meta-analysis of genetic association studies. Mol Psychiatry. 2013;18:799–805.
91. Cappi C, Oliphant ME, Péter Z, et al. De novo damaging coding mutations are strongly associated with obsessive-compulsive disorder and overlap with autism. 2017. https://doi.org/10.1101/127712.
92. Cappi C, Brentani H, Lima L, et al. Whole-exome sequencing in obsessive-compulsive disorder identifies rare mutations in immunological and neurodevelopmental pathways. Transl Psychiatry. 2016; https://doi.org/10.1038/tp.2016.30.
93. Hayes S, Strosahl K, Wilson K. Acceptance and commitment therapy: an experiential approach to behavior change. New York: Guilford Press; 1999.
94. Twohig MP, Hayes SC, Plumb JC, Pruitt LD, Collins AB, Hazlett-Stevens H, et al. A randomized clinical trial of acceptance and commitment therapy versus progressive relaxation training for obsessive compulsive disorder. J Consult Clin Psychol. 2010;78:705–16.
95. Strauss C, Rosten C, Hayward M, Lea L, Forrester E, Jones AM. Mindfulness-based exposure and response prevention for obsessive compulsive disorder: study protocol for a pilot randomised controlled trial. Trials. 2015; https://doi.org/10.1186/s13063-015-0664-7.
96. Gasnier M, Pelissolo A, Bondolfi G, Pelissolo S, Tomba M, Mallet L, et al. Mindfulness-based interventions in obsessive-compulsive disorder: mechanisms of action and presentation of a pilot study. Encéphale. 2017;43:594–9.
97. Lafleur D, Pittenger C, Klemendi B, Gardner T, Wasylink S, Malison R, et al. N-acetylcysteine augmentation in serotonin reuptake inhibitor refractory obsessive-compulsive disorder. Psychopharmacology. 2006;164:254–6.
98. Stewart SE, Jenike EA, Hezel DM, Stack DE, Dodman NH, Shuster L, et al. A single-blinded case-control study of memantine in severe obsessive-compulsive disorder. J Clin Psychopharmacol. 2010;30:34–9.
99. Rodriguez C, Bender J, Marcus S, Snape M, Rynn M, Simpson HB. Minocycline augmentation of pharmacotherapy in Obsessive Compulsive Disorder: an open-label trial. J Clin Psychiatry. 2010;71:1247–9.
100. Rodriguez CI, Kegeles LS, Levinson A, Feng T, Marcus SM, Vermes D, et al. Randomized controlled crossover trial of ketamine in obsessive-compulsive disorder: proof-of-concept. Neuropsychopharmacology. 2013;38:2475–83.
101. Pittenger C, Bloch MH, Wasylink S, Billingslea E, Simpson R, Jakubovski E, et al. Riluzole augmentation in treatment-refractory obsessive-compulsive disorder: a pilot randomized placebo-controlled trial. J Clin Psychiatry. 2015;76:1075–84.
102. Gremel CM, Chancey J, Atwood B, et al. Habit formation. 2017;90:1312–24.
103. Lutz B, Marsicano G, Maldonado R, Hillard C. The endocannabinoid system in guarding against fear, anxiety and stress. Nat Rev Neurosci. 2015;16:705–18.
104. Nardo M, Casarotto P, Gomes F, Guimarães F. Cannabidiol reverses the mCPP-induced increase in marble-burying behavior. Fundam Clin Pharmacol. 2014;28:544–50.
105. Deiana S, Watanabe A, Yamasaki Y, et al. Plasma and brain pharmacokinetic profile of cannabidiol (BD), cannabidivarine (CBDV), Δ^9-tetrahydrocannabivarin (THCV) and cannabigerol (CBG) in rats and mice following oral and intraperitoneal administration and CBD action on obsessive-compulsive behavio. Pychopharmacology (Berl). 2019;219:859–73.
106. Casarotto P, Gomes F, Resstel L, Guimaraes F. Cannabidiol inhibitory effect on marble-burying behavior: involvement of CB1 receptors. Behav Pharmacol. 2010;21:353–8.
107. Gomes F, Casarotto P, Resstel L, Guimarães F. Facilitation of CB1 receptor-mediated neurotransmission decreases marble burying behavior in mice. Prog Neuro-Psychopharmacology Biol Psychiatry. 2011;35:434–8.
108. Schindler F, Anghelescu I, Regen F, Jockers-Scherubl M. Improvement in refractory obsessive compulsive disorder with dronabinol. 2Am J Psychiatr. 2008;165:536–7.
109. Paydary K, Akamaloo A, Ahmadipour A, Pishgar F, Emamzadehfard S, Akhondzadeh S. N-acetylcysteine augmentation therapy for moderate-to-severe obsessive–compulsive disorder: randomized, double-blind, placebo-controlled trial. J Clin Pharm Ther. 2016;41:214–9.

110. Shalbafan M, Mohammadinejad P, Shariat S-V, Alavi K, Zeinoddini A, Salehi M, et al. Celecoxib as an adjuvant to fluvoxamine in moderate to severe obsessive-compulsive disorder: a double-blind, placebo-controlled. Randomized Trial Pharmacopsychiatr. 2015;48:136–40.
111. Narayanaswamy JC, Jose D, Chhabra H, Agarwal SM, Shrinivasa B, Hegde A, et al. Successful application of add-on transcranial direct current stimulation (tDCS) for treatment of SSRI resistant OCD. Brain Stimul. 2015; https://doi.org/10.1016/j.brs.2014.12.003.
112. Sundar Arumugham S, Ravi M, Sharma E, Thirthalli J, Janardhan Reddy Y. Augmentation effect of low frequency-repetitive transcranial magnetic stimulation over pre-supplementary motor area in obsessive compulsive disorder: a randomized controlled trial. Brain Stimul. 2015;8:391.
113. Mantione M, Nieman DH, Figee M, Denys D. Cognitive–behavioural therapy augments the effects of deep brain stimulation in obsessive–compulsive disorder. Psychol Med. 2014;44:3515–22.

Treatment of Opioid Dependence

12

Michael Soyka

For many substance use disorders, such as cocaine, amphetamine and cannabis use disorder, there are no approved medications or standard therapy. This is not the case for opioid dependence, however, for which some gold standards for treatment have been defined [1] and novel medications are available for otherwise treatment refractory individuals and for those with side effects or severe adverse events.

In ICD-10 [2] and DSM-IV [3], opioid dependence is defined by various somatic, psychological and behavioural symptoms (three out of six or seven criteria must be fulfilled). It is a chronic, relapsing disorder [4] with high mortality rates from comorbid psychiatric and physical diseases (hepatitis, HIV, carcinoma, etc.), particularly in untreated individuals [5, 6]. The rates of cardiovascular and respiratory disorders, suicide and traffic accidents are also high [7]. Worldwide, 33 million people misuse opioids [8]. In the European Union, the number of opioid users is estimated at 1.3 million people. Opioids account for and can be detected in 82% of fatal drug intoxications [9]. Mortality from overdose is high and was found to be higher in patients who receive psychosocial support alone than in those who receive opioid agonist therapy [10].

In recent years, the USA in particular has experienced an epidemic of misuse of opioid prescription drugs (painkillers), such as oxycodone. In the USA, 2.6 people per 1000 use heroin [11] and in Europe, 4 per 1000 [9]. In 2015, about half of the 33,091 opioid overdoses involved opioid prescription drugs [12], and about two million individuals in the USA had an opioid use disorder associated with prescription opioids [13]. Prognosis and treatment adherence are often poor in opioid use disorders, with only about a third of patients successfully completing treatment [14]. Apart from psychosocial therapies, which often have only a limited effect on abstinence rates in opioid dependence, opioid maintenance treatment is a well-proven, first-line approach [15]. Oral methadone (MET), buprenorphine (BUP) and a combination of BUP and the opioid antagonist naloxone (BUP/naloxone) are frequently used for treatment [1, 16–18]. All three treatments have been studied extensively in opioid dependence [1, 15, 19–21], and numerous studies and meta-analyses have demonstrated the efficacy of both MET and BUP [17, 22, 23]. For comprehensive reviews, see Mammen and Bell [16] and Yokell et al. [24]. Meanwhile, a number of pharmacological options are available or on the horizon for the treatment of opioid dependence (see Table 12.1).

M. Soyka
Medical Park Chiemseeblick, Bernau, Germany

Psychiatric Hospital, University of Munich, Munich, Germany
e-mail: m.soyka@medicalpark.de

Y.-K. Kim (ed.), *Treatment Resistance in Psychiatry*, https://doi.org/10.1007/978-981-10-4358-1_12

Table 12.1 Available and potential pharmacotherapies for opioid dependence

Drug name	Method of administration
Available treatments	
Methadone	Oral, i.m.
Buprenorphine/naloxone	
Buprenorphine film	Sublingual
Buprenorphine	Depot (implant)
Naloxone	i.v., nasal
Naltrexone	oral, Depot
Morphine sulphate	oral
Diacetylmorphine	i.v.
Potential treatment	
Hydromorphone	i.v.

Most studies on MET and BUP have been short or medium term (of several months of duration), but a few long-term studies have also been performed [25, 26]. Studies comparing MET and BUP have shown that both drugs have comparable effects on opioid use, but the retention rate is somewhat lower in BUP-treated patients [27–29]. In our large naturalistic 6-year follow-up study [30], we found high overall retention rates in both MET- and BUP-treated patients and no differences in retention rates between the two medications.

12.1 Methadone and Buprenorphine Pharmacology:

MET is a long-acting synthetic opioid that, in combination with psychosocial interventions, effectively treats opioid dependence [15]. It addresses symptoms of opioid withdrawal and reduces craving and opioid-induced euphoria. It is a full agonist at the mu- and all other opioid receptors, whereas BUP is an agonist at the mu-opioid receptor and an antagonist at the kappa-opioid receptor.

MET can be ingested in a liquid form or as a tablet and is orally active. BUP, on the other hand, has low bioavailability after oral administration because it is subject to extensive first-pass metabolism in the liver. Consequently, BUP tablets are administered sublingually. Both MET and BUP have a long half-life and bind to opioid receptors for at least a day. BUP is available in two tablet forms: BUP only and BUP/naloxone. Because naloxone has poor sublingual but good parenteral bioavailability, it precipitates opioid withdrawal only when administered intravenously. Thus, the combination tablet aims to prevent patients from dissolving and injecting the tablet and consequently to reduce the risk for misuse and diversion. Naloxone has a short elimination half-life in plasma of about 30 min [31]. Further information on the emergency treatment of opioid overdose with naloxone is given below (under "Alternative Treatments in Treatment-Refractory Patients").

The induction phase is important for and predictive of treatment outcome, especially for BUP, and thus requires special attention [32].

MET is orally absorbed and basically metabolized in the liver by CYP3A4 (demethylation) to the inactive metabolite EDDP. There is a strong genetic variability of CYP3A4 activity among individuals. CYP2D6 and possibly CYP1A2 also play a role. CYP3A4 inducers such as many antiretrovirals may reduce methadone concentrations possibly causing withdrawal symptoms.

BUP is absorbed sublingually; CYP3A4 and to a lesser extent CYP2C8 convert and N-dealkylate it in the liver to the active metabolite norbuprenorphine. Both BUP and norbuprenorphine are metabolized further by uridine diphosphate glucuronosyltransferases (UGTs). Similar to MET, BUP does not significantly induce or inhibit P450 enzymes, but it may compete with drugs that are metabolized by the same pathways. BUP is only a weak inhibitor of CYP3A4.

12.2 Dosage

The usual dosage of MET is 60–120 mg/day, but higher dosages may be given, especially in rapid metabolizers. BUP is usually started at 2–4 mg/day [15] and can be increased by 2–4 mg/day. The typical BUP dosage for maintenance treatment is 8–16 mg/day, and the Food and Drug Administration (FDA) limits the dose to a maximum of 24 mg/day [15]. A dose of 16 mg/day of BUP suppresses 80% of the opioid receptor. The

BUP/naloxone tablet contains BUP and naloxone in a 4:1 ratio, i.e. BUP 2 mg/naloxone 0.5 mg or BUP 8 mg/naloxone 2 mg.

Dosing issues are critical for treatment retention and outcome, and numerous studies have shown the extreme importance of administering an adequate dose in opioid-dependent individuals. Many patients are underdosed and may experience opioid withdrawal or craving as a consequence. A meta-analysis of 21 randomized clinical studies showed that the retention rate for BUP is better at a higher dose (16–32 mg/day) than at a lower one (<16 mg/day). Similar results have been published for MET [33]. The results of a 24-week randomized multicentre study comparing the effects and treatment retention rates of MET and BUP in 1267 patients [34] found a higher retention rate with MET than with BUP (74% vs 46%) and a retention rate of up to 80% in the MET group when the maximum dose reached or exceeded 60 mg/day. In BUP patients, the completion rate also increased and reached a 60% retention rate at doses of 30–32 mg/day. A lower dose (BUP <16 mg/day, MET <60 mg/day) was associated with dropout. The induction phase for BUP is crucial: in patients with more severe withdrawal symptoms, a lower dropout rate was found if the dose was increased more rapidly in the induction phase [35].

12.3 Safety

A comprehensive review on 58 prospective studies of people with opioid dependence [36] indicated high mortality rates (all-cause mortality: 2.09 per 100 person-years [PY]) but confirmed that maintenance treatment significantly lowers rates compared with untreated heroin dependence The review found that most patients died from overdose and the risk was higher in males and in patients during out-of-treatment periods.

Both MET and BUP may cause respiratory depression, but at higher concentrations, BUP has a ceiling effect for respiratory depression [37], i.e. higher doses of BUP >24–32 mg/day do not further increase its respiratory depressant effect.

Both drugs cause typical opioid-related side effects. The side effects of MET include sedation, respiratory depression, constipation, decreased appetite, sweating (which may be a reason for switching to other medications) and fatigue [38]. Caution is required when MET is taken in combination with other CNS "downers", such as alcohol and psychotropic drugs. In addition to respiratory depression, BUP can also cause anxiety, sweating, constipation, headache, insomnia, nausea, dizziness, asthenia and somnolence. Liver enzyme elevations or hepatotoxic effects may occur with buprenorphine [39], although they are rare [40].

12.3.1 Cardiotoxicity

Opioid-induced QT prolongation or arrhythmias (torsade des pointes) have been repeatedly described in opioids [41], especially with MET and other full opioid agonists when given at higher doses [42, 43], and may limit clinical use. The cardiac side effects increase the risk of sudden cardiac death.

The first step in patients with cardiotoxic side effects is to reconsider the dosage and possible interactions with other drugs; the second step is to change the opioid being given. With respect to cardiotoxicity, BUP appears to be safer than MET and to have fewer or no cardiotoxic effects and no risk of cardiac arrhythmias [44, 45]. Another alternative is to use morphine sulphate (see below).

12.4 Alternative Treatments in Treatment-Refractory Patients

The first approach in treatment-resistant patients is to switch from MET to BUP or vice versa. No precautions are necessary when switching from BUP to MET, but switching MET to BUP may be more difficult. Because BUP can induce precipitated withdrawal, opioid-dependent patients should wait until they experience mild to moderate opioid withdrawal (tremor, mydriasis, restlessness, vomiting, anxiety, rhinorrhoea, etc.) before taking the first MET dose. Many guidelines suggest reducing the MET dose to 30–40 mg/day before initiating treatment with BUP [15].

12.4.1 Other Opioids

12.4.1.1 Slow-Release Morphine Sulphate

Slow-release oral morphine sulphate is available in some countries [46] and is especially helpful in treatment-resistant patients. It has been evaluated in a few studies, including randomized clinical trials [46, 47]. Although an initial Cochrane analysis on three relevant studies failed to find sufficient evidence for its use [48], some additional open-label studies have been published since then [49, 50]. The abuse potential of morphine sulphate seems to be rather high [51, 52]. Morphine sulphate is frequently used in Austria and is a second-line medication for individuals with severe craving and opioid use that does not respond to conventional treatment. The advantages of morphine sulphate over other full agonists are its lack of QT prolongation, less sweating and no metabolisation via CYP450.

12.4.1.2 Diacetylmorphine

Diacetylmorphine is the active ingredient in heroin. A number of studies have been conducted on supervised diacetylmorphine treatment in severe opioid dependence [53] (for a review, see [54]). The use of diacetylmorphine may be limited by its overdose and diversion risk, the fact that it is highly addictive, the i.v. route of administration and its relatively short half-life, which necessitates several injections a day or concomitant MET treatment. Nevertheless, in otherwise treatment-resistant patients, diacetylmorphine has been shown to be effective, and in many countries, it has been approved for use in this indication. In a systematic review of six randomized controlled trials, Strang et al. [54] showed that diacetylmorphine is effective in patients refractory to standard treatment. However, the group also found that the drug is less safe than MET and therefore requires "more clinical attention to manage greater safety issues" [54]. In most countries, significant regulatory restrictions limit the use of diacetylmorphine, and it is available only in special supervised treatment settings.

12.4.1.3 Hydromorphone

The opioid analgesic hydromorphone may emerge as a further alternative for treatment-refractory opioid dependence. The Canadian "Study to Assess Longer-term Opioid Medication Effectiveness" (SALOME), a phase 3 double-blind study, compared injectable hydromorphone with injectable diacetylmorphine in 202 randomized chronic injection opioid users [55, 56]. Medications were adjusted individually up to a maximum of 400 mg/dose diacetylmorphine and 1000 mg/day of hydromorphone. The study confirmed noninferiority of hydromorphone. Interestingly, 29 severe adverse events occurred (24 in the diacetylmorphine group, 5 in the hydromorphone group), mostly seizures and overdoses. Hydromorphone is not yet available for treatment of opioid use disorders.

12.4.2 Naloxone for Overdose Prevention

Naloxone is a non-selective, rapid-acting full opioid receptor antagonist and an established and rapid-acting medication to prevent overdose deaths; take-home emergency naloxone is a possible strategy to prevent such deaths [57, 58]. Naloxone is not active when orally administered. Routes of administration include i.v. and non-injectable routes such as nasal naloxone, which has already been approved in some countries [59].

12.4.3 Naltrexone and Extended-Release Naltrexone

Oral naltrexone 50 mg/day or two 100 mg doses three times weekly followed by 150 mg/day can be considered for patients for whom adherence can be supervised. The treatment is appropriate for patients who seek abstinence. However, this treatment carries a special risk: after opioid antagonist therapy, patients who resume opioid use lack opioid tolerance and consequently are at increased risk of overdose and death after opioid (heroin) use; patients must be made aware of this risk when entering treatment. Side effects include nausea, malaise and gastrointestinal problems. There is no dependence risk.

As an alternative to opioid agonist treatment, extended-release naltrexone may be used to prevent opioid relapse in some patients [60] (for a review, see [61]), such as criminal justice offenders [62] or those who have problems with adherence. A recent study indicated non-inferiority of injectable extended-release naltrexone vs daily buprenorphine in a 12-week randomized clinical trial [63]. Common side effects include hepatic enzyme abnormalities, insomnia, hypertension and injection side pain [61]. As is the case with oral naltrexone, after extended-release naltrexone treatment, opioid tolerance is reduced and opioid relapse may result in severe intoxications. Patients must be told about this risk.

12.4.4 Novel Depot Formulations/Implants

Novel and longer-lasting opioids and opioid formulations are needed to improve retention and treatment adherence. A longer-acting MET formulation (levo-alpha-acetylmethadol, LAAM) unfortunately had to be withdrawn because of cardiotoxic side effects. Different formulations of BUP have been tested and developed. In 2016, a 6-month BUP subdermal implant (Probuphine®) was approved by the FDA for the maintenance treatment of opioid dependence in people who showed sustained, prolonged clinical stability at doses of no more than 8 mg/day sublingual BUP. The available studies [63–66] indicate that the BUP implant shows noninferiority or equal effects to sublingual BUP. The hope is that a long-acting depot formulation may lower the risk of diversion and facilitate treatment of stable opioid-dependent patients as a suitable alternative to daily sublingual BUP (for a review, see [67]). This formulation is not yet available in Europe.

Data on a weekly BUP depot preparation, CAM 20038 (24 mg and 32 mg), have recently been published showing that the drug is safely tolerated and produces immediate and sustained opioid blockade and opioid withdrawal suppression [68]. In the near future, both depot (injection) and implant formulations of long-acting BUP may be available to further improve maintenance treatment in opioid-dependent people. BUP depot or implant preparations will probably be suitable mainly in stable rather than treatment-refractory individuals [68].

12.4.5 Psychotherapy

The dropout rate for drug therapies is significant and estimated to be about 40% by Gossop and Marsden [69], who also reported abstinence rates of 51% at 6 months after discharge from inpatient treatment. Most other studies indicate abstinence rates of 20% to a maximum of 30% [70–72]. Depending on the definition, in the first year of treatment, 30–50% of the patients were drug-free.

Concomitant psychotherapy is useful in treatment-resistant patients, but the optimal approach is a matter of debate and the number of studies limited [73, 74]. Motivational interviewing, contingency management and cognitive behavioural therapy (CBT) are important evidence-based psychotherapies. Long-term studies [70, 71] and meta-analyses have evaluated the efficacy of psychosocial therapies. Dutra et al. [75] found that contingency management, relapse prevention, general CBT and treatments combining CBT and contingency management have moderate effect sizes. Two Cochrane analyses [76, 77] have examined the efficacy of psychosocial therapies in combination with substitution treatment, whereby most of the studies were in patients receiving MET; evidence was best for CBT and contingency management. A meta-analysis of 24 studies on the treatment of opioid dependence by Berglund et al. [19] found that psychotherapies have moderately large effect sizes in comparison with the control groups.

Fewer studies are available for CBT patients in BUP treatment [78–80] and the results are mixed. In a systematic review, Dugosh et al. [74] found that the evidence for the efficacy of psychosocial interventions in BUP treatment is less clear than for MET. Recently a study comparing CBT, contingency management and the combination of both with no additional treatment in BUP-maintained patients failed to show any differences between the groups [79].

Conclusions

A broad spectrum of pharmacological and non-pharmacological interventions is now available for treatment-refractory opioid dependence. In addition to opioid maintenance treatment with partial or full opioid agonists, treatment with opioid antagonists is a realistic treatment option. Whether novel dopamine antagonists or partial agonists can be used for treatment of opioid dependence, as indicated by some preclinical studies [81, 82], remains to be seen. In sum, in contrast to the situation for other substance use disorders, treatment of opioid dependence is an emerging and promising field with different treatment options.

Disclosure For the past 5 years, MS has worked as a consultant or has received research grants from Lundbeck, Sanofi Aventis, Camurus, Reckitt Benckiser/Indivior, Servier and Novartis. No funding was used in the preparation of this review.

References

1. Soyka M, Kranzler HR, van den Brink W, Krystal J, Moller HJ, Kasper S. The World Federation of Societies of Biological Psychiatry (WFSBP) guidelines for the biological treatment of substance use and related disorders. Part 2: Opioid dependence. World J Biol Psychiatry. 2011;12(3):160–87.
2. World Health Organization. International classification of diseases, 10th revision (ICD-10). Geneva: World Health Organization; 2010.
3. American Psychiatric Association. Diagnostic and statistical manual of mental disorders, Text Revision. 4th ed. Washington, DC: American Psychiatric Publishing; 2000.
4. Schuckit MA. Treatment of opioid-use disorders. N Engl J Med. 2016;375(4):357–68.
5. Lieb M, Wittchen HU, Palm U, Apelt SM, Siegert J, Soyka M. Psychiatric comorbidity in substitution treatment of opioid-dependent patients in primary care: prevalence and impact on clinical features. Heroin Addict Relat Clin Probl. 2010;12(4):5–16.
6. Mattick RP, Breen C, Kimber J, Davoli M. Methadone maintenance therapy versus no opioid replacement therapy for opioid dependence. Cochrane Database Syst Rev. 2009;3:CD002209.
7. Kelty E, Hulse G. Morbidity and mortality in opioid dependent patients after entering an opioid pharmacotherapy compared with a cohort of non-dependent controls. J Public Health (Oxf). 2018;40:409–14.
8. United Nations Office on Drugs and Crime. World drug report 2016. New York: United Nations; 2016.
9. EMCDDA. European drug report 2016: trends and developments. Lisbon: EMCDDA; 2016. Available from: http://www.emcdda.europa.eu/publications/edr/trends-developments/2014
10. Pierce M, Bird SM, Hickman M, Marsden J, Dunn G, Jones A, et al. Impact of treatment for opioid dependence on fatal drug-related poisoning: a national cohort study in England. Addiction. 2016;111(2):298–308.
11. Jones CM, Logan J, Gladden RM, Bohm MK. Vital signs: demographic and substance use trends among heroin users – United States, 2002–2013. MMWR Morb Mortal Wkly Rep. 2015;64(26):719–25.
12. Rudd RA, Aleshire N, Zibbell JE, Gladden RM. Increases in drug and opioid overdose deaths – United States, 2000–2014. MMWR Morb Mortal Wkly Rep. 2016;64(50–51):1378–82.
13. Schuchat A, Houry D, Guy GP Jr. New data on opioid use and prescribing in the United States. JAMA. 2017;318(5):425–6.
14. Eastwood B, Strang J, Marsden J. Effectiveness of treatment for opioid use disorder: a national, five-year, prospective, observational study in England. Drug Alcohol Depend. 2017;176:139–47.
15. Kampman K, Jarvis M. American Society of Addiction Medicine (ASAM) national practice guideline for the use of medications in the treatment of addiction involving opioid use. J Addict Med. 2015;9(5):358–67.
16. Mammen K, Bell J. The clinical efficacy and abuse potential of combination buprenorphine-naloxone in the treatment of opioid dependence. Expert Opin Pharmacother. 2009;10(15):2537–44.
17. Mattick RP, Breen C, Kimber J, Davoli M. Buprenorphine maintenance versus placebo or methadone maintenance for opioid dependence. Cochrane Database Syst Rev. 2014;2:CD002207.
18. Soyka M, Trader A, Klotsche J, Backmund M, Buhringer G, Rehm J, et al. Six-year mortality rates of patients in methadone and buprenorphine maintenance therapy: results from a nationally representative cohort study. J Clin Psychopharmacol. 2011;31(5):678–80.

19. Berglund M, Thelander S, Jonsson E. Treating alcohol and drug abuse: an evidence based review. Weinheim: Wiley-VCH; 2003.
20. Kleber HD, Weiss RD, Anton RF Jr, George TP, Greenfield SF, Kosten TR, et al. Treatment of patients with substance use disorders, second edition. American Psychiatric Association. Am J Psychiatry. 2007;164(4 Suppl):5–123.
21. World Health Organization. Guidelines for the psychosocially assisted pharmacological treatment of opioid dependence. Geneva: World Health Organization; 2009.
22. Connock M, Juarez-Garcia A, Jowett S, Frew E, Liu Z, Taylor RJ, et al. Methadone and buprenorphine for the management of opioid dependence: a systematic review and economic evaluation. Health Technol Assess. 2007;11(9):1–171. iii–iv
23. Kakko J, Svanborg KD, Kreek MJ, Heilig M. 1-year retention and social function after buprenorphine-assisted relapse prevention treatment for heroin dependence in Sweden: a randomised, placebo-controlled trial. Lancet. 2003;361(9358):662–8.
24. Yokell MA, Zaller ND, Green TC, Rich JD. Buprenorphine and buprenorphine/naloxone diversion, misuse, and illicit use: an international review. Curr Drug Abuse Rev. 2011;4(1):28–41.
25. Hser YI, Evans E, Grella C, Ling W, Anglin D. Long-term course of opioid addiction. Harv Rev Psychiatry. 2015;23(2):76–89.
26. Hser YI, Evans E, Huang D, Weiss R, Saxon A, Carroll KM, et al. Long-term outcomes after randomization to buprenorphine/naloxone versus methadone in a multi-site trial. Addiction. 2016;111(4):695–705.
27. Kakko J, Gronbladh L, Svanborg KD, von Wachenfeldt J, Ruck C, Rawlings B, et al. A stepped care strategy using buprenorphine and methadone versus conventional methadone maintenance in heroin dependence: a randomized controlled trial. Am J Psychiatry. 2007;164(5):797–803.
28. Schottenfeld RS, Pakes JR, Oliveto A, Ziedonis D, Kosten TR. Buprenorphine vs methadone maintenance treatment for concurrent opioid dependence and cocaine abuse. Arch Gen Psychiatry. 1997;54(8):713–20.
29. Soyka M, Zingg C, Koller G, Kuefner H. Retention rate and substance use in methadone and buprenorphine maintenance therapy and predictors of outcome: results from a randomized study. Int J Neuropsychopharmacol. 2008;11(5):641–53.
30. Soyka M, Strehle J, Rehm J, Buhringer G, Wittchen HU. Six-year outcome of opioid maintenance treatment in heroin-dependent patients: results from a naturalistic study in a nationally representative sample. Eur Addict Res. 2017;23(2):97–105.
31. Chiang CN, Hawks RL. Pharmacokinetics of the combination tablet of buprenorphine and naloxone. Drug Alcohol Depend. 2003;70(2 Suppl):S39–47.
32. Apelt SM, Scherbaum N, Soyka M. Induction and switch to buprenorphine-naloxone in opioid dependence treatment: predictive value of the first four weeks. Heroin Addict Relat Clin Probl. 2014;16:87–98.
33. Fareed A, Vayalapalli S, Casarella J, Drexler K. Effect of buprenorphine dose on treatment outcome. J Addict Dis. 2012;31(1):8–18.
34. Hser YI, Saxon AJ, Huang D, Hasson A, Thomas C, Hillhouse M, et al. Treatment retention among patients randomized to buprenorphine/naloxone compared to methadone in a multi-site trial. Addiction. 2014;109(1):79–87.
35. Jacobs P, Ang A, Hillhouse MP, Saxon AJ, Nielsen S, Wakim PG, et al. Treatment outcomes in opioid dependent patients with different buprenorphine/naloxone induction dosing patterns and trajectories. Am J Addict. 2015;24(7):667–75.
36. Degenhardt L, Bucello C, Mathers B, Briegleb C, Ali H, Hickman M, et al. Mortality among regular or dependent users of heroin and other opioids: a systematic review and meta-analysis of cohort studies. Addiction. 2011;106(1):32–51.
37. Walsh SL, Preston KL, Stitzer ML, Cone EJ, Bigelow GE. Clinical pharmacology of buprenorphine: ceiling effects at high doses. Clin Pharmacol Ther. 1994;55(5):569–80.
38. Haber PS, Elsayed M, Espinoza D, Lintzeris N, Veillard AS, Hallinan R. Constipation and other common symptoms reported by women and men in methadone and buprenorphine maintenance treatment. Drug Alcohol Depend. 2017;181:132–9.
39. Saxon AJ, Ling W, Hillhouse M, Thomas C, Hasson A, Ang A, et al. Buprenorphine/Naloxone and methadone effects on laboratory indices of liver health: a randomized trial. Drug Alcohol Depend. 2013;128(1–2):71–6.
40. Soyka M, Backmund M, Schmidt P, Apelt S. Buprenorphine-naloxone treatment in opioid dependence and risk of liver enzyme elevation: results from a 12-month observational study. Am J Addict. 2014;23(6):563–9.
41. Katz DF, Sun J, Khatri V, Kao D, Bucher-Bartelson B, Traut C, et al. QTc interval screening in an opioid treatment program. Am J Cardiol. 2013;112(7):1013–8.
42. Ehret GB, Voide C, Gex-Fabry M, Chabert J, Shah D, Broers B, et al. Drug-induced long QT syndrome in injection drug users receiving methadone: high frequency in hospitalized patients and risk factors. Arch Intern Med. 2006;166(12):1280–7.
43. Westermeyer J, Adabag S, Anand V, Thuras P, Yoon G, Batres YCT. Methadone maintenance dose/weight ratio, long QTc, and EKG screening. Am J Addict. 2016;25(6):499–507.
44. Kao DP, Haigney MC, Mehler PS, Krantz MJ. Arrhythmia associated with buprenorphine and methadone reported to the Food and Drug Administration. Addiction. 2015;110(9):1468–75.
45. Wedam EF, Bigelow GE, Johnson RE, Nuzzo PA, Haigney MC. QT-interval effects of methadone, levomethadyl, and buprenorphine in a randomized trial. Arch Intern Med. 2007;167(22):2469–75.
46. Beck T, Haasen C, Verthein U, Walcher S, Schuler C, Backmund M, et al. Maintenance treatment for opioid dependence with slow-release oral morphine: a

randomized cross-over, non-inferiority study versus methadone. Addiction. 2014;109(4):617–26.
47. Jegu J, Gallini A, Soler P, Montastruc JL, Lapeyre-Mestre M. Slow-release oral morphine for opioid maintenance treatment: a systematic review. Br J Clin Pharmacol. 2011;71(6):832–43.
48. Ferri M, Minozzi S, Bo A, Amato L. Slow-release oral morphine as maintenance therapy for opioid dependence. Cochrane Database Syst Rev. 2013;6:CD009879.
49. Falcato L, Beck T, Reimer J, Verthein U. Self-reported cravings for heroin and cocaine during maintenance treatment with slow-release oral morphine compared with methadone: a randomized, crossover clinical trial. J Clin Psychopharmacol. 2015;35(2):150–7.
50. Hammig R, Kohler W, Bonorden-Kleij K, Weber B, Lebentrau K, Berthel T, et al. Safety and tolerability of slow-release oral morphine versus methadone in the treatment of opioid dependence. J Subst Abus Treat. 2014;47(4):275–81.
51. Peyriere H, Eiden C, Micallef J, Lapeyre-Mestre M, Faillie JL, Blayac JP. Slow-release oral morphine sulfate abuse: results of the postmarketing surveillance systems for psychoactive prescription drug abuse in France. Eur Addict Res. 2013;19(5):235–44.
52. Peyriere H, Nogue E, Eiden C, Frauger E, Charra M, Picot MC. Evidence of slow-release morphine sulfate abuse and diversion: epidemiological approaches in a French administrative area. Fundam Clin Pharmacol. 2016;30(5):466–75.
53. Oviedo-Joekes E, Brissette S, Marsh DC, Lauzon P, Guh D, Anis A, et al. Diacetylmorphine versus methadone for the treatment of opioid addiction. N Engl J Med. 2009;361(8):777–86.
54. Strang J, Groshkova T, Uchtenhagen A, van den Brink W, Haasen C, Schechter MT, et al. Heroin on trial: systematic review and meta-analysis of randomised trials of diamorphine-prescribing as treatment for refractory heroin addictiondagger. Br J Psychiatry. 2015;207(1):5–14.
55. Oviedo-Joekes E, Brissette S, MacDonald S, Guh D, Marchand K, Jutha S, et al. Safety profile of injectable hydromorphone and diacetylmorphine for long-term severe opioid use disorder. Drug Alcohol Depend. 2017;176:55–62.
56. Oviedo-Joekes E, Guh D, Brissette S, Marchand K, MacDonald S, Lock K, et al. Hydromorphone compared with diacetylmorphine for long-term opioid dependence: a randomized clinical trial. JAMA Psychiat. 2016;73(5):447–55.
57. McDonald R, Campbell ND, Strang J. Twenty years of take-home naloxone for the prevention of overdose deaths from heroin and other opioids-conception and maturation. Drug Alcohol Depend. 2017;178:176–87.
58. Parmar MK, Strang J, Choo L, Meade AM, Bird SM. Randomized controlled pilot trial of naloxone-on-release to prevent post-prison opioid overdose deaths. Addiction. 2017;112(3):502–15.
59. Strang J, McDonald R, Alqurshi A, Royall P, Taylor D, Forbes B. Naloxone without the needle – systematic review of candidate routes for non-injectable naloxone for opioid overdose reversal. Drug Alcohol Depend. 2016;163:16–23.
60. Krupitsky E, Nunes EV, Ling W, Illeperuma A, Gastfriend DR, Silverman BL. Injectable extended-release naltrexone for opioid dependence: a double-blind, placebo-controlled, multicentre randomised trial. Lancet. 2011;377(9776):1506–13.
61. Syed YY, Keating GM. Extended-release intramuscular naltrexone (VIVITROL(R)): a review of its use in the prevention of relapse to opioid dependence in detoxified patients. CNS Drugs. 2013;27(10):851–61.
62. Lee JD, Friedmann PD, Kinlock TW, Nunes EV, Boney TY, Hoskinson RA Jr, et al. Extended-release naltrexone to prevent opioid relapse in criminal justice offenders. N Engl J Med. 2016;374(13):1232–42.
63. Tanum L, Solli KK, Latif ZE, Benth JS, Opheim A, Sharma-Haase K, Krajci P, Kunoe N. Effectiveness of injectable extended-release naltrexone vs daily buprenorphine-naloxone for opioid dependence: a randomized clinical noninferiority trial. JAMA Psychiatry. 2017;74:11097–205.
64. Rosenthal RN, Ling W, Casadonte P, Vocci F, Bailey GL, Kampman K, et al. Buprenorphine implants for treatment of opioid dependence: randomized comparison to placebo and sublingual buprenorphine/naloxone. Addiction. 2013;108(12):2141–9.
65. Ling W, Casadonte P, Bigelow G, Kampman KM, Patkar A, Bailey GL, et al. Buprenorphine implants for treatment of opioid dependence: a randomized controlled trial. JAMA. 2010;304(14):1576–83.
66. White J, Bell J, Saunders JB, Williamson P, Makowska M, Farquharson A, et al. Open-label dose-finding trial of buprenorphine implants (Probuphine) for treatment of heroin dependence. Drug Alcohol Depend. 2009;103(1–2):37–43.
67. Barnwal P, Das S, Mondal S, Ramasamy A, Maiti T, Saha A. Probuphine(R) (buprenorphine implant): a promising candidate in opioid dependence. Ther Adv Psychopharmacol. 2017;7(3):119–34.
68. Walsh SL, Comer SD, Lofwall MR, Vince B, Levy-Cooperman N, Kelsh D, et al. Effect of buprenorphine weekly depot (CAM2038) and hydromorphone blockade in individuals with opioid use disorder: a randomized clinical trial. JAMA Psychiat. 2017;74:894–902.
69. Gossop M, Marsden J. Assessment and treatment of opiate problems. Baillieres Clin Psychiatry. 1996;2:445–59.
70. Simpson DD, Sells SB. Effectiveness of treatment for drug abuse: an overview of the DARP Research Program. Adv Alcohol Subst Abuse. 1982;2:27–9.
71. Simpson DD, Sells SBe. Opioid addiction and treatment: a 12-year follow-up. Malabar: Robert E. Kreiger; 1990.
72. Hubbard RL, Marsden ME, Rachal JV, Harwood HJ, Cavanaugh ER, Ginzburg HM. Drug abuse treatment: a national study of effectiveness. Chapel Hill: The University of North Carolina Press; 1989.
73. Day E, Mitcheson L. Psychosocial interventions in opiate substitution treatment services: does the

evidence provide a case for optimism or nihilism? Addiction. 2017;112:1329–36.
74. Dugosh K, Abraham A, Seymour B, McLoyd K, Chalk M, Festinger DA. Systematic review on the use of psychosocial interventions in conjunction with medications for the treatment of opioid addiction. J Addict Med. 2016;10(2):93–103.
75. Dutra L, Stathopoulou G, Basden SL, Leyro TM, Powers MB, Otto MW. A meta-analytic review of psychosocial interventions for substance use disorders. Am J Psychiatry. 2008;165(2):179–87.
76. Amato L, Minozzi S, Davoli M, Vecchi S. Psychosocial combined with agonist maintenance treatments versus agonist maintenance treatments alone for treatment of opioid dependence. Cochrane Database Syst Rev. 2011;10:CD004147.
77. Amato L, Minozzi S, Davoli M, Vecchi S. Psychosocial and pharmacological treatments versus pharmacological treatments for opioid detoxification. Cochrane Database Syst Rev. 2011;9:CD005031.
78. Fiellin DA, Barry DT, Sullivan LE, Cutter CJ, Moore BA, O'Connor PG, et al. A randomized trial of cognitive behavioral therapy in primary care-based buprenorphine. Am J Med. 2013;126(1):74. e11-7
79. Ling W, Hillhouse M, Ang A, Jenkins J, Fahey J. Comparison of behavioral treatment conditions in buprenorphine maintenance. Addiction. 2013;108(10):1788–98.
80. Moore BA, Barry DT, Sullivan LE, O'Connor PG, Cutter CJ, Schottenfeld RS, et al. Counseling and directly observed medication for primary care buprenorphine maintenance: a pilot study. J Addict Med. 2012;6(3):205–11.
81. Kumar V, Bonifazi A, Ellenberger MP, Keck TM, Pommier E, Rais R, et al. Highly selective dopamine D3 receptor (D3R) antagonists and partial agonists based on eticlopride and the D3R crystal structure: new leads for opioid dependence treatment. J Med Chem. 2016;59(16):7634–50.
82. You ZB, Gao JT, Bi GH, He Y, Boateng C, Cao J, et al. The novel dopamine D3 receptor antagonists/partial agonists CAB2-015 and BAK4-54 inhibit oxycodone-taking and oxycodone-seeking behavior in rats. Neuropharmacology. 2017;126:190–9.

13 Treatment-Resistant Panic Disorder

Mu-Hong Chen and Shih-Jen Tsai

Panic disorder is one of the most frequently observed mental illnesses with a chronic or a remitting-relapsing condition [1–3]. Panic disorder includes two symptomatic domains: somatic/physical domain and cognitive domain. The somatic/physical domain expresses repetitive panic attacks with various somatic/physical symptoms, such as palpitation, dyspnea, chest pain, sweating, numbness, nausea, and dizziness; as for the cognitive domain, panic disorder manifests in the development of phobic avoidance, behavioral changes due to panic attacks, and persistent worries and concerns for the future attacks [1–5]. In the human population, the prevalence of panic disorder is approximately 2.7% at 12 months and 4.7% during one's lifetime [6–8].

An American national survey reported that panic disorder individuals had around a doubling risk of 1-month work impairment than that of mood disorders, causing 1.7 working day absence [9]. The World Health Organization survey demonstrated that around 1% of all disability-adjusted life years and 3.5% of all years lived with disability worldwide were due to anxiety disorders, including panic disorder [10, 11]. Although international reports were able to suggest the severe disease burdens due to panic disorder, panic disorder treatments in the real world remained frustrating. Only about one-third of the patients with panic disorder have treatment contact in the first year of onset [12, 13].

Increasing evidence indicated that panic disorder is a remitting-relapsing or a chronic or mental illness, significantly interfering with the individual's functions and life qualities [14–19]. With recommended treatment methods from current clinical guidelines [20–25], only about one-third of the patients with panic disorder could be symptom free at long-term follow-up, and yet over 50% of patients did not achieve remission, with threshold or subthreshold panic symptoms, particularly in terms of cognitive and phobic avoidance [14, 15, 17, 18, 26, 27]. A recent cross-national study further reported that, among individuals with experiences of panic attacks, the majority (66.5%) had recurrent panic attacks [28]. Relapses of panic disorder commonly occur in life among half of the panic disorder patients [15, 16, 18, 19, 29–31]. However, the definition of treatment-resistant panic disorder (TRPD) remains unclear despite that several studies stated the need to elaborate this clinical phenomenon in this decade [32–35]. In this chapter, we wish to address the concept, psychopathology, pathogenesis, and potential treatment strategies for TRPD.

M.-H. Chen · S.-J. Tsai (✉)
Department of Psychiatry, Taipei Veterans General Hospital, Taipei, Taiwan

School of Medicine, National Yang-Ming University, Taipei, Taiwan

Y.-K. Kim (ed.), *Treatment Resistance in Psychiatry*, https://doi.org/10.1007/978-981-10-4358-1_13

13.1 Idea of Remission and Treatment Resistance in Panic Disorder

In past decades, treatment-resistant depression had been frequently studied despite many existing clinical and diagnostic debates [36–38]. Yet, much less attention was paid to the TRPD. Before defining TRPD, we ought to know the definition of response, remission, and recovery of panic disorder which inversely associates with treatment resistance [33].

Panic disorder treatment response was generally defined as a minimal reduction that exceeds 50% from baseline score on Hamilton Anxiety Scale (HAM-A), a Clinical Global Impressions Scale-Severity scale (CGI-S) score of "mild" or better, no panic attacks in the past week, and Mobility Inventory-unaccompanied subscale <1.8 [39, 40] or defined as a 40% reduction of the Panic Disorder Severity Scale (PDSS) score and a CGI- Improvement scale (CGI-I) score of "much" or "very much" improved relative to pretreatment assessments [41, 42]. Treatment responses were measured in two dimensions, including symptomatic and functional aspects. HAMA-A or PDSS was the index for the symptomatic aspect; CGI was the index for the functional aspect. When a patient achieved the response after an optimal treatment, we would further assess whether he or she may achieve the remission state. In fact, the nonappearance of physical and autonomic symptoms of panic disorder may not indicate a real remission and recovery. For instance, a subject with panic disorder had no panic attacks but yet the patient persistently ruminated about the catastrophic incidences that he or she experienced in previous panic attacks. Thus, in panic disorder, panic-free condition (symptomatic remission) and the functional remission (recovery) are not identical. Furthermore, the presence of panic attacks could be a normal stress response, and this may not always be regarded as a psychopathology [33]. The multidimensional assessment for the remission and recovery is highly recommended and thus should always consider not just somatic symptoms but also its cognitive and functional condition.

We summarize two potential remission criteria for panic disorder in this chapter based on previous studies and expert opinions [43–46] (Table 13.1). An almost complete resolution of panic attacks (core symptom of panic disorder), cognitive and phobic avoidance, anticipatory anxiety, and functional and social impairment was defined as the first criteria [43]. A HAM-A score <7 indicated no/minimal anxiety; a Sheehan Disability Scale score <1 on each item indicated no/mild functional and social impairment [43, 44]. Furthermore, depression-free condition, defined as a Hamilton Rating Scale for Depression (HAM-D) scoring ≤7, was included in the remission criteria of panic disorder [43, 44]. Second criteria were defined as a PDSS score <3 with one individual item more than 1 and HAM-D scoring ≤7 [44]. PDSS assessed the core symptoms of panic disorder (panic frequency, distress levels during panic, panic-focused anticipatory anxiety, phobic avoidance of situations and of physical sensations) and also assessed impairment in social and occupational functioning [41]. Briefly speaking, when we would define the full remission of panic disorder in the clinical

Table 13.1 Proposed remission criteria of panic disorder

Criteria 1	Criteria 2
Essentially free of panic attacks	PDSS total score ≤3 and no individual item score >1
No or mild agoraphobic avoidance	
No or minimal anxiety:	HAM-D score ≤7
HAM-A score ≤7–10	
No functional impairment:	
Sheehan Disability Scale score ≤1 on each item	
No or minimal symptoms of depression	
HAM-D score ≤7	

HAM-A Hamilton Rating Scale for Anxiety, *HAM-D* Hamilton Rating Scale for Depression, *PDSS* Panic Disorder Severity Scale practice, we should assess the panic disorder condition from symptomatic and functional views. The symptomatic criteria (i.e., HAM-A or PDSS) and the functional criteria (i.e., Sheehan Disability Scale score or CGI) should be integrated together for defining the remission of panic disorder [47, 48]. In addition, the symptom severity should be positively correlated to the functional impairment, indicating a greater symptom severity correlating with higher functional impairment and vice versa [47, 48]. For example, the HAM-A score ≤7–10 is approximately equal to a CGI-severity score <2 [47, 48]. The scores of 2–5 and 0–1 in PDSS corresponds to the CGI-S score of "borderline mentally" and "not at all ill," respectively [41].

TRPD should be defined as the failure to achieve remission according to the previously mentioned criteria after at least 9–12 months of optimal treatment [43, 44]. The follow-up studies assessing the long-term prognosis of panic disorder indicated that approximately 1/3 of panic patients would be free from panic disorder with the standard treatments, another 1/3 would improve and partially respond to treatment, and yet the last 1/3 would be considered the TRPD group by the current treatments [15, 17–19, 33, 49].

13.2 Factors Related to Treatment Resistance

Factors associated with the failure to achieve response and remission in panic disorder could be the representatives of factors associated with TRPD. We proposed five major risk factors for TRPD, including the characteristic essence of panic disorder, personal demographic characteristics, comorbid medical illnesses, comorbid psychiatric disorders, and psychosocial factors, in the following text (Table 13.2).

Table 13.2 Predictors for the treatment resistance of panic disorder

Characteristics of panic disorder	**Medical comorbidities**
Greater severity of panic symptoms	Cardiovascular diseases
Higher frequency of panic attacks	Cardiac dysrhythmia
Longer course of panic disorder	Cerebrovascular disease
Persistent existence of anticipatory anxiety and panic-related phobias	Asthma
	Hay fever
Younger age of panic attack onset	Migraine
Personal demographic factors	Epilepsy
Male	Pheochromocytoma
Old age	**Medications**
Ethnic minority	Rifampin
Lower level of individual functioning	Vicodin
Low social economic state	Trimethoprim-sulfamethoxazole
Past history of panic disorder	Interferon
Family history of psychiatric disorders	Corticosteroids
Psychiatric comorbidities	Isotretinoin
Agoraphobia	**Psychosocial factors**
Other anxiety disorders (i.e., separation anxiety disorder, generalized anxiety disorder, social phobia)	Social support problems
Major depression	Occupational problems
Bipolar disorder	Economic problems/poverty
Post-traumatic stress disorder	Sexual maltreatment and abuse
Obsessive-compulsive disorder	Childhood maltreatment
Alcohol and substance use disorders	
Personality disorders	

13.3 Traits Defining Panic Disorder

Symptomatic manifestations of panic disorder, such as severe panic and anxiety symptoms, greater severity in panic-related distress, higher panic attack frequency, higher degree of agoraphobic avoidance, more persistence of anticipatory anxiety and phobic avoidance, panic attacks with fear of dying or going crazy, nocturnal panic attacks, and non-respiratory subtype of panic disorder, were associated with TRPD. Furthermore, earlier panic disorder onset age, longer clinical course, relapse of panic attack, greater residual functional and social difficulties, and continued use of anxiolytics have also been suggested as the susceptibility to TRPD [14, 16, 17, 19, 26, 30, 50–60].

13.4 Personal Demographic Characteristics

Sex and ethnicity may have a role in the treatment responses or resistance of panic disorder. Low social economic status or ethnic minority had been reported to be associated with treatment resistance in panic disorder [52, 61–63]. Women reported a later onset and achieved significantly greater improvement than men [14, 16, 19, 30, 53, 62, 64]. Age may be another factor. Both pharmacotherapy and psychotherapy for anxiety disorders, including panic disorder, may not be as effective for older patients as they are for younger patients [65]. Furthermore, family history of bipolar disorder, major depression, and anxiety disorders may be also related to treatment resistance of panic disorder [66–69].

13.5 Other Personal Characteristics

Personality traits, self-concepts, and motivations for treatment, as well as therapeutic alliance between patients and psychiatrists/therapists, were associated with the treatment response or resistance of panic disorder [54, 70–80]. The higher impulsivity, the more neuroticism, the lower extraversion, the higher levels of harm avoidance, the lower levels of persistence, and borderline personality traits may be related to TRPD [73–76, 78, 79]. Furthermore, the higher the expectations for the treatment effect, the higher the confidence in the treatment rationale and the stronger the beliefs about the manageability of panic disorder contributing to the better therapeutic response [54, 80]. On the contrary, the psychological and behavioral resistance to therapy and the therapeutic alliance increased the likelihood of treatment resistance of panic disorder [72, 73, 77]. In addition, sensitivity toward personal anxiety was another predicting factor for the treatment response of panic disorder [81–86]. Reduced anxiety sensitivity indicated treatment response of panic disorder, but high anxiety sensitivity was linked to subsequent panic attacks and relapse of panic disorder [83].

13.6 Psychiatric Comorbidities

Comorbid psychiatric diseases, such as bipolar disorder, obsessive-compulsive disorder, major depression, agoraphobia, other anxiety disorders (social phobia, generalized anxiety disorder), personality disorders, as well as substance use disorders, would be associated with increased symptom severity of panic disorder and decreased individual functioning. The psychiatric comorbidities were also related to the deterioration in the clinical course and poor prognosis of panic disorder [1, 14–18, 30, 53, 64, 87, 88]. Psychiatric comorbidities would increase the risk of treatment resistance in panic disorder.

13.7 Medical Comorbidities

Panic disorder was frequently comorbid with medical diseases, such as cerebrovascular diseases, cardiovascular diseases, cardiac arrhythmia, respiratory diseases, hay fever, migraine, and pheochromocytoma [89–97]. Panic disorder was also regarded as an independent risk factor for other physical diseases, such as ischemic heart disease and cerebrovascular diseases [96, 98–100]. Previous studies reported that panic disorder may worsen in postpartum and menopause [101–103]. In addition, panic disorder occurred less frequently in the aged than in younger adults and rarely had onset in old age [104]. Panic attacks that began in old age should prompt a detail search for physical diseases or medications that could be contributing to their presence [104]. Some symptoms of medical comorbidities were very similar with symptoms of panic attacks, such as palpitation, dyspnea, chest tightness, nausea, and dizziness. In addition, some medical comorbidities may induce the onset of panic attacks and disrupt the clinical course of panic disorder and were also associated with the impaired individual functions. When atypical panic symptoms, such as changes in consciousness, additional physical symptoms, and longer panic attack, are noted during panic attack, prompt intervention for medical comorbidities should be suggested. Furthermore, some medications, such as rifampin, Vicodin, interferon, mefloquine, isotretinoin, rimonabant, corticosteroids, and trimethoprim-sulfamethoxazole, may trigger or worsen the panic attacks [105–109]. The comprehensive scrutiny for physical conditions and medication use was warranted. Panic patients with a greater burden of physical disease were more psychiatrically ill, with higher severity of anxiety symptoms, greater disability, and more psychiatric comorbidities [94].

13.8 Psychosocial Factors

Stressful life events and childhood adversities may be related to the age of onset, persistence, and the relapses of panic disorder [52, 53, 110–117]. Psychosocial stressors included issues in social support, social environment, occupation, economy, personal loss, legal issues, and instability in interpersonal relationships, as well as childhood adversities including sexual abuse and physical and/or emotional ill-treatment. Early childhood adversities would increase likelihood of developing panic disorder after exposure to stressful life events [118]. Patients with panic disorder who had more psychosocial stresses would be more severely ill, with higher severity of panic disorder, increased medical and psychiatric comorbidity, and also greater disability and functional impairment [52, 53, 110–117].

13.9 Potential Pathophysiology of TRPD

13.9.1 Genetic Factors

Several monoamine-related neurotransmitter pathway genes, such as *serotonin transporter* and *monoamine oxidase A* (*MAOA*) genes, have been found to be related to the onset age, persistence, and therapeutic response of panic disorder [40, 119–123]. Individuals who carry the high-expression alleles of a promoter repeat polymorphism in *MAOA* (*MAOA-uVNTR*) were susceptible to panic disorder, had greater panic symptom severity, and poorly responded to standard antidepressant treatment [40, 122]. The inhibitory anterior cingulate cortex-amygdala coupling during fear conditioning was modulated by the L/L genotype of the serotonin transporter-linked polymorphic region (*5-HTTLPR*) and has been regarded as a biomarker to predict treatment responses in panic disorder [121]. The *5-HTTLPR* S allele was related to poor treatment responses in panic disorder patients [123]. Homozygote GG carriers of serotonin 1A receptor (*HTR1A*) -1019C/G polymorphism responded poorly to treatment with antidepressants and were more likely to become resistant to medication treatment [123, 124]. In addition, several *serotonin transporters* and *HTR1A* and *MAOA* polymorphisms have been found to modulate activity in specific brain regions, such as amygdala and prefrontal cortex, which play significant roles in panic disorder and its treatment response [125, 126]. Furthermore, the genetic variants affecting pharmacodynamics or pharmacokinetics of medications for panic disorder may have a potential role in the treatment response of panic disorder [127, 128]. For example, CYP2C19 genetic polymorphism *1/*1 as an extensive metabolizer was associated with poor outcome of escitalopram treatment for panic disorders [128]. However, pharmacogenetic studies investigating the genetic contribution to treatment response of panic disorder were still limited and thus require further genome-wide association studies to clarify this issue.

13.9.2 Brain Circuit Dysfunction

A number of specific brain regions, such as the prefrontal/orbitofrontal region, cingulum, hippocampus, amygdala, striatum, and insular cortex, play crucial roles in anxiety sensitivity and are implicated in the gating, processing, and integration of threat information based on functional neuroimaging studies [1, 33, 86, 129–133]. The chronic anticipatory anxiety and phobic avoidance in panic disorder were mediated by interoceptive fear conditioning of internal physical cues such as palpitation and dyspnea of panic attack and have been found to be a predictor for poor therapeutic response [1, 33, 86, 131–134]. The decoupling processing between amygdala and anterior cingulate cortex and increased activations in the anterior insula, orbitofrontal cortex, dorsal anterior cingulate cortex, amygdala, and dorsomedial prefrontal cortex may contribute to the threat anticipation of somatic symptoms and anxiety sensitivity and were associated with the treatment outcome of panic disorder [130–132, 135–138]. Enhanced activation in the anterior cingulate cortex, the amygdala, and the hippocampus in response to a safety signal was noted in panic disorder patients who have poor response to cognitive-behavioral therapy (CBT) [137], and on the contrary, increased activation in dorsolateral prefrontal cortex and insula during threat processing was related to improved response [133]. Voxel-based morphometry studies determined a relative increase in insula and a reduction in anterior cingulate cortex in panic disorder [139, 140].

In summary, the persistence and maintenance of conditioning fear and cognitive and phobic avoidance were mediated by the dysregulation in bottom-up excitement of the limbic system (i.e., insular cortex, amygdala), top-down inhibition from cortical level (i.e., prefrontal cortex), and the modulation of the hippocampus for the above brain circuits, which played a critical role in TRPD.

13.9.3 Hypothalamus-Pituitary-Adrenal (HPA) Axis Dysregulation

HPA axis plays a crucial role in the physiology of fear conditioning and fear- and anxiety-related behaviors, which are the core psychopathology of panic disorder [141–146]. Several studies suggested that dexamethasone, which suppressed the cortisol levels in a negative feedback manner, may facilitate the fear extinction and reduced fear-associated physical symptoms [147, 148]. Panic disorder patients demonstrated increased overnight cortisol secretion and greater amplitude of ultradian secretory episodes relative to healthy controls, and those with high frequent panic attacks had shifted corticotropin circadian cycles [141, 142]. The hypercortisol state was still noted in the remitted, drug-free panic disorder [149]. In addition, similar with the findings in post-traumatic stress disorder patients and much different with the findings in major depressive patients, panic disorder patients showed a cortisol hypo-responsiveness after the Trier Social Stress Test, independent of comorbid depression [150]. Furthermore, panic disorder patients who had the non-suppression of dexamethasone suppression test had more anxious symptoms, more work and social dysfunction, and more likely to develop major depression as well as a more disabling chronic panic conditions [151]. Those patients who had complete remissions after medication treatment had less evidence of overactivity of HPA axis at baseline than those who did not achieve remission [152]. Another hypothesis for the influence of HPA axis in patients with panic disorder was the dissociation between the HPA axis response in panic disorder and the subjective stress response, which might be the outcome of an overfocused self-monitoring leading to an increased stress perception in spite of normal or only mild HPA axis activation [145].

The modulation of HPA axis may be one of the critical treatment strategies for panic disorder. The levels of cortisol and corticotropin significantly decreased after cognitive intervention in panic disorder patients who were treated with cholecystokinin-B agonist pentagastrin (a pharmacological trigger of panic attacks) [153]. However, antidepressant treatment had no substantial effect on cortisol response to cholecystokinin tetrapeptide (CCK-4), although antidepressants could also reduce 50% of full panic attack frequency induced by injection of CCK-4 in panic disorder patients [154]. The above findings may implicate the different underlying mechanisms for treating panic disorder between pharmacotherapy and psychotherapy.

13.9.4 Brain-Derived Neurotrophic Factor (BDNF)

BDNF plays an important role in the amygdala-dependent fear conditioning [155–159] and may play a role in the pathophysiology of panic disorder [159–163]. Animal studies suggested that BDNF had a panicolytic-like effect [164, 165]. Subjects who had a lower serum BDNF level had an increased risk of developing panic disorder and were more likely to have a poor therapeutic response [159, 161]. In addition, individuals who had *BDNF* 196G-1175C haplotype were prone to developing panic disorder [161, 166]. Potential effects of BDNF in the pathophysiology and treatment prognosis of panic disorder may motivate further studies to clarify the role of other neurotrophic factors in the clinical manifestation, course, and prognosis in panic disorder.

13.9.5 Chronic Systemic Inflammation

Chronic systemic inflammation and related changes of inflammatory cytokines may play crucial roles in the mental illnesses (including panic disorder) as well as in many physical diseases, including metabolic diseases and cardiovascular diseases [167–173]. Low-grade systemic inflammation was also related to psychosocial stresses. Acute and chronic stresses may induce alterations in sensitivity of inflammatory pathways to multiple stress signals [170, 171, 174]. Previous reports have demonstrated the link between systemic inflammation and anxiety disorders [173, 175]. Higher level of interleukin (IL)-6 was associated with current panic disorder compared to remitted panic disorder and was related to higher scores of PDSS [176]. Increased level of C-reactive protein (CRP) was found in the late-onset anxiety disorders [173]. Particularly, higher levels of CRP, tumor necrosis factor (TNF)-α, and IL-6 were related to the somatic symptoms of anxiety disorder, whereas only CRP level was associated with cognitive anxiety symptoms [177].

Stress axis dysregulation, including autonomic nervous system imbalance and alternation in HPA axis, was related to panic disorder and would further support systemic inflammation and contribute to increased panic symptoms by having effects on fear- and anxiety-related brain regions (i.e., the prefrontal cortex, hippocampus, amygdala, and insula) [172]. Furthermore, interferon treatment may reduce and interfere with the panic disorder treatment response of cognitive therapy [108]. Therapeutic cell-mediated immunity intervention may relieve the anxiety symptoms [178]. The treatment-resistant panic disorder may be associated with the cumulative impacts of systemic inflammation due to psychiatric comorbidities, psychosocial stressors, and physical disease.

13.9.6 Biopsychosocial Model Hypothesis

Bringing the above evidences together, we proposed a biopsychosocial hypothesis to explain the potential pathophysiology of the treatment-resistant panic disorder. Individuals who carry some risk alleles (i.e., *serotonin transporter* and *HTR1A* and *MAOA* genes) for panic disorder and have family members having panic disorder or other major psychiatric disorders may exhibit an early onset, a higher symptom severity, and a poor prognosis of panic disorder, further suffered from some psychosocial stresses and childhood adversities, and also manifested the dysregulated

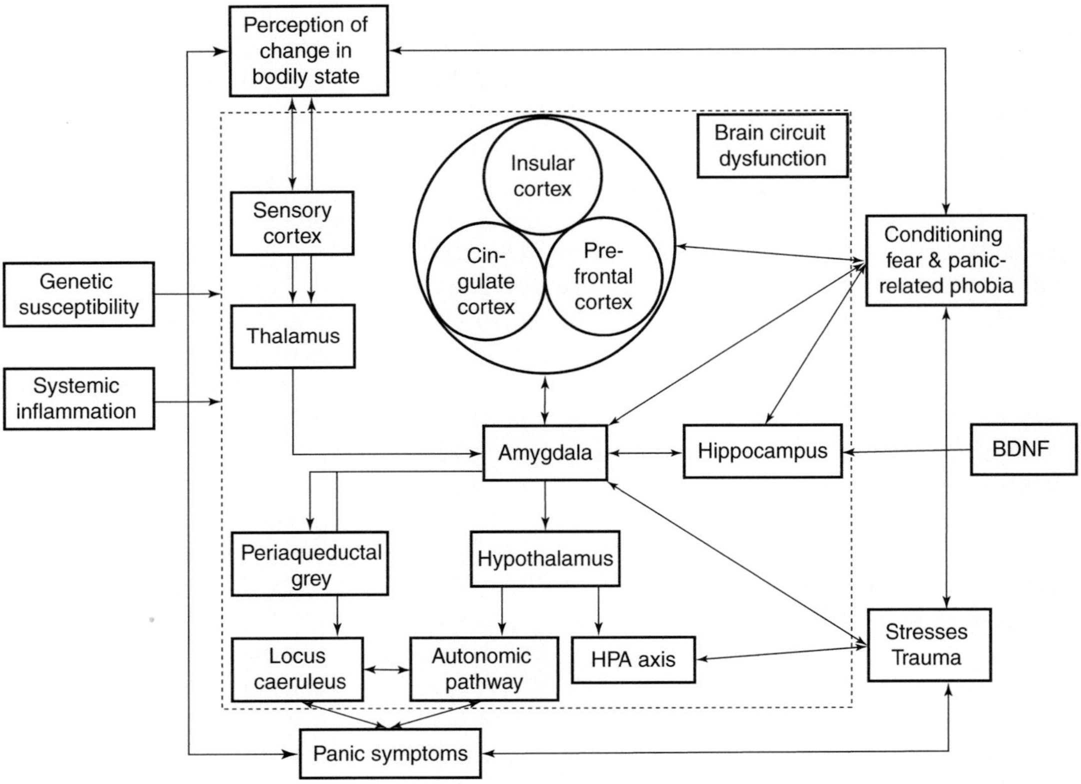

Fig. 13.1 Biopsychosocial and cognitive model for treatment-resistant panic disorder

top-down inhibition from cortical levels and increased bottom-up excitement of the limbic system, as well as the long-term systemic inflammation, resulting in a higher propensity for the treatment resistance (Fig. 13.1).

Because the definition of remission and treatment resistance in panic disorder did not achieve a clinical consensus, the underlying mechanisms for treatment-resistant panic disorder were less investigated and remained unclear. Here, we proposed the potential biopsychosocial model to explain the treatment resistance in panic disorder, but the exact pathophysiology required more investigation in the future.

13.10 Therapeutic Strategies for TRPD

13.10.1 Pharmacological Intervention

Combination treatment of atypical antipsychotics, benzodiazepines, or buspirone and azapirone with antidepressants has shown a better therapeutic response in patients with panic disorder compared with antidepressant treatment alone [179–186] (Table 13.3), despite a recent meta-analysis which failed to support the medication augmentation in treatment-resistant anxiety disorders [187]. However, atypical antipsychotics-related metabolic syndrome and benzodiazepine-associated risk of dependence should be thoroughly taken into consideration, and a comprehensive risk and benefit assessment should be made for the combination treatment [188, 189]. The chronic use of benzodiazepines may indicate a poor treatment response of panic disorder. Antidepressants are usually the preferable agents than benzodiazepines as the first-line treatment for elderly patients with panic disorder [104]. Other potential agents for TRPD included GABA-ergic anticonvulsants (i.e., gabapentin, pregabalin), anti-inflammatory agents, antihistamine, low-dose ketamine infusion, xenon, metabotropic glutamate II receptor agonists, and D-cycloserine [190–197].

Table 13.3 Treatment for treatment-resistant panic disorder

Pharmacological intervention (combined with antidepressants)	Non-pharmacological intervention (combined with pharmacological intervention)
Atypical antipsychotics	Psychotherapy
Risperidone	Cognitive-behavioral therapy
Olanzapine	Interpersonal psychotherapy
Quetiapine	Exposure therapy
Aripiprazole	Mindfulness-based cognitive therapy
Ziprasidone	Eye movement desensitization and reprocessing therapy
Benzodiazepines	Psychodynamic psychotherapy
Buspirone	Neuro-stimulation therapy
Azapirone	Repetitive transcranial magnetic stimulation
GABA-ergic antiepileptics	Transcranial direct current stimulation
Gabapentin	Vagus nerve stimulation
Pregabalin	Alternative therapy
Tiagabine	Exercise
Topiramate	Yoga
D-cycloserine	Light therapy
Anti-inflammatory agents (i.e., immunotherapy)	Omega-3
Antihistamine (i.e., chlorpheniramine, meclizine)	Acupuncture
Low-dose ketamine infusion	

13.10.2 Non-pharmacological Intervention

13.10.2.1 Psychotherapy

Increasing evidence supported the efficacy of CBT for panic disorder in this decade. CBT only and CBT combined with medication treatment could improve panic disorder especially for patients who have strong sense about self-control of panic disorder [80]. A combination of CBT and medication treatment has also been beneficial for TRPD [25, 188, 189, 198–203]. Interpersonal psychotherapy, psychodynamic psychotherapy, eye movement desensitization and reprocessing (EMDR), mindfulness-based therapy, and coping skills and exposure therapy may have also been used in the treatment of panic disorder [199, 204–210].

13.10.2.2 Neuro-stimulation Therapy

Both repetitive trans-cranial magnetic stimulation (r-TMS) and vagus nerve stimulation (VNS) have been reported to have potential therapeutic efficacy in the treatment of anxiety and panic disorder [33, 211–213]. However, available data were insufficient to conclude the efficacy of r-TMS and VNS for panic disorder. Transcranial direct current stimulation (tDCS), which has been used for the treatment of depressive disorder patients, was still rarely investigated in the treatment of panic disorder [212, 214]. The effectiveness of r-TMS, tDCS, and VNS for panic disorder treatment requires future research with adequate sample size and sound methodology.

13.10.2.3 Alternatives Therapy

Because of high comorbidity between depression and panic disorder, some alternative therapies for depression, such as exercise, yoga, light therapy, S-adenosylmethionine, herbal remedy, fish oil supplements, and tryptophan supplements, may have a potential therapeutic efficacy for panic disorder treatment. However, only exercise augmentation has Level 3 support in panic disorder treatment [215, 216]. Acupuncture could have potential efficacy of generalized anxiety disorder treatment, but no research has test the therapeutic effect of acupuncture for panic disorder [216].

Finally, based on the current treatment guidelines of panic disorder, pharmacotherapy or CBT should be the first-line treatment strategy for panic disorder, with a combination of both treatments as the second-line treatment strategy, which may be effective for TRPD. The augmentation treatment with neuro-stimulation therapy or alternative therapy may be considered if the above strategies still failed. Of course, the patients' individual characteristics may be related to the clinical decision-making to select the most favorable treatment option for patients. For example, CBT may be used as first choice for a patient who concerned or cannot withstand the medication's side effects, and pharmacotherapy may be the first-line treatment strategy for patients who have more physical symptoms rather than cognitive symptoms, such as persistent worries for additional panic attacks.

Conclusion

Panic disorder, in its chronic, remitting, relapsing, and treatment-resistant forms, significantly affects individuals' functions and life qualities, resulting in prominent personal, familial, and societal burdens. Treatment-resistant panic disorder was associated with multidimensional factors, including characteristic of panic disorder, comorbidities with physical illnesses and mental diseases, and psychosocial stressors. The prompt and optimal interventions, especially the combination of medication treatment and CBT and the well intervention for psychosocial stresses, could benefit panic disorder sufferers and reduce the risk of chronic morbidity and disability.

References

1. Roy-Byrne PP, Craske MG, Stein MB. Panic disorder. Lancet. 2006;368(9540):1023–32.
2. Klein DF. Panic disorder. Lancet. 1999;353(9149):326–7.
3. Association AP. Diagnostic and statistical manual of mental disorders. 3rd ed. Washington, DC: American Psychiatric Association; 1980. p. 230–2.
4. Asmundson GJ, Taylor S, Smits JA. Panic disorder and agoraphobia: an overview and commentary on DSM-5 changes. Depress Anxiety. 2014;31(6):480–6.
5. Association AP. Diagnostic and statistical manual of mental disorders. 5th ed. Washington, DC: American Psychiatric Association; 2013. p. 119–21.
6. Kessler RC, Berglund P, Demler O, Jin R, Merikangas KR, Walters EE. Lifetime prevalence and age-of-onset distributions of DSM-IV disorders in the National Comorbidity Survey Replication. Arch Gen Psychiatry. 2005;62(6):593–602.
7. Kessler RC, Chiu WT, Demler O, Merikangas KR, Walters EE. Prevalence, severity, and comorbidity of 12-month DSM-IV disorders in the National Comorbidity Survey Replication. Arch Gen Psychiatry. 2005;62(6):617–27.
8. Kessler RC, Chiu WT, Jin R, Ruscio AM, Shear K, Walters EE. The epidemiology of panic attacks, panic disorder, and agoraphobia in the National Comorbidity Survey Replication. Arch Gen Psychiatry. 2006;63(4):415–24.
9. Kessler RC, Greenberg PE, Mickelson KD, Meneades LM, Wang PS. The effects of chronic medical conditions on work loss and work cutback. J Occup Environ Med/Am Coll Occup Environ Med. 2001;43(3):218–25.
10. Whiteford HA, Degenhardt L, Rehm J, Baxter AJ, Ferrari AJ, Erskine HE, et al. Global burden of disease attributable to mental and substance use disorders: findings from the Global Burden of Disease Study 2010. Lancet. 2013;382(9904):1575–86.
11. Lynskey MT, Strang J. The global burden of drug use and mental disorders. Lancet. 2013;382(9904):1540–2.
12. Wang PS, Angermeyer M, Borges G, Bruffaerts R, Tat Chiu W, DE Girolamo G, et al. Delay and failure in treatment seeking after first onset of mental disorders in the World Health Organization's World Mental Health Survey Initiative. World Psychiatry. 2007;6(3):177–85.
13. Wang PS, Berglund P, Olfson M, Pincus HA, Wells KB, Kessler RC. Failure and delay in initial treatment contact after first onset of mental disorders in the National Comorbidity Survey Replication. Arch Gen Psychiatry. 2005;62(6):603–13.
14. Batelaan NM, de Graaf R, Spijker J, Smit JH, van Balkom AJ, Vollebergh WA, et al. The course of panic attacks in individuals with panic disorder and subthreshold panic disorder: a population-based study. J Affect Disord. 2010;121(1–2):30–8.
15. Cowley DS, Flick SN, Roy-Byrne PP. Long-term course and outcome in panic disorder: a naturalistic follow-up study. Anxiety. 1996;2(1):13–21.
16. Hirschfeld RM. Panic disorder: diagnosis, epidemiology, and clinical course. J Clin Psychiatry. 1996;57(Suppl 10):3–8. discussion 9–10
17. Katschnig H, Amering M. The long-term course of panic disorder and its predictors. J Clin Psychopharmacol. 1998;18(6 Suppl 2):6S–11S.
18. Swoboda H, Amering M, Windhaber J, Katschnig H. The long-term course of panic disorder – an 11 year follow-up. J Anxiety Disord. 2003;17(2):223–32.
19. Yonkers KA, Bruce SE, Dyck IR, Keller MB. Chronicity, relapse, and illness – course of panic disorder, social phobia, and generalized anxiety disorder: findings in men and women from 8 years of follow-up. Depress Anxiety. 2003;17(3):173–9.
20. Practice guideline for the treatment of patients with panic disorder. Work group on panic disorder. American Psychiatric Association. Am J Psychiatry. 1998;155(5 Suppl):1–34.

21. Baldwin DS, Anderson IM, Nutt DJ, Allgulander C, Bandelow B, den Boer JA, et al. Evidence-based pharmacological treatment of anxiety disorders, post-traumatic stress disorder and obsessive-compulsive disorder: a revision of the 2005 guidelines from the British Association for Psychopharmacology. J Psychopharmacol. 2014;28(5):403–39.
22. Baldwin DS, Anderson IM, Nutt DJ, Bandelow B, Bond A, Davidson JR, et al. Evidence-based guidelines for the pharmacological treatment of anxiety disorders: recommendations from the British Association for Psychopharmacology. J Psychopharmacol. 2005;19(6):567–96.
23. Bandelow B, Sher L, Bunevicius R, Hollander E, Kasper S, Zohar J, et al. Guidelines for the pharmacological treatment of anxiety disorders, obsessive-compulsive disorder and posttraumatic stress disorder in primary care. Int J Psychiatry Clin Pract. 2012;16(2):77–84.
24. Bandelow B, Zohar J, Hollander E, Kasper S, Moller HJ. World Federation of Societies of Biological Psychiatry (WFSBP) guidelines for the pharmacological treatment of anxiety, obsessive-compulsive and posttraumatic stress disorders. World J Biol Psychiatry. 2002;3(4):171–99.
25. Bandelow B, Zohar J, Hollander E, Kasper S, Moller HJ, Allgulander C, et al. World Federation of Societies of Biological Psychiatry (WFSBP) guidelines for the pharmacological treatment of anxiety, obsessive-compulsive and post-traumatic stress disorders – first revision. World J Biol Psychiatry. 2008;9(4):248–312.
26. Batelaan NM, de Graaf R, Penninx BW, van Balkom AJ, Vollebergh WA, Beekman AT. The 2-year prognosis of panic episodes in the general population. Psychol Med. 2010;40(1):147–57.
27. Wittchen HU, Nocon A, Beesdo K, Pine DS, Hofler M, Lieb R, et al. Agoraphobia and panic. Prospective-longitudinal relations suggest a rethinking of diagnostic concepts. Psychother Psychosom. 2008;77(3):147–57.
28. de Jonge P, Roest AM, Lim CC, Florescu SE, Bromet EJ, Stein DJ, et al. Cross-national epidemiology of panic disorder and panic attacks in the world mental health surveys. Depress Anxiety. 2016;33(12):1155–77.
29. Bruce SE, Yonkers KA, Otto MW, Eisen JL, Weisberg RB, Pagano M, et al. Influence of psychiatric comorbidity on recovery and recurrence in generalized anxiety disorder, social phobia, and panic disorder: a 12-year prospective study. Am J Psychiatry. 2005;162(6):1179–87.
30. Francis JL, Weisberg RB, Dyck IR, Culpepper L, Smith K, Orlando Edelen M, et al. Characteristics and course of panic disorder and panic disorder with agoraphobia in primary care patients. Prim Care Companion J Clin Psychiatry. 2007;9(3):173–9.
31. Katon WJ. Clinical practice. Panic disorder. N Engl J Med. 2006;354(22):2360–7.
32. Ammar G, Naja WJ, Pelissolo A. Treatment-resistant anxiety disorders: a literature review of drug therapy strategies. Encephale. 2015;41(3):260–5.
33. Bystritsky A. Treatment-resistant anxiety disorders. Mol Psychiatry. 2006;11(9):805–14.
34. Menezes GB, Fontenelle LF, Mululo S, Versiani M. Treatment-resistant anxiety disorders: social phobia, generalized anxiety disorder and panic disorder. Rev Bras Psiquiatr. 2007;29(Suppl 2):S55–60.
35. Stein DJ, Seedat S. Unresolved questions about treatment-resistant anxiety disorders. CNS Spectr. 2004;9(10):715.
36. Gaynes BN. Identifying difficult-to-treat depression: differential diagnosis, subtypes, and comorbidities. J Clin Psychiatry. 2009;70(Suppl 6):10–5.
37. Papakostas GI, Ionescu DF. Towards new mechanisms: an update on therapeutics for treatment-resistant major depressive disorder. Mol Psychiatry. 2015;20:1142–50.
38. Souery D, Papakostas GI, Trivedi MH. Treatment-resistant depression. J Clin Psychiatry. 2006;67(Suppl 6):16–22.
39. Gloster AT, Wittchen HU, Einsle F, Lang T, Helbig-Lang S, Fydrich T, et al. Psychological treatment for panic disorder with agoraphobia: a randomized controlled trial to examine the role of therapist-guided exposure in situ in CBT. J Consult Clin Psychol. 2011;79(3):406–20.
40. Reif A, Richter J, Straube B, Hofler M, Lueken U, Gloster AT, et al. MAOA and mechanisms of panic disorder revisited: from bench to molecular psychotherapy. Mol Psychiatry. 2014;19(1):122–8.
41. Furukawa TA, Katherine Shear M, Barlow DH, Gorman JM, Woods SW, Money R, et al. Evidence-based guidelines for interpretation of the Panic Disorder Severity Scale. Depress Anxiety. 2009;26(10):922–9.
42. Payne LA, White KS, Gallagher MW, Woods SW, Shear MK, Gorman JM, et al. Second-stage treatments for relative nonresponders to cognitive behavioral therapy (Cbt) for panic disorder with or without agoraphobia-continued Cbt versus Ssri: a randomized controlled trial. Depress Anxiety. 2016;33(5):392–9.
43. Ballenger JC. Clinical guidelines for establishing remission in patients with depression and anxiety. J Clin Psychiatry. 1999;60(Suppl 22):29–34.
44. Ballenger JC. Treatment of anxiety disorders to remission. J Clin Psychiatry. 2001;62(Suppl 12):5–9.
45. Ballenger JC, Davidson JR, Lecrubier Y, Nutt DJ, Baldwin DS, den Boer JA, et al. Consensus statement on panic disorder from the International Consensus Group on Depression and Anxiety. J Clin Psychiatry. 1998;59(Suppl 8):47–54.
46. Doyle AC, Pollack MH. Establishment of remission criteria for anxiety disorders. J Clin Psychiatry. 2003;64(Suppl 15):40–5.
47. Bandelow B. Defining response and remission in anxiety disorders: toward an integrated approach. CNS Spectr. 2006;11(10 Suppl 12):21–8.

48. Bandelow B, Baldwin DS, Dolberg OT, Andersen HF, Stein DJ. What is the threshold for symptomatic response and remission for major depressive disorder, panic disorder, social anxiety disorder, and generalized anxiety disorder? J Clin Psychiatry. 2006;67(9):1428–34.
49. Brown C, Schulberg HC, Madonia MJ, Shear MK, Houck PR. Treatment outcomes for primary care patients with major depression and lifetime anxiety disorders. Am J Psychiatry. 1996;153(10):1293–300.
50. Ginsburg GS, Kendall PC, Sakolsky D, Compton SN, Piacentini J, Albano AM, et al. Remission after acute treatment in children and adolescents with anxiety disorders: findings from the CAMS. J Consult Clin Psychol. 2011;79(6):806–13.
51. Ramsawh HJ, Weisberg RB, Dyck I, Stout R, Keller MB. Age of onset, clinical characteristics, and 15-year course of anxiety disorders in a prospective, longitudinal, observational study. J Affect Disord. 2011;132(1–2):260–4.
52. Sibrava NJ, Beard C, Bjornsson AS, Moitra E, Weisberg RB, Keller MB. Two-year course of generalized anxiety disorder, social anxiety disorder, and panic disorder in a longitudinal sample of African American adults. J Consult Clin Psychol. 2013;81(6):1052–62.
53. Kelly JM, Jakubovski E, Bloch MH. Prognostic subgroups for remission and response in the Coordinated Anxiety Learning and Management (CALM) trial. J Clin Psychiatry. 2015;76(3):267–78.
54. Dow MG, Kenardy JA, Johnston DW, Newman MG, Taylor CB, Thomson A. Prognostic indices with brief and standard CBT for panic disorder: I. Predictors of outcome. Psychol Med. 2007;37(10):1493–502.
55. Song HM, Kim JH, Heo JY, Yu BH. Clinical characteristics of the respiratory subtype in panic disorder patients. Psychiatry Investig. 2014;11(4):412–8.
56. Roberson-Nay R, Kendler KS. Panic disorder and its subtypes: a comprehensive analysis of panic symptom heterogeneity using epidemiological and treatment seeking samples. Psychol Med. 2011;41(11):2411–21.
57. Chen J, Tsuchiya M, Kawakami N, Furukawa TA. Non-fearful vs. fearful panic attacks: a general population study from the National Comorbidity Survey. J Affect Disord. 2009;112(1–3):273–8.
58. Goodwin RD, Hamilton SP. The early-onset fearful panic attack as a predictor of severe psychopathology. Psychiatry Res. 2002;109(1):71–9.
59. Nakamura M, Sugiura T, Nishida S, Komada Y, Inoue Y. Is nocturnal panic a distinct disease category? Comparison of clinical characteristics among patients with primary nocturnal panic, daytime panic, and coexistence of nocturnal and daytime panic. J Clin Sleep Med. 2013;9(5):461–7.
60. Craske MG, Tsao JC. Assessment and treatment of nocturnal panic attacks. Sleep Med Rev. 2005;9(3):173–84.
61. Beidas RS, Suarez L, Simpson D, Read K, Wei C, Connolly S, et al. Contextual factors and anxiety in minority and European American youth presenting for treatment across two urban university clinics. J Anxiety Disord. 2012;26(4):544–54.
62. Clayton AH, Stewart RS, Fayyad R, Clary CM. Sex differences in clinical presentation and response in panic disorder: pooled data from sertraline treatment studies. Arch Womens Ment Health. 2006;9(3):151–7.
63. Safren SA, Gonzalez RE, Horner KJ, Leung AW, Heimberg RG, Juster HR. Anxiety in ethnic minority youth. Methodological and conceptual issues and review of the literature. Behav Modif. 2000;24(2):147–83.
64. Nay W, Brown R, Roberson-Nay R. Longitudinal course of panic disorder with and without agoraphobia using the National Epidemiologic Survey on Alcohol and Related Conditions (NESARC). Psychiatry Res. 2013;208(1):54–61.
65. Wetherell JL, Petkus AJ, Thorp SR, Stein MB, Chavira DA, Campbell-Sills L, et al. Age differences in treatment response to a collaborative care intervention for anxiety disorders. Br J Psychiatry. 2013;203(1):65–72.
66. Biederman J, Faraone SV, Hirshfeld-Becker DR, Friedman D, Robin JA, Rosenbaum JF. Patterns of psychopathology and dysfunction in high-risk children of parents with panic disorder and major depression. Am J Psychiatry. 2001;158(1):49–57.
67. Biederman J, Rosenbaum JF, Bolduc EA, Faraone SV, Hirshfeld DR. A high risk study of young children of parents with panic disorder and agoraphobia with and without comorbid major depression. Psychiatry Res. 1991;37(3):333–48.
68. Hirshfeld-Becker DR, Biederman J, Henin A, Faraone SV, Dowd ST, De Petrillo LA, et al. Psychopathology in the young offspring of parents with bipolar disorder: a controlled pilot study. Psychiatry Res. 2006;145(2–3):155–67.
69. Pilowsky DJ, Wickramaratne PJ, Rush AJ, Hughes CW, Garber J, Malloy E, et al. Children of currently depressed mothers: a STAR*D ancillary study. J Clin Psychiatry. 2006;67(1):126–36.
70. Dow MG, Kenardy JA, Johnston DW, Newman MG, Taylor CB, Thomson A. Prognostic indices with brief and standard CBT for panic disorder: II. Moderators of outcome. Psychol Med. 2007;37(10):1503–9.
71. Weck F, Grikscheit F, Hofling V, Kordt A, Hamm AO, Gerlach AL, et al. The role of treatment delivery factors in exposure-based cognitive behavioral therapy for panic disorder with agoraphobia. J Anxiety Disord. 2016;42:10–8.
72. Huppert JD, Kivity Y, Barlow DH, Gorman JM, Shear MK, Woods SW. Therapist effects and the outcome-alliance correlation in cognitive behavioral therapy for panic disorder with agoraphobia. Behav Res Ther. 2014;52:26–34.
73. Zickgraf HF, Chambless DL, McCarthy KS, Gallop R, Sharpless BA, Milrod BL, et al. Interpersonal factors are associated with lower therapist adherence in cognitive-behavioural therapy for panic disorder. Clin Psychol Psychother. 2016;23(3):272–84.

74. Carrera M, Herran A, Ramirez ML, Ayestaran A, Sierra-Biddle D, Hoyuela F, et al. Personality traits in early phases of panic disorder: implications on the presence of agoraphobia, clinical severity and short-term outcome. Acta Psychiatr Scand. 2006;114(6):417–25.
75. Vohma U, Raag M, Toru I, Aluoja A, Maron E. Association between personality traits and escitalopram treatment efficacy in panic disorder. Nord J Psychiatry. 2017;71(6):433–40.
76. Marchesi C, De Panfilis C, Cantoni A, Fonto S, Giannelli MR, Maggini C. Personality disorders and response to medication treatment in panic disorder: a 1-year naturalistic study. Prog Neuro-Psychopharmacol Biol Psychiatry. 2006;30(7):1240–5.
77. Haug T, Nordgreen T, Ost LG, Tangen T, Kvale G, Hovland OJ, et al. Working alliance and competence as predictors of outcome in cognitive behavioral therapy for social anxiety and panic disorder in adults. Behav Res Ther. 2016;77:40–51.
78. Marchesi C, Cantoni A, Fonto S, Giannelli MR, Maggini C. The effect of temperament and character on response to selective serotonin reuptake inhibitors in panic disorder. Acta Psychiatr Scand. 2006;114(3):203–10.
79. Wachleski C, Salum GA, Blaya C, Kipper L, Paludo A, Salgado AP, et al. Harm avoidance and self-directedness as essential features of panic disorder patients. Compr Psychiatry. 2008;49(5):476–81.
80. Dusseldorp E, Spinhoven P, Bakker A, van Dyck R, van Balkom AJ. Which panic disorder patients benefit from which treatment: cognitive therapy or antidepressants? Psychother Psychosom. 2007;76(3):154–61.
81. Hazen AL, Walker JR, Eldridge GD. Anxiety sensitivity and treatment outcome in panic disorder. Anxiety. 1996;2(1):34–9.
82. Ino K, Ogawa S, Kondo M, Imai R, Ii T, Furukawa TA, et al. Anxiety sensitivity as a predictor of broad dimensions of psychopathology after cognitive behavioral therapy for panic disorder. Neuropsychiatr Dis Treat. 2017;13:1835–40.
83. McNally RJ. Anxiety sensitivity and panic disorder. Biol Psychiatry. 2002;52(10):938–46.
84. Park HJ, Kim EJ, Ku JI, Woo JM, Lee SH, Chung SK, et al. Psychological characteristics of early remitters in patients with panic disorder. Psychiatry Res. 2012;197(3):237–41.
85. Plehn K, Peterson RA. Anxiety sensitivity as a predictor of the development of panic symptoms, panic attacks, and panic disorder: a prospective study. J Anxiety Disord. 2002;16(4):455–74.
86. Poletti S, Radaelli D, Cucchi M, Ricci L, Vai B, Smeraldi E, et al. Neural correlates of anxiety sensitivity in panic disorder: a functional magnetic resonance imaging study. Psychiatry Res. 2015;233(2):95–101.
87. Lecrubier Y. The impact of comorbidity on the treatment of panic disorder. J Clin Psychiatry. 1998;59(Suppl 8):11–4. discussion 5–6
88. Skodol AE, Geier T, Grant BF, Hasin DS. Personality disorders and the persistence of anxiety disorders in a nationally representative sample. Depress Anxiety. 2014;31(9):721–8.
89. Batelaan NM, ten Have M, van Balkom AJ, Tuithof M, de Graaf R. Anxiety disorders and onset of cardiovascular disease: the differential impact of panic, phobias and worry. J Anxiety Disord. 2014;28(2):252–8.
90. Carr RE. Panic disorder and asthma: causes, effects and research implications. J Psychosom Res. 1998;44(1):43–52.
91. Chen YH, Lin HC. Patterns of psychiatric and physical comorbidities associated with panic disorder in a nationwide population-based study in Taiwan. Acta Psychiatr Scand. 2011;123(1):55–61.
92. Player MS, Peterson LE. Anxiety disorders, hypertension, and cardiovascular risk: a review. Int J Psychiatry Med. 2011;41(4):365–77.
93. Smitherman TA, Kolivas ED, Bailey JR. Panic disorder and migraine: comorbidity, mechanisms, and clinical implications. Headache. 2013;53(1):23–45.
94. Roy-Byrne P, Stein MB, Russo J, Craske M, Katon W, Sullivan G, et al. Medical illness and response to treatment in primary care panic disorder. Gen Hosp Psychiatry. 2005;27(4):237–43.
95. Goodwin RD. Self-reported hay fever and panic attacks in the community. Ann Allergy Asthma Immunol. 2002;88(6):556–9.
96. Smoller JW, Pollack MH, Wassertheil-Smoller S, Jackson RD, Oberman A, Wong ND, et al. Panic attacks and risk of incident cardiovascular events among postmenopausal women in the Women's Health Initiative Observational Study. Arch Gen Psychiatry. 2007;64(10):1153–60.
97. Meuret AE, Kroll J, Ritz T. Panic disorder comorbidity with medical conditions and treatment implications. Annu Rev Clin Psychol. 2017;13:209–40.
98. Chou PH, Lin CH, Loh el W, Chan CH, Lan TH. Panic disorder and risk of stroke: a population-based study. Psychosomatics. 2012;53(5):463–9.
99. Tully PJ, Turnbull DA, Beltrame J, Horowitz J, Cosh S, Baumeister H, et al. Panic disorder and incident coronary heart disease: a systematic review and meta-regression in 1131612 persons and 58111 cardiac events. Psychol Med. 2015;45(14):2909–20.
100. Weissman MM, Markowitz JS, Ouellette R, Greenwald S, Kahn JP. Panic disorder and cardiovascular/cerebrovascular problems: results from a community survey. Am J Psychiatry. 1990;147(11):1504–8.
101. Claudia P, Andrea C, Chiara C, Stefano L, Giuseppe M, Vincenzo DL, et al. Panic disorder in menopause: a case control study. Maturitas. 2004;48(2):147–54.
102. Bandelow B, Sojka F, Broocks A, Hajak G, Bleich S, Ruther E. Panic disorder during pregnancy and postpartum period. Eur Psychiatry. 2006;21(7):495–500.
103. Northcott CJ, Stein MB. Panic disorder in pregnancy. J Clin Psychiatry. 1994;55(12):539–42.

104. Flint AJ, Gagnon N. Diagnosis and management of panic disorder in older patients. Drugs Aging. 2003;20(12):881–91.
105. Kukoyi O, Argo TR, Carnahan RM. Exacerbation of panic disorder with rifampin therapy in a patient receiving citalopram. Pharmacotherapy. 2005;25(3):435–7.
106. Sansone RA, Sansone LA. Exacerbation of panic disorder symptoms following Vicodin exposure. Gen Hosp Psychiatry. 2002;24(6):448–9.
107. Zealberg JJ, Lydiard RB, Christie S. Exacerbation of panic disorder in a woman treated with trimethoprim-sulfamethoxazole. J Clin Psychopharmacol. 1991;11(2):144–5.
108. Farber GA, Levin T, White CA. A cognitive therapy conceptualization of panic disorder exacerbated by interferon treatment. Gen Hosp Psychiatry. 2005;27(5):329–37.
109. Abadie D, Essilini A, Fulda V, Gouraud A, Yelehe-Okouma M, Micallef J, et al. Drug-induced panic attacks: analysis of cases registered in the French pharmacovigilance database. J Psychiatr Res. 2017;90:60–6.
110. Barrera TL, Graham DP, Dunn NJ, Teng EJ. Influence of trauma history on panic and posttraumatic stress disorder in returning veterans. Psychol Serv. 2013;10(2):168–76.
111. Liebowitz MR. Panic disorder as a chronic illness. J Clin Psychiatry. 1997;58(Suppl 13):5–8.
112. Moreno-Peral P, Conejo-Ceron S, Motrico E, Rodriguez-Morejon A, Fernandez A, Garcia-Campayo J, et al. Risk factors for the onset of panic and generalised anxiety disorders in the general adult population: a systematic review of cohort studies. J Affect Disord. 2014;168:337–48.
113. Pollack MH. Long-term management of panic disorder. J Clin Psychiatry. 1990;51(Suppl):11–3. discussion 50–3
114. Pollack MH, Allgulander C, Bandelow B, Cassano GB, Greist JH, Hollander E, et al. WCA recommendations for the long-term treatment of panic disorder. CNS Spectr. 2003;8(8 Suppl 1):17–30.
115. Scheibe G, Albus M. Predictors and outcome in panic disorder: a 2-year prospective follow-up study. Psychopathology. 1997;30(3):177–84.
116. Roy-Byrne P, Sherbourne C, Miranda J, Stein M, Craske M, Golinelli D, et al. Poverty and response to treatment among panic disorder patients in primary care. Am J Psychiatry. 2006;163(8):1419–25.
117. Roy-Byrne PP, Russo J, Cowley DS, Katon WJ. Unemployment and emergency room visits predict poor treatment outcome in primary care panic disorder. J Clin Psychiatry. 2003;64(4):383–9.
118. Asselmann E, Stender J, Grabe HJ, Konig J, Schmidt CO, Hamm AO, et al. Assessing the interplay of childhood adversities with more recent stressful life events and conditions in predicting panic pathology among adults from the general population. J Affect Disord. 2017;225:715–22.
119. Cannon DM, Klaver JM, Klug SA, Carlson PJ, Luckenbaugh DA, Ichise M, et al. Gender-specific abnormalities in the serotonin transporter system in panic disorder. Int J Neuropsychopharmacol. 2013;16(4):733–43.
120. Jacob C, Domschke K, Gajewska A, Warrings B, Deckert J. Genetics of panic disorder: focus on association studies and therapeutic perspectives. Expert Rev Neurother. 2010;10(8):1273–84.
121. Lueken U, Straube B, Wittchen HU, Konrad C, Strohle A, Wittmann A, et al. Therapygenetics: anterior cingulate cortex-amygdala coupling is associated with 5-HTTLPR and treatment response in panic disorder with agoraphobia. J Neural Transm. 2015;122(1):135–44.
122. Reif A, Weber H, Domschke K, Klauke B, Baumann C, Jacob CP, et al. Meta-analysis argues for a female-specific role of MAOA-uVNTR in panic disorder in four European populations. Am J Med Genet Part B, Neuropsychiatr Genet. 2012;159B(7):786–93.
123. Saeki Y, Watanabe T, Ueda M, Saito A, Akiyama K, Inoue Y, et al. Genetic and pharmacokinetic factors affecting the initial pharmacotherapeutic effect of paroxetine in Japanese patients with panic disorder. Eur J Clin Pharmacol. 2009;65(7):685–91.
124. Yevtushenko OO, Oros MM, Reynolds GP. Early response to selective serotonin reuptake inhibitors in panic disorder is associated with a functional 5-HT1A receptor gene polymorphism. J Affect Disord. 2010;123(1–3):308–11.
125. Domschke K, Braun M, Ohrmann P, Suslow T, Kugel H, Bauer J, et al. Association of the functional -1019C/G 5-HT1A polymorphism with prefrontal cortex and amygdala activation measured with 3 T fMRI in panic disorder. Int J Neuropsychopharmacol. 2006;9(3):349–55.
126. Domschke K, Ohrmann P, Braun M, Suslow T, Bauer J, Hohoff C, et al. Influence of the catechol-O-methyltransferase val158met genotype on amygdala and prefrontal cortex emotional processing in panic disorder. Psychiatry Res. 2008;163(1):13–20.
127. Greenblatt DJ, von Moltke LL, Harmatz JS, Ciraulo DA, Shader RI. Alprazolam pharmacokinetics, metabolism, and plasma levels: clinical implications. J Clin Psychiatry. 1993;54(Suppl):4–11. discussion 2–4
128. He Q, Yuan Z, Liu Y, Zhang J, Yan H, Shen L, et al. Correlation between cytochrome P450 2C19 genetic polymorphism and treatment response to escitalopram in panic disorder. Pharmacogenet Genomics. 2017;27(8):279–84.
129. Fonzo GA, Ramsawh HJ, Flagan TM, Sullivan SG, Letamendi A, Simmons AN, et al. Common and disorder-specific neural responses to emotional faces in generalised anxiety, social anxiety and panic disorders. Br J Psychiatry: J Ment Sci. 2015;206(3):206–15.
130. Hahn T, Kircher T, Straube B, Wittchen HU, Konrad C, Strohle A, et al. Predicting treatment response to

cognitive behavioral therapy in panic disorder with agoraphobia by integrating local neural information. JAMA Psychiat. 2015;72(1):68–74.
131. Holtz K, Pane-Farre CA, Wendt J, Lotze M, Hamm AO. Brain activation during anticipation of interoceptive threat. NeuroImage. 2012;61(4):857–65.
132. Mechias ML, Etkin A, Kalisch R. A meta-analysis of instructed fear studies: implications for conscious appraisal of threat. NeuroImage. 2010;49(2):1760–8.
133. Reinecke A, Thilo K, Filippini N, Croft A, Harmer CJ. Predicting rapid response to cognitive-behavioural treatment for panic disorder: the role of hippocampus, insula, and dorsolateral prefrontal cortex. Behav Res Ther. 2014;62:120–8.
134. De Cort K, Schroijen M, Hurlemann R, Claassen S, Hoogenhout J, Van den Bergh O, et al. Modeling the development of panic disorder with interoceptive conditioning. Eur Neuropsychopharmacol. 2017;27(1):59–69.
135. de Carvalho MR, Dias GP, Cosci F, de-Melo-Neto VL, Bevilaqua MC, Gardino PF, et al. Current findings of fMRI in panic disorder: contributions for the fear neurocircuitry and CBT effects. Expert Rev Neurother. 2010;10(2):291–303.
136. de Carvalho MR, Rozenthal M, Nardi AE. The fear circuitry in panic disorder and its modulation by cognitive-behaviour therapy interventions. World J Biol Psychiatry. 2010;11(2 Pt 2):188–98.
137. Lueken U, Straube B, Konrad C, Wittchen HU, Strohle A, Wittmann A, et al. Neural substrates of treatment response to cognitive-behavioral therapy in panic disorder with agoraphobia. Am J Psychiatry. 2013;170(11):1345–55.
138. Melzig CA, Michalowski JM, Holtz K, Hamm AO. Anticipation of interoceptive threat in highly anxiety sensitive persons. Behav Res Ther. 2008;46(10):1126–34.
139. Asami T, Hayano F, Nakamura M, Yamasue H, Uehara K, Otsuka T, et al. Anterior cingulate cortex volume reduction in patients with panic disorder. Psychiatry Clin Neurosci. 2008;62(3):322–30.
140. Uchida RR, Del-Ben CM, Busatto GF, Duran FL, Guimaraes FS, Crippa JA, et al. Regional gray matter abnormalities in panic disorder: a voxel-based morphometry study. Psychiatry Res. 2008;163(1):21–9.
141. Abelson JL, Curtis GC. Hypothalamic-pituitary-adrenal axis activity in panic disorder. 24-hour secretion of corticotropin and cortisol. Arch Gen Psychiatry. 1996;53(4):323–31.
142. Abelson JL, Khan S, Liberzon I, Young EA. HPA axis activity in patients with panic disorder: review and synthesis of four studies. Depress Anxiety. 2007;24(1):66–76.
143. de Oliveira AR, Reimer AE, Reis FM, Brandao ML. Conditioned fear response is modulated by a combined action of the hypothalamic-pituitary-adrenal axis and dopamine activity in the basolateral amygdala. Eur Neuropsychopharmacol. 2013;23(5):379–89.
144. Herman JP, McKlveen JM, Solomon MB, Carvalho-Netto E, Myers B. Neural regulation of the stress response: glucocorticoid feedback mechanisms. Braz J Med Biol Res. 2012;45(4):292–8.
145. Ising M, Hohne N, Siebertz A, Parchmann AM, Erhardt A, Keck M. Stress response regulation in panic disorder. Curr Pharm Des. 2012;18(35):5675–84.
146. Petrowski K, Wintermann GB, Kirschbaum C, Bornstein SR. Dissociation between ACTH and cortisol response in DEX-CRH test in patients with panic disorder. Psychoneuroendocrinology. 2012;37(8):1199–208.
147. Jovanovic T, Phifer JE, Sicking K, Weiss T, Norrholm SD, Bradley B, et al. Cortisol suppression by dexamethasone reduces exaggerated fear responses in posttraumatic stress disorder. Psychoneuroendocrinology. 2011;36(10):1540–52.
148. Michopoulos V, Norrholm SD, Stevens JS, Glover EM, Rothbaum BO, Gillespie CF, et al. Dexamethasone facilitates fear extinction and safety discrimination in PTSD: a placebo-controlled, double-blind study. Psychoneuroendocrinology. 2017;83:65–71.
149. Leyton M, Belanger C, Martial J, Beaulieu S, Corin E, Pecknold J, et al. Cardiovascular, neuroendocrine, and monoaminergic responses to psychological stressors: possible differences between remitted panic disorder patients and healthy controls. Biol Psychiatry. 1996;40(5):353–60.
150. Wichmann S, Kirschbaum C, Bohme C, Petrowski K. Cortisol stress response in post-traumatic stress disorder, panic disorder, and major depressive disorder patients. Psychoneuroendocrinology. 2017;83:135–41.
151. Coryell W, Noyes R Jr, Reich J. The prognostic significance of HPA-axis disturbance in panic disorder: a three-year follow-up. Biol Psychiatry. 1991;29(2):96–102.
152. Abelson JL, Curtis GC. Hypothalamic-pituitary-adrenal axis activity in panic disorder: prediction of long-term outcome by pretreatment cortisol levels. Am J Psychiatry. 1996;153(1):69–73.
153. Abelson JL, Liberzon I, Young EA, Khan S. Cognitive modulation of the endocrine stress response to a pharmacological challenge in normal and panic disorder subjects. Arch Gen Psychiatry. 2005;62(6):668–75.
154. Shlik J, Aluoja A, Vasar V, Vasar E, Podar T, Bradwejn J. Effects of citalopram treatment on behavioural, cardiovascular and neuroendocrine response to cholecystokinin tetrapeptide challenge in patients with panic disorder. J Psychiatry Neurosci. 1997;22(5):332–40.
155. Monfils MH, Cowansage KK, LeDoux JE. Brain-derived neurotrophic factor: linking fear learning to memory consolidation. Mol Pharmacol. 2007;72(2):235–7.
156. Ou LC, Yeh SH, Gean PW. Late expression of brain-derived neurotrophic factor in the amygdala is

required for persistence of fear memory. Neurobiol Learn Mem. 2010;93(3):372–82.
157. Rattiner LM, Davis M, French CT, Ressler KJ. Brain-derived neurotrophic factor and tyrosine kinase receptor B involvement in amygdala-dependent fear conditioning. J Neurosci. 2004;24(20):4796–806.
158. Yamada K, Nabeshima T. Brain-derived neurotrophic factor/TrkB signaling in memory processes. J Pharmacol Sci. 2003;91(4):267–70.
159. Kobayashi K, Shimizu E, Hashimoto K, Mitsumori M, Koike K, Okamura N, et al. Serum brain-derived neurotrophic factor (BDNF) levels in patients with panic disorder: as a biological predictor of response to group cognitive behavioral therapy. Prog Neuro-Psychopharmacol Biol Psychiatry. 2005;29(5):658–63.
160. Han EJ, Kim YK, Hwang JA, Kim SH, Lee HJ, Yoon HK, et al. Evidence for association between the brain-derived neurotrophic factor gene and panic disorder: a novel haplotype analysis. Psychiatry Investig. 2015;12(1):112–7.
161. Suliman S, Hemmings SM, Seedat S. Brain-Derived Neurotrophic Factor (BDNF) protein levels in anxiety disorders: systematic review and meta-regression analysis. Front Integr Neurosci. 2013;7:55.
162. Chen K, Wang N, Zhang J, Hong X, Xu H, Zhao X, et al. Is the Val66Met polymorphism of the brain-derived neurotrophic factor gene associated with panic disorder? A meta-analysis. Asia Pac Psychiatry. 2017;9(2). https://doi.org/10.1111/appy.12228. Epub 2015 Dec 21.
163. Lam P, Cheng CY, Hong CJ, Tsai SJ. Association study of a brain-derived neurotrophic factor (Val66Met) genetic polymorphism and panic disorder. Neuropsychobiology. 2004;49(4):178–81.
164. Casarotto PC, de Bortoli VC, Correa FM, Resstel LB, Zangrossi H Jr. Panicolytic-like effect of BDNF in the rat dorsal periaqueductal grey matter: the role of 5-HT and GABA. Int J Neuropsychopharmacol. 2010;13(5):573–82.
165. Casarotto PC, Santos PC, Lucas GA, Biojone C, Pobbe RL, Vilela-Costa HH, et al. BDNF-TRKB signaling system of the dorsal periaqueductal gray matter is implicated in the panicolytic-like effect of antidepressant drugs. Eur Neuropsychopharmacol. 2015;25(6):913–22.
166. Strohle A, Stoy M, Graetz B, Scheel M, Wittmann A, Gallinat J, et al. Acute exercise ameliorates reduced brain-derived neurotrophic factor in patients with panic disorder. Psychoneuroendocrinology. 2010;35(3):364–8.
167. Candore G, Caruso C, Jirillo E, Magrone T, Vasto S. Low grade inflammation as a common pathogenetic denominator in age-related diseases: novel drug targets for anti-ageing strategies and successful ageing achievement. Curr Pharm Des. 2010;16(6):584–96.
168. Esser N, Legrand-Poels S, Piette J, Scheen AJ, Paquot N. Inflammation as a link between obesity, metabolic syndrome and type 2 diabetes. Diabetes Res Clin Pract. 2014;105(2):141–50.
169. Rana JS, Nieuwdorp M, Jukema JW, Kastelein JJ. Cardiovascular metabolic syndrome – an interplay of, obesity, inflammation, diabetes and coronary heart disease. Diabetes Obes Metab. 2007;9(3):218–32.
170. Rohleder N. Acute and chronic stress induced changes in sensitivity of peripheral inflammatory pathways to the signals of multiple stress systems – 2011 Curt Richter Award Winner. Psychoneuroendocrinology. 2012;37(3):307–16.
171. Rohleder N. Stimulation of systemic low-grade inflammation by psychosocial stress. Psychosom Med. 2014;76(3):181–9.
172. Michopoulos V, Powers A, Gillespie CF, Ressler KJ, Jovanovic T. Inflammation in fear- and anxiety-based disorders: PTSD, GAD, and beyond. Neuropsychopharmacology. 2017;42(1):254–70.
173. Vogelzangs N, Beekman AT, de Jonge P, Penninx BW. Anxiety disorders and inflammation in a large adult cohort. Transl Psychiatry. 2013;3:e249.
174. Tsigos C, Chrousos GP. Hypothalamic-pituitary-adrenal axis, neuroendocrine factors and stress. J Psychosom Res. 2002;53(4):865–71.
175. Hoge EA, Brandstetter K, Moshier S, Pollack MH, Wong KK, Simon NM. Broad spectrum of cytokine abnormalities in panic disorder and posttraumatic stress disorder. Depress Anxiety. 2009;26(5):447–55.
176. Belem da Silva CT, Costa MA, Bortoluzzi A, Pfaffenseller B, Vedana F, Kapczinski F, et al. Cytokine levels in panic disorder: evidence for a dose-response relationship. Psychosom Med. 2017;79(2):126–32.
177. Duivis HE, Vogelzangs N, Kupper N, de Jonge P, Penninx BW. Differential association of somatic and cognitive symptoms of depression and anxiety with inflammation: findings from the Netherlands Study of Depression and Anxiety (NESDA). Psychoneuroendocrinology. 2013;38(9):1573–85.
178. Koh KB, Lee Y. Reduced anxiety level by therapeutic interventions and cell-mediated immunity in panic disorder patients. Psychother Psychosom. 2004;73(5):286–92.
179. Freire RC, Machado S, Arias-Carrion O, Nardi AE. Current pharmacological interventions in panic disorder. CNS Neurol Disord Drug Targets. 2014;13(6):1057–65.
180. Gao K, Muzina D, Gajwani P, Calabrese JR. Efficacy of typical and atypical antipsychotics for primary and comorbid anxiety symptoms or disorders: a review. J Clin Psychiatry. 2006;67(9):1327–40.
181. Nardi AE, Machado S, Almada LF, Paes F, Silva AC, Marques RJ, et al. Clonazepam for the treatment of panic disorder. Curr Drug Targets. 2013;14(3):353–64.
182. Offidani E, Guidi J, Tomba E, Fava GA. Efficacy and tolerability of benzodiazepines versus antidepressants in anxiety disorders: a systematic review and meta-analysis. Psychother Psychosom. 2013;82(6):355–62.

183. Ravindran LN, Stein MB. The pharmacologic treatment of anxiety disorders: a review of progress. J Clin Psychiatry. 2010;71(7):839–54.
184. Wang HR, Woo YS, Bahk WM. The potential role of atypical antipsychotics in the treatment of panic disorder. Hum Psychopharmacol. 2014;29(5):405–13.
185. Apter JT, Allen LA. Buspirone: future directions. J Clin Psychopharmacol. 1999;19(1):86–93.
186. Imai H, Tajika A, Chen P, Pompoli A, Guaiana G, Castellazzi M, et al. Azapirones versus placebo for panic disorder in adults. Cochrane Database Syst Rev. 2014;(9):CD010828. https://doi.org/10.1002/14651858.CD010828.pub2.
187. Patterson B, Van Ameringen M. Augmentation strategies for treatment-resistant anxiety disorders: a systematic review and meta-analysis. Depress Anxiety. 2016;33(8):728–36.
188. Simon NM, Otto MW, Worthington JJ, Hoge EA, Thompson EH, Lebeau RT, et al. Next-step strategies for panic disorder refractory to initial pharmacotherapy: a 3-phase randomized clinical trial. J Clin Psychiatry. 2009;70(11):1563–70.
189. Zamorski MA, Albucher RC. What to do when SSRIs fail: eight strategies for optimizing treatment of panic disorder. Am Fam Physician. 2002;66(8):1477–84.
190. Murrough JW, Yaqubi S, Sayed S, Charney DS. Emerging drugs for the treatment of anxiety. Expert Opin Emerg Drugs. 2015:1–14.
191. Perna G, Guerriero G, Caldirola D. Emerging drugs for panic disorder. Expert Opin Emerg Drugs. 2011;16(4):631–45.
192. Perna G, Schruers K, Alciati A, Caldirola D. Novel investigational therapeutics for panic disorder. Expert Opin Investig Drugs. 2015;24(4):491–505.
193. Hellbom E, Humble M. Panic disorder treated with the antihistamine chlorpheniramine. Ann Allergy Asthma Immunol. 2003;90(3):361. author reply -2
194. Sansone RA, Sears CD. The successful use of meclizine in panic disorder. J Clin Psychiatry. 2004;65(9):1285–6.
195. Mataix-Cols D, Fernandez de la Cruz L, Monzani B, Rosenfield D, Andersson E, Perez-Vigil A, et al. D-Cycloserine augmentation of exposure-based cognitive behavior therapy for anxiety, obsessive-compulsive, and posttraumatic stress disorders: a systematic review and meta-analysis of individual participant data. JAMA Psychiat. 2017;74(5):501–10.
196. Ray SM, Kious BM. Sustained resolution of panic disorder, agoraphobia, and generalized anxiety disorder with a single ketamine infusion: a case report. Prim Care Companion CNS Disord. 2016;18(4).
197. Dobrovolsky A, Ichim TE, Ma D, Kesari S, Bogin V. Xenon in the treatment of panic disorder: an open label study. J Transl Med. 2017;15(1):137.
198. McHugh RK, Smits JA, Otto MW. Empirically supported treatments for panic disorder. Psychiatr Clin North Am. 2009;32(3):593–610.
199. Ougrin D. Efficacy of exposure versus cognitive therapy in anxiety disorders: systematic review and meta-analysis. BMC Psychiatry. 2011;11:200.
200. Rodrigues H, Figueira I, Goncalves R, Mendlowicz M, Macedo T, Ventura P. CBT for pharmacotherapy non-remitters – a systematic review of a next-step strategy. J Affect Disord. 2011;129(1–3):219–28.
201. Roshanaei-Moghaddam B, Pauly MC, Atkins DC, Baldwin SA, Stein MB, Roy-Byrne P. Relative effects of CBT and pharmacotherapy in depression versus anxiety: is medication somewhat better for depression, and CBT somewhat better for anxiety? Depress Anxiety. 2011;28(7):560–7.
202. Wang Z, Whiteside SPH, Sim L, Farah W, Morrow AS, Alsawas M, et al. Comparative effectiveness and safety of cognitive behavioral therapy and pharmacotherapy for childhood anxiety disorders: a systematic review and meta-analysis. JAMA Pediatr. 2017;171:1049–56.
203. Campbell-Sills L, Roy-Byrne PP, Craske MG, Bystritsky A, Sullivan G, Stein MB. Improving outcomes for patients with medication-resistant anxiety: effects of collaborative care with cognitive behavioral therapy. Depress Anxiety. 2016;33(12):1099–106.
204. Markowitz JC, Lipsitz J, Milrod BL. Critical review of outcome research on interpersonal psychotherapy for anxiety disorders. Depress Anxiety. 2014;31(4):316–25.
205. Meuret AE, Wolitzky-Taylor KB, Twohig MP, Craske MG. Coping skills and exposure therapy in panic disorder and agoraphobia: latest advances and future directions. Behav Ther. 2012;43(2):271–84.
206. Kim B, Lee SH, Kim YW, Choi TK, Yook K, Suh SY, et al. Effectiveness of a mindfulness-based cognitive therapy program as an adjunct to pharmacotherapy in patients with panic disorder. J Anxiety Disord. 2010;24(6):590–5.
207. Kim YW, Lee SH, Choi TK, Suh SY, Kim B, Kim CM, et al. Effectiveness of mindfulness-based cognitive therapy as an adjuvant to pharmacotherapy in patients with panic disorder or generalized anxiety disorder. Depress Anxiety. 2009;26(7):601–6.
208. Horst F, Den Oudsten B, Zijlstra W, de Jongh A, Lobbestael J, De Vries J. Cognitive behavioral therapy vs. eye movement desensitization and reprocessing for treating panic disorder: a randomized controlled trial. Front Psychol. 2017;8:1409.
209. Pompoli A, Furukawa TA, Imai H, Tajika A, Efthimiou O, Salanti G. Psychological therapies for panic disorder with or without agoraphobia in adults: a network meta-analysis. Cochrane Database Syst Rev. 2016;4:CD011004.
210. Milrod B, Leon AC, Busch F, Rudden M, Schwalberg M, Clarkin J, et al. A randomized controlled clinical trial of psychoanalytic psychotherapy for panic disorder. Am J Psychiatry. 2007;164(2):265–72.
211. Li H, Wang J, Li C, Xiao Z. Repetitive transcranial magnetic stimulation (rTMS) for panic disorder in adults. Cochrane Database Syst Rev. 2014;9:CD009083.
212. George MS, Padberg F, Schlaepfer TE, O'Reardon JP, Fitzgerald PB, Nahas ZH, et al. Controversy:

repetitive transcranial magnetic stimulation or transcranial direct current stimulation shows efficacy in treating psychiatric diseases (depression, mania, schizophrenia, obsessive-compulsive disorder, panic, posttraumatic stress disorder). Brain Stimul. 2009;2(1):14–21.
213. Mantovani A, Aly M, Dagan Y, Allart A, Lisanby SH. Randomized sham controlled trial of repetitive transcranial magnetic stimulation to the dorsolateral prefrontal cortex for the treatment of panic disorder with comorbid major depression. J Affect Disord. 2013;144(1–2):153–9.
214. Ironside M, O'Shea J, Cowen PJ, Harmer CJ. Frontal cortex stimulation reduces vigilance to threat: implications for the treatment of depression and anxiety. Biol Psychiatry. 2016;79(10):823–30.
215. Ravindran AV, da Silva TL. Complementary and alternative therapies as add-on to pharmacotherapy for mood and anxiety disorders: a systematic review. J Affect Disord. 2013;150(3):707–19.
216. Pilkington K, Kirkwood G, Rampes H, Cummings M, Richardson J. Acupuncture for anxiety and anxiety disorders – a systematic literature review. Acupunct Med. 2007;25(1–2):1–10.

14 Treatment Resistance in Anxiety Disorder: Generalized Anxiety Disorder and Social Anxiety Disorder

Kang Soo Lee and Sang Hyuk Lee

14.1 Introduction

Anxiety disorder may be the most frequent common mental disorder, with a combined lifetime prevalence of 28% [1]. In addition, anxiety is an important symptom when considered as a comorbid diagnosis as well as primary diagnostic anxiety disorder. In recent years, remarkable developments have been forthcoming in the field of treating anxiety disorders [2]. Evidence-based treatments are widely used to treat and prevent a variety of anxiety disorder with efficacies from 60% to 80% [3–5]. In the case of pharmacological treatments, selective serotonin reuptake inhibitors (SSRIs) are chosen as first-line therapy according to several clinical practice guidelines. Randomized, controlled trials report response rates of 40–70% and remission rates of 20–47% [6]. Psychological treatment, including cognitive-behavioral treatment, has also become an accepted first-line therapy with anxiety disorders. However, many patients do not improve, despite successful delivery of standard therapeutic interventions.

The definition of treatment resistance is that standard treatments have been effectively delivered, but the results are ineffective [7]. Treatment resistance is reversely associated with remission. The definition of treatment resistance in anxiety disorders is not universally accepted, but neither is there worldwide consensus on the adequate treatment for persistent anxiety disorders. Nonetheless, the treatment goals in anxiety disorder would include not only an absence of symptoms but also functional parameters. Considering the chronic wax and wane course of anxiety disorder, remission criteria would be applied more flexibly as restoration of functional status with tolerable treatment. If we applied this criterion, we could intuitively assume that approximately one-third of patients with anxiety disorders would be considered in remission, and one-third would be considered in partial remission. The remaining one-third would be considered treatment-resistant in terms of the standard treatments [8]. This chapter will review treatment resistance in anxiety disorder, with a particular focus on two diseases: generalized anxiety disorder (GAD) and social anxiety disorder (SAD). It will review the factors that contribute to treatment resistance, novel pharmacological approaches for treatment resistance in GAD and SAD, and potential new targets for drug development.

14.2 Pathophysiology of Treatment Resistance

Many studies have analyzed moderators or clinical predictors of treatment response or nonresponse in anxiety disorders. The contributing

K. S. Lee · S. H. Lee (✉)
Department of Psychiatry, School of Medicine, CHA University, CHA Bundang Medical Center, Seongnam, South Korea

Y.-K. Kim (ed.), *Treatment Resistance in Psychiatry*, https://doi.org/10.1007/978-981-10-4358-1_14

factors in treatment resistance can be classified as treatment- and patient-related factors. Treatment-related factors include incorrect diagnosis and inappropriate treatment such as inadequate dosing schedules and insufficient maintenance duration. Patient-related factors include such comorbidities as personality disorders, substance abuse, and poor adherence. Factors associated with treatment resistance according to Bystritsky are divided into aspects related to the pathology (lack of knowledge on the pathophysiology, inaccurate diagnosis, limitation of the biological treatment), patient (symptom severity, comorbidities, nonadherence), professional (lack of CBT skills, cost), and environment (stress, childhood experiences, life cycles) [9]. Pollcak listed factors associated with treatment resistance as related to the patient (comorbidity, lack of adherence), related to the treatment (incomplete diagnosis, inadequate treatment), and related to the logistics (lack of training, inadequate health system) [10].

The exact biological mechanisms of treatment-resistant GAD and SAD are unknown. GAD shares substantial genetic variation with major depression and the personality trait neuroticism. An alarm reaction mediated by activation of neuronal circuits including amygdale and other limbic structures is most often found in neuroimaging studies of GAD. Right hemispheric involvement and a variety of abnormalities in the amygdala and superior temporal gyrus were also observed in GAD. Abnormalities in the limbic-medial prefrontal circuit shown in functional neuroimaging studies may be critical for the pathophysiology of SAD which has dysfunctional emotion regulation by reappraisal of social criticism. Some studies suggested that reduced resting-state functional connectivity between the amygdala and orbitofrontal cortex predicted treatment resistance in SAD [11, 12]. Psychosocial theories of treatment resistance in GAD and SAD underestimate environmental factors associated with severe persistent stressors. Another important factor of treatment resistance in GAD and SAD is comorbidity such as major depressive disorder, personality disorder, bipolar disorder, substance use disorder, and attention deficit hyperactivity disorder, which can lead to non-compliance and maladapted behavioral coping strategies.

14.3 Strategies for Treatment Resistance

Correct and complete diagnostic workup of anxiety disorders and comorbidities, as well as the appropriate delivery of pharmacological and psychological treatment, is crucial to maximize therapeutic benefits for anxiety disorders. For patient engagement, psychoeducation, including the clinical course of the illness and the consequences of optimal treatment, is important. Finally, comprehensive assessment and appropriate targeted interventions are needed to achieve remission or recovery [13].

The first step in overcoming treatment resistance is reassessment of diagnosis and reevaluation of the treatment effectiveness [9]. Patients who fail to respond to at least two SSRIs, one serotonin-norepinephrine reuptake inhibitor (SNRI), and cognitive behavior therapy (CBT) should be reappraised, and the presence of comorbidities, including personality disorder, should be reevaluated. Treatment compliance and adequacy of medication treatment must be explored. In terms of pharmacotherapy, augmentation or combination strategies have been attempted in treatment-resistant anxiety disorders. Examples of augmentation or combination strategies for treatment resistance include using buspirone, lithium, or other mood stabilizers as add-on therapy, combining two SSRIs or an SSRI with an SNRI, or using tricyclic antidepressants with SSRIs. Although the scientific data do not report any good efficacy for polypharmacy, the use of multiple drugs with different mechanisms is not unusual in treatment-resistant anxiety patients. Augmentation with medication is one of the best strategies for patients who are treatment-resistant. Antipsychotics, anticonvulsants, and other novel medications have been studied for patients who fail to respond to standard treatment. The use of long-term benzodiazepines for treatment-resistant anxiety disorder is debated due to high comorbidity rate of anxiety disorders with substance use disorders. The use of g-aminobutyric acid (GABA)-ergic anticonvulsants involving gabapentin, pregabalin, and tiagabine leads to less dependency but also is less effective [14, 15]. Several medications show better efficacy than SSRI monotherapy. One of the most valuable findings was the combination treatment of SSRI and atypical antipsychotics for anxiety disorders, including social anxiety disorders without psychotic symptoms.

Several pharmacological agents with novel mechanisms of action such as substance P, NK, and corticotropin-releasing factor (CRF) antagonists have recently been tested but have failed to prove their efficacy [16, 17]. The most attractive targets for new anxiolytic development include non-serotonin, dopamine, norepinephrine, and non-GABA neurotransmitters that have been implicated in the development of anxiety disorders as shown in preclinical studies. Neuropeptides are short-chain amino acids that act as neurotransmitters and are involved in a wide range of brain functions, including reward, food intake, social behaviors, mood, and stress response. The most prominent groups of these small neuropeptide receptor ligands are substance P, CRF-1, CRF-2, neuropeptide Y, cholecystokinin (CCK)-2, and galanin [18, 19]. A CCK-B antagonist which has known reduced potentiated states of anxiety has been studied in patients with GAD but was not more effective than a placebo [20].

Recently, psychotherapeutic modalities such as mindfulness, meditation, interpersonal, and psychodynamic therapies have been tested in various anxiety disorders [21, 22]. It is apparent that a complicated patient may require long-term consistent treatments. Combining CBT and pharmacotherapy for patients who do not respond to either treatment alone indicates the need for an alternative treatment strategy. Few randomized trials comparing combined pharmacotherapy and CBT, with either modality alone or with a placebo, have been conducted with treatment-resistant anxiety disorders. A more definitive advantage for combined treatment has been shown in SAD and other anxiety disorders. Although a study conducted for resistant SAD did not show the superiority of combination treatment over either treatment modality alone [23], the most common first action by most clinicians when a patient does not respond to one of the two initial treatment modalities is to combine two treatment modalities. A newer approach to combined treatment for treatment of anxiety disorders is that pharmacotherapy is used not to attenuate symptoms but to enhance extinction learning [24]. The N-methyl-D-aspartate (NMDA) partial agonist D-cycloserine contributes consolidation of conditioned fear and extinction memory in animal models [25]. In a proof-of-concept study, 28 patients with phobia were randomized to exposure therapy plus D-cycloserine or placebo, administered before each of two weekly exposure sessions. D-Cycloserine resulted in significantly fewer anxiety symptoms compared with placebo during the trial as well as long-term follow-up. In a replication study of the D-cycloserine effect, it has shown better treatment effectiveness in 27 patients with SAD [26].

14.4 Generalized Anxiety Disorder

Most of the patients with GAD follow the chronic wax and wane course. Effective management of treatment-resistant GAD has not yet been determined, and there are few studies suggesting available options for treatment-resistant GAD. Some evidence-based pharmacological and psychotherapeutic treatments for GAD include SSRIs, SNRIs, and CBT. However, despite appropriate treatments, many patients with GAD fail to achieve remission in both short- and long-term follow-up studies [27, 28], and as few as 38% of patients have achieved remission at 5 years [29]. Treatment options for patients who failed to respond to pharmacotherapy suggest the need for augmentation with other antidepressants, benzodiazepines, or pregabalin, despite their own limitations [30]. Until now, few studies have investigated the efficacy of pharmacological treatment and/or psychotherapeutic modalities in combination treatment for treatment-resistant GAD.

Including the Canadian Psychiatric Association and National Institute for Health and Clinical Excellence, clinical practice guidelines suggest that the SSRIs, SNRIs, and CBT could be chosen as first-line treatments for GAD [27, 31–33]. There was conflict regarding the use of atypical antipsychotics treatment across guidelines. Antipsychotics are not suggested in the National Institute for Health and Clinical Excellence and British Association for Psychopharmacology guidelines, but the Canadian guidelines suggested atypical antipsychotics augmentation as consistent with third-line treatments. Augmentation with atypical antipsychotics working at dopaminergic and serotonin receptors appears to be an efficacious strategy for patients with treatment-resistant GAD [34] as evidenced by randomized controlled trials [35, 36]. In the first study, patients who did not achieve remission after the use of fluoxetine were randomized to small doses of olanzapine or placebo. The augmentation with atypical antipsychotic olanzapine significantly reduced symptoms of GAD. In the second study, patients who had not responded to the standard treatment for GAD showed significant improvement of their symptoms by augmentation of a mean dose of 1 mg risperidone. One open-label study reported that augmentation with low-dose risperidone may be an alternative strategy for patients with treatment-resistant GAD after standard treatment with antidepressants and benzodiazepines [37]. However, a systematic review and meta-analysis of treatment-resistant GAD suggests a lack of benefit for atypical antipsychotics augmentation in terms of overall response [38]. However, a modest effect was observed in the improvement of symptom severity compared with baseline results. In four open-label studies, aripiprazole was added to an antidepressant until 2 months; the results were encouraging, with improvement of residual anxiety symptoms [39–42]. One open study suggested the efficacy of a mean dose of 40 mg ziprasidone used as monotherapy for 7 weeks in treatment-resistant GAD patients [43]. When quetiapine was used as monotherapy, it was efficacious compared to placebo, despite problems with adverse events and tolerability. Based on current evidence, quetiapine monotherapy at 150 mg dose would be the useful option, as it may provide symptomatic relief for treatment-resistant GAD patients.

Case reports suggest the efficacy of GABAergic anticonvulsants in treatment-resistant GAD, including gabapentin and tiagabine [44, 45]. Open-label case series suggest the augmentation of GABAergic anticonvulsants is efficacious for treatment-resistant GAD. Although the precise action mechanisms of gabapentin have not been fully understood, gabapentin was found to increase GABA synthesis [46]. Levetiracetam modulates the voltage-gated calcium channel, and tiagabine acts as a selective GABA reuptake inhibitor [47, 48]. Though it should be noted that pregabalin was not specifically tested in treatment-resistant cases, it has been suggested to be effective for GAD in controlled trials [49, 50], with side effects generally well-tolerated and an efficacy comparable to benzodiazepine. Short- and long-term GAD treatments with pregabalin at doses up to 600 mg/day were challenging [51–53]. The World Federation of Biological Psychiatry recommends pregabalin as one of several first-line agents for the treatment of GAD. Pregabalin appears to be effective in psychic and somatic symptoms of GAD similar to benzodiazepines, but with less risk of tolerance or dependence. Long-term trials have shown continuous effectiveness and less severe cognitive and psychomotor impairments compared to benzodiazepines.

14.5 Social Anxiety Disorder

Meta-analyses and clinical practice guidelines have recommended SSRIs and the SNRI venlafaxine as first-line pharmacotherapy and CBT as first-line psychotherapeutic modalities for SAD. Nevertheless, many patients do not respond to the first-line pharmacotherapy or CBT, and even fewer achieve remission [54]. Treatment-resistant SAD has been assessed by means of remission criteria on the Liebowitz Social Anxiety Scale

[55]. It is remarkable that in some patients, drug response occasionally starts only after 8–12 weeks [56].

Although there are few studies about SAD, there is weak evidence that other SSRIs or venlafaxine may be effective in patients with SAD who have failed to achieve a remission to an initial SSRI treatment [57–59]. Despite the adverse effects and dietary restrictions, monoamine oxidase inhibitors (MAOIs) are also thought to be alternative agents in the treatment-resistant SAD [60]. A number of open studies have suggested preliminary efficacy of MAOIs in treatment-resistant SAD. The use of escitalopram and citalopram in patients who have failed to respond to other SSRIs showed also positive results [34, 61]. In open studies describing the use of SNRI or MAOIs in treatment-resistant SAD patients, therapeutic outcomes have also been improved [60, 62]. Based on evidence suggesting anxiolytic properties of the olanzapine, an olanzapine monotherapy warrants new approaches for the treatment-resistant patients with SAD [63]. Likewise, efficacy was suggested for an anticonvulsant topiramate, valproic acid, and levetiracetam in open-label trials in SAD [64–67].

A few studies have suggested the possibilities of augmentation strategies for treatment-resistant SAD [37, 68]. In an open study, the buspirone augmentation in patients with SAD who have an inadequate response to the initial SSRI treatment was effective in relieving anxiety symptoms, but the small sample size and the lack of control limit the interpretation and generalizability of the study. In a placebo-controlled study for SAD, pindolol augmentation with paroxetine was not superior to placebo [69]. Clonazepam has also been studied as an augmentation option for SAD. Clonazepam showed an improvement in clinical global impression (CGI) scale compared with placebo, but the effect only approximated significance [70]. Although there were limited data about treatment-resistant SAD, MAOIs, buspirone, and clonazepam are thought to have useful roles as augmentations or alternatives in treatment-resistant SAD patients. The augmentation with atypical antipsychotics was investigated using aripiprazole with SSRIs [40] and risperidone with SSRIs or benzodiazepines [66]. In both studies, the augmentation strategies were proven to be successful, although placebo-controlled studies are necessary to confirm those observations. Further, in one small randomized controlled trial, olanzapine monotherapy also showed a possible option for SAD [63].

Delivering CBT for treatment-resistant SAD seems to be a reasonable strategy, as supported by studies suggesting that the combination of MAOI and CBT is superior to either treatment alone [71, 72]. A partial NMDA agonist, D-cycloserine, was studied as a newer treatment option with exposure therapy in anxiety disorders [25]. Preliminary evidence has suggested that D-cycloserine significantly enhances the effectiveness of an attenuated exposure therapy for SAD [73]. Although meta-analyses have demonstrated significant effects of CBT, as well as pharmacotherapy, a significant proportion of patients does not achieve remission from these treatments [74]. Treatment-resistant SAD may be very common in clinical practice but currently has no systematic studies [75].

References

1. Kessler RC, Berglund P, Demler O, Jin R, Merikangas KR, Walters EE. Lifetime prevalence and age-of-onset distributions of DSM-IV disorders in the National Comorbidity Survey Replication. Arch Gen Psychiatry. 2005;62(6):593–602.
2. Ballenger JC. Treatment of anxiety disorders to remission. J Clin Psychiatry. 2001;62:5–9.
3. Barlow DH, Lehman CL. Advances in the psychosocial treatment of anxiety disorders. Implications for national health care. Arch Gen Psychiatry. 1996;53(8):727–35.
4. Ballenger JC, Davidson JR, Lecrubier Y, Nutt DJ, Bobes J, Beidel DC, et al. Consensus statement on social anxiety disorder from the International Consensus Group on Depression and Anxiety. J Clin Psychiatry. 1998;59:54–60.
5. Ballenger JC, Davidson JR, Lecrubier Y, Nut DJ, Borkovec TD, Rickels K, et al. Consensus statement on generalized anxiety disorder from the International Consensus Group on Depression and Anxiety. J Clin Psychiatry. 2001;62:53–8.
6. Ballenger JC. Current treatment of the anxiety disorders in adults. Biol Psychiatry. 1999;46(11):1579–94.
7. Roy-Byrne P. Treatment-refractory anxiety; definition, risk factors, and treatment challenges. Dialogues Clin Neurosci. 2015;17(2):191–206.

8. Brown C, Schulberg HC, Madonia MJ, Shear MK, Houck PR. Treatment outcomes for primary care patients with major depression and lifetime anxiety disorders. Am J Psychiatry. 1996;153(10):1293–300.
9. Bystritsky A. Treatment-resistant anxiety disorders. Mol Psychiatry. 2006;11(9):805–14.
10. Pollack MH, Otto MW, Roy-Byrne PP, Coplan JD, Rothbaum BO, Simon NM, et al. Novel treatment approaches for refractory anxiety disorders. Depress Anxiety. 2008;25(6):467–76.
11. Klumpp H, Keutmann MK, Fitzgerald DA, Shankman SA, Phan KL. Resting state amygdala-prefrontal connectivity predicts symptom change after cognitive behavioral therapy in generalized social anxiety disorder. Biol Mood Anxiety Disord. 2014;4(1):14.
12. Roy-Whitfield-Gabrieli S, Ghosh SS, Nieto-Castanon A, Saygin Z, Doehrmann O, Chai XJ, et al. Brain connectomics predict response to treatment in social anxiety disorder. Mol Psychiatry. 2016;21(5):680–5.
13. Byrne P, Cowley DS. Clinical approach to treatment-resistant panic disorder. In: Rosenbaum JF, Pollack MH, editors. Panic disorder and its treatment. New York: Marcel Dekker; 1998. p. 205–27.
14. Blanco C, Raza MS, Schneier FR, Liebowitz MR. The evidence-based pharmacological treatment of social anxiety disorder. Int J Neuropsychopharmacol. 2003;6(4):427–42.
15. Lauria-Horner BA, Pohl RB. Pregabalin: a new anxiolytic. Expert Opin Investig Drugs. 2003;12(4):663–72.
16. McDougle CJ, Barr LC, Goodman WK, Price LH. Possible role of neuropeptides in obsessive compulsive disorder. Psychoneuroendocrinology. 1999;24(1):1–24.
17. Nemeroff CB. New vistas in neuropeptide research in neuropsychiatry: focus on corticotrophin releasing factor. Neuropsychopharmacology. 1992;6:69–75.
18. Herranz R. Cholecystokinin antagonists: pharmacological and therapeutic potential. Med Res Rev. 2003;23(5):559–605.
19. Holmes A, Heilig M, Rupniak NMJ, Steckler T, Griebel G. Neuropeptide systems as novel therapeutic targets for depression and anxiety disorders. Trends Pharmacol Sci. 2003;24(11):580–8.
20. Adams JB, Pyke RE, Costa J, Cutler NR, Schweizer E, Wilcox CS, et al. A double blind, placebo controlled study of a CCK-B receptor antagonist, CI-988, in patients with generalized anxiety disorder. J Clin Psychopharmacol. 1995;15(6):428–34.
21. Borkovec TD, Ruscio AM. Psychotherapy for generalized anxiety disorder. J Clin Psychiatry. 2001;62:37–42.
22. Krisanaprakornkit T, Sriraj W, Piyavhatkul N, Laopaiboon M. Meditation therapy for anxiety disorders. Cochrane Database Syst Rev. 2006;1:CD004998.
23. Hambrick JP, Weeks JW, Harb GC, Heimberg RG. Cognitive behavioral therapy for social anxiety disorder: supporting evidence and future directions. CNS Spectr. 2003;8(5):373–81.
24. Ressler KJ, Rothbaum BO, Tannenbaum L, Anderson P, Graap K, Zimand E, et al. Cognitive enhancers as adjuncts to psychotherapy: use of D-cycloserine in phobic individuals to facilitate extinction of fear. Arch Gen Psychiatry. 2004;61(11):1136–44.
25. Walker DL, Ressler KJ, Lu KT, Davis M. Facilitation of conditioned fear extinction by systemic administration of intraamygdala infusions of D-cycloserine as assessed with fear potentiated startle in rats. J Neurosci. 2002;22(6):2343–51.
26. Hofmann SG, Meuret AE, Smits JA, Simon NM, Pollack MH, Eisenmenger K, et al. Augmentation of exposure therapy for social anxiety disorder with D-Cycloserine. Arch Gen Psychiatry. 2006;63(3):298–304.
27. Canadian Psychiatric Association. Clinical practice guidelines: management of anxiety disorders. Can J Psychiatr. 2006;51(8 Suppl 2):9S.
28. Rubio G, Lopez-Ibor JJ. Generalized anxiety disorder: a 40-year follow-up study. Acta Psychiatr Scand. 2007;115(5):372–9.
29. Yonkers KA, Warshaw MG, Massion AO, Keller MB. Phenomenology and course of generalized anxiety disorder. Br J Psychiatry. 1996;168(3):308–13.
30. Pollack MH. Refractory generalized anxiety disorder. J Clin Psychiatry. 2009;70(Suppl 2):32–8.
31. National Institute for Health and Clinical Excellence. Clinical guideline 22 (Amended). Anxiety: management of anxiety (panic disorder, with or without agoraphobia, and generalised anxiety disorder) in adults in primary, secondary and community care. Available from at: http://www.nice.org.uk/CG022NICEguideline.
32. Baldwin DS, Anderson IM, Nutt DJ, Bandelow B, Bond A, Davidson JR, et al. Evidence-based guidelines for the pharmacological treatment of anxiety disorders: recommendations from the British Association for Psychopharmacology. J Psychopharmacol. 2005;19(6):567–96.
33. Bandelow B, Zohar J, Hollander E, Kasper S, Moller HJ. World Federation of Societies of Biological Psychiatry (WFSBP) guidelines for the pharmacological treatment of anxiety, obsessive-compulsive and posttraumatic stress disorders. World J Biol Psychiatry. 2008;9(4):248–312.
34. Ipser JC, Carey P, Dhansay Y, Fakier N, Seedat S, Stein DJ. Pharmacotherapy augmentation strategies in treatment-resistant anxiety disorders. Cochrane Database Syst Rev. 2006;4:CD005473.
35. Brawman-Mintzer O, Knapp RG, Nietert PJ. Adjunctive risperidone in generalized anxiety disorder: a double-blind, placebo-controlled study. J Clin Psychiatry. 2005;66(10):1321–5.
36. Pollack MH, Simon NM, Zalta AK, Worthington JJ, Hoge EA, Mick E, et al. Olanzapine augmentation of fluoxetine for refractory generalized anxiety disorder: a placebo controlled study. Biol Psychiatry. 2006;59:211–5.
37. Simon NM, Hoge EA, Fischmann D, Worthington JJ, Christian KM, Kinrys G, et al. An open-label trial of risperidone augmentation for refractory anxiety disorders. J Clin Psychiatry. 2006;67(3):381–5.

38. Patterson B, Van Ameringen M. Augmentation strategies for treatment-resistant anxiety disorders: a systematic review and meta-analysis. Depress Anxiety. 2016;33(8):728–36.
39. Adson DE, Kushner MG, Fahnhorst TA. Treatment of residual anxiety symptoms with adjunctive aripiprazole in depressed patients taking selective serotonin reuptake inhibitors. J Affect Disord. 2005;86(1):99–104.
40. Worthington JJ III, Kinrys G, Wygant LE, Pollack MH. Aripiprazole as an augmentor of selective serotonin reuptake inhibitors in depression and anxiety disorder patients. Int Clin Psychopharmacol. 2005;20(1):9–11.
41. Menza MA, Dobkin RD, Marin H. An open label trial of aripiprazole augmentation for treatment-resistant generalized anxiety disorder. J Clin Psychopharmacol. 2007;27(2):207–10.
42. Hoge EA, Worthington IIIJJ, Kaufman RE, Delong HR, Pollack MH, Simon NM. Aripiprazole as augmentation treatment of refractory generalized anxiety disorder and panic disorder. CNS Spectr. 2008;13(6):522–7.
43. Snyderman SH, Rynn MA, Rickels K. Open-label pilot study of ziprasidone for refractory generalized anxiety disorder. J Clin Psychopharmacol. 2005;25(5):497–9.
44. Schwartz TL. The use of tiagabine augmentation for treatment-resistant anxiety disorders: a case series. Psychopharmacol Bull. 2002;36(2):53–7.
45. Pollack MH, Matthews J, Scott EL. Gabapentin as a potential treatment for anxiety disorders. Am J Psychiatry. 1998;155(7):992–3.
46. Pollack M. Levetiracetam (Keppra) for anxiety. Curbside Consult. 2002;1(4):4.
47. Crane D. Tiagabine for the treatment of anxiety. Depress Anxiety. 2003;18(1):51–2.
48. Feltner DE, Pollack MH, Davidson JR, Stein MB, Fulterer R, Jefferson JW, et al. A placebo-controlled, double-blind study of pregabalin treatment of social phobia: outcome and predictors of response. J Eur Coll Neuropsychopharmacol. 2000;10:344–5.
49. Rickels K, Pollack MH, Feltner DE, Lydiard RB, Zimbroff DL, Bielski RJ, et al. Pregabalin for treatment of generalized anxiety disorder: a 4-week, multicenter, double-blind, placebo-controlled trial of pregabalin and alprazolam. Arch Gen Psychiatry. 2005;62(9):1022–30.
50. Montgomery S, Chatamra K, Pauer L, Whalen E, Baldinetti F. Efficacy and safety of pregabalin in elderly people with generalised anxiety disorder. Br J Psychiatry. 2008;193(5):389–94.
51. Feltner DE, Crockatt JG, Dubovsky SJ, Cohn CK, Shrivastava RK, Targum SD, et al. A randomized, double-blind, placebo controlled, fixed-dose, multicenter study of pregabalin in patients with generalized anxiety disorder. J Clin Psychopharmacol. 2003;23(3):240–9.
52. Pande AC, Crockatt JG, Feltner DE, Janney CA, Smith WT, Weisler R, et al. Pregabalin in generalized anxiety disorder: a placebo-controlled trial. Am J Psychiatry. 2003;160(3):533–40.
53. Montgomery SA, Tobias K, Zornberg GL, Kasper S, Pande AC. Efficacy and safety of pregabalin in the treatment of generalized anxiety disorder: a 6-week, multicenter, randomized, double-blind, placebo-controlled comparison of pregabalin and venlafaxine. J Clin Psychiatry. 2006;67(5):771–82.
54. Stein MB, Stein DJ. Social anxiety disorder. Lancet. 2008;371(9618):1115–25.
55. Bandelow B, Baldwin DS, Dolberg OT, Andersen HF, Stein DJ. What is the threshold for symptomatic response and remission for major depressive disorder, panic disorder, social anxiety disorder, and generalized anxiety disorder. J Clin Psychiatry. 2006;67(9):1428–34.
56. Stein DJ, Stein MB, Pitts CD, Kumar R, Hunter B. Predictors of response to pharmacotherapy in social anxiety disorder: an analysis of 3 placebo-controlled paroxetine trials. J Clin Psychiatry. 2002;63:152–5.
57. Pallanti S, Quercioli L. Resistant social anxiety disorder response to escitalopram. Clin Pract Epidemiol Ment Health. 2006;2(1):35.
58. Kelsey JE. Venlafaxine in social phobia. Psychopharmacol Bull. 1995;31:767–71.
59. Altamura AC, Pioli R, Vitto M, Mannu P. Venlafaxine in social phobia: a study in selective serotonin reuptake non-responders. Int Clin Psychopharmacol. 1999;14(4):239–45.
60. Aarre TF. Phenelzine efficacy in refractory social anxiety disorder: a case series. Nord J Psychiatry. 2003;57(4):313–5.
61. Simon NM, Korbly NB, Worthington JJ, Kinrys G, Pollack MH. Citalopram for social anxiety disorder: an open-label pilot study in refractory and nonrefractory patients. CNS Spectr. 2002;7(9):655–7.
62. Altamura AC, Pioli R, Vitto M, Mannu P. Venlafaxine in social phobia: a study in selective serotonin reuptake inhibitor non-responders. Int Clin Psychopharmacol. 1999;14(4):239–45.
63. Barnett SD, Kramer ML, Casat CD, Connor KM, Davidson JR. Efficacy of olanzapine in social anxiety disorder: a pilot study. J Psychopharmacol. 2002;16(4):365–8.
64. Shaywitz JE, Liebowitz MR. Antiepileptic treatment of anxiety disorders. Prim Psychiatry. 2003:51–6.
65. Van Ameringen M, Mancini C, Pipe B, Oakman J, Bennett M. An open-label trial of topiramate in the treatment of generalized social phobia. J Clin Psychiatry. 2004;65(12):1674–8.
66. Kinrys G, Pollack MH, Simon NM, Worthington JJ, Nardi AE, Versiani M. Valproic acid for the treatment of social anxiety disorder. Int Clin Psychopharmacol. 2003;18(3):169–72.
67. Simon NM, Worthington JJ, Doyle AC, Hoge EA, Kinrys G, Fischmann D, et al. An open-label study of levetiracetam for the treatment of social anxiety disorder. J Clin Psychiatry. 2004;65(9):1219–22.
68. Van Ameringen M, Mancini C, Wilson C. Buspirone augmentation of selective serotonin reuptake

inhibitors (SSRIs) in social phobia. J Affect Disord. 1996;39(2):115–21.
69. Stein MB, Sareen J, Hami S, Chao J. Pindolol potentiation of paroxetine for generalized social phobia: a double-blind, placebo-controlled, crossover study. Am J Psychiatry. 2001;158(10):1725–7.
70. Seedat S, Stein MB. Double-blind, placebo-controlled assessment of combined clonazepam with paroxetine compared with paroxetine monotherapy for generalized social anxiety disorder. J Clin Psychiatry. 2004;65(2):244–8.
71. Blanco C, Heimberg RG, Schneier FR, Fresco DM, Chen H, Turk CL, et al. A placebo-controlled trial of phenelzine, cognitive behavioral group therapy, and their combination for social anxiety disorder. Arch Gen Psychiatry. 2010;67(3):286–95.
72. Blanco C, Okuda M, Markowitz JC, Liu SM, Grant BF, Hasin DS. The epidemiology of chronic major depressive disorder and dysthymic disorder: results from the National Epidemiologic Survey on Alcohol and Related Conditions. J Clin Psychiatry. 2010;71(12):1645–56.
73. Guastella AJ, Richardson R, Lovibond PF, et al. A randomized controlled trial of D-cycloserine enhancement of exposure therapy for social anxiety disorder. Biol Psychiatry. 2008;63:544–9.
74. Mayo WE, Dias S, Mavranezouli I, Kew K, Clark DM, Ades AE, et al. Psychological and pharmacological interventions for social anxiety disorder in adults: a systematic review and network meta analysis. Lancet Psychiatry. 2014;1(5):368–76.
75. Craske MG, Golinelli D, Stein MB, Roy-Byrne P, Bystritsky A, Sherbourne C. Does the addition of cognitive behavioral therapy improve panic disorder treatment outcome relative to medication alone in the primary care setting? Psychol Med. 2005;35(11):1645–54.

Treatment Resistance in Attention-Deficit/Hyperactivity Disorder

15

Amber D. Hunt, David W. Dunn, Hillary S. Blake, and Jennifer Downs

15.1 Introduction

Attention-deficit/hyperactivity disorder (ADHD) is one of the most common and widely researched disorders of childhood [1]. According to the DSM-5, it is a neurodevelopmental disorder characterized by at least six of nine inattention symptoms and/or at least six of nine hyperactivity/impulsivity symptoms. Specifiers include predominantly inattentive presentation and predominantly hyperactive/impulsive presentation, and the disorder can be categorized as mild, moderate, or severe. Symptoms must interfere with functioning or development and must be present prior to the age of 12 to qualify for ADHD (Table 15.1) [2].

15.2 Epidemiology

US prevalence estimates of attention-deficit/hyperactivity disorder in youth ages 4–17 range from 5% to 11% [3], with the childhood male to female ratio estimated to be 3–4:1 in epidemiological samples [4]. Worldwide prevalence of ADHD/hyperkinetic disorder is estimated to be 5.3% for children and adolescents [5]. The male to female ratio becomes more evenly distributed in adulthood [6]. Inattention symptoms tend to persist, while hyperactivity symptoms decline with age [3]. ADHD persists into adulthood for up to 60–65% of cases [7, 8]. In both children and adults with ADHD, a larger percentage of females are diagnosed with ADHD-inattentive type than males, but males are more likely to be diagnosed with ADHD-combined presentation, as well as with ADHD overall [9].

15.3 Impact

The economic and psychosocial costs of ADHD are significant for patients, their families, and the society. In 2000, the annual estimated economic cost of ADHD in the United States alone was estimated to exceed $30 billion [10]. ADHD is associated with a higher risk for substance use disorders and other comorbid psychiatric disorders, increased mortality due to accidents, unwanted pregnancies, lower academic achievement and occupational performance, adult antisocial behavior, and poor social functioning, including higher divorce rates [1, 11, 12]. Bernardi et al. presented the results from the National Epidemiological Survey on Alcohol and Related Conditions and reported that adults with ADHD were more likely to be diagnosed with histrionic, borderline, narcissistic, schizo-

A. D. Hunt · D. W. Dunn (✉) · H. S. Blake
J. Downs
Indiana University School of Medicine,
Indianapolis, IN, USA
e-mail: adhunt@iupui.edu; ddunn@iupui.edu;
hcstanle@iupui.edu; downsjl@iupui.edu

Y.-K. Kim (ed.), *Treatment Resistance in Psychiatry*, https://doi.org/10.1007/978-981-10-4358-1_15

Table 15.1 Comparison of DSM-IV and DSM-5 ADHD criteria

DSM-IV	DSM-5
Symptoms of inattention: Must meet ≥6/9 criteria	Symptoms of inattention: Those under 17 must meet ≥ 6/9 criteria **Those 17 and older must meet 5**
Symptoms of hyperactivity-impulsivity: Must meet ≥ 6/9 criteria	Symptoms of hyperactivity-impulsivity: Those under 17 must meet ≥ 6/9 criteria **Those 17 and older must meet 5**
Some symptoms causing **impairment** prior to **age 7**	**Several** symptoms **present** prior to **age 12**
Impairment in two or more settings	**Present** in two or more settings
Clinically significant impairment in social, academic, or occupational function	Symptoms **interfere with** or **reduce the quality** of social, academic, or occupational function
Unable to diagnose in setting of pervasive developmental disorder	**Able** to diagnose in setting of autism spectrum disorder
Specify "**type**": combined vs. predominantly impulsive or hyperactive-impulsive	Specify "**presentation**": combined vs. predominately impulsive or hyperactive-impulsive
ADHD **not otherwise specified**	**Other specified** ADHD **Unspecified** ADHD

typal as well as posttraumatic stress disorder, generalized anxiety disorder, specific phobia, and bipolar disorder. They were also more likely to engage in high-risk impulsive behaviors and experience less social support, higher perceived stress, and higher number of traumas, independent of comorbid psychiatric disorders. The average age of first treatment (counseling/psychotherapy and/or medications) for the population in this review was 18, and the lifetime rate of treatment seeking was less than half (44%) [13]. Untreated ADHD is associated with poorer self-esteem and social outcomes versus treated ADHD [14]. And finally, Hechtman et al. compared MTA outcomes 16 years following childhood diagnosis of ADHD and found educational, occupational, legal, emotional, substance use disorder, and sexual behavior outcomes to be significantly worse for young adults with persisting ADHD symptoms versus those with desisting symptoms [15].

15.4 Etiology

The etiology of ADHD is complex and involves multiple factors. The literature base suggests a bidirectional relationship between genetic, neurobiological, and environmental factors resulting in a heterogeneous phenotype of the disorder.

15.4.1 Genetics

ADHD is thought to be one of the most heritable psychiatric conditions, with a heritability estimate of 0.6–0.75 [16–19]. Although no specific gene has been identified as of yet, some genome-wide association studies suggest involvement of chromosome regions 16q22–24 [19]. Due to the established success of methylphenidate (MPH) in treating ADHD, a good deal of research has concentrated on a catecholaminergic hypothesis to explain the etiology of ADHD, since MPH increases dopamine and norepinephrine actions [20]. Several studies suggest genetic polymorphisms that result in lower dopaminergic and alpha-2A receptor densities are associated with ADHD symptoms, which fit with the mechanisms of action of stimulants and alpha-2 agonists such as guanfacine [21]. Dopaminergic receptor gene variants include DRD4, DRD5, and the dopamine transporter (DAT-1) [21–23] as well as the genes encoding the serotonin transporter and the serotonin 1B receptor [23]. Other genome-wide association studies have identified several possible genes involved in the etiology of ADHD including a gene involved in cell adhesion (CDH13), protein kinase genes (PRKG-1 and CAMK1D), integrin genes (ITGAE and ITGA11), and genes involved in the cell signaling process (SLC9A9) and serotonin synthesis (TPH2) [6].

15.4.2 Brain Structure

Multiple studies have established abnormalities in the fronto-striatal-cerebellar circuit in children with ADHD, including cortical thinning and reduction in gray matter volumes. A meta-analysis of MRI voxel-based morphometry (VBM) studies highlighted consistent abnormalities in basal ganglia and limbic regions [24]. Studies finding morphological abnormalities in the amygdala and thalamus shed new light on the sensory and emotional abnormalities of children with ADHD. More recent studies have also suggested there is a delay in cortical maturation in areas associated with attention and motor planning in children with ADHD versus controls [23, 25].

Diffuse tensor imaging (DTI) studies are a relatively new advancement and have allowed researchers to examine not just white matter volume but white matter tracts connecting gray matter regions [23]. In order to identify the most consistent microstructural white matter abnormalities in ADHD, Chen et al. performed a systematic review and meta-analysis of the existing DTI studies that use tract-based spatial statistics. The authors found that fractional anisotropy (FA), the most commonly used parameter of directional diffusion, was consistently reduced in the interhemispheric communication, posterior brain circuitries, and the limbic system. Taken together, these abnormalities may explain some of the inattention, distractibility, and deficits in visual processing in patients with ADHD [26].

15.4.3 Brain Function

Cortese et al. performed a meta-analysis of 55 task-based functional MRI studies (including 39 children and 16 adults) [27]. Children with ADHD demonstrated significant hypoactivation in the frontoparietal network and ventral attentional network versus controls. These networks are primarily responsible for goal-directed executive processes and attention, respectively. Conversely, hyperactivation was seen in the networks responsible for sensorimotor processes, including the visual and somatomotor systems. It is thought that the deficits in the frontoparietal network (specifically anterior cingulate and prefrontal cortices) lead to overcompensation with areas associated with visual, spatial, and motor processing in patients with ADHD [27].

15.4.4 Environment

A number of prenatal, perinatal, and postnatal environmental insults have been linked to the etiology of ADHD. However, it must be cautioned that the available data only provides evidence for association and not causation. Prenatal risk factors include exposure to toxins in utero such as tobacco, alcohol, prescription drugs, and illicit drugs, lead, organophosphate pesticides, polychlorinated biphenyls, and maternal stress. Perinatal risk factors include prematurity and low birthweight, although quasi-experimental designs suggest there are unknown confounding variables contributing to this association [4]. Dietary factors such as artificial food coloring, low/high IgG foods, and dietary deficiencies in iron, zinc, magnesium, and polyunsaturated fatty acids have been associated with ADHD in children [16, 28, 29].

Psychosocial risk factors such as family adversity, parent-child hostility and conflict, and low income are thought to be associated with, but do not directly cause, ADHD. Severe and early neglect is a likely causal risk factor for development of ADHD [28], whereas parental factors, including parental ADHD and adverse parenting styles, likely have a bidirectional relationship on externalizing behaviors and severity of ADHD symptoms [16].

15.5 Assessment

In 2011, the American Academy of Pediatrics (AAP) published updated guidelines that allow for diagnosis of ADHD in children ages 4–18 [30]. The primary care physician plays an essential role in the initial evaluation and treatment of ADHD in children and adolescents. According to the CDC's National Health Statistics Report, half of children with ADHD are diagnosed by primary care physicians, and three quarters of patients with ADHD were diagnosed by age 9 [31]. The assessment and diagnosis of ADHD requires a thorough history, ideally from multiple sources, including caregivers, teachers, and other relevant adults in the child's life, and mental status examination. As much as possible, the patient should also be included in providing history, keeping in mind that young children provide less reliable history. Diagnosis should be based on DSM-5 criteria and incorporate data from at least two settings.

There are currently no medical tests or biomarkers that can definitively diagnose ADHD. As mentioned above, ADHD is a highly heterogeneous disorder, and there is a wide variety of core symptom presentation, degree of severity, and psychiatric comorbidities. The AAP recommends standardized rating scales be used as part of a comprehensive diagnostic assessment. Several rating scales with good sensitivity and specificity include the Conners' Rating Scale-Revised (CRS), the Conners Abbreviated Symptom Questionnaire (ASQ), the Child Behavior Checklist-Attention Problem (CBCL-AP) [32], and the Vanderbilt Parent and Teacher Rating Scales [33, 34]. Screening scales are best used in conjunction with a thorough history taking and mental status examination and are most helpful when used to assess response to treatment over time. Review of academic records, such as psychoeducational testing and reports cards, may also be useful in evaluating school functioning.

An essential component of assessment for ADHD includes evaluating for differential diagnoses and psychiatric comorbidities. Several disorders include symptoms that overlap with the core symptoms of ADHD and can cloud the clinical picture. For example, children and adolescents with anxiety disorders can present with psychomotor agitation, inattention and distractibility, externalizing behaviors, and poor academic functioning. Depressive disorders can likewise cause poor attention and concentration and psychomotor agitation. Other mental illnesses that can mimic ADHD include learning disorders, oppositional defiant disorder, conduct disorder, and substance abuse. Social factors such as bullying, familial conflict, rigorous academic and extracurricular schedules, and frequent changes in school can lead to academic problems and confound the ADHD diagnosis [35].

Further complicating the picture is the fact that ADHD is associated with a wide variety of psychiatric comorbidities. In a study of US children ages 6–17 years with ADHD, about a third of subjects had at least one comorbid psychiatric disorder [36]. Oppositional defiant disorder is the most common comorbidity, with some estimates ranging from 54% to 67% [35]. The comorbidity of learning disorders can reach as high as 45% when writing disorders are included with reading and math disorders [37]. Other common comorbidities include mood disorders, anxiety disorders, tic disorders, sleep disorders, substance abuse disorders, autism spectrum disorder, posttraumatic stress disorder, circadian rhythm disorders, and sleep disorders [38–41].

15.6 Treatment of ADHD

The treatment of ADHD should involve a systematic approach targeting the predominant clinical symptoms with the goal of minimizing the negative impact on social and academic functioning. An evidence-based risk-benefit analysis should always be undertaken when choosing pharmacologic and/or nonpharmacologic intervention(s). The original Multimodal Treatment Study of Children with ADHD study examined the short-term (14 months) outcome of different arms of treatment, including intensive behavioral, medication, and multimodal treatment versus community care only. The study found superior outcomes for medication versus other treatment arms. However, a more recent analysis of long-term outcomes suggests the superiority of medication is diminished over time and indicates superiority of combined treatment for long-term positive outcomes, such as academic and social functioning and parenting styles [42]. Parents of subjects in the combined treatment group showed the greatest reduction in negative/ineffective discipline styles. Furthermore, only in the combined treatment group (and not with intensive behavioral intervention alone) was the normalization of teacher-reported disruptive behavior scores seen [43]. Combined behavioral and medication treatment may be especially effective for those with ADHD and comorbid anxiety and for patients of lower socioeconomic status [44, 45]. When treating patients with medications, the AAP recommends vitals (height, weight, blood pressure, and heart rate) be performed at each visit and that monthly visits occur until the medication dose is stabilized. If the youth is on a stimulant, he or she should be seen every 3 months.

The patient's age should be considered when formulating a treatment plan. For preschool-aged children (4–5 years of age), parent management training is considered the first-line intervention [46]. If parental training is unsuccessful, or unavailable in the patient's area, monotherapy is methylphenidate and is the next option following careful weighing of risks and benefits. A study looking at long-term pharmacotherapy of preschool children with ADHD found methylphenidate was successful in treating preschool ADHD but with higher rates of adverse effects and discontinuation [47]. Evidence from this age group suggests starting at lower doses and increasing in smaller increments [30]. In certain cases in which safety is a concern, such as the patient exhibiting co-occurring severe aggression or dangerous, impulsive behaviors, the risk of not treating with medication may outweigh the risk of adverse effects [30, 47]. For the school-age child [6–12], stimulants are more efficacious than non-stimulants, although both have good evidence. Behavioral treatments are also effective in this age group, especially if there is only a partial response to medications and/or adverse effects [48]. For adolescents (ages 12–18), the evidence suggests both stimulant and non-stimulant medications are efficacious for ADHD core symptoms, and psychosocial interventions can have a small to moderate effect on parent-rated ADHD symptoms, as well as co-occurring behavioral, emotional, or interpersonal problems [49].

15.6.1 Pharmacologic

15.6.1.1 Stimulants

A wealth of evidence supports stimulants as the first-line treatment of the core symptoms of ADHD in children and adolescents, namely, methylphenidates and amphetamines. The mechanism of action is proposed to be increased dopamine and norepinephrine transmission in brain regions associated with attention and concentration, executive functioning, and motor activity, such as the prefrontal cortex and basal ganglia. Functional MRI studies have shown cerebral blood flow to the prefrontal/frontal areas normalizes following administration of methylphenidate [12]. In a meta-analysis of psychostimulant effects on brain structure and function, Spencer et al. found that stimulant use in subjects with ADHD (child and adolescent, ages 4–20) attenuated previous abnormalities of brain structure and function in certain regions [50]. Comparison studies of stimulants have not shown one stimulant class to be superior over another [51]. The response rate of initial treatment with any stimulant is estimated to be 70% and up to 90% will respond to some form of stimulant with careful titration [52]. Newer formulations of stimulants include long-acting forms that may help improve adherence by decreasing the burden and stigma of multiple daily administrations, reduce risk of side effects associated with peak in dosage, and reduce abuse potential [52]. Chewable or liquid formulations are also designed to improve adherence for patients who have difficulty swallowing pills. Table 15.2 summarizes the current FDA-approved list of stimulants for use in children and adolescents with ADHD, as well as formulations and dosing range [20, 53, 54]. Most reports generally indicate the adverse effects of stimulants to be mild and transient [55], and the possible benefit of treatment is higher than the risk of adverse effects. However, as with most medications, side effects can occur. Table 15.3 shows commonly occurring stimulant-related adverse effects and current best practice in managing them [56].

Some common concerns patients and their families may have about long-term adverse effects of stimulants in children and adolescents include

Table 15.2 FDA-approved ADHD medications for children/adolescents

Class	Generic name	Brand name	Age (years)	Initial dose (mg/day)	FDA max dose (mg/day)	Duration of action (hours)	Dosage formulation
Stimulants	Amphetamine mixed salts	Adderall	3–5	2.5	40	4–6	Immediate-release tablet
			6+	5–10			
		Adderall XR	6–12	5–10	30	10–12	Extended-release capsules, can be opened
			13+	10			
		Adzenys ER*	6+	6.3	18.8	10–12	Extended-release suspension
		Adzenys XR	6+	6.3	18.8	10–12	Extended-release ODT, orange
		Evekeo	3–5	2.5	40	4–6	Immediate-release tablet
			6+	5			
		Dyanavel XR	6+	2.5	20	12	Extended-release suspension, bubblegum
		Mydayis	13+	12.5	25	16	Extended-release capsules, can be opened
	Dextroamphetamine	Dexedrine	3–5	2.5	No approval for age 3–5	4–6	Immediate-release tablet
			6+	5	40		
		Dexedrine Spansule	6+	5	40	6–10	Extended-release capsule
		ProCentra	3–5	2.5	40	4–6	Immediate-release suspension, bubblegum
			6+	5			
		Zenzedi	3–5	2.5	40	4–6	Immediate-release tablet
			6+	5			
	Lisdexamphetamine	Vyvanse	6+	30	70	12–14	Extended-release capsule
	Methylphenidate	Ritalin	3–5	2.5	No approval for age 3–5	3–4	Immediate-release tablet
			6+	5	60		
		Ritalin SR	6+	20	60	6–8	Sustained-release tablet
		Ritalin LA	6+	20	60	8–10	Extended-release capsule, can be opened
		Metadate ER	6+	10	60	6–8	Extended-release tablet
		Metadate CD	6+	10	60	8–10	Extended-release capsule, can be opened
		Methylin	6+	5	60	3–4	Immediate-release chewable and suspension

		Methylin ER	6+	10	60	6–8	Extended-release chewable, grape
		Concerta	6–12	18	54	10–14	Extended-release capsule
			13+	18	72		
		Daytrana TD	6+	10	30	8–12	Transdermal patch
		Aptensio XR	6+	10	60	8–12	Extended-release capsules, can be opened
		Cotempla	6+	17.3	51.8	6–8	Extended-release ODT
		Quillivant XR	6+	20	60	6–8	Extended-release suspension, banana
		QuilliChew ER	6+	20	60	6–8	Extended-release chewable, cherry
	Dexmethylphenidate	Focalin	6+	2.5	20	3–4	Immediate-release tablet
		Focalin XR	6+	5	30	8–10	Extended-release capsule, can be opened
Non-stimulants	Atomoxatine	Strattera	6+		100	24	Capsule
	Clonidine	Catapres		0.05	No approval for ADHD	3–6	Immediate-release tablet, transdermal patch
		Kapvay	6+	0.1	0.4	12–16	Extended-release tablet
	Guanfacine	Tenex		0.5	No approval for age < 18	6–12	Immediate-release tablet
		Intinuv	6+	1	4	14–18	Extended-release tablet

Sources: Stahl [20]; Adesman A. The ADHD Medication Guide [53]; Spencer et al. [54]

Table 15.3 Current best practices in managing stimulant adverse effects

	Stimulants	Alpha agonists	Atomoxetine
Common	GI distress – often resolves; reassurance Loss of appetite – decr dose, give after meals, or high-calorie, high-protein supplemental nutrition	GI distress – often resolves; reassurance	GI distress – give with meal/snack
	Headaches – often resolves; reassurance	Headaches – often resolves; reassurance	Headaches – often resolves; reassurance
	Insomnia – administer earlier if possible	Decr BP/HR – if asymptomatic, reassurance; consider dosing at bedtime	Transient growth effects – as with stimulants
	Elevated BP/HR* – if <95th%ile, offer reassurance; if >95th%ile, "drug holiday" and/or cardiology referral	Sedation – often resolves; administer at bedtime	Elevated BP/HR – as with stimulants
	Tics** – if mild, reassurance; if mod-sev, decr dose, d/c, or add guanfacine Mood disturbance/agitation – if present during peak medication effect, decr dose or d/c Rebound effects – if IR, change to ER; if ER, consider adding IR during wear-off Transient growth effects – suggest "drug holidays" on weekends/summer; referral to endocrine specialist for values below critical thresholds		Sedation – often resolves, administer at bedtime
Rare but serious	Priapism – medical emergency; d/c	If d/c abruptly, rebound hypertension; wean slowly	Hepatotoxicity – d/c medication if signs/sx of hepatotoxicity occur
			Increased SI – d/c

Source: Cortese et al. [23], https://doi.org/10.1111/jcpp.12036

*Despite Black Box Warning of sudden cardiac death, evidence does not support this and baseline EKG is only required in patients with medical history of cardiac arrhythmias/preexisting cardiac structural defects and/or family history of sudden cardiac death at young age

**Not causative but can unmask/exacerbate

Abbreviations: decr decrease, *mod-sev* moderate-severe, *d/c* discontinue, *SI* suicidal ideation/thoughts

decreased appetite and poor growth and increased risk for stimulant addiction or other substance use disorders. Concerning growth deficits, most available research suggests short-term minimal impact on growth parameters (height and weight) that normalizes by late adolescence or adulthood [57–59]. Regarding stimulant treatment of ADHD and substance use disorder, stimulants do not appear to increase risk for later substance use disorders [60, 61]. Families and practitioners may also be concerned about seizure risk with stimulants as methylphenidate product information states there is a risk of lowering seizure threshold. However, review of the literature does not support a link between methylphenidate use and increased seizure rates [62, 63].

15.6.1.2 Non-stimulants

Common non-stimulant pharmacologic treatment includes the alpha-2 agonists clonidine and guanfacine and the noradrenaline reuptake inhibitor atomoxetine. It is thought that these three agents are effective due to regulation of the noradrenergic neurotransmitter system in the prefrontal cortex (PFC). Atomoxetine is thought to increase extracellular availability of norepinephrine (NE) in the PFC by blocking norepinephrine reuptake pumps, indirectly causing increased dopamine transmission in the PFC [20, 21, 56]. The alpha-2 agonists are thought to work by improving noradrenergic transmission in the PFC as well by stimulating postsynaptic alpha-2A receptors, with guanfacine being more selective for the alpha-2A receptor than is clonidine [20, 21, 56]. Table 15.2 contains the non-stimulant pharmacologic treatments and dosing guidelines. Table 15.3 lists commonly occurring adverse effects with non-stimulants and best practice in managing them.

15.6.1.3 Treatment Algorithm

In 2006, the Texas Children's Revised Medication Algorithm Project (TMAP) [64] outlines an evidence-based approach to stepwise treatment of ADHD in children and adolescents. An open trial of the feasibility of and adherence to the first algorithm developed in 1998 showed physicians demonstrated good adherence to the first two stages of the algorithm and that adherence to the algorithm predicted better outcomes and less polypharmacy than historical controls. However, developing a treatment algorithm, the authors noted, is difficult due to expanding knowledge in the field of child and adolescent psychiatry [64].

The TMAP algorithm is based on a well-established diagnosis of ADHD, and entry into the algorithm excludes certain psychiatric disorders such as a manic episode, psychotic disorders, and autism spectrum disorder. Stage 1 includes trialing a stimulant from the methylphenidate or amphetamine and stage 2 involves choosing from the alternative stimulant category or changing the formulation (short-acting versus long-acting formulation) within the same category. In stage 3, atomoxetine should be trialed. Families should be cautioned that it may take 2–6 weeks for beneficial effects [56]. Substage 3 was added for low-dose atomoxetine combined with a stimulant (if atomoxetine monotherapy is not as effective as stimulants but stimulants could not control evening or early morning symptoms) based on clinical consensus. It should be noted that atomoxetine combined with a stimulant significantly increases the risk of adverse effects such as appetite loss, insomnia, and irritability [35]. Stage 4 stipulates trial of bupropion or a tricyclic antidepressant (nortriptyline or imipramine), and stage 5 is the alternative not used in stage 4. The alpha agonists are trialed in stage 6 [64].

The TMAP review also outlines treatment of ADHD and comorbidities. For ADHD and comorbid depression, the most severe disorder is treated first, and the secondary disorder is treated if remission does not occur for both disorders with monotherapy. Anxiety and ADHD are treated by using atomoxetine to treat both disorders or first treating ADHD with a stimulant and then adding an SSRI for anxiety. In stage 2 the alternative strategy is chosen. ADHD and tic disorders are treated with stimulant monotherapy in stage 1 and in stage 2 adding an alpha agonist for continued impairing tics. In stage 3, an atypical antipsychotic is added, although more recent data suggests using HRT and C-BIT prior to antipsychotics [65]. If this fails, stage 4 consists of adding haloperidol or pimozide only if an atypical antipsychotic fails. In aggression and co-occurring ADHD, it is recommended to follow the ADHD treatment algorithm first, and if aggression does not resolve, stage 2 stipulates adding behavioral intervention to a stimulant. In stage 3 an atypical antipsychotic is tried, and in stage 4, lithium or divalproex sodium is suggested. The agent not used in stage 4 is tried in stage 5 [64].

15.6.2 Nonpharmacologic

In addition to medication management, studies have shown that behavioral therapy further improves ADHD symptoms and ADHD-related impairments such as oppositional and defiant behavior [66, 67], conduct problems, poor social skills [67, 68], and academic achievement [68]. Behavioral interventions can be implemented at home and/or school, each with the goal of increasing desirable behaviors and decreasing problem behaviors.

15.6.2.1 Behavioral Parent Training

Behavioral parent training is an empirically supported treatment to address ADHD symptoms [66, 67, 69, 70], where parents learn behavior modification techniques [69]. Typically, BPT is a manualized treatment that ranges from 8 to 12 sessions [71]. It can be implemented in a group or individualized treatment [70, 72]. During BPT, parents are provided instruction by his/her therapist, the therapist models the skills, and then the parent practices the skill with his/her child while receiving feedback from the therapist. Problem-solving, using behavioral techniques outside the home, and planning for future misbehavior is also covered during BPT [70, 72, 73].

15.6.2.2 Behavior Classroom Management

Teachers should implement behavioral strategies in their classroom to reduce ADHD symptoms and ADHD-related behaviors [74]. Classroom management increases academic productivity, peer relations, and adaptive behavior while decreasing oppositional behavior and aggression [75]. Behavioral classroom interventions are similar to those implemented with BPT. Specifically, teachers implement classroom rules, time-outs, and other response cost interventions to decrease negative behaviors [75, 76]. Additionally, teachers use positive reinforcement strategies such as a point system, token economy, and positive praise [77]. Clinicians can provide consultations with teachers in order to assist with implementing classroom management procedures [68, 72].

15.6.2.3 Social Skills Training

Children with ADHD often have poor social skills and are rejected by their peers [78]. Studies indicate that behavioral treatments help improve social skills in individuals with ADHD [65, 79, 80]. Social skills training are often taught in a group setting [80]. In social skills training, children are taught skills such as good sportsmanship, assertiveness, dealing with teasing, making friends, playing with others [81], conversational skills [82], contacts with adults at home and school, handling problem situations [82], sharing, listening skills, giving and receiving compliments, and accepting negative consequences [80]. After children are taught these skills and instructors model how to use them, children practice these skills in session and receive feedback from the instructor and/or peers [80, 83]. To assist with generalization, children are assigned homework. Some programs implement reinforcement such as point systems, positive praise [82], and tangible rewards [79] to further increase utilization of skills.

15.6.2.4 Skills Training for Executive Functioning Deficits

Children with ADHD often have poor executive functioning, resulting in difficulty with organization and planning [84]. Impaired executive functioning results in misplacing homework assignments, failure to turn in completed assignments [85, 86], forgetting to bring materials home [85], careless mistakes, poor planning for tests [86], difficulty tracking assignments, poor time management, and forgetting class materials which in turn negatively impacts academic performance [82]. A combination of skills training and behavioral techniques has been shown in the literature to improve organizational and planning skills.

In addition to having planning and organizational problems, individuals with ADHD often have deficits in their working memory, which is the ability to hold information in one's mind and manipulate it [87, 88]. Working memory deficits are associated with lower academic achievement and behavioral problems [88]. As such, studies have examined how to improve working memory deficits through working memory training (WMT). The most common working memory training program used in studies, Cogmed, has been shown to improve working memory [89–91]. However, long-term studies suggest that the increase in working memory do not persist past 24 months [89]. Despite the improvement in working memory, studies indicate that Cogmed does not increase academic achievement [89, 90] or improve ADHD symptoms of inattention, impulsivity, or hyperactivity [90, 92].

15.6.2.5 Multimodal Treatments

When children with ADHD do not respond to BPT, behavior classroom management, organization skills training, or social skills training alone, clinicians can combine multiple behavioral treatments in order to target treatment-resistant ADHD. In fact, multimodal treatments are the most effective treatment for ADHD [74]. The most well-known multimodal treatment is the summer treatment program (STP). STP is an intensive program that combines behavioral therapy and medication management that has strong empirical support to reduce symptoms of ADHD

[67, 68, 77, 93]. STP ranges from 6 to 9 weeks and is for individuals between the ages of 5 and 16 years old.

15.6.3 Investigational/Complementary

Current conventional treatments for ADHD in children and adolescents have limitations. Although stimulants are known to be significantly efficacious, it is estimated that 10–30% of patients will not respond or cannot tolerate adverse effects [94, 95]. Stimulants also do not provide 24-h coverage. Non-stimulants can provide all-day coverage but are generally less effective [96]. Additionally, many geographic areas lack availability of behavioral therapy providers, or families and teachers have difficulty committing the amount of time required for behavioral interventions [97]. These limitations have prompted research to identify additional therapies. Parents, families, and patients are often interested in nontraditional therapies and may be utilizing one or more without physician awareness. One study found 54% of parents reported using complementary and alternative medicines to treat their child with ADHD, but only 11% of parents reported discussing CAM use with their child's physician. The most frequent CAM therapies were expressive therapies (sensory integration, occupational therapy, art, music, etc.), vitamins, and dietary restrictions such as the elimination of sugar and food additives [98]. Families and patients not using CAM may often be curious about such therapies but reluctant to broach the subject with the physician. Information that is not always accurate is widely disseminated through the Internet and social media. It behooves the practitioner to be prepared to discuss the topic of CAM and be well-informed regarding the potential benefits and risks of investigational and complementary treatments.

15.6.3.1 Dietary/Nutritional

A 2014 review by Hurt et al. found that some children with ADHD have documented deficiencies, or more commonly insufficiencies, of minerals such as iron, magnesium, and zinc and vitamins such as vitamin D. Review of data from the US Department of Agriculture suggests that the average American consumes less than the recommended daily intake of vitamin E, calcium, folate, vitamin A, and magnesium. If a deficiency/insufficiency of vitamins and minerals is suspected, a careful dietary history should be performed, especially in children who do not have well-balanced diets and/or stimulant-related appetite suppression. If a thorough history, physical examination, and laboratory testing indicate deficiencies/insufficiencies, supplementation is recommended with careful monitoring for adverse effects such as constipation and diarrhea [99].

Dietary treatments have been commonly used by parents and families in treating children with ADHD. Two common therapies include restricted elimination diets (RED) and artificial food color elimination (AFCE). These diets rely on careful control of dietary ingestion of food ingredients to which the child may have demonstrated hypersensitivity with worsening of ADHD symptoms. The results of the efficacy of RED are somewhat promising, but more large-scale trials using unselected (those not already suspected of being responders) subjects and blinded assessments and examining long-term outcomes will need to be performed before recommending this therapy. Similarly, the evidence for AFCE is currently limited, but further research using unselected subjects and blinded assessments is required before using as a standardized treatment [100].

15.6.3.2 Natural Supplements/Herbal Remedies

A number of systematic reviews have found small to moderate effect sizes for polyunsaturated fatty acids (PUFA), with the thought that omega-3 fatty acids protect against neuro-inflammation and by the modulation of dopamine and serotonin neurotransmission in the frontal cortex [101]. In these reviews, eicosapentaenoic acid (EPA) was highly associated with efficacy [102]. Limitations in studies looking at omega-3 fatty acids include many studies being underpowered and the lack of consistent dosing and formula [103]. Efficacy with PUFA is still inferior to conventional medications. The current data suggests use of PUFA for treatment of ADHD should be limited to mild cases and as adjunct treatment with conventional pharmacologic agents in severe cases [99, 102, 103].

Although a number of studies have examined the safety and efficacy of natural supplements and herbal remedies, the results are mixed. Ahn et al. reviewed clinical studies evaluating the safety and efficacy of a variety of nutritional and herbal supplements. This review of studies included botanical agents, vitamins, minerals, amino acids, essential fatty acids, and emerging natural product-derived treatments from preclinical studies. A major limitation of comparing these agents to standard medications in clinical trials is the lack of standardization of herbal supplements that make it difficult to determine purity, safety, and toxicity profiles. Although many of the botanical agents showed promise, the authors conclude that due to the complexity and heterogeneity of ADHD, a combination therapy of standard pharmacologic agents, a botanical or nutritional supplement, and behavioral therapy may yield the most positive outcomes. It should be noted that naturally derived supplements can still have bothersome side effects, and some agents, such as St. John's wort, can have significant interactions with psychotropic medications [97, 102].

15.6.3.3 Investigational Drugs

A number of novel stimulant and non-stimulant drugs are currently being examined. New stimulant delayed- and extended-release preparations being investigated are designed to improve early morning symptoms and extend coverage throughout the day [96], including HLD200, a methylphenidate formulation with combination delayed- and extended-release delivery allowing for evening administration with release beginning in the morning (after an 8- or 9-h delay) and occurring throughout the day [104]. Investigational non-stimulants include drugs that target reuptake and transportation of serotonin, norepinephrine, and dopamine and agents targeting novel receptors such as betahistine hydrochloride (H1 agonist and H3 antagonist), V81444 (adenosine A2a antagonist), and tipepidine hibenzate (inhibits G-protein coupled inwardly rectifying potassium [GIRK]-channel currents) [96].

15.6.3.4 Noninvasive Brain Stimulation

Noninvasive brain stimulation consists of transcranial magnetic stimulation (TMS) and transcranial direct current stimulation (repetitive transcranial magnetic stimulation [rTMS]) and has potential diagnostic and therapeutic application in a number of neuropsychiatric disorders in children, including Tourette's syndrome and autism spectrum disorder [105]. However, there are limited well-designed trials examining the safety and efficacy of noninvasive brain stimulation in children and adolescents with ADHD. Although the highly neuroplastic developing brain has the potential for responding to neuromodulation, there are potential risks associated with this intervention, including seizure risk, as well as potential for commercial misuse [106]. In 2009, a consensus conference committee reviewed safety and ethical issues in TMS clinical use and recommended that single- and paired-pulse TMS is likely safe in patients aged 2 and older, but there is not enough data to recommend safe use of rTMS in pediatric patients [107]. Further research will need to be performed before noninvasive brain stimulation becomes a standard treatment for ADHD in children and adolescents.

15.6.3.5 Neurofeedback

Neurofeedback training (NFT) is gaining support after a number of clinical trials have demonstrated improvement in behavior, attention, and neuropsychological test performance [108]. NFT involves self-regulation of brain activity patterns by utilizing EEG biofeedback of brain waves. The improvement with neurofeedback training rests on theorized neurophysiological changes occurring in children and adolescents with ADHD. These trials have been criticized, however, for lack of control groups and low power [109]. Despite this, neurofeedback training appears to be a promising and valid option for treating ADHD, but further studies illuminating treatment protocol and predictors of response are necessary [110].

15.7 Treatment Resistance

ADHD is considered to be one of the most highly treatable psychiatric disorders. Approximately 75–90% of patients will respond to some form of pharmacotherapy, although not necessarily on the first trial [111]. However, despite the wealth of evidence of a number of treatments for children and adolescents with ADHD, not every child or teen will respond. There is no standard definition of ADHD treatment resistance in the literature, but as noted previously, it is estimated that 10–30% of patients may not respond to any stimulant treatment [94]. Although it is difficult to define "inadequate response" to treatment in clinical research, it may best be thought of as a response that does not sufficiently improve core ADHD symptoms to the point of improving overall functioning [112]. Additionally, treatment failure may best be defined as failure to reach treatment goals despite the maximum, therapeutic dose of medication or experiencing intolerable side effects [63]. If the treating physician determines that a patient is not responding well to pharmacologic treatment, a few factors may need to be addressed before moving forward.

Firstly, the issue of adherence should be discussed. Child nonadherence to ADHD medications can range from 15% to 87% [113]. A different review found that in community samples, only a third to two-thirds of children and adolescents with ADHD consistently take stimulant medications and that, on average, families do not persist in medication use beyond 1 year [114]. Rates of adherence appear higher in clinical research samples. For example, in the 3-year follow-up of the NIH MTA study, 71% of the sample continued immediate-release stimulant medication for up to 3 years [115]. Long-acting stimulants are generally associated with higher rates of adherence [113, 116], but more research is needed to assess adherence over an extended period of time [114]. Many factors impact adherence including, but not limited to, adverse effects, parent-child dynamics, comorbid oppositional defiant disorder, and perceived lack of effectiveness, and these factors will need to be addressed before progressing in the treatment algorithm.

Diversion or misuse of stimulants should also be considered in cases of apparent treatment resistance. In a recent study, 16% of parents reported diverting their child's stimulants, predominantly to themselves but sometimes to other household family members, and another 13% reported being tempted to self-administer their child's stimulant medication [117]. The prevalence of nonmedical use of stimulants is believed to be approximately 5–10% of high school students [118]. If parent or peer diversion is a strong concern, it is recommended that the prescriber closely monitor prescription refills or switch to a long-acting stimulant or non-stimulant [61, 119].

If a patient is deemed to be adherent to medications, the dosing may need to be optimized for weight, and, if a patient is on an IR formulation, the number of administrations may need to be increased. Table 15.2 lists dosage guidelines per weight and administration schedule for each ADHD medication, including stimulants and non-stimulants. Considering duration of treatment time is also important, especially if the patient is using atomoxetine. One review of open-label studies found a median response time of 4 weeks of treatment with atomoxetine with full remission (defined as an ADHD-RS-IV score ≤ 18) having a median response time of 8 weeks and probability of remission reaching 85% at 52 weeks [120]. Although stimulants can provide relatively immediate benefits, observation of symptoms should take place over at least a week to fully assess any pattern changes in behavior. Again, core symptom rating scales completed by caregivers and other adults across settings can provide a more objective appraisal of medication response. If not already done so, it may also be beneficial to educate families regarding realistic expectations for improvement and developmentally appropriate symptoms versus pathological symptoms.

If symptoms have not responded to a therapeutic medication dose and/or schedule, it may be worthwhile at this point to reassess diagnosis and rule out alternative causes of symptoms [30]. ADHD, and even more, ADHD plus stimulants, may impair sleep, and sleep deprivation can negatively affect attention. Other behavioral effects may occur such as irritability with amphetamines. Possible comorbid diagnoses may also need to be reconsidered as co-occurring conditions can have an impact on response to treatment. For example, a review of the literature suggests fewer subjects with autism spectrum disorder are considered "responders" to stimulant medication, treatment effects are slightly smaller, and adverse effects are more common than in the non-ASD population [38]. However, effect sizes with stimulants are still statistically significant. If ADHD is the predominant, established diagnosis, treatment can proceed in a stepwise progression, preferably with only one medication change at a time.

Several factors have been identified in treatment-refractory patients including caregiver psychiatric illness. In a study examining moderators of treatment response in the MTA, parental depression was associated with decreased response in the medication management group but not combined or behavioral treatment only [121]. The authors theorize that since the behavioral treatment groups involve group and individual parent training, parental depression is, in a sense, treated. For patients in families requiring public assistance, the MTA data suggests evidence-based medication management plus intensive home- and school-based behavioral therapy may be necessary to see benefits in social skills and peer relationships [43].

Patient characteristics such as subaverage IQ, higher baseline symptom severity, and medical comorbidities that impair fronto-striatal function (e.g., TBI, epilepsy, etc.) are also associated with treatment-resistant ADHD. For patients with higher baseline symptom severity, early nonpharmacologic intervention, such as parent training programs through Head Start or other public prekindergarten programs, may help reduce ADHD symptom severity [30, 121]. However, the MTA data found only 10% of patients with the combination of parental depression, lower IQ, and higher symptom severity achieved an excellent response to treatment [121]. Emotional lability has also been linked with worse outcomes and multiple modality treatments [122].

Despite the use of medication and behavioral treatments, some youth with ADHD and comorbid disruptive behavior disorders will continue to exhibit aggressive behaviors. In patients with comorbid ODD, a stimulant plus behavioral therapy is considered first-line treatment, and alpha agonists may be added if symptoms persist [35]. Several studies have shown the combination of a stimulant with the extended-release formulations of clonidine and guanfacine was significantly effective for patients with complicated ADHD [94]. For ADHD with comorbid conduct disorder, multisystemic therapy is the only behavioral intervention determined to be effective [35]. Atypical antipsychotics should only be considered for ADHD with disruptive behavior disorders if behavioral interventions plus standard ADHD treatments (stimulants, atomoxetine, and alpha agonists) have failed and significant aggressive behaviors are present [123].

There has been much interest in examining pharmacogenetic factors in ADHD treatment resistance, and a relatively large number of studies have examined ADHD pharmacogenomics compared to other mental health disorders [124]. Bruxel et al. performed a systematic review of ADHD pharmacogenetics studies. Most genes studied involved the catecholamine pathway and have focused on methylphenidate response. The most studied polymorphism involves the dopamine transporter gene (DAT1 or SLC6A3) [123]. The authors found that there were conflicting results and that, overall, findings did not consistently support a gene-drug interaction for this polymorphism. Other genes studied in the child population included the dopamine receptor D4 (DRD4), the COMT enzyme, the norepinephrine transporter (NET1), the adrenergic alpha-2A receptor, the serotonin transporter (5HTT), the synaptosomal-associated protein 25 (SNAP-25), the brain-derived neurotrophic factor (BDNF), and, a relatively recent gene studied, the latrophilin 3 (LPHN3). Findings for these polymorphisms again were inconsistent, and the authors conclude that polymorphisms have small effect sizes in predicting methylphenidate response. However, the results from gene candidate studies and genome-wide association studies for NET1 and LPHN3 were promising and should be further investigated [124, 125].

Some early studies on gene-environment interactions found evidence for an association between maternal stress and maternal smoking during pregnancy and reduced response to methylphenidate in patients with gene variants involved in the dopamine pathway [124, 126]. Studies have also examined interactions between drug metabolism genes and medications. A systematic review of candidate genes associated with methylphenidate-related adverse effects was conducted by Joensen et al. and found a number of genes associated with significant adverse effects, including appetite reduction, emotionality, irritability, and picking. However, methodology of these studies was limited by small sample sizes, lack of standardization of treatment regimens, and short-term outcome assessments. More randomized, controlled studies of significant power examining long-term outcomes are needed [127].

Additionally, neuroimaging studies have examined association between neurobiological structure and function and treatment response, specifically involving the prefrontal circuitry, the corpus callosum, and the caudate and accumbens nuclei. Some studies have reported association of homozygosity of the 10-repeat allele form of DAT1 with higher DAT density and better response with methylphenidate than in those without 10-repeat homozygosity [125, 128, 129]. The emerging evidence appears promising for identifying biomarkers predicting treatment response; however, further research will need to be performed to recommend pharmacogenomics and/or neuroimaging as a standard component of treatment planning.

15.8 Conclusion/Future Directions

ADHD in children and adolescents is a widely prevalent and potentially chronic, debilitating disorder, affecting 5–10% of US youth and resulting in poorer functioning compared to youth without ADHD. Its etiology is complex and multifactorial, and there is impressive heterogeneity in clinical presentation of the disorder. This can lead to overdiagnosis in some populations and underdiagnosis in others. Therefore, assessment of ADHD requires a thorough history from multiple adults involved in the youth's care, should be based on DSM-5 criteria, and ideally incorporates rating scales at baseline and periodically to monitor response to treatment. Psychiatric conditions that mimic ADHD symptoms as well as co-occurring psychiatric disorders should be considered at initial assessment and if patients show minimal or only partial response to standard treatments.

Treatment of ADHD in preschool-aged children should start with behavioral interventions such as parent management training, and methylphenidate can be added if an adequate trial of therapy fails. In older children, a stimulant is considered first-line therapy, and if a trial with one stimulant fails, a stimulant from a different category should be trialed. Atomoxetine can be trialed as monotherapy, or in combination with a stimulant in select cases, if stimulants fail. The alpha-2 agonists can be used in combination with stimulants for patients who do not respond to stimulant or atomoxetine monotherapy. Bupropion and tricyclic antidepressants are reserved for the most treatment-resistant cases, although data for these agents in ADHD is limited and the risk of adverse effects may outweigh treatment benefits (see Fig. 15.1 for an evidence-based treatment algorithm by severity). For youth with co-occurring anxiety disorders, disruptive behavior disorders with aggression, and/or lower socioeconomic status, intensive behavioral interventions combined with medications may have better long-term outcomes. In youth with co-occurring ODD and CD with aggression, agents such as atypical antipsychotics and

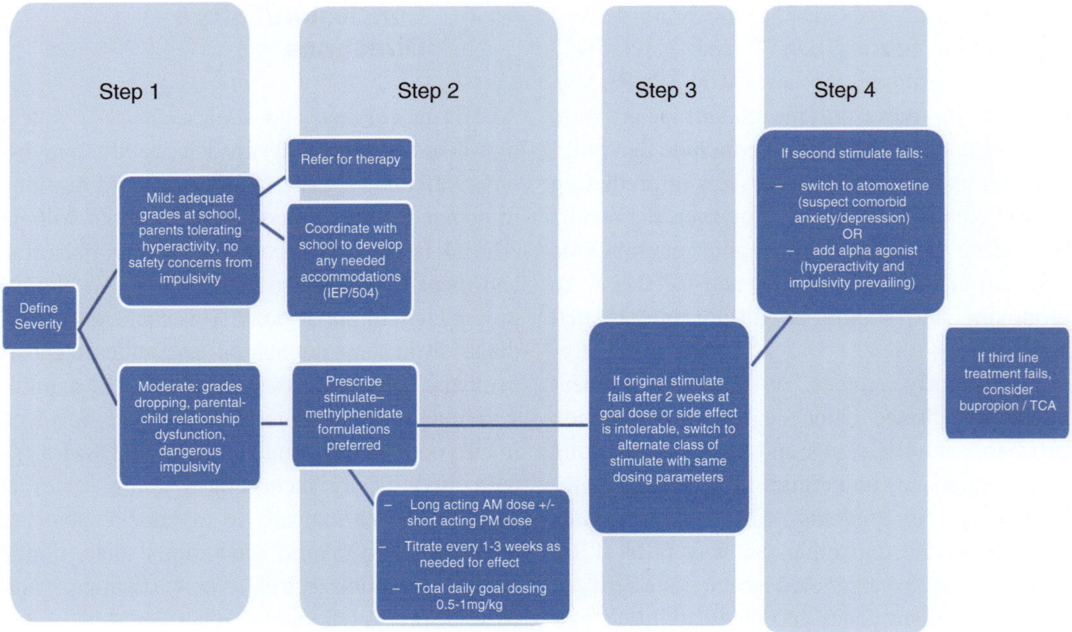

Fig. 15.1 Evidence-based treatment by severity

divalproex sodium can sometimes be used to treat the aggression separately.

Standard pharmacologic and nonpharmacologic treatments will not benefit a minority of patients. Factors that have been associated with worse pharmacologic treatment outcomes include caregiver depression and higher baseline ADHD symptom severity, and, when both of those factors were combined, subaverage IQ may be an additional factor. For these treatment-resistant patients, well-delivered evidence-based medication management combined with psychosocial interventions may be necessary to see responses to treatment. Other moderating factors may be the presence of co-occurring anxiety disorders and conduct disorder symptoms as these patients have shown significant benefit with behavioral therapy alone or in combination with medication management. Investigational therapies such as cognitive training, noninvasive brain stimulation, and neurofeedback training have limited evidence currently and are not recommended as standard treatment. Studies examining pharmacogenomic and/or neurobiological factors have shown promise in the potential for using personalized medicine in treating ADHD, but further studies are needed to incorporate these tools as part of a standardized treatment plan.

References

1. Pliszka S, Bernet W, Bukstein O, Walter HJ, Arnold V, Beitchman J, et al. Practice parameter for the assessment and treatment of children and adolescents with attention-deficit/hyperactivity disorder. J Am Acad Child Adolesc Psychiatry. 2007;46(7):849–921.
2. American Psychiatric Association. Diagnostic and statistical manual of mental disorders: DSM-5. 5th ed. Arlington: American Psychiatric Publishing. p. 59–60.
3. Visser SN, Danielson ML, Bitsko RH, Holbrook JR, Kogan MD, Ghandour RM, et al. Trends in the parent-report of health care provider-diagnosed and medicated attention-deficit/hyperactivity disorder: United States, 2003–2011. J Am Acad Child Adolesc Psychiatry. 2014;53(1):14–6.
4. Thapar A, Cooper M. Attention deficit hyperactivity disorder. Lancet. 2016;387:1240–50.
5. Polanczyk G, de Lima MS, Horta BL, Biederman J, Rohde LA. The worldwide prevalence of ADHD: a systematic review and metaregression analysis. Am J Psychiatry. 2007;164:942–8.
6. Akutagava-Martins GC, Rohde LA, Hutz MH. Genetics of attention-deficit/hyperactivity disorder: an update. Expert Rev Neurother. 2016;16(2):145–56.

7. Biederman J, Mick E, Faraone SV. Age-dependent decline of symptoms of attention deficit hyperactivity disorder: impact of remission definition and symptom type. Am J Psychiatry. 2000;157:816–8.
8. Faraone SV, Biederman J, Mick E. The age-dependent decline of attention deficit hyperactivity disorder: a meta-analysis of follow-up studies. Psychol Med. 2006;36(2):159–65.
9. Willcutt EG. The prevalence of DSM-IV attention-deficit/hyperactivity disorder: a meta-analytic review. Neurotherapeutics. 2012;9:490–9.
10. Birnbaum HG, Kessler RC, Lowe SW, Secnik K, Greenberg PE, Leong SA, et al. Costs of attention deficit-hyperactivity disorder (ADHD) in the US: excess costs of persons with ADHD and their family members in 2000. Curr Med Res Opin. 2005;21(2):195–206.
11. Usami M. Functional consequences of attention-deficit hyperactivity disorder on children and their families. Psychiatry Clin Neurosci. 2016;70:303–17.
12. Martin A, Volkmar FR. Lewis's child and adolescent psychiatry: a comprehensive textbook. 4th ed. Philadelphia: Wolters Kluwer; 2007. p. 441.
13. Bernard S, Faraone SV, Cortese S, Kerridge BT, Pallanti S, Wang S, et al. The lifetime impact of attention-deficit hyperactivity disorder: results from the national epidemiologic survey on alcohol and related conditions. Psychol Med. 2012;42(4):875–87.
14. Harpin V, Mazzone L, Raynaud JP, Kahle J, Hodgkins P. Long-term outcomes of ADHD: a systematic review of self-esteem and social function. J Atten Disord. 2016;20(4):295–305.
15. Hechtman L, Swanson JM, Sibley MH, Stehli A, Owens EB, Mitchell JT, et al. Functional adult outcomes 16 years after childhood diagnosis of attention-deficit/hyperactivity disorder: MTA results. J Am Acad Child Adolesc Psychiatry. 2016;55(11):945–52.
16. Tarver J, Daley D, Sayal K. Attention-deficit hyperactivity disorder (ADHD): an updated review of the essential facts. Child Care Health Dev. 2014;40(6):762–74.
17. Faraone SV, Perlis RH, Doyle AE, Smoller JW, Goralnick JJ, Holmgren MA, et al. Molecular genetics of attention-deficit/hyperactivity disorder. Biol Psychiatry. 2005;57:1313–23.
18. Faraone SV, Mick E. Molecular genetics of attention deficit hyperactivity disorder. Psychiatr Clin N Am. 2010;33:159–80.
19. Zhou K, Dempfle A, Arcos-Burgos M, Bakker SC, Banaschewski T, Biederman J. Meta-analysis of genome-wide linkage scans of attention deficit hyperactivity disorder. Am J Med Genet B Neuropsychiatr Genet. 2008;147B(8):1392–8.
20. Stahl SM. Stahl's essential psychopharmacology: prescriber's guide. 6th ed. San Diego: Cambridge University Press; 2017. p. 449–55.
21. Sharma A, Couture J. A review of the pathophysiology, etiology, and treatment of attention-deficit hyperactivity disorder (ADHD). Ann Pharmacother. 2014;48(2):209–25.
22. Gizer IR, Ficks C, Waldman ID. Candidate gene studies of ADHD: a meta-analytic review. Hum Genet. 2009;126:51–90.
23. Cortese S. The neurobiology and genetics of attention-deficit/hyperactivity disorder (ADHD): what every clinician should know. Eur J Paediatr Neurol. 2012;16:422–33.
24. Frodl T, Skokauskas N. Meta-analysis of structural MRI studies in children and adults with attention deficit hyperactivity disorder indicates treatment effects. Acta Psychiatr Scand. 2012;125:114–26.
25. Shaw P, Eckstrand K, Sharp W, Blumenthal J, Lerch JP, Greenstein D, et al. Attention-deficit/hyperactivity disorder is characterized by a delay in cortical maturation. PNAS. 2007;104(49):19649–54.
26. Chen L, Hu X, Ouyang L, He N, Liao Y, Liu Q, et al. A systematic review and meta-analysis of tract-based spatial statistics studies regarding attention-deficit/hyperactivity disorder. Neurosci Biobehav Rev. 2016;68:838–47.
27. Cortese S, Kelly C, Chabernaud C, Proal E, Di Martino A, Milham MP, et al. Towards systems neuroscience of ADHD: a meta-analysis of 55 fMRI studies. Am J Psychiatry. 2012;169(10):1038–55.
28. Thapar A, Cooper M, Eyre O, Langley K. Practitioner review: what have we learnt about the causes of ADHD? J Child Psychol Psychiatry. 2013;54(1):3–16.
29. Cortese S, Angriman M, Lecendreux M, Konofal E. Iron and attention deficit/hyperactivity disorder: what is the empirical evidence so far? A systematic review of the literature. Expert Rev Neurother. 2012;12(10):1227–40.
30. American Academy of Pediatrics. ADHD: clinical practice guideline for the diagnosis, evaluation, and treatment of attention-deficit/hyperactivity disorder in children and adolescents. Pediatrics. 2011;128(5):1007–22.
31. Visser S, Zablotsky B, Holbrook JR, Danielson ML, Bitsko RH. Diagnostic experiences of children with attention deficit/hyperactivity disorder. Hyattsville: Natl Health Stat Report; 2015. 8 p. Report no.: 81
32. Chang LY, Wang MY, Tsai PS. Diagnostic accuracy of rating scales for attention-deficit/hyperactivity disorder: a meta-analysis. Pediatrics. 2016;137(3):e20152749.
33. Xiao ZH, Wang QH, Luo TT, Zhong L. Diagnostic value of Vanderbilt ADHD parent rating scale in attention deficit hyperactivity disorder. Zhongguo Dang Dai Er Ke Za Zhi. 2013;15(5):348–52. Chinese
34. Wolraich ML, Bard DE, Neas B, Doffing M, Beck L. The psychometric properties of the Vanderbilt attention-deficit hyperactivity disorder diagnostic teacher rating scale in a community population. J Dev Behav Pediatr. 2013;34:83–93.
35. Austerman J. ADHD and behavioral disorders: assessment, management, and an update from DSM-5. Cleve Clin J Med. 2015;82(11 Suppl 1):S2–7.

36. Larson K, Russ SA, Kahn RS, Halfon N. Patterns of comorbidity, functioning, and service use for US children with ADHD, 2007. Pediatrics. 2011;127:462–70.
37. DuPaul GJ, Gormley MJ, Laracey SD. Comorbidity of LD and ADHD: implications of DSM-5 for assessment and treatment. J Learn Disabil. 2013;46(1):43–51.
38. Antshel KM, Zhang-James Y, Faraone SV. The comorbidity of ADHD and autism spectrum disorder. Expert Rev Neurother. 2013;13(10):1117–28.
39. Coogan AN, Baird AL, Popa-Wagner A, Thome J. Circadian rhythms and attention deficit hyperactivity disorder: the what, the when and the why. Prog Neuro-Psychopharmacol Biol Psychiatry. 2016;67:74–81.
40. El Malhaney N, Gulisano M, Rizzo R, Curatolo P. Tourette syndrome and comorbid ADHD: causes and consequences. Eur J Pediatr. 2015;174:279–88.
41. Spencer AE, Faraone SV, Bogucki OE, Pope AL, Uchida M, Milad MR, et al. Examining the association between posttraumatic stress disorder and attention deficit hyperactivity disorder: a systematic review and meta-analysis. J Clin Psychiatry. 2016;77(1):72–83.
42. Hinshaw SP, Arnold LE. Multimodal treatment study of children with ADHD (MTA) Cooperative Group. WIREs Cogn Sci. 2015;6:39–52.
43. Hinshaw SP, Owens EB, Wells KC, Kraemer HC, Abikoff HB, Arnold LE, et al. Family processes and treatment outcome in the MTA: negative/ineffective parenting practices in relation to multimodal treatment. J Abnorm Child Psychol. 2000;28(6):555–68.
44. MTA Cooperative Group. Moderators and mediators of treatment response for children with ADHD: the MTA study. Arch Gen Psychiatry. 1999;56:1088–96.
45. Feldman HM, Reiff MI. Attention-deficit hyperactivity disorder in children and adolescents. N Engl J Med. 2014;370:838–46.
46. Greenhill L, Kollins S, Abikoff H, et al. Efficacy and safety of immediate-release methylphenidate treatment for preschoolers with ADHD. JAACAP. 2006;45:1284–93.
47. Gleason MM, Egger HL, Emslie GJ, Greenhill LL, Kowatch RA, Lieberman AF, et al. Psychopharmacological treatment for very young children: contexts and guidelines. J Am Acad Child Adolesc Psychiatry. 2007;46(12):1532–72.
48. Felt BT, Christner JG, Kochhar P. Diagnosis and management of ADHD in children. Am Fam Physician. 2014;90(7):456–64.
49. Chan E, Fogler JM, Hammerness PG. Treatment of attention deficit hyperactivity disorder in adolescents: a systematic review. JAMA. 2016;315(18):1997–2008.
50. Spencer TJ, Brown A, Seidman LJ, Valera EM, Makris N, Lomedico A, et al. Effect of psychostimulants on brain structure and function in ADHD: a qualitative literature review of MRI-based neuroimaging studies. J Clin Psychiatry. 2013;74(9):902–17.
51. Brown RT, Amler RW, Freeman WS, Perrin JM, Stein MT, Feldman HM, et al. Treatment of attention-deficit/hyperactivity disorder: overview of the evidence. Pediatrics. 2005;115(6):749–57.
52. Connor DF, Steingard RJ. New formulations of stimulants for attention-deficit hyperactivity disorder. CNS Drugs. 2004;18(14):1011–30.
53. Adesman A. The ADHD Medication Guide [Internet]. Adhdmedicationguide.com. 2018 [cited 29 October 2017]. Available from: http://www.adhdmedicationguide.com/.
54. Spencer TJ, Biederman J, Wilens TE. Medications used for attention-deficit/hyperactivity disorder. In: Dulcan MK, editor. Dulcan's textbook of child and adolescent psychiatry. 2nd ed. American Psychiatric Association Publishing. 2016; p. 711–26.
55. Cortese S, Holtmann M, Banaschewski T, Buitelaar J, Coghill D, Danckaerts M, European ADHD Guidelines Group, et al. Practitioner review: current best practice in the management of adverse events during treatment with ADHD medications in children and adolescents. J Child Psychol Psychiatry. 2013;54(3):227–46.
56. Warikoo N, Faraone SV. Background, clinical features and treatment of attention deficit hyperactivity disorder in children. Expert Opin Pharmacother. 2013;14(14):1885–906.
57. Faraone SV, Biederman J, Morley CP, Spencer TJ. Effect of stimulants on height and weight: a review of the literature. J Am Acad Child Adolesc Psychiatry. 2008;47(9):994–1009.
58. Spencer TJ, Biederman J, Harding M, O'Donnell D, Faraone SV, Wilens TE. Growth deficits in ADHD children revisited: evidence for disorder-associated growth delays? J Am Acad Child Adolesc Psychiatry. 1996;35(11):1460–9.
59. Zachor DA, Roberts AW, Hodgens JB, Isaacs JS, Merrick J. Effects of long-term psychostimulant medication on growth of children with ADHD. Res Dev Disabil. 2006;27(2):162–74.
60. Molina BSG, Hinshaw SP, Arnold LE, Swanson JM, Pelham WE, Hechtman L, MTA Cooperative Group, et al. Adolescent substance use in the Multimodal Treatment Study of attention-deficit/hyperactivity disorder (MTA) (ADHD), as a function of childhood ADHD, random assignment to childhood treatments, and subsequent medication. J Am Acad Child Adolesc Psychiatry. 2013;52(3):250–63.
61. Chang Z, Lichtenstein P, Halldner L, D'Onofrio B, Serlachius A, Fazel S, et al. Stimulant ADHD medication and risk for substance abuse. J Child Psychol Psychiatry. 2014;55(8):878–85.
62. Groenman AP, Schweren LJS, Dietrich A, Hoekstra PJ. An update on the safety of psychostimulants for the treatment of attention-deficit/hyperactivity disorder. Expert Opin Drug Saf. 2017;16(4):455–64.
63. Ravi M, Ickowicz A. Epilepsy, attention-deficit/hyperactivity disorder and methylphenidate: critical

examination of guiding evidence. J Can Acad Child Adolesc Psychiatry. 2016;25:50–8.
64. Pliszka SR, Crismon ML, Hughes CW, Conners CK, Emslie GJ, Jensen PS. The Texas children's medication algorithm project: revision of the algorithm for pharmacotherapy of ADHD. J Am Acad Child Adolesc Psychiatry. 2006;45(6):642–57.
65. Budman CL. The role of atypical antipsychotics for treatment of Tourette's syndrome: an overview. Drugs. 2014;74:1177–93.
66. Pelham WJ, Fabiano GA, Waxmonsky JG, Greiner AR, Gnagy EM, Pelham WI, et al. Treatment sequencing for childhood ADHD: a multiple-randomization study of adaptive medication and behavioral interventions. J Clin Child Adolesc Psychol. 2016;45(4):396–415.
67. MTA Cooperative Group. A 14-month randomized clinical trial of treatment strategies for attention-deficit/hyperactivity disorder. Arch Gen Psychiatry. 1999;56(12):1073–86.
68. Daley D, Van Der Oord S, Ferrin M, Danckaerts M, Doepfner M, Cortese S, et al. Behavioral interventions in attention-deficit/hyperactivity disorder: a meta-analysis of randomized controlled trials across multiple outcome domains. J Am Acad Child Adolesc Psychiatry. 2014;53(8):835–47.
69. Chronis AM, Chacko A, Fabiano GA, Wymbs BT, Pelham WJ. Enhancements to the behavioral parent training paradigm for families of children with ADHD: review and future directions. Clin Child Fam Psychol Rev. 2004;7(1):1–27.
70. Fabiano GA, Pelham WJ, Coles EK, Gnagy EM, Chronis-Tuscano A, O'Connor BC. A meta-analysis of behavioral treatments for attention-deficit/hyperactivity disorder. Clin Psychol Rev. 2009;29(2):129–40.
71. Evans SW, Owens JS, Bunford N. Evidence-based psychosocial treatments for children and adolescents with attention-deficit/hyperactivity disorder. J Clin Child Adolesc Psychol. 2014;43(4):527–51.
72. Barkley RA. Defiant children. New York: The Guilford Press; 2013.
73. Pfiffner LJ, Haack LM. Behavior management for school-aged children with ADHD. Child Adolesc Psychiatr Clin N Am. 2014;23(4):731–46.
74. Pelham WJ, Wheeler T, Chronis A. Empirically supported psychosocial treatments for attention deficit hyperactivity disorder. J Clin Child Psychol. 1998;27(2):190–205.
75. Schoenfelder EN, Sasser T. Skills versus pills: psychosocial treatments for ADHD in children and adolescents. Pediatr Ann. 2016;45(10):367–72.
76. Carlson CL, Pelham WE, Milich R, Dixon J. Single and combined effects of methylphenidate and behavior therapy on the classroom performance of children with attention-deficit hyperactivity disorder. J Abnorm Child Psychol. 1992;20(2):213–32.
77. Fabiano GA, Schatz NK, Pelham WJ. Summer treatment programs for youth with ADHD. Child Adolesc Psychiatr Clin N Am. 2014;23(4):757–73.
78. Landau S, Moore LA. Social skill deficits in children with attention-deficit hyperactivity disorder. School Psych Rev. 1991;20(2):235–51.
79. Sheridan SM, Dee CC, Morgan JC, McCormick ME, Walker D. A multimethod intervention for social skills deficits in children with ADHD and their parents. School Psych Rev. 1996;25(1):57–76.
80. De Boo GM, Prins PM. Social incompetence in children with ADHD: possible moderators and mediators in social-skills training. Clin Psychol Rev. 2007;27(1):78–97.
81. Haack LM, Villodas M, McBurnett K, Hinshaw S, Pfiffner LJ. Parenting as a mechanism of change in psychosocial treatment for youth with ADHD, predominantly inattentive presentation. J Abnorm Child Psychol. 2017;45(5):841–55.
82. Abikoff H, Hechtman L, Klein RG, Gallagher R, Fleiss K, Etcovitch J, et al. Social functioning in children with ADHD treated with long-term methylphenidate and multimodal psychosocial treatment. J Am Acad Child Adolesc Psychiatry. 2004;43(7):820–9.
83. Hantson J, Wang PP, Grizenko-Vida M, Ter-Stepanian M, Harvey W, Joober R, et al. Effectiveness of a therapeutic summer camp for children with ADHD: phase I clinical intervention trial. J Atten Disord. 2012;16(7):610–7.
84. Bikic A, Reichow B, McCauley SA, Ibrahim K, Sukhodolsky DG. Meta-analysis of organizational skills interventions for children and adolescents with attention deficit/hyperactivity disorder. Clin Psychol Rev. 2017;52:108–23.
85. Langberg JM, Epstein JN, Girio-Herrera E, Becker SP, Vaughn AJ, Altaye M. Materials organization, planning, and homework completion in middle-school students with ADHD: impact on academic performance. Sch Ment Heal. 2011;3(2):93–101.
86. Langberg JM, Epstein JN, Urbanowicz CM, Simon JO, Graham AJ. Efficacy of an organization skills intervention to improve the academic functioning of students with attention-deficit/hyperactivity disorder. Sch Psychol Q. 2008;23(3):407–17.
87. Baddeley A. The fractionation of working memory. Proc Nat Acad Sci USA. 1996;93(24):13468–72.
88. Alloway TP, Gathercole SE, Elliott J. Examining the link between working memory behaviour and academic attainment in children with ADHD. Dev Med Child Neurol. 2010;52(7):632–6.
89. Roberts G, Quach J, Spencer-Smith M, Anderson PJ, Gathercole S, Gold L. Academic outcomes 2 years after working memory training for children with low working memory a randomized trial. JAMA Pediatr. 2016;170(5):1–10.
90. Chacko A, Bedard AC, Marks DJ, Feirsen N, Uderman JZ, Chimiklis A, et al. A randomized clinical trial of Cogmed working memory training in school-age children with ADHD: a replication in a diverse sample using a control condition. J Child Psychol Psychiatry. 2014;55(3):247–55.

91. Dunning DL, Holmes J, Gathercole SE. Does working memory training lead to generalized improvements in children with low working memory? A randomized controlled trial. Dev Sci. 2013;16(6):915–25.
92. Dongen-Boomsma M, Vollebregt MA, Buitelaar JK, Slaats-Willemse D. Working memory training in young children with ADHD: a randomized placebo-controlled trial. J Child Psychol Psychiatry. 2014;55(8):886–96.
93. Pelham WJ, Gnagy EM, Greiner AR, Hoza B, Hinshaw SP, Swanson JM, et al. Behavioral versus behavioral and pharmacological treatment in ADHD children attending a summer treatment program. J Abnorm Child Psychol. 2000;28(6):507–25.
94. Sallee FR. The role of alpha 2-adrenergic agonists in attention-deficit/hyperactivity disorder. Postgrad Med. 2010;122(5):78–87.
95. Barbaresi WJ1, Katusic SK, Colligan RC, Weaver AL, Leibson CL, Jacobsen SJ. Long-term stimulant medication treatment of attention-deficit/hyperactivity disorder: results from a population-based study. J Dev Behav Pediatr. 2014;35(7):448–57.
96. Childress A, Tran C. Current investigational drugs for the treatment of attention-deficit/hyperactivity disorder. Expert Opin Investig Drugs. 2016;25(4):463–74.
97. Ahn J, Seok Ahn H, Hoon Cheong J, dela Pena I. Natural product-derived treatments for attention-deficit/hyperactivity disorder: safety, efficacy, and therapeutic potential of combination therapy. Neural Plast. 2016;2016:1320423.
98. Chan E, Rappaport LA, Kemper KJ. Complementary and alternative therapies in childhood attention and hyperactivity problems. J Dev Behav Pediatr. 2003;24(1):4–8.
99. Hurt EA, Arnold LE. An integrated dietary/nutritional approach to ADHD. Child Adolesc Psychiatr Clin N Am. 2014;23:955–64.
100. Stevenson J, Buitelaar J, Cortese S, Ferrin M, Konofal E, Lecendreux M, European ADHD Guidelines Group, et al. Research review: the role of diet in the treatment of attention-deficit/hyperactivity disorder – an appraisal of the evidence on efficacy and recommendations on the design of future studies. J Child Psychol Psychiatry. 2014;55(5):416–27.
101. Chalon S. Omega-3 fatty acids and monoamine neurotransmission. Prostaglandins Leukot Essent Fat Acids. 2006;75:259–69.
102. Bloch MH, Mulqueen J. Nutritional supplements for the treatment of ADHD. Child Adolesc Psychiatr Clin N Am. 2014;23:883–97.
103. Gow RV, Hibbeln JR, Parletta N. Current evidence and future directions for research with omega-3 fatty acids and attention-deficit/hyperactivity disorder. Curr Opin Clin Nutr Metab Care. 2015;18:133–8.
104. Jain R, Katic A. Current and investigational medication delivery systems for treating attention-deficit/hyperactivity disorder. Prim Care Companion CNS Disord. 2016;18(4) https://doi.org/10.4088/PCC.16r01979.
105. Hameed MQ, Dhamne SC, Gersner R, Kaye HL, Oberman LM, Pascual-Leone A, et al. Transcranial magnetic and direct current stimulation in children. Curr Neurol Neurosci Rep. 2017;17(2):11.
106. Rubio B, Boes AD, Laganiere S, Rotenberg A, Jeurissen D, Pascual-Leone A. Noninvasive brain stimulation in pediatric attention-deficit/hyperactivity disorder: a review. J Child Neurol. 2016;31(6):784–96.
107. Rossi S, Hallett M, Rossini P, Pascual-Leone A, The Safety of TMS Consensus Group. Safety, ethical considerations, and application guidelines for the use of transcranial magnetic stimulation in clinical practice and research. J Clin Neurophysiol. 2009;120:2008–39.
108. Hodgson K, Hutchinson AD, Denson L. Nonpharmacological treatments for ADHD: a meta-analytical review. J Atten Disord. 2014;18(4):275–82.
109. Holtmann M, Pniewski B, Wachtlin D, Worz S, Strehl U. Neurofeedback in children with attention-deficit/hyperactivity disorder (ADHD) – a controlled multicenter study of a non-pharmacological treatment approach. BMC Pediatr. 2014;14:202.
110. Moriyama TS, Polanczyk G, Caye A, Banaschewski T, Brandeis D, Rohde L. Evidence-based information on the clinical use of neurofeedback for ADHD. Neurotherapeutics. 2012;9:588–98.
111. Connolly JJ, Glessner JT, Elias J, Hakonarson H. ADHD & pharmacotherapy: past, present and future: a review of the changing landscape of drug therapy for attention deficit hyperactivity disorder. Ther Innov Regul Sci. 2015;49(5):632–42.
112. Childress AC, Sallee FR. Attention-deficit/hyperactivity disorder with inadequate response to stimulants: approaches to management. CNS Drugs. 2014;28:121–9.
113. Ahmed R, Aslani P. Attention-deficit/hyperactivity disorder: an update on medication adherence and persistence in children, adolescents and adults. Expert Rev Pharmacoecon Outcomes Res. 2013;13(6):791–815.
114. Chacko A, Newcorn JH, Feirsen N, Uderman JZ. Improving medication adherence in chronic pediatric health conditions: a focus on ADHD in youth. Curr Pharm Des. 2010;16:2416–23.
115. Jensen PS, Arnold LE, Swanson JM, Vitiello B, Abikoff HB, Greenhill LL, et al. 3-year follow-up of the NIMH MTA study. J Am Acad Child Adolesc Psychiatry. 2007;46(8):989–1002.
116. Palli SR, Kamble PS, Chen H, Aparasu RR. Persistence of stimulants in children and adolescents with attention-deficit/hyperactivity disorder. J Child Adolesc Psychopharmacol. 2012;22(2):139–48.
117. Pham T, Milanaik R, Kaplan A, Papaioannou H, Adesman A. Household diversion of prescription stimulants: medication misuse by parents of children

with attention-deficit/hyperactivity disorder. J Child Adolesc Psychopharmacol. 2017;27(8):741–6.
118. Clemow DB, Walker DJ. The potential for misuse and abuse of medications in ADHD: a review. Postgrad Med. 2014;126(5):64–81.
119. Martinez-Raga J, Ferreros A, Knecht C, de Alvaro R, Carabal E. Attention-deficit hyperactivity disorder medication use: factors involved in prescribing, safety aspects and outcomes. Ther Adv Drug Saf. 2017;8(3):87–99.
120. Dickson RA, Macki E, Gibbins C, Gutkin SW, Turgay A, Weiss MD. Time courses of improvement and symptom remission in children treated with atomoxetine for attention-deficit/hyperactivity disorder: analysis of Canadian open-label studies. Child Adolesc Psychiatry Ment Health. 2011;11(5):14.
121. Owens EB, Hinshaw SP, Arnold LE, Cantwell DP, Elliot G, Hechtman L. Which treatment for whom for ADHD? Moderators of treatment response in the MTA. J Consult Clin Psychol. 2003;71(3):540–52.
122. van Stralen J. Emotional dysregulation in children with attention-deficit/hyperactivity disorder. ADHD Atten Def Hyp Disord. 2016;8:175–87.
123. Patel BD, Barzman DH. Pharmacology and pharmacogenetics of pediatric ADHD with associated aggression: a review. Psychiatry Q. 2013;84:407–15.
124. Bruxel EM, Akutagava-Martins GC, Salatino-Oliveira A, Contini V, Kieling C, Hutz MH. ADHD pharmacogenetics across the life cycle: new findings and perspectives. Am J Med Genet Part B. 2014;165B:263–82.
125. Shim SH, Yoon HJ, Bak J, Hahn SW, Kim YK. Clinical and neurobiological factors in the management of treatment refractory attention-deficit hyperactivity disorder. Prog Neuro-Psychopharmacol Biol Psychiatry. 2016;70:237–44.
126. Pagerols M, Richarte V, Sanchez-Mora C, Garcia-Martinez I, Corrales M, Corominas M, et al. Pharmacogenetics of methylphenidate response and tolerability in attention-deficit/hyperactivity disorder. Pharm J. 2017;17:98–104.
127. Joensen B, Meyer M, Aagaard L. Specific genes associated with adverse events of methylphenidate use in the pediatric population: a systematic literature review. J Res Pharm Pract. 2017;6(2):65–72.
128. Rohde LA, Roman T, Szobot C, Cunha RD, Hutz MH, Biederman J. Dopamine transporter gene, response to methylphenidate and cerebral blood flow in attention-deficit/hyperactivity disorder: a pilot study. Synapse. 2003;48(2):87–9.
129. Cheon KA1, Ryu YH, Kim JW, Cho DY. The homozygosity for 10-repeat allele at dopamine transporter gene and dopamine transporter density in Korean children with attention deficit hyperactivity disorder: relating to treatment response to methylphenidate. Eur Neuropsychopharmacol. 2005;15(1):95–101.

16 Treatment Resistance in Tourette Syndrome

Renata Rizzo and Mariangela Gulisano

16.1 Introduction

According to the fifth edition of the *Diagnostic and Statistical Manual of Mental Disorders* (*DSM-5*), tics are defined as "sudden, rapid, recurrent, but non-rhythmical motor movements/ and or vocalizations, generally preceded by premonitory urges, that could be simple or complex. The pattern of their severity, intensity, and frequency is typically 'waxing/waning'" [1]. Tics are usually easily recognizable and are preceded by distressing, irresistible sensations/urges (premonitory urges) that typically disappear following tic performance. Nonetheless, these premonitory urges are often experienced as more disturbing than the tics themselves. Tics also vary in severity according to the situation: Boredom or stress is known to increase symptoms, while absorption in a task (e.g. sports, music) is known to reduce symptoms. Tics are suggestible, suppressible, and distractible. In most cases, tics are associated with a transient condition known as provisional tic disorder, as defined in the *DSM-5*. However, when symptoms persist for longer than 12 months, there is a risk of transition to chronicity, at which point patients are diagnosed with persistent tic disorder (Table 16.1).

R. Rizzo (✉) · M. Gulisano
Child and Adolescent Neurology and Psychiatry Clinics, Policlinico, Catania, Italy
e-mail: rerizzo@unict.it

Tourette syndrome (TS)—the most debilitating tic disorder—is a childhood-onset neurodevelopmental disorder characterized by motor and phonic tics lasting for more than 1 year [2]. Motor tics often begin between the ages of 3 and 8, several years before the appearance of vocal tics. Although TS follows a developmental time course in which the frequency of tics tends to decrease by early adulthood [3], many of the most severe and debilitating cases of TS occur in adulthood. Adult-onset tics usually represent recurrences of childhood tics, although some tic disorders other than TS can initially manifest during adulthood [4, 5]. TS can involve echolalia, palilalia, echopraxia, coprophenomena, and involuntary utterances of obscenities, which occur in approximately 10% of clinical cases.

The majority of patients with TS present with psychiatric comorbidities such as attention-deficit/hyperactivity disorder (ADHD), obsessive-compulsive disorder (OCD), and autism spectrum disorders (ASD). Such patients may also present with psychopathologies such as mood disorders, anxiety, substance abuse, childhood conduct disorder, or adult personality disorder [6, 7]. While recent genetic studies have suggested that there are various endophenotypes of TS, more precise clinical and genetic definitions are necessary [8, 9].

Y.-K. Kim (ed.), *Treatment Resistance in Psychiatry*, https://doi.org/10.1007/978-981-10-4358-1_16

Table 16.1 Diagnostic criteria for tic disorders *DSM-5*

Tourette's disorder 307.23 (F95.2)
A. Both multiple motor and one or more vocal tics have been present at some time during the illness, although not necessarily concurrently
B. The tics may wax and wane in frequency but have persisted for more than 1 year since first tic onset
C. Onset is before age 18 years
D. The disturbance is not attributable to the physiological effects of a substance (e.g. cocaine) or another medical condition (e.g. Huntington's disease, postviral encephalitis)
Persistent (chronic) motor or vocal tic disorder 307.22 (F95.1)
A. Single or multiple motor or vocal tics have been present during the illness, but not both motor and vocal
B. The tics may wax and wane in frequency but have persisted for more than 1 year since first tic onset
C. Onset is before age 18 years
D. The disturbance is not attributable to the physiological effects of a substance (e.g. cocaine) or another medical condition (e.g. Huntington's disease, postviral encephalitis)
E. Criteria have never been met for Tourette's disorder
Specify if:
With motor tics only
With vocal tics only
Provisional tic disorder 307.21 (F95.0)
A. Single or multiple motor and/or vocal tics
B. The tics have been present for less than 1 year since first tic onset
C. Onset is before age 18 years
D. The disturbance is not attributable to the physiological effects of a substance (e.g. cocaine) or another medical condition (e.g. Huntington's disease, postviral encephalitis)
E. Criteria have never been met for Tourette's disorder or persistent (chronic) motor or vocal tic disorder
Specifiers: The "motor tics only"or "vocal tics only" specifier is only required for persistent (chronic) motor or vocal tic disorder

16.2 Epidemiology

TS has long been considered relatively rare, with initial prevalence estimates of approximately 5 per 10,000 individuals [10]. However, these early prevalence studies analysed data from severely affected children only. Over the past two decades, there has been a marked increase recognition of TS among paediatricians, neurologists, and psychiatrists. This increase has in turn led to increased awareness regarding the broader spectrum of TS severity. Recent estimates suggest that the prevalence of TS among the general paediatric population (ages 5–18 years) is approximately 1% [11].

16.3 Comorbidity

Only 10–15% of individual patients with TS present with tics only (pure TS) in both clinical [12] and community settings [6, 13, 14], while the remaining patients (approximately 85%) present with comorbid OCD, ADHD, ASD, or other psychopathologies such as conduct disorder, oppositional defiant disorder, and depression [15].

International databases have revealed that tics are strongly associated with additional symptoms and neuropsychiatric comorbidities, with ADHD and OCD being the most common, occurring in approximately 60% and 30% of patients, respectively [12]. Hirschtritt et al. [6] estimated the lifetime prevalence of any psychiatric comorbidity among 1374 individuals with TS to be 85.7%, with 57.7% of patients exhibiting two or more disorders and a mean of 2.1 comorbid disorders. The presence of comorbidities is a challenge for the clinician from both diagnostic and therapeutic points of view [16]. Although the long-term prognosis of pure TS is largely good, outcomes are more severe for patients with comorbid conditions [17]. Among patients with TS, diagnoses of ADHD are associated with increases in maladaptive behaviour and decreased cognitive functioning [18]. Additional studies have indicated that the presence of comorbidities associated with poorer quality of life (QoL) [19]. Eddy et al. [20] reported that high ADHD symptom scores were associated with poorer QoL within the Self and Relationship domains, whereas high OCD symptom scores were associated with more widespread difficulties across the Self, Relationship, Environment, and General domains. Significant differences in QoL may be most likely when both comorbidities are present, and features of OCD and ADHD may exert a differential impact on QoL across individual domains [20].

The endophenotype of OCD in the context of tic disorders differs from that of OCD without tics: The former is associated with more frequent counting, aggressive thoughts, symmetry, and touching, while the latter is associated with more frequent contamination compulsions. Indeed, such obsessive-compulsive tic disorders are associated with earlier symptom onset, male sex, sensory phenomena, and ADHD [21].

Self-injurious behaviour occurs in a minority of patients with TS and has been associated with obsessive tendencies. Likewise, non-obscene socially inappropriate behaviours are more common in adult TS and may be associated with impulse control disorder [7]. In addition, conduct disorders and other disruptive behaviours, such as those associated with oppositional defiant disorder, are strongly linked to comorbid ADHD and impulsivity [22, 23].

Chou et al. [24] reported that patients with TS have a significantly higher risk of developing depression than individuals without TS. More recently, Rizzo et al. [22, 23] demonstrated that depression is common among patients with TS (41.8%) and is associated with tic severity, comorbid ADHD, coexisting anxiety, CDs, and behavioural problems.

ASD has been diagnosed in 5–15% of TS cohorts [22, 23]. In a recent study, Darrow et al. [8, 9] utilized the Social Responsiveness Scale to demonstrate that 2.8% of patients met ASD criteria, although this was primarily due to higher scores on the repetitive and restricted behaviours subscale, highlighting the importance of social communication impairments when diagnosing ASD in children with TS.

16.4 Neurobiology

TS represents a complex and heterogeneous disorder with an equally heterogeneous aetiology. Previous studies have suggested that several genes associated with multiple neural systems—including the dopaminergic, serotonergic, and histaminergic pathways—are involved in the pathogenesis of TS (*DRD2*, *DRD4*, *5-HT2C*, *SERT*). More recent studies have identified several new candidate genes, such as *SLITRK1*, *IMMP2L*, *CNTNAP2*, and *NLGN4* [25].

Although abnormal dopaminergic transmission is involved in the aetiology of tics, it does not explain the presence of comorbidities, suggesting that the noradrenergic and serotoninergic systems are also involved. Neuroimaging studies involving heterogenous patient groups as well as animal studies support the pathological involvement of cortico-striato-thalamo-cortical circuits TS. Recent studies have identified alterations in several brain regions in patients with TS, including the lateral prefrontal cortex (inferior, middle, and superior frontal gyri), anterior cingulate cortex, lateral premotor cortex (precentral gyrus), supplementary motor area (SMA), posterior superior temporal sulcus, supramarginal gyrus, retrosplenial cortex, secondary somatosensory cortex (postcentral gyrus), and lingual gyrus [26]. Such studies have indicated that premonitory urges likely result from altered structure and functional connectivity in the cortico-striatal-thalamic-cortical loop. Evidence from volumetric MRI studies, functional MRI (fMRI), and isotope neurochemical ligand studies also suggests that TS is associated with structural and functional abnormalities in the basal ganglia. However, functional imaging and postmortem studies have failed to identify dopaminergic dysfunction in patients with TS [27, 28], leading some researchers to speculate that imbalances in the serotoninergic, glutamatergic, GABAergic, cholinergic, and opioid systems may be involved.

16.5 Pharmacological Therapy

The current treatment guidelines for the management of TS first recommend psychological education and supportive management, followed by the addition of psychological therapy. Cognitive behavioural therapy (CBT) should be considered as first-line treatment for patients with TS. Psychopharmacological treatments for TS aim to diminish the frequency of tics and improve psychosocial functioning while minimizing adverse effects. Practical management of TS should focus on evaluating tics as well as comorbidities and coexistent conditions (ADHD, OCD, ASD, depression, anxiety, etc.), as these may be more disabling for the patient than the tics themselves. Moreover, it is important to discuss treatment priorities with patients and families to ensure appropriate, individualized treatment for the most disabling symptoms.

The 2011 European guidelines for the pharmacological management of TS recommend the use of the second-generation antipsychotic risperidone as a first-line treatment option [29]. However, despite their efficacy, Canadian and US guidelines only weakly recommend the use of antipsychotics due to their high rates of adverse events, instead recommending first-line treatment with alpha-2 (α_2) adrenergic agonists [30].

To date, three classes of drugs have exhibited efficacy in the treatment of TS: (i) dopamine receptor blockers, which include both typical and atypical antipsychotics (e.g. haloperidol, tiapride, sulpiride, pimozide, risperidone, aripiprazole, etc.), (ii) non-dopaminergic agents (α_2-adrenergic agonists (e.g. clonidine and guanfacine), baclofen, and topiramate), and (iii) vesicular monoamine transporter-2 (VMAT2) inhibitors (tetrabenazine, deutetrabenazine, valbenazine) [31].

16.5.1 Dopamine Receptor Blockers

Antipsychotics such as dopamine-blocking agents and partial agonists have been used in the treatment of TS for several decades. Both typical and atypical antipsychotics are effective treatment options with different efficacy profiles and side effects.

The efficacy of typical antipsychotics (e.g. haloperidol and pimozide) is supported by randomized controlled trials (RCTs), as well as broad clinical experience in treating TS with dopamine-blocking agents [32–34]. However, their use is limited due to severe side effects such as sedation, somnolence, metabolic disturbances, dystonic reaction, hyperprolactinaemia, and menstrual disorders. RCTs have revealed that the atypical antipsychotics risperidone and aripiprazole are as effective in reducing tics as typical antipsychotics [35], with fewer adverse effects [36]. Indeed, a meta-analysis of antipsychotics used for the treatment of TS reported no differences in efficacy among risperidone, haloperidol, pimozide, and ziprasidone [37]. More recently, a comprehensive systematic review of four trials investigating treatments for tics in children and young people with TS and persistent tic disorder found no significant differences in effect sizes among specific antipsychotic drugs (aripiprazole (SMD = −0.62), haloperidol (SMD = 0.50), pimozide (SMD = −0.81), risperidone (SMD = −1.18), ziprasidone (SMD = −0.74)) [35].

Research has indicated that tics also respond to neuroleptic drugs, often using smaller dosages than required for antipsychotics. However, responses vary among patients, and treatment with several agents may be necessary before the most appropriate drug is identified. Pharmacological treatment of tics should be initiated at the lowest doses possible and increased slowly.

16.5.2 Non-dopaminergic Agents

Non-dopaminergic agents such as α_2-adrenergic agonists, clonidine, and guanfacine are often preferred over neuroleptics for first-line treatment in children with TS. Several RCTs have demonstrated that such agents exhibit similar efficacy to that of risperidone [38] and haloperidol [35]. In a meta-analysis regarding the efficacy of α_2-adrenergic agonists on tic suppression in patients with TS, Weisman et al. [37]

concluded that the efficacy of such agents is associated with the presence of ADHD: Patients without ADHD were less responsive to treatment. When prescribing α_2-adrenergic agonists, clinicians must remain aware of the potential for the following side effects: hypotension, sedation, bradycardia, dizziness, sleep problems, and irritability [39].

Baclofen has been used to treat tics since 1999 [40], and its efficacy has been associated with its GABAergic properties, although this remains somewhat controversial. A double-blind placebo-controlled study revealed that patients treated with baclofen exhibited significant decreases in Yale Global Tic Severity Scale (YGTSS) scores, relative to placebo-treated patients [41]. However, a subsequent RCT failed to demonstrate the same results (Jancovic 2010). The following adverse events have also been associated with baclofen treatment: sedation, constipation, nausea, anxiety, and depression.

One positive-controlled trial of the anticonvulsant topiramate, a GABAergic agent that blocks AMA/kainite receptors, reported that patients treated with the agent exhibited significant decreases in YGTSS scores with only mild side effects (weight loss, paraesthesia, headache, and diarrhoea) [4, 5].

16.5.3 Vesicular Monoamine Transporter-2 Inhibitors

The dopamine-depleting agent tetrabenazine blocks the transport of dopamine, norepinephrine, and serotonin from synaptic vesicles to synapses. Currently, three VMAT2 inhibitors have exhibited efficacy in the treatment of TS: tetrabenazine, deutetrabenazine, and valbenazine.

Several long-term and open-label studies have reported that tetrabenazine is effective in reducing tics and improving Clinical Global Impression ratings in patients with TS, with only mild side effects (e.g. sedation, fatigue, nausea, insomnia, parkinsonism, depression, drowsiness) (Porta et al. [42]). Unfortunately, 93% of studies included patients taking concomitant medications [43]. To our knowledge, no RCTs have examined the efficacy of tetrabenazine alone in patients with TS. Nonetheless, evidence indicates that adjunct treatment with tetrabenazine may improve the efficacy of other medications in reducing tics.

Conventional pharmacological treatment options for tics associated with TS are summarized in Table 16.2.

Table 16.2 Conventional treatment options available for tics in TS

Drug	Daily/dosage mg	Efficacy	Adverse events
Haloperidol	0.5–3	Level A	Extrapyramidal effects, anxiety, depression, sedation, anxiety, fatigue, constipation, QTc prolongation, hyperprolactinaemia
Pimozide	0.5–4	Level A	Less extrapyramidal than haloperidol, sedation, moderate weight gain, and QTc prolongation
Aripiprazole	2–20	Level C	Moderate weight gain, metabolic syndrome, extrapyramidal effects, sleep problems, nausea, fatigue, sedation, hypertension
Risperidone	0.25–4	Level A	Weight gain, metabolic syndrome, extrapyramidal effects, somnolence, QTc prolongation
Tiapride and Sulpiride	50–200	Level B	Sedation, hyperprolactinaemia, sleep problems, weight gain
Ziprasidone	20–40	Level B	Sedation, anxiety, sleep problems, akathisia, QTc prolongation
Olanzapine	2.5–10	Level B	Weight gain, metabolic syndrome, extrapyramidal effects, somnolence, QTc prolongation, hypoglycaemia
Quetiapine	50–250	Level C	Weight gain, metabolic syndrome, extrapyramidal effects, somnolence, QTc prolongation
Clonidine	0.025–0.3	Level A	Sedation, bradycardia, hypotension, dry mouth, irritability, headache

(continued)

Table 16.2 (continued)

Drug	Daily/dosage mg	Efficacy	Adverse events
Guanfacine	0.5–3	Level A	Sedation, bradycardia, hypotension, dry mouth, irritability, headache, stomach ache, sleep disturbances
Baclofen	10–60	Not provided	Sedation, constipation, nausea, anxiety, and depression
Topiramate	<200	Not provided	Weight loss, paresthesias
Tetrabenazine	12.5–50	Not provided	Sedation, fatigue, nausea, insomnia, parkinsonism, depression, drowsiness

[a]Modified from Ganos et al. [44]
Efficacy based on the level of evidence established from the European Society for the Study of Tourette Syndrome Treatment Guidelines

16.6 Novel Pharmacological Treatment Options

16.6.1 Cannabinoids

Cannabinoids predominantly act through the CB1 receptor in the central nervous system and the CB2 receptor in immune tissues. Endocannabinoids modulate the activity of excitatory neurotransmitters such as glutamate, inhibitory transmitters such as GABA and glycine, and several monoamines such as dopamine, serotonin, noradrenaline, acetylcholine, and neuropeptides (NOTA). Several case studies and two small controlled trials (NOTE) have documented improvements in TS symptoms and comorbid conditions (i.e. associated behavioural problems such as OCD, attention deficits, impulsivity, and aggression) following cannabinoid use [45]. Evidence suggests that these benefits are due to the specific effects of cannabinoids, rather than secondary mechanisms associated with sedation or decreased general activity. CB1 receptors are highly localized in brain regions thought to be involved in TS pathology and exhibit complex interactions with the dopaminergic system, suggesting that the beneficial effects of cannabinoids are directly mediated via the central CB1 receptor system. Many experts recommend cannabinoids for the treatment of refractory TS.

16.6.2 D1/D5 Receptor Antagonist: Ecopipam

Ecopipam is a selective D1/D5 receptor agonist currently being investigated for its efficacy in the treatment of TS. An 8-week, open-label trial reported that ecopipam treatment resulted in a mean reduction in YGTSS score of 5.2. The principle side effects reported included sedation, fatigue, and insomnia [46]. Recently, Gilbert et al. [47] presented the preliminary results of an ongoing multicentre, double-blind, placebo-controlled trial of ecopipam in children with TS (NCT02102690), reporting decreases in YGTSS scores at 2 and 4 weeks, with moderate side effects.

16.6.3 VMAT2 Inhibitors: Deutetrabenazine (SD-809) and Valbenazine (NBI-98854)

The VMAT2 inhibitors deutetrabenazine and valbenazine are isomers of tetrabenazine that exhibit a longer half-life and have been associated with fewer adverse effects. In a prospective, open-label study, Jankovic et al. [48] evaluated the safety and efficacy of deutetrabenazine in children and adolescents with TS, observing significant decreases in the frequency of tics accompanied by the following side effects: irritability, fatigue, and headache.

Valbenazine is the only VMAT2 inhibitor specifically investigated for its role in the treatment of TS. One open-label phase Ib study, one open-label phase II study, and one randomized placebo-controlled phase IIc study were completed in the USA (NCT02679079, NCT02581865, and NCT02256475), although their results have yet to be reported. A phase II placebo-controlled study is now recruiting in the USA (NCT03325010). Preliminary results indicate that valbenazine treatment significantly improves tic symptoms as measured using the YGTSS, as well as Clinical Global Impression. No serious or severe adverse events have been reported. These preliminary findings suggest that deutetrabenazine and valbenazine are preferable to tetrabenazine with regard to side effects, although further studies of safety and efficacy are required.

16.6.4 Histamine H3 Receptor Antagonist: AZD5213

AZD5213 was developed following the identification of the brain's histaminergic dysregulation in TS [49]. The H3R receptor, which is expressed primarily in the central nervous system, represents a promising pharmacotherapeutic target. In one recently completed placebo-controlled study (NCT01904773), AZD5213 significantly reduced total YGTSS scores in patients treated with high doses (2.0 mg), while no significant effects were observed in patients treated with low doses (0.5 mg). Mild adverse events including palpitations, gastrointestinal disorders, headache, dizziness, constipation, nausea, fatigue, asthenia, vomiting, and irritability have also been associated with AZD5213 treatment (NCT1904773).

Novel pharmacological treatment options for TS are summarized in Table 16.3.

16.7 Treatment of Comorbidity

When present, comorbid symptoms are often more disruptive than tics, and screening for comorbidity is essential for determining therapeutic priorities according to functional impairment.

ADHD is the most common comorbid disorder in children and adolescents with TS. The most effective treatment for ADHD and related oppositional and aggressive behaviours involves the use of psychostimulants. Psychostimulants block the reuptake of dopamine and norepinephrine into presynaptic neurons (methylphenidate) or increase the release of these monoamines into the extraneuronal space (amphetamine). One research group in the USA has demonstrated that methylphenidate is effective in the treatment of ADHD in patients with tics. Although 20% of patients exhibited worsening of tics, no significant difference was observed between methylphenidate and placebo treatment [50]. Psychostimulants should be used as second-line treatment for ADHD symptoms in children with tics, although literature regarding the efficacy of dexamphetamine in patients with tics is lacking. Clonidine or guanfacine rather than psychostimulants can be given as first-line treatment because the α_2 agonists are effective in alleviating symptoms of both disorders, as well as related oppositional behaviour (Rizzo et al. 2017).

First-line treatment for anxiety, depression, and OCD involves CBT, followed by the addition of selective serotonin reuptake inhibitors (SSRIs) if necessary. Treatment recommendations are similar for children with OCD alone. However, patients with TS and comorbid OCD may also benefit from the addition of atypical antipsychotics [51].

16.8 Definition of Treatment Resistance

Although the term treatment-refractory TS is commonly used in research and clinical practice, there has been no consensus regarding its definition. Storch et al. [52] defined optimal treatment response as a decrease in total YGTSS score of at least 35% or a reduction in raw total tic severity score of six to seven points [52]. Severe tics may

Table 16.3 Novel pharmacological treatment options

Drug	Year or status	Age range (years)	Daily dosage (mg)	Length	Phase	Type of study	Clinical trial number
Cannabis	Recruiting	18–65	Not stated	–	II	Double-blind, randomized, placebo-controlled crossover pilot trial	NCT03247244
Nabiximols	Not yet recruiting	>18	Starting dose:	13 weeks	III	Randomized, double-blind, placebo-controlled parallel-group	NCT03087201
			2.7 THC 2.5 CBD maximum dose:				
			32.4 THC 30 CBD				
Dronabinol	Recruiting	18–60	2.5–10	12 weeks	III	Open label	NCT03066193
Deutetrabenazine	Completed	12–18	Not stated	8 weeks	I	Open label	NCT02674321
Valbenazine	Recruiting	6–17	Not stated	12 weeks	IIb	Randomized, double-blind, placebo-controlled	NCT03325010
Valbenazine	Completed	18–64	High and low fix dosage, not stated	8 weeks	II	Randomized, double-blind, placebo-controlled	NCT02581865
Valbenazine	Completed	6–11	3 dosing cohorts	21 days	Ib	Open label	NCT02256475
		12–18	Not stated				
Valbenazine	Completed	6–17	2 dosing cohorts dosage not stated	6 weeks	II	Randomized, double-blind, placebo-controlled	NCT02679079
Ecopipam	2014	>18	50–100	8 weeks	I/II	Open label	NCT01244633
Ecopipam	Ongoing	7–17	Not stated	30 days	II	Randomized, double-blind, placebo-controlled	NCT02102698
AZD5213	2016	12–17	2	6 months	II	Randomized, double-blind, placebo-controlled	NCT01904773
			0.5				

Efficacy measured with statistically significant decrease of YGTSS total score and/or statistically significant improvement of Clinical Global Impression Improvement
THC delta-9-tetrahydro cannabinol, *CBD* cannabidiol

not only lead to serious social problems but also represent a danger to the patient's health, as they may cause repeated trauma to the involved body parts. Several life-threatening TS symptoms have been reported in the literature: death following subdural haematoma due to head banging, paralyses secondary to neck jerking, infections of the oral muscles secondary to biting, and permanently impaired vision due to self-inflicted injuries.

However, the presence of comorbidities is also frequently associated with refractory TS. Cheung et al. [53] reviewed data from a series of 333 patients with TS, 5% of whom had ≥2 emergency room visits or ≥1 hospitalization. Such patients were described as having "malignant TS". When prescribing treatments for TS, clinicians should emphasize the achievement of adequate functioning in the social, occupational, and educational domains, despite the presence of residual tics [54]. It is important to identify patients with refractory TS, as the condition may represent a significant source of disability. A standardised definition of refractoriness to pharmacological treatment of tics in TS and persistent tic disorder would aid in making decisions regarding medication use, psychological treatment, or invasive treatments such as functional surgery [55]. In a European survey by Macerollo et al. [55], a panel of seven expert clinicians judged the following items as "essential" for the definition of refractoriness: dichotomous judgement of improvements in tic severity (improved/not improved), documented changes in the YGTSS severity score, maximum dose reached and reasons for dose increases, and number of single doses missed on average over a 10-day period. In addition, the panel argued that refractoriness should primarily be judged based on lack of efficacy at the highest tolerated dose or lack of tolerability at the initial or effective dose. This survey provides preliminary information that may aid in the development of a consensus-based definition of refractoriness to tic treatment. Lack of tolerability at the initial or effective medication dose resulted in a judgement of refractoriness in at least a third of cases. The authors also reported that a minority of patients could be judged as treatment refractory even when treatment reduced the baseline YGTSS severity sub-score by ≥20%, suggesting that other clinical measures should be considered when evaluating treatment efficacy. Indeed, in some patients, seemingly relevant decreases in tic severity as indicated using an assessment tool may be insufficient for improving QoL and functioning [55].

Over the last 10 years, several guidelines for defining refractory TS and selecting candidates for deep brain stimulation have been proposed by expert medical associations.

In 2006, the Tourette Syndrome Association (TSA) suggested that the term refractory should be applied to patients in whom the following have failed or produced severe side effects: (1) alpha-adrenergic agonists, typical and atypical antipsychotics, and benzodiazepines, (2) concomitant CBT for at least 6 months, and (3) 12 consecutive sessions of habit reversal training (HRT) or exposure prevention (EP). However, the dosage and duration of therapy were not reported. The TSA also recommended adequate, stable, and optimized treatment of concomitant disorders for at least 6 months [56].

The Dutch/Flemish guidelines recommend that at least three medications (including typical and atypical antipsychotics) should be tried at adequate doses for 12 weeks, while other groups have suggested a minimum treatment period of 6 months for TS to be considered medication-refractory. Porta et al. [57] defined "treatment refractoriness" in potential candidates for DBS as failure of the following drugs or severe adverse events after at least 2 years of psychological treatment: typical or atypical antipsychotics, SSRIs, and catecholamine-depleting agents. The Müller-Vahl KR et al. [58] suggested that TS can be considered "treatment resistant" upon the occurrence of adverse events or failure of at least three appropriate pharmacological treatment options (including both typical and atypical antipsychotics) after at least 12 sessions of CBT.

Recently, the Tourette Syndrome Association International Deep Brain Stimulation (DBS) Database and Registry Study Group [59] provided updated opinions and recommendations for the definition of "refractory patient", suggesting the following recruitment criteria for DBS: (a) primary diagnosis of TS in accordance with *DSM-5* criteria; (b) YGTSS >35/50; (c) blinded video-based ratings and assessments of comorbidities over the previous year using validated rating scales for OCD, ADHD, depression, anxiety, and self-injurious behaviour; and (d) failed treatment with alpha-adrenergic agonists, two typical and/or atypical antipsychotics, clonazepam/topiramate/tetrabenazine, and concomitant CBT despite treatment adherence.

In AA opinion, however, several issues must be considered before defining a patient as resistant to pharmacological treatment (Fig. 16.1: Flow chart for refractory TS):

- Clinicians must be sure that the diagnosis of TS is correct and that other symptoms are not incorrectly classified as tics. Differential diagnosis should be performed to exclude paediatric autoimmune neuropsychiatric disorders associated with streptococcal infections (PANDAS), secondary tics, myoclonic jerks, dystonic dyskinesias, paroxysmal dyskinesias, compulsive behaviour, stereotypies, and functional movement disorders [60] (see Table 16.4).
- Treatment failure or severe adverse events for three different pharmacological agents, including both typical and atypical antipsychotics, despite adequate duration and dosage of treatment [29].
- Some individuals who fail to exhibit improvement after adequate treatment at correct doses may respond after additional months of continued treatment.
- Clinicians should remain aware that medical or psychiatric comorbidities may affect treatment responses (e.g. OCD, anxiety, ADHD, etc.) [54].
- Clinicians should ensure that the patient is engaged in appropriate concomitant behavioural therapy (CBT, HRT, and/or EP) with regard to the number of sessions and treatment adherence.

Emerging therapy, including transcranial magnetic stimulation and DBS, may be recommended for patients with correctly identified "refractory" TS (Fig. 16.1).

16.9 Transcranial Magnetic Stimulation

Repetitive transcranial magnetic stimulation (rTMS) is an unintrusive procedure characterized by electrical cortical stimulation generated by small coils positioned over the scalp. Indeed, rTMS has been licenced by several regulatory agencies for the treatment of movement disorders and mood disorder in adults. Recent studies have investigated the use of rTMS in children with neurological and psychiatric diseases whose pathophysiology is associated with cortical over-activation or under-activation [62]. Research has indicated that the SMA is involved in producing voluntary movements, playing a key role in preparing for intentional movements [63]. In the past, fMRI studies have shown that activation of the SMA is responsible for voluntary movements and producing the urge to move [64]. Patients with TS exhibit increased activation in the SMA during motor tasks, and bilateral activation of the SMA is observed before tic performance [65]. Moreover, several fMRI and magnetoencephalography studies involving patients with TS have reported increased connectivity between the SMA and motor cortex prior to tic performance [66]. By utilizing different intensities, frequencies, pulse numbers, and durations of stimulation, rTMS can correct abnormal excitability in patients with TS. In general, frequencies higher than 5 Hz (high) increase cortical excitability, while lower frequencies decrease or inhibit cortical excitability.

Previous studies have demonstrated that rTMS exerts its effects by inhibiting the excitability of interneurons and reducing connectivity between interneurons and cortical neurons. Moreover, rTMS facilitates the production of the inhibitory neurotransmitter GABA, thereby reducing neural

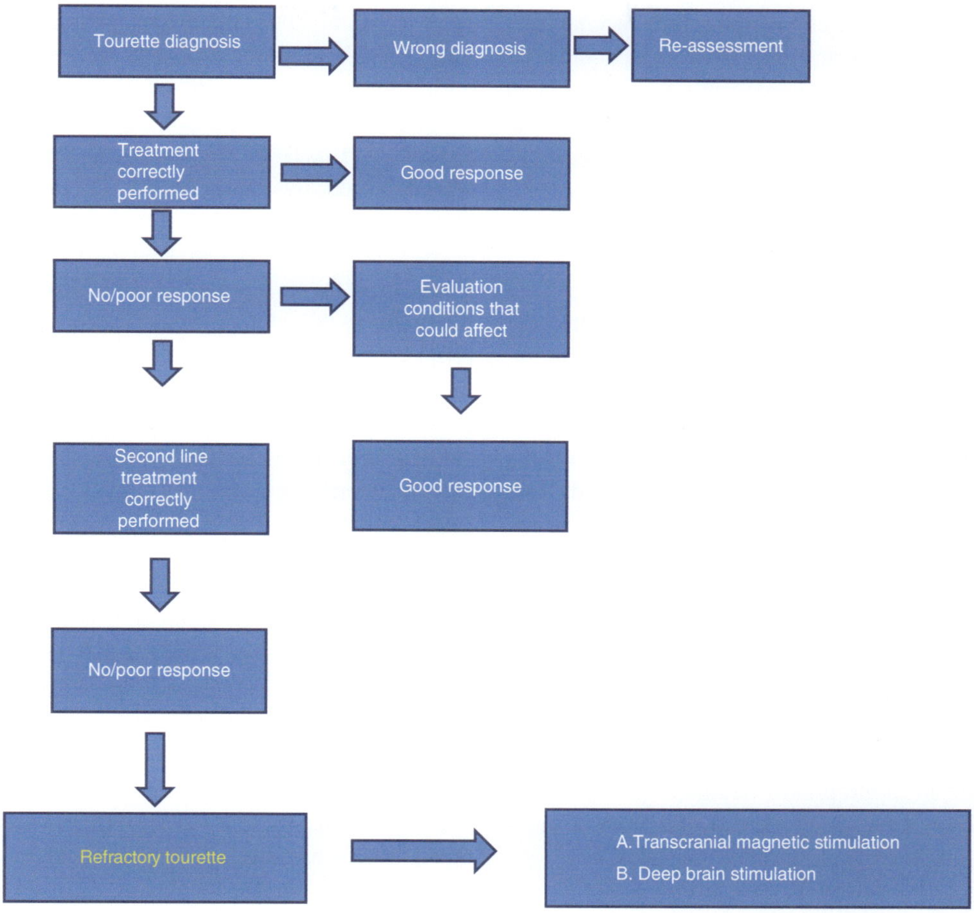

Fig. 16.1 Flow chart for refractory TS

Table 16.4 Differential diagnosis with Tourette syndrome

Disorder	Differences with tics in Tourette syndrome
Other kind of tics	
PANS Chang et al. [61]	(1) Sudden onset (<72 h) of OCD or eating restriction
	(2) At least two qualifying attributes (anxiety, mood or behaviour disturbances, irritability or aggression, developmental regression, deterioration in school performance, sensory or motor abnormalities (tic), and somatic symptoms)
	(3) Lack of a known medical or neurologic disorder to better explain symptoms
Secondary tic disorder	Neurodegenerative conditions (e.g. Wilson's disease, Huntington's disease, neuroacanthocytosis, etc.)
Other symptoms	
Dystonic dyskinesias	Not associated with premonitory urge and not suppressible. Generally simple movement
Stereotypies	Long-lasting/continuous, without premonitory urge, incapacity of suppression
Paroxysmal dyskinesias	Without urge, incapacity of suppression, sudden movement or exercise
Compulsion behaviour	Repetitive movement to complete ritual

Roth [60]
PANS paediatric acute-onset neuropsychiatric syndrome, *OCD* obsessive-compulsive disorder

activity and nerve conduction. Such mechanisms explain the efficacy of rTMS in reducing tic symptoms (as measured using the YGTSS) in both children and adults [67] and in improving comorbid behavioural and depressive symptoms.

16.10 Deep Brain Stimulation

DBS is a good, established chirurgical intervention for patients with severely impairing motor and vocal tics that have been refractory to medical and behavioural therapy. Although DBS is advantageous in that it is non-destructive, reversible, and adjustable [59], data obtained from patients with TS may be difficult to interpret. Given the great phenotypic variability of TS, the selection of the DBS target is particularly complicated and heterogeneous. The potential for DBS to improve patient QoL should be determined on a strictly individual basis while bearing in mind the natural course of the disease as well as the risk/benefit ratio [68]. Although DBS seems an appropriate treatment solution for refractory patients affected by TS, critical questions remain regarding the following:

- Definitions of medication-refractory TS and the selection of candidates for DBS treatment
- Patient age
- Brain regions to be targeted based on different clusters of symptoms
- Stimulation parameters
- Post-operative complications

In order to reach a consensus, experts on DBS in TS have created the International Tourette Syndrome Deep Brain Stimulation Public Database and Registry to share pertinent information regarding DBS. One year after the development of this database, the authors reported that the most effective DBS targets were the (i) anterior globus pallidus internus within the thalamus and the (ii) centromedian-parafascicular complex (both with level A evidence) [69]. Moreover, decreases of 50.5% and 46.3% were observed in YGTSS scores following DBS, respectively. The study revealed that patients treated with DBS were predominantly male and within the age range of 13–58 years, although they presented with complex phenotypes. OCD was the most frequent comorbidity, followed by depression, anxiety, and ADHD. High rates of side effects were reported: dysarthria (6.3%, due to stimulation), paraesthesia (8.2%), and haemorrhage (1.3%). However, rates of adverse events were lower than those reported in previous studies, likely due to the relatively short follow-up period [70]. Implanted patients exhibited higher rates of infection and hardware-related complications [71]. Common adverse events associated with the surgical procedures for DBS included intracerebral haemorrhage (1%) [72], infection (18%) (most commonly *Staphylococcus aureus*), and seroma/haematoma (19.3%) [73].

Adverse events due to stimulation vary depending on the target of stimulation. The most commonly reported adverse events include changes in sexual behaviour (centromedial nucleus, substantia periventricularis nucleo ventro oralis internus) (Temel and Visser-Vandewalle 2003); weight loss (anteromedial globus pallidus internal) [74]; nausea, vertigo, anxiety, and social avoidance (ventromedial globus pallidus internus) [75]; and transient paresthesias (thalamus) [70]).

Although there are multiple ongoing studies investigating the most effective DBS targets for improving tics and comorbid symptoms in patients with TS, further large-scale multicentre studies are required to increase statistical power. Such studies should include systematic assessment of social outcomes as well as longer follow-up periods. The first-year data within the multinational DBS registry support the notion that DBS represents a surgical treatment option for select patients with TS. Clinicians should remain aware of the high number of stimulation-related adverse events, most of which are likely reversible [70].

Conclusions

Although several studies and meta-analyses have reported moderate-to-high efficacy in reducing tics and comorbid symptoms in patients with TS, there are limitations associated with treating patients with refractory TS. To date, evidence-based studies have failed to identify reliable neurobiological factors or clinical markers that contribute to or may aid in the prediction of treatment-refractory TS. The efficacy of treatment for refractory TS is related to several factors: pharmacological efficacy and tolerability, therapist ability, and the patient's capacity to adhere to the treatment. Understanding the differences between patients with TS who experience better treatment outcomes and those with treatment-refractory TS may aid in elucidating the heterogeneity of the disorder. Additional studies should focus on identifying genetic or neuroimaging factors that can be used to determine the most appropriate medications and on developing novel pharmacological interventions to optimize the treatment of patients with TS. Among these novel strategies, rTMS and DBS represent valid therapeutic options for improving QoL in patients with refractory TS.

Acknowledgements and Conflicts of Interest Prof. Rizzo has nothing to disclose. Dr. Gulisano has nothing to disclose.

References

1. Robertson MM. Corrections. A personal 35 year perspective on Gilles de la Tourette syndrome: prevalence, phenomenology, comorbidities, and coexistent psychopathologies. Lancet Psychiatry. 2015;2(4):291.
2. American Psychiatric Association. The fifth edition of the diagnostic and statistical manual of mental disorders (DSM-5). Washington, DC: American Psychiatric Association; 2013. p. 947.
3. Bloch MH, Peterson BS, Scahill L, Otka J, Katsovich L, Zhang H, Leckman JF. Adulthood outcome of tic and obsessive-compulsive symptom severity in children with Tourette syndrome. Arch Pediatr Adolesc Med. 2006;160(1):65–9.
4. Jankovic J, Gelineau-Kattner R, Davidson A. Tourette's syndrome in adults. Mov Disord. 2010a;25(13):2171–5.
5. Jankovic J, Jimenez-Shahed J, Brown LW. A randomised, double-blind, placebo-controlled study of topiramate in the treatment of Tourette syndrome. J Neurol Neurosurg Psychiatry. 2010b;81(1):70–3.
6. Hirschtritt ME, Lee PC, Pauls DL, Dion Y, Grados MA, Illmann C, King RA, Sandor P, McMahon WM, Lyon GJ, Cath DC, Kurlan R, Robertson MM, Osiecki L, Scharf JM, Mathews CA, Tourette Syndrome Association International Consortium for Genetics. Lifetime prevalence, age of risk, and genetic relationships of comorbid psychiatric disorders in Tourette syndrome. JAMA Psychiat. 2015;72(4):325–33.
7. Robertson MM, Eapen V, Singer HS, Martino D, Scharf JM, Paschou P, Roessner V, Woods DW, Hariz M, Mathews CA, Črnčec R, Leckman JF. Gilles de la Tourette syndrome. Nat Rev Dis Primers. 2017;3:16097.
8. Darrow SM, Grados M, Sandor P, Hirschtritt ME, Illmann C, Osiecki L, Dion Y, King R, Pauls D, Budman CL, Cath DC, Greenberg E, Lyon GJ, McMahon WM, Lee P, Delucchi KL, Scharf JM, Mathews CA. Autism spectrum symptoms in a Tourette's disorder sample. J Am Acad Child Adolesc Psychiatry. 2017a;56(7):610–7.
9. Darrow SM, Hirschtritt ME, Davis LK, Illmann C, Osiecki L, Grados M, Sandor P, Dion Y, King R, Pauls D, Budman CL, Cath DC, Greenberg E, Lyon GJ, Yu D, McGrath LM, McMahon WM, Lee PC, Delucchi KL, Scharf JM, Mathews CA, Tourette Syndrome Association International Consortium for Genetics. Identification of two heritable cross-disorder endophenotypes for Tourette syndrome. Am J Psychiatry. 2017b;174(4):387–96. https://doi.org/10.1176/appi.ajp.2016.16020240.
10. Scharf JM, Miller LL, Gauvin CA, Alabiso J, Mathews CA, Ben-Shlomo Y. Population prevalence of Tourette syndrome: a systematic review and meta-analysis. Mov Disord. 2015;30(2):221–8.
11. Robertson MM. The prevalence and epidemiology of Gilles de la Tourette syndrome. Part 1: the epidemiological and prevalence studies. J Psychosom Res. 2008;65(5):461–72.
12. Freeman RD, Fast DK, Burd L, Kerbeshian J, Robertson MM, Sandor P. An international perspective on Tourette syndrome: selected findings from 3,500 individuals in 22 countries. Dev Med Child Neurol. 2000;42(7):436–47.
13. Khalifa N, von Knorring AL. Prevalence of tic disorders and Tourette syndrome in a Swedish school population. Dev Med Child Neurol. 2003;45(5):315–9.
14. Khalifa N, von Knorring AL. Tourette syndrome and other tic disorders in a total population of children: clinical assessment and background. Acta Paediatr. 2005;94(11):1608–14.
15. Robertson MM, Eapen V. Tourette's: syndrome, disorder or spectrum? Classificatory challenges and an appraisal of the DSM criteria. Asian J Psychiatr. 2014;11:106–13.
16. Rizzo R, Gulisano M, Calì PV, Curatolo P. Tourette syndrome and comorbid ADHD: current pharmacological treatment options. Eur J Paediatr Neurol. 2013;17(5):421–8.
17. Rizzo R, Gulisano M, Calì PV, Curatolo P. Long term clinical course of Tourette syndrome. Brain and Development. 2012;34(8):667–73.
18. Rizzo R, Curatolo P, Gulisano M, Virzì M, Arpino C, Robertson MM. Disentangling the effects of Tourette syndrome and attention deficit hyperactivity disorder on cognitive and behavioral phenotypes. Brain and Development. 2007;29(7):413–20.

19. Eddy CM, Cavanna AE, Gulisano M, Agodi A, Barchitta M, Calì P, Robertson MM, Rizzo R. Clinical correlates of quality of life in Tourette syndrome. Mov Disord. 2011;26(4):735–8.
20. Eddy CM, Cavanna AE, Gulisano M, Calì P, Robertson MM, Rizzo R. The effects of comorbid obsessive-compulsive disorder and attention-deficit hyperactivity disorder on quality of life in Tourette syndrome. J Neuropsychiatry Clin Neurosci. 2012;24(4):458–62.19.
21. Dell'Osso B, Marazziti D, Albert U, Pallanti S, Gambini O, Tundo A, Zanaboni C, Servello D, Rizzo R, Scalone L, Benatti B, Altamura AC, Porta M. Parsing the phenotype of obsessive-compulsive tic disorder (OCTD): a multidisciplinary consensus. Int J Psychiatry Clin Pract. 2017;21(2):156–9.
22. Rizzo R, Gulisano M, Domini CN, Ferro MC, Curatolo P. The relationship between autism spectrum disorder and Tourette syndrome in childhood: an overview of shared characteristics. J Pediatr Neurol JPN. 2017a;15(3)
23. Rizzo R, Gulisano M, Martino D, Robertson MM. Gilles de la Tourette syndrome, depression, depressive illness, and correlates in a child and adolescent population. J Child Adolesc Psychopharmacol. 2017b;27(3):243–9.
24. Chou IC, Lin HC, Lin CC, Sung FC, Kao CH. Tourette syndrome and risk of depression: a population-based cohort study in Taiwan. J Dev Behav Pediatr. 2013;34(3):181–5.
25. Qi Y, Zheng Y, Li Z, Xiong L. Progress in genetic studies of Tourette's syndrome. Brain Sci. 2017;7(10):E134. https://doi.org/10.3390/brainsci7100134.
26. Polyanska L, Critchley HD, Rae CL. Centrality of prefrontal and motor preparation cortices to Tourette syndrome revealed by meta-analysis of task-based neuroimaging studies. NeuroImage. 2017;16(3):257–67.
27. Albin RL, Koeppe RA, Wernette K, Zhuang W, Nichols T, Kilbourn MR, Frey KA. Striatal [11C]dihydrotetrabenazine and [11C]methylphenidate binding in Tourette syndrome. Neurology. 2009;72(16):1390–6.
28. Singer HS. The neurochemistry of Tourette syndrome. In: Martino D, Leckmann JF, editors. Tourette syndrome. Oxford: Oxford University Press; 2013. p. 276–300.
29. Roessner V, Plessen KJ, Rothenberger A, Ludolph AG, Rizzo R, Skov L, Strand G, Stern JS, Termine C, Hoekstra PJ, ESSTS Guidelines Group. European clinical guidelines for Tourette syndrome and other tic disorders. Part II: pharmacological treatment. Eur Child Adolesc Psychiatry. 2011;20(4):173–96.
30. Pringsheim T, Doja A, Gorman D, McKinlay D, Day L, Billinghurst L, Carroll A, Dion Y, Luscombe S, Steeves T, Sandor P. Canadian guidelines for the evidence-based treatment of tic disorders: pharmacotherapy. Can J Psychiatr. 2012;57(3):133–43.
31. Martino D, Macerollo A, Leckman JF. Neuroendocrine aspects of Tourette syndrome. Int Rev Neurobiol. 2013;112:239–79.
32. Bloch M, State M, Pittenger C. Recent advances in Tourette syndrome. Curr Opin Neurol. 2011;24(2):119–25.
33. Mogwitz S, Buse J, Ehrlich S, Roessner V. Clinical pharmacology of dopamine-modulating agents in Tourette's syndrome. Int Rev Neurobiol. 2013;112:281–349.
34. Roessner V, Schoenefeld K, Buse J, Bender S, Ehrlich S, Münchau A. Pharmacological treatment of tic disorders and Tourette syndrome. Neuropharmacology. 2013;68:143–9.
35. Whittington C, Pennant M, Kendall T, Glazebrook C, Trayner P, Groom M, Hedderly T, Heyman I, Jackson G, Jackson S, Murphy T, Rickards H, Robertson M, Stern J, Hollis C. Practitioner review: treatments for Tourette syndrome in children and young people – a systematic review. J Child Psychol Psychiatry. 2016;57(9):988–1004.
36. Yang C, Hao Z, Zhu C, Guo Q, Mu D, Zhang L. Interventions for tic disorders: an overview of systematic reviews and meta analyses. Neurosci Biobehav Rev. 2016;63:239–55.
37. Weisman H, Qureshi IA, Leckman JF, Scahill L, Bloch MH. Systematic review: pharmacological treatment of tic disorders—efficacy of antipsychotic and alpha-2 adrenergic agonist agents. Neurosci Biobehav Rev. 2013;37(6):1162–71.
38. Gaffney G, Perry P, Lund B, Bever-Stille K, Arndt S, Kuperman S. Risperidone versus clonidine in the treatment of children and adolescents with Tourette's disorder. J Am Acad Child Adolesc Psychiatry. 2002;41:330–6.
39. Rizzo R, Gulisano M. Clinical pharmacology of comorbid attention deficit hyperactivity disorder in Tourette syndrome. Int Rev Neurobiol. 2013;112:415–44.
40. Awaad Y. Tics in Tourette syndrome: new treatment options. J Child Neurol. 1999;14:316–9.
41. Singer HS, Wendlandt J, Krieger M, Giuliano J. Baclofen treatment in Tourette syndrome: a double-blind, placebo-controlled, crossover trial. Neurology. 2001;56(5):599–604.
42. Porta M, Sassi M, Ali F, Cavanna AE, Servello D. Neurosurgical treatment for Gilles de la Tourette syndrome: the Italian perspective. J Psychosom Res. 2009;67(6):585–90.
43. Quezada J, Coffman KA. Current approaches and new developments in the pharmacological management of Tourette syndrome. CNS Drugs. 2018;32:33–45.
44. Ganos C, Martino D, Pringsheim T. Tics in the pediatric population: pragmatic management. Mov Disord Clin Pract. 2017;4(2):160–72. https://doi.org/10.1002/mdc3.12428. Epub 2016 Nov 11. Review
45. Lim K, See YM, Lee J. A systematic review of the effectiveness of medical cannabis for psychiatric, movement and neurodegenerative disorders. Clin Psychopharmacol Neurosci. 2017;15(4):301–12.
46. Gilbert DL, Budman CL, Singer HS, Kurlan R, Chipkin RE. A D1 receptor antagonist, Ecopipam, for treatment of tics in Tourette syndrome. Clin Neuropharmacol. 2014;37:26–30.

47. Gilbert D, Murphy T, Jankovic J, Budman C, Black K, Kurlan R, Coffman K, McCracken J, Juncos J, Grant J, Chipkin R. A randomized, double-blind, placebo-controlled study of the D1 receptor antagonist ecopipam for children and adolescents with Tourette syndrome. Mov Disord. 2017;32
48. Jankovic J, Jimenez-Shahed J, Budman C, Coffey B, Murphy T, Shprecher D, Stamler D. Deutetrabenazine in tics associated with Tourette syndrome. Tremor Other Hyperkinet Mov. 2016;7(6):422. (eCollection 2016)
49. Karagiannidis I, Dehning S, Sandor P, Tarnok Z, Rizzo R, Wolanczyk T, Madruga-Garrido M, Hebebrand J, Nöthen MM, Lehmkuhl G, Farkas L, Nagy P, Szymanska U, Anastasiou Z, Stathias V, Androutsos C, Tsironi V, Koumoula A, Barta C, Zill P, Mir P, Müller N, Barr C, Paschou P. Support of the histaminergic hypothesis in Tourette syndrome: association of the histamine decarboxylase gene in a large sample of families. J Med Genet. 2013;50(11):760–4.
50. Tourette's Syndrome Study Group. Treatment of ADHD in children with tics: a randomized controlled trial. Neurology. 2002;58:527–36.
51. Rizzo R, Pellico A, Silvestri R, Chiarotti F, Cardona F. A randomized controlled trial comparing behavioral, educational, and pharmacological treatments in youths with chronic tic disorder or Tourette syndrome. Front Psych. 2018; https://doi.org/10.3389/fpsyt.2018.00100.
52. Storch E, De Nadai AS, Lewin AB, McGuire JF, Jones AM, Mutch PJ, Shytle RD, Murphy TK. Defining treatment response in pediatric tic disorders: a signal detection analysis of the Yale Global Tic Severity Scale. J Child Adolesc Psychopharmacol. 2011;21(6):621–7.
53. Cheung MYC, Shahed J, Jankovic J. Malignant Tourette syndrome. Mov Disord. 2007;22(12):1743–50.
54. Kious BM, Jimenez-Shahed J, Shprecher DR. Treatment-refractory Tourette syndrome. Prog Neuro-Psychopharmacol Biol Psychiatry. 2016;70:227–36.
55. Macerollo A, Martino D, Cavanna AE, Gulisano M, Hartmann A, Hoekstra PJ, Hedderly T, Debes NM, Muller-Vahl K, Neuner I, Porta M, Rickards H, Rizzo R, Cardona F, Roessner V. Refractoriness to pharmacological treatment for tics: a multicentre European audit. J Neurol Sci. 2016;366:136–8.
56. Mink JW, Walkup J, Frey KA, Como P, Cath D, Delong MR, Erenberg G, Jankovic J, Juncos J, Leckman JF, Swerdlow N, Visser-Vandewalle V, Vitek JL, Tourette Syndrome Association, Inc. Patient selection and assessment recommendations for deep brain stimulation in Tourette syndrome. Mov Disord. 2006;21(11):1831–8.
57. Porta M, Sassi M, Menghetti C, Servello D. The need for a proper definition of a "treatment refractoriness" in Tourette syndrome. Front Integr Neurosci. 2011;5:22.
58. Müller-Vahl KR, Cath DC, Cavanna AE, Dehning S, Porta M, Robertson MM, Visser-Vandewalle V, ESSTS Guidelines Group. European clinical guidelines for Tourette syndrome and other tic disorders. Part IV: deep brain stimulation. Eur Child Adolesc Psychiatry. 2011;20(4):209–17. https://doi.org/10.1007/s00787-011-0166-4.
59. Schrock LE, Mink JW, Woods DW, Porta M, Servello D, Visser-Vandewalle V, Silburn PA, Foltynie T, Walker HC, Shahed-Jimenez J, Savica R, Klassen BT, Machado AG, Foote KD, Zhang JG, Hu W, Ackermans L, Temel Y, Mari Z, Changizi BK, Lozano A, Auyeung M, Kaido T, Agid Y, Welter ML, Khandhar SM, Mogilner AY, Pourfar MH, Walter BL, Juncos JL, Gross RE, Kuhn J, Leckman JF, Neimat JA, Okun MS, Tourette Syndrome Association International Deep Brain Stimulation (DBS) Database and Registry Study Group. Tourette syndrome deep brain stimulation: a review and updated recommendations. Mov Disord. 2015;30(4):448–71.
60. Roth J. The colorful spectrum of Tourette syndrome and its medical, surgical and behavioral therapies. Parkinsonism Relat Disord. 2018;46(Suppl 1):S75–9.
61. Chang K, Frankovich J, Cooperstock M, Cunningham MW, Latimer ME, Murphy TK, Pasternack M, Thienemann M, Williams K, Walter J, Swedo SE, PANS Collaborative Consortium. Clinical evaluation of youth with pediatric acute-onset neuropsychiatric syndrome (PANS): recommendations from the 2013 PANS consensus conference. J Child Adolesc Psychopharmacol. 2015;1:3–13.
62. Hameed MQ, Dhamne SC, Gersner R, Kaye HL, Oberman LM, Pascual-Leone A, Rotenberg A. Transcranial magnetic and direct current stimulation in children. Curr Neurol Neurosci Rep. 2017;17:11. https://doi.org/10.1007/s11910-017-0719-0.
63. Cunnington R, Windischberger C, Moser E. Premovement activity of the pre-supplementary motor area and the readiness for action: studies of time-resolved event-related functional MRI. Hum Mov Sci. 2005;24(5–6):644–56.
64. Leckman. In: Martino D, Leckmann JF, editors. Tourette syndrome. Oxford: Oxford University Press; 2013. p. 276–300.
65. Bohlhalter S, Goldfine A, Matteson S, Garraux G, Hanakawa T, Kansaku K, Wurzman R, Hallett M. Neural correlates of tic generation in Tourette syndrome: an event-related functional MRI study. Brain. 2006;129(Pt 8):2029–37.
66. Orth M, Kirby R, Richardson MP, Snijders AH, Rothwell JC, Trimble MR, Robertson MM, Münchau A. Subthreshold rTMS over pre-motor cortex has no effect on tics in patients with Gilles de la Tourette syndrome. Clin Neurophysiol. 2005;116:764–8.
67. Wu YJ, Tseng P, Chang CF, Pai MC, Hsu KS, Lin CC, Juan CH. Modulating the interference effect on spatial working memory by applying transcranial direct current stimulation over the right dorsolateral prefrontal cortex. Brain Cogn. 2014;91:87–94.
68. Di Biase L, Munhoz RP. Deep brain stimulation for the treatment of hyperkinetic movement disorders. Expert Rev Neurother. 2016;16(9):1067–78.

69. Budman E, Deeb W, Martinez-Ramirez D, Pilitsis JG, Peng-Chen Z, Okun MS, Ramirez-Zamora A. Potential indications for deep brain stimulation in neurological disorders: an evolving field. Eur J Neurol. 2018;25:434–e30.
70. Martinez-Ramirez D, Jimenez-Shahed J, Leckman JF, Porta M, Servello D, Meng FG, Kuhn J, Huys D, Baldermann JC, Foltynie T, Hariz MI, Joyce EM, Zrinzo L, Kefalopoulou Z, Silburn P, Coyne T, Mogilner AY, Pourfar MH, Khandhar SM, Auyeung M, Ostrem JL, Visser-Vandewalle V, Welter ML, Mallet L, Karachi C, Houeto JL, Klassen BT, Ackermans L, Kaido T, Temel Y, Gross RE, Walker HC, Lozano AM, Walter BL, Mari Z, Anderson WS, Changizi BK, Moro E, Zauber S, Schrock LE, Zhang JG, Hu W, Rizer K, Monari EH, Foote KD, Malaty IA, Deeb W, Gunduz A, Okun MS. Efficacy and safety of deep brain stimulation in Tourette syndrome. The international Tourette syndrome deep brain stimulation public database and registry. JAMA Neurol. 2018;75(3):353–9.
71. Marceglia S, Servello D, Foffani G, Porta M, Sassi M, Mrakic-Sposta S, Rosa M, Barbieri S, Priori A. Thalamic single-unit and local field potential activity in Tourette syndrome. Mov Disord. 2010;25(3):300–8.
72. Fraint A, Pal G. Deep brain stimulation in Tourette's syndrome. Front Neurol. 2015;4(6):170.
73. Servello D, Sassi M, Gaeta M, Ricci C, Porta M. Tourette syndrome (TS) bears a higher rate of inflammatory complications at the implanted hardware in deep brain stimulation (DBS). Acta Neurochir. 2011;153(3):629–32.
74. Temel Y, Visser-Vandewalle V. Surgery in Tourette syndrome. Mov Disord. 2004;19(1):3–14. Review
75. Houeto JL, Karachi C, Mallet L, Pillon B, Yelnik J, Mesnage V, Welter ML, Navarro S, Pelissolo A, Damier P, Pidoux B, Dormont D, Cornu P, Agid Y. Tourette's syndrome and deep brain stimulation. J Neurol Neurosurg Psychiatry. 2005;76(7):992–5.
76. Shahed J, Poysky J, Kenney C, Simpson R, Jankovic J. GPi deep brain stimulation for Tourette syndrome improves tics and psychiatric comorbidities. Neurology. 2007;68(2):159–60.

Treatment-Resistant Eating Disorders

17

Youl-Ri Kim and Jione Kim

17.1 Clinical Aspects

Eating disorders (ED) affect roughly 2% of the population, and anorexia nervosa accounts for 1% [1]. The mean duration of anorexia nervosa is 7 years; 25% remain ill for life [2], depending on benefits, families, and repeated hospital care [3] and featuring premature deaths [4]. The criteria for anorexia nervosa include restraint eating, weight loss, and an acute sense of fear of weight gain according to the *Diagnostic and Statistical Manual of Mental Disorders*, fifth edition (*DSM-5* [5]), although a substantial proportion of persons with anorexia nervosa also binge eat and/or use compensatory behaviors. The *DSM-5* [5] accepted bulimia nervosa in 1979 and has recently accepted binge eating disorder as a diagnostic category; bulimia nervosa and binge eating disorder are characterized by a loss of control over eating and the rapid consumption of large amounts of food. People with bulimia nervosa use compensatory behaviors to prevent weight gain (e.g., self-induced vomiting, compulsive exercising). These disorders often share similar risk and maintaining factors[5]. Eating disorders as life-threatening conditions for many run a protracted course, which causes profound impacts on health and psychosocial functioning [6].

Half of patients with anorexia and three quarters of patients with bulimia will be in remission at 10 years. Anorexia nervosa in particular has high mortality rates, and all disorders can have significant physical and psychosocial costs for sufferers and their families. One third inpatient cases of anorexia and one in ten cases of bulimia will have a chronic course. Illness severity and duration predict anorexia nervosa outcomes, and the severity of other psychiatric difficulties predicts the outcomes in bulimia nervosa.

In the Oxford Record Linkage Study of females age 10–44 in the UK, age-standardized hospital admission rates for eating disorders increased, whereas admissions for most other psychiatric disorders had been declining [7]. This finding means that eating disorders have become a greater burden on secondary care.

17.2 Staging Models for Eating Disorders

The staging model of psychiatric disorders is based on the fact that many psychiatric disorders may follow a severe and enduring trajectory across the life course, being resistant to treatment and being associated with significant physical

Y.-R. Kim (✉)
Department of Psychiatry, Seoul Paik Hospital, Inje University, Seoul, South Korea

Institute of Eating Disorders and Mental Health, Inje University, Gimhae, South Korea

J. Kim
Institute of Eating Disorders and Mental Health, Inje University, Gimhae, South Korea

Y.-K. Kim (ed.), *Treatment Resistance in Psychiatry*, https://doi.org/10.1007/978-981-10-4358-1_17

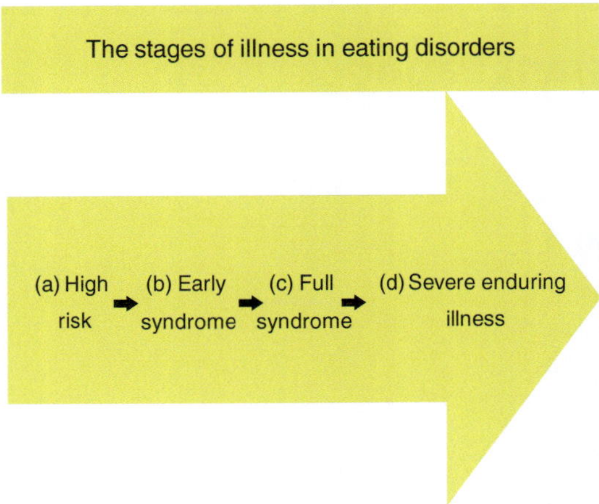

Fig. 17.1 A longitudinal staging model for eating disorders. (**a**) High risk; the common childhood antecedents to an eating disorder; (**b**) early form, including partial (subsyndromal) forms; (**c**) full syndrome; and (d) the severe and enduring forms

and psychiatric comorbidity over time [8]. Despite the decreased odds in later stages, remission and recovery can occur at any stage. Over the course of the psychopathology, biological features are modified and shaped via neuroprogression or neuro-adaptation [8, 9]; therefore, it may be possible to provide what could be called "neuroprotection" with early intervention strategies. There is uncertainty about the time frames attached to the different stages. Prof. Treasure described maintenance of anorexia nervosa causes an enduring form of illness [10], and severe and enduring anorexia nervosa is usually described as lasting for 7 years or more [11]. For bulimia nervosa and binge eating disorder, there are insufficient data to accurately describe time frames. Figure 17.1 shows a longitudinal staging model for eating disorders.

17.3 Severe and Enduring Eating Disorders

17.3.1 Treatment-Resistant Model of Anorexia Nervosa

Because of the relative rarity of anorexia nervosa, there are very few prospective designs to define risk factors. As a result, most of the evidence for models of AN are correlational, whereas a longitudinal perspective is essential for treating eating disorders [8]. Anorexia nervosa typically develops gradually and progresses with subsequent reductions in food intake, resulting in severe restriction and, finally, extreme emaciation. Repeated over time, these behaviors become fixed [6].

The cognitive interpersonal model of anorexia nervosa [10] illustrates how the visible aspects of the disorder that are relevant for interpersonal processes add to the valued elements, such as feelings of control, adherence to rules, and channeling negative emotions and lack of connection to others into food as a form of emotional regulation [10, 12]. Vulnerabilities in social processing and emotional regulation may increase the influence of social pressures during adolescence, a critical stage of eating disorder development, which if combined with reduced set shifting allow the illness to take hold [12]. These difficulties are accentuated by the secondary outcomes of the illness including intra- and interpersonal characteristics, and these contribute to maintaining the illness.

A somewhat unique consequence of eating disorders is that the symptoms themselves have an impact on brain and body health. Starvation reduces brain plasticity, and the consequences of habitual abnormal patterns of eating and digestive processes on brain-gut synchrony disturb the process of appetite. In Treasure's maintenance model [13], biological traits and circuits of brain are key factors in eating disorder maintenance.

Figure 17.2 shows a simplified diagram illustrating development of severe enduring eating disorders based on Treasure's model. In the model, the consequences of starvation on brain function caused by reduced brain plasticity in anorexia nervosa are regarded as crucial mechanisms that maintain the disorder, accentuating obsessive-compulsive traits (weak central coherence, set shifting), and further impair social and emotional processing (e.g., anxiety) [10, 12]. Another consequence of starvation is the impact it has on close others, who grow highly anxious [14]. Carer anxiety is mirrored by patient anxiety, which in turn induces more eating disorder symptoms [10, 12]. Accommodating and enabling

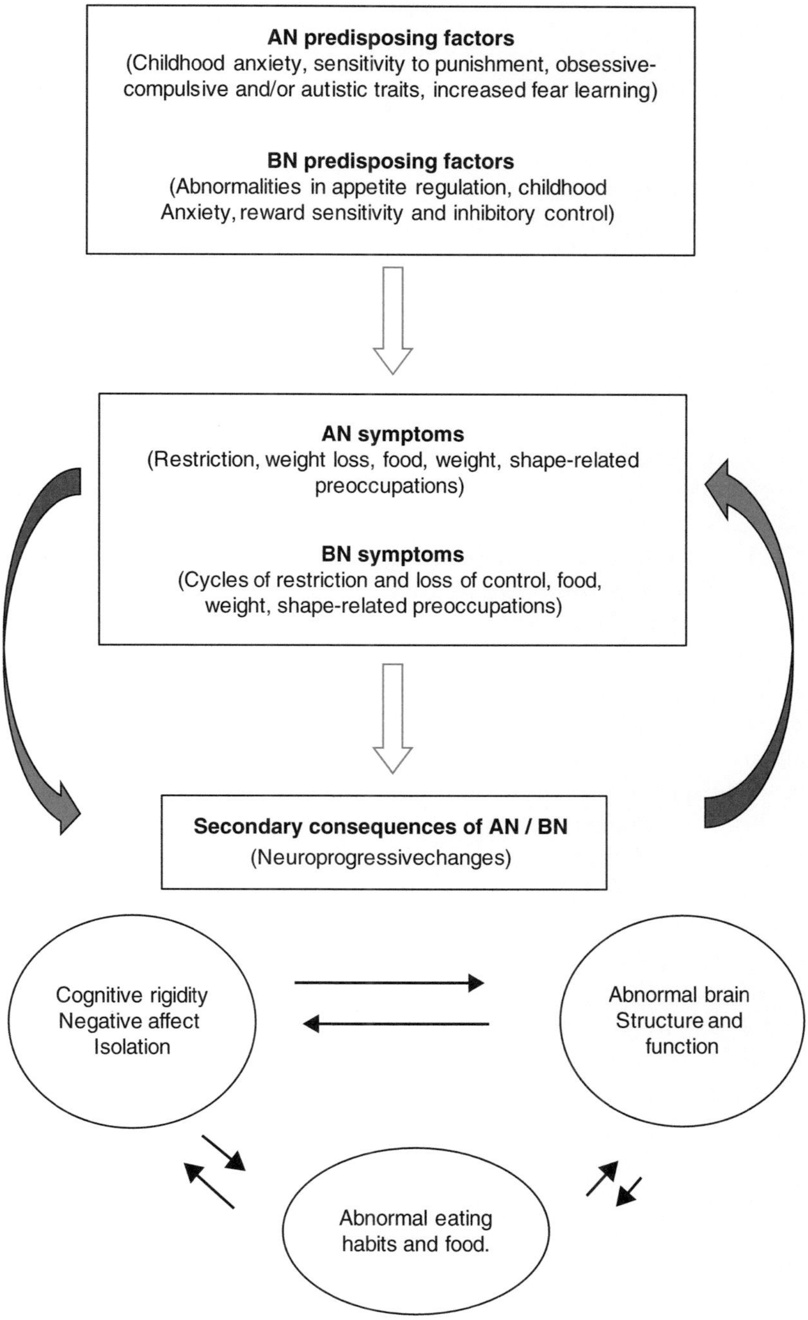

Fig. 17.2 The development of severe and enduring anorexia nervosa (AN) and bulimia nervosa (BN) based on Treasure's maintenance model

behaviors or highly expressed emotions mediate this process [15]. Carer anxiety (professionals, family members) can cause struggles during mealtime [16], and negative experiences related to meals can decrease appetite [17]. This can in turn increase negative associations with food [18]. A series of vicious circles develops, which adversely affects outcomes.

17.3.2 Treatment-Resistant Model of Loss of Control over Eating

Animal models of binge eating illustrate how a fasting and feasting pattern of eating highly palatable foods can affect the brain and cause addiction-like changes in neural circuits and neurotransmitters with changes in reward systems

[19]. The concept of food addiction [20] in obesity and overeating is controversial [20], but it might explain why bulimia nervosa persists. As shown in Fig. 17.2, Treasure's maintenance model of bulimia nervosa illustrates that similar changes provide the mechanism for chronicity in bulimia nervosa [13]. Within the addiction model, impulsive behaviors become compulsive habits particularly in the context of the rebound low, anxious mood in the withdrawal state [21, 22]; urge impulsivity overrides cognitive control, and so binge eating persists. In Fig. 17.2, a simplified diagram illustrates Treasure's maintenance model of bulimia nervosa.

17.4 The Recovery Approach for Treatment-Resistant Eating Disorders

There has been a shift toward *recovery*-based in mainstream psychiatry, in particular for schizophrenia [23]. This *recovery* approach moves beyond the focus on a cure or absence of symptoms to how patients can be helped to build meaningful and valued lives across a number of life domains. This approach has guiding principles that emphasize treatments that promote autonomy, self-management, and the reclaiming of identity, and it supports patients in meaningful activity. Thereby, it could reduce the stigma of mental illness and increase self-awareness, self-esteem, and self-acceptance; in the process of this approach, patients are not discouraged if they are not "cured" after their first treatment episode; this approach might be useful for all people with ED but of most benefit and relevance to those with long-standing disorders.

From a traditional clinical perspective, recovery was described as remission of symptoms and other deficits associated with psychiatric disorders to a sufficient degree that they no longer restrict daily functioning. Moreover, recovered patients are expected to resume daily personal, social, and vocational functioning within what is regarded as a normal range. More recently, the mental health consumer/survivor movement has given a new meaning for *recovery* [24]. The "new" recovery does not require amelioration of symptoms or other deficits and does not simply involve a return to a previous state; it is also not synonymous with cure and does not constitute a return to normal functioning. Rather, it is a lifelong process that involves an indefinite number of incremental steps in various life domains. It views mental illness as only one aspect of an otherwise whole person. This new *recovery* emphasizes accepting and living well with the illness; assuming responsibility in treatment goals and plans; expanding and redefining sense of self, renewed hope, meaningful activity, and autonomy; overcoming stigma; becoming empowered and exercising citizenship; and rebuilding personal, social, and environmental connections.

There have been discussions about how to define and measure *recovery* from EDs. Studies of patient perspectives on *recovery* highlight having a relaxed attitude toward the body and food, having a functioning social environment, accepting oneself, and seeing oneself as an individual. Crucially, these studies' authors have also highlighted that patients' common view is that recovery does not depend entirely on symptom absence. Despite these findings in other domains of mental illness, there have been very few studies on the *recovery* from EDs. Because of the long illness durations and poor outcomes in some individuals, there might exist questions whether recovery can apply to EDs.

Turton et al. [25] conducted an interview-based study of adults with an ED to investigate the meaning of *recovery*. In the project, analysis of interviews generated ten broad domains: the future, process, social inclusion, treatment, self, "clinical" recovery, ambivalence, physical health, practical matters, and rights. That study's findings showed that *recovery* is meaningful and relevant to people with eating disorders. However, themes also emerged that corresponded to a move convention understanding of recovery such as ambivalence or "clinical." The authors emphasized acknowledging the struggles of *recovery* as well as the positives and understanding how painful the *recovery* process can be. In that study, "conventional" recovery and patients' desire to be symptom-free were also important, and the value of peer support programs was highlighted.

17.5 Treatments

17.5.1 Treatment Approaches at the Different Stages of Illness

There is limited evidence from high-quality trials to answer questions on the enduring state of eating disorders regarding which treatments are effective and how much treatments can be beneficial [6]. Currently, there are few recommendations for first-line therapy for patients in the later stages of anorexia nervosa [26], although the limited evidence on patients with severe, enduring illness suggests that remission rates are modest and treatment effectiveness is poor [66]. Additional research is needed that explores treatment approaches for less responsive patients. For eating disorders, many treatments have been adapted from those used to treat other illnesses, whereas it is possible that a more targeted approach to treating key ED symptoms can improve outcomes [6].

17.5.2 New Perspectives on Treatment for Treatment-Resistant EDs

In over 50% of patients, EDs run a protracted trajectory and become severe and enduring [27], and once this occurs, the illness becomes less responsive to any form of treatment, and there is uncertainty about clinical management [28, 29]. In the 2000s, a group of clinicians and researchers began to question traditional treatments and identified a need for a different paradigm. Some studies showed the possibility of new perspectives on treating severe and enduring eating disorders focusing more on improving quality of life, keeping individuals in treatment, and reducing the number of "failed" treatment experiences [25]. Authors refined existing treatments by tailoring for the requirements of different groups and adding adjunctive treatments such as cognitive remediation therapy [30]. This approach has guiding principles including seeing treatment as part of a recovery journey; improving quality of life; working on specific issues; supporting the decision to engage in other treatments; maintaining hope; emphasizing reassurance, support, and encouragement; being aware of medical concerns and possible risk of destabilization; accepting that pace of change may be slow; emphasizing engagement and reducing premature ending; collaboratively agreeing on goals; and acknowledging losses and gains as a result of long-term illness [31]. In the research conducted by Touyz et al. [11], patients with severe and enduring anorexia nervosa participated in one of the tailored therapies for long-standing eating disorders for 30 sessions. Patients in each group experienced improvements in quality of life, depression, social functioning, and eating-related pathologies. New treatment approaches are recommended that could target the neuro-progressive changes that occur with EDs.

17.6 Cognitive Remediation Therapy

Cognitive remediation therapy (CRT) for eating disorders is an innovative therapy that was developed by Dr. Tchanturia [32]; it can be conducted as individual, group [32], or family-based treatment [33]. CRT consists of fun and entertaining activities to retrain thinking patterns in set shifting, achieving central coherence, and enhancing meta-cognitive skills; it aims to reduce the obsessive-compulsive cognitive styles that are related to poor AN recovery.

The feasibility and acceptability of CRT have been demonstrated in case studies and pilot studies of adults, children, and adolescents with anorexia nervosa [33]. It can help patients with anorexia nervosa to reduce rigid cognitive styles, learn more global processing styles, and enhance visual-spatial memory. In randomized controlled trials, patients who received CRT showed lower dropout rates and improvements in set shifting and quality of life; however, these findings focused on anorexia nervosa. Although there is evidence that suggested CRT can enhance treatment for obesity, adapting it for other eating disorders such as bulimia nervosa or binge eating disorder needs additional research.

17.7 Cognitive Bias Modification

Cognitive bias modification (CBM) aims at adjusting maladaptive cognitive biases in interpretations and attention among clinical populations such as affective disorders, obsessive-compulsive disorder, and substance abuse. CBM is composed of two computerized main variants, one of which was developed for the purpose of shifting negative biases in attention with a modified visual version of the dot-probe task [34]. On the dot-probe task, positive or negative valenced stimuli appear onscreen; a probe then appears briefly onscreen and patients must press a computer key as soon as possible. The other CBM approach can be useful for improving negative biases in interpretation; patients listen to ambiguous scenarios that can be interpreted negatively but are given positive decisions.

Some studies suggested that CBM can ameliorate negative biases toward emotional stimuli or stimuli associated with anxiety or depression, and there is also evidence that a CBM intervention to remediate maladaptive self-beliefs was associated with a decrease in eating-related pathologies in subclinical and clinical samples [35, 36]. Furthermore, a recent study on therapy that combined trainings for attentional and interpretation bias showed improvements in attention to smiling faces and fewer biased interpretations of ambiguous social stimuli. This finding indicates that CBM may improve negative cognitions in eating disorders [6].

17.8 Repetitive Transcranial Magnetic Stimulation

Anorexia nervosa is associated with changes in the brain; in particular, alterations have been found in systems implicated in reward processing, mood, symptom plasticity, and inhibitory control [13]. Repetitive transcranial magnetic stimulation (rTMS) was described as a therapeutic approach that stimulates the brain areas [35, 36]. Unlike electroconvulsive therapy, rTMS is noninvasive and already used in depression, obsessive-compulsive disorder, and schizophrenia. It can be helpful for improving feeding behaviors, controlling serotonergic processing, and augmenting brain-derived neurotrophic factor [6]. Thus, rTMS can be a novel form of therapy for eating disorders because of its possibility for improving maladaptive eating patterns and its regulation. In one study, rTMS for 20 sessions aimed at the dorsolateral prefrontal cortex (DLPFC) improved eating-related pathologies and affected severe and enduring AN [37]. rTMS also showed promising findings for the DMPFC treatment-resistant patients with BN [38].

17.9 Oxytocin

Oxytocin, a neuropeptide, plays an important role in neural circuits associated with social behavior, appetite, anxiety, and stress [39, 40]. Because these features are core characteristics of people with eating disorders, anomalies in oxytocin functioning might be involved in these disorders [41, 42].

Study authors have found that the bias toward attention on food-related stimuli and body image improved [43], as did biases toward negative emotional expression [44]. These results indicate that oxytocin can be helpful for moderating fear and avoidance related to a protracted trajectory in anorexia nervosa. Intranasal oxytocin led to a reduction in caloric intake in the 24 h after administration in patients with bulimia nervosa [45]. These results indicate that intranasal oxytocin can change abnormalities in attentional processes to specific and general aversive stimuli in anorexia nervosa and may change eating behaviors.

ED symptoms produce neuro-adaptive changes that cause chronicity and severely impaired quality of life. Oxytocin is a key central regulator of appetite, stress, and social functions, and translational pilot work suggests that it can moderate the automatic processes that underpin treatment resistance.

Conclusion

Evidence from epidemiological studies, neuropsychological findings, treatment responsivity, and prognosis supports a specific staging trajectory for anorexia nervosa in that there is a longitudinal trajectory with evidence of neurobiological progression and evidence that interventions matched to stage of illness may optimize the treatment benefits. Early and effective interventions appear crucial because the prognosis sharply declines the longer the illness persists. There is little information at the moment to support such a model for bulimia nervosa and binge eating disorder [8].

References

1. Hudson JI, Hiripi E, Pope HG, Kessler RC. The prevalence and correlates of eating disorders in the national comorbidity survey replication. Biol Psychiatry. 2007;61(3):348–58.
2. Vos T, Mathers C, Herrman H, et al. The burden of mental disorders in Victoria, 1996. Soc Psychiatry Psychiatr Epidemiol. 2001;36(2):53–62.
3. Hjern A, Lindberg L, Lindblad F. Outcome and prognostic factors for adolescent female in-patients with anorexia nervosa: 9-to 14-year follow-up. Br J Psychiatry. 2006;189:428–32.
4. Harris EC, Barraclough B. Excess mortality of mental disorder. Br J Psychiatry. 1998;173:11–53.
5. American Psychiatric Association. Diagnostic and statistical manual of mental disorders. 5th ed. Washington, DC: American Psychiatric Association; 2013.
6. Treasure J, Cardi V, Leppanen J, Turton R. New treatment approaches for severe and enduring eating disorders. Physiol Behav. 2015;152:456–65.
7. Holland J, Hall N, Yeates DGR, Goldacre M. Trends in hospital admission rates for anorexia nervosa in Oxford (1968–2011) and England (1990–2011): database studies. J R Soc Med. 2016;109(2):59–66.
8. Treasure J, Stein D, Maguire S. Has the time come for a staging model to map the course of eating disorders from high risk to severe enduring illness? An examination of the evidence. Early Intervent Psychiatry. 2015;9(3):173–84.
9. Berk M, Conus P, Kapczinski F, et al. From neuroprogression to neuroprotection: implications for clinical care. Med J Aust. 2010;193(4):S36–40.
10. Schmidt U, Treasure J. Anorexia nervosa: valued and visible. A cognitive-interpersonal maintenance model and its implications for research and practice. Br J Clin Psychol. 2006;45:343–66.
11. Touyz S, Le Grange D, Lacey H, et al. Treating severe and enduring anorexia nervosa: a randomized controlled trial. Psychol Med. 2013;43(12):2501–11.
12. Treasure J, Schmidt U. The cognitive-interpersonal maintenance model of anorexia nervosa revisited: a summary of the evidence for cognitive, socio-emotional and interpersonal predisposing and perpetuating factors. J Eat Disord. 2013;1(13):1–10.
13. Treasure J, Cardi V, Schmidt U. Moving to establish the mechanisms underpinning the biopsychiatric models of eating disorders with brain-based translational treatments: from paradigm clash to paradigm complementarity. Adv Eat Disord: Theory, Res Pract. 2014;2(2):171–9.
14. Zabala MJ, Macdonald P, Treasure J. Appraisal of caregiving burden, expressed emotion and psychological distress in families of people with eating disorders: a systematic review. Eur Eat Disord Rev. 2009;17(5):338–49.
15. Sepulveda AR, Kyriacou O, Treasure J. Development and validation of the accommodation and enabling scale for eating disorders (AESED) for caregivers in eating disorders. BMC Health Serv Res. 2009;9:171.
16. Long S, Wallis D, Leung N, Meyer C. "All eyes are on you": anorexia nervosa patient perspectives of in-patient mealtimes. J Health Psychol. 2012;17(3):419–28.
17. Wyrwicka W. Anorexia nervosa as a case of complex instrumental conditioning. Exp Neurol. 1984;84(3):579–89.
18. Treasure J, Cardi V, Kan C. Eating in eating disorders. Eur Eat Disord Rev. 2012;20(1):e42–e9.
19. Avena NM, Bocarsly ME. Dysregulation of brain reward systems in eating disorders: neurochemical information from animal models of binge eating, bulimia nervosa, and anorexia nervosa. Neuropharmacology. 2012;63(1):87–96.
20. Volkow ND, Wang GJ, Fowler JS, Tomasi D. Addiction circuitry in the human brain. In: Insel PA, Amara SG, Blaschke TF, editors. Annual review of pharmacology and toxicology, vol. 52. Palo Alto: Annual Reviews; 2012. p. 321–36.
21. Gladwin TE, Figner B, Crone EA, Wiers RW. Addiction, adolescence, and the integration of control and motivation. Dev Cogn Neurosci. 2011;1(4):364–76.
22. Everitt BJ, Belin D, Economidou D, Pelloux Y, Dalley JW, Robbins TW. Neural mechanisms underlying the vulnerability to develop compulsive drug-seeking habits and addiction. Trans Royal Soc B-Biol Sci. 2008;363(1507):3125–35.
23. Department of Health. The NHS improvement plan. 2004. www.dh.gov.uk/publications.
24. Nelson G, Ochocka J, Janzen R, Trainor J. A longitudinal study of mental health consumer/survivor initiatives: Part 1 – literature review and overview of the study. J Community Psychol. 2006;34(3):247–60.

25. Turton P, Demetriou A, Boland W, et al. One size fits all: or horses for courses? Recovery-based care in specialist mental health services. Soc Psychiatry Psychiatr Epidemiol. 2011;46(2):127–36.
26. Hay P, Chinn D, Forbes D, et al. Royal Australian and New Zealand College of Psychiatrists Clinical practice guidelines for the treatment of eating disorders. Aust N Z J Psychiatry. 2014;48(11):977–1008.
27. Stoving RK, Andries A, Brixen K, Bilenberg N, Horder K. Gender differences in outcome of eating disorders: a retrospective cohort study. Psychiatry Res. 2011;186(2–3):362–6.
28. Hay PJ, Touyz S, Sud R. Treatment for severe and enduring anorexia nervosa: a review. Aust N Z J Psychiatry. 2012;46(12):1136–44.
29. Wonderlich S, Mitchell JE, Crosby RD, et al. Minimizing and treating chronicity in the eating disorders: a clinical overview. Int J Eat Disord. 2012;45(4):467–75.
30. Harrison A, Mountford VA, Tchanturia K. Social anhedonia and work and social functioning in the acute and recovered phases of eating disorders. Psychiatry Res. 2014;218(1–2):187–94.
31. Bamford BH, Mountford VA. Cognitive behavioural therapy for individuals with longstanding anorexia nervosa: adaptations, clinician survival and system issues. Eur Eat Disord Rev. 2012;20(1):49–59.
32. Tchanturia K, Lloyd S, Lang K. Cognitive remediation therapy for anorexia nervosa: current evidence and future research directions. Int J Eat Disord. 2013;46(5):492–5.
33. Lang K, Treasure J, Tchanturia K. Acceptability and feasibility of self-help cognitive remediation therapy for anorexia nervosa delivered in collaboration with carers: a qualitative preliminary evaluation study. Psychiatry Res. 2015;225(3):387–94.
34. Mathews A, MacLeod C. Cognitive vulnerability to emotional disorders. Annu Rev Clin Psychol. 2005;1:167–95.
35. Brockmeyer T, Schmidt U, Friederich HC. The ABBA study – approach bias modification in bulimia nervosa and binge eating disorder: study protocol for a randomised controlled trial. Trials. 2016;17:466.
36. Cardi V, Esposito M, Bird G, et al. A preliminary investigation of a novel training to target cognitive biases towards negative social stimuli in Anorexia Nervosa. J Affect Disord. 2015;188:188–93.
37. McClelland J, Bozhilova N, Nestler S, et al. Improvements in symptoms following neuronavigated repetitive transcranial magnetic stimulation (rTMS) in severe and enduring anorexia nervosa: findings from two case studies. Eur Eat Disord Rev. 2013;21(6):500–6.
38. Downar J, Bakker N, Geraci J, et al. RTMS of the dorsomedial prefrontal cortex FFR binge and purge behaviours in refractory anorexia and bulimia nervosa: a case series. Biol Psychiatry. 2013;73(9):99S.
39. Blevins JE, Schwartz MW, Baskin DG. Evidence that paraventricular nucleus oxytocin neurons link hypothalamic leptin action to caudal brain stem nuclei controlling meal size. Am J Phys Regul Integr Comp Phys. 2004;287(1):R87–96.
40. Insel TR. The challenge of translation in social neuroscience: a review of oxytocin, vasopressin, and affiliative behavior. Neuron. 2010;65(6):768–79.
41. Maguire S, O'Dell A, Touyz L, Russell J. Oxytocin anorexia nervosa: a review of the emerging literature. Eur Eat Disord Rev. 2013;21:475–8.
42. Sabatier N, Leng G, Menzies J. Oxytocin, feeding, and satiety. Front Endocrinol. 2013;35(4):1–10.
43. Kim YR, Kim CH, Cardi V, Eom JS, Seong Y, Treasure J. Intranasal oxytocin attenuates attentional bias for eating and fat shape stimuli in patients with anorexia nervosa. Psychoneuroendocrinology. 2014;44:133–42.
44. Kim YR, Kim CH, Park JH, Pyo J, Treasure J. The impact of intranasal oxytocin on attention to social emotional stimuli in patients with anorexia nervosa: a double blind within-subject cross-over experiment. PLoS One. 2014;9(3):e90721.
45. Kim YR, Eom JS, Yang JW, Kang J, Treasure J. The impact of oxytocin on food intake and emotion recognition in patients with eating disorders: a double blind single dose within-subject cross-over design. PLoS One. 2015;10(9):e0137514.

18 Comorbid Sleep and Wake Problems in Treatment-Resistant Psychiatric Conditions

Seung-Gul Kang, Heon-Jeong Lee, Yong-Ku Kim, and Leen Kim

18.1 Introduction

Sleep and wake problems are the major cause of treatment resistance and dissatisfaction with treatment in psychiatric patients. Psychiatric patients feel sleep and wake problems more painfully and express them more often. Patients are more susceptible to sleep and wake disturbances because those symptoms are relatively objective and quantitative, and impairment of their quality of life is considered to be more direct than other psychiatric symptoms.

In many psychiatric disorders, sleep problems are very common and important symptoms. In the case of depression, one of the most common mental illnesses, the subjective complaint of sleep problems (insomnia or hypersomnia) is one of the most consistently reported symptoms associated with major depression. Previous studies have reported that approximately 75% of patients with major depression have sleep symptoms [1, 2]. Furthermore, the disruption of sleep patterns (insomnia or hypersomnia) is one of the diagnostic criteria for depressive episodes in the diagnostic criteria of mental disorders, such as the *Diagnostic and Statistical Manual of Mental Disorders 5th edition* (*DSM-5*) [3]. Such situations are similar in anxiety disorders and trauma-related disorders. Symptoms such as insomnia and abrupt nocturnal awakening are common in panic disorder and post-traumatic stress disorder (PTSD) [4]. In addition, sleep disturbance is one of the diagnostic criteria for generalized anxiety disorder, separation anxiety disorder, and PTSD [3]. Many patients experience insomnia and anxiety disorder at the same time. They are bidirectional risk factors to each other since insomnia is sometimes caused by anxiety disorder and sometimes the opposite is the case [5, 6]. Sleep disturbance is a very important and prominent symptom in bipolar disorder and may be a risk factor for relapses of mood episodes [7]. In addition, several types of sleep disturbances are described as diagnostic criteria for manic and depressive mood episodes [3]. Sleep disturbance of bipolar disorders persists even during the inter-episode period. Up to 70% of patients with bipolar disorder experience a clinically significant sleep disturbance, even during periods without mood episodes [8].

Sleep symptoms or polysomnographic findings are sometimes considered to be biologic markers of psychiatric illness or are associated with the treatment response. The typical

S.-G. Kang (✉)
Department of Psychiatry, Gil Medical Center, College of Medicine, Gachon University, Incheon, Republic of Korea
e-mail: kangsg@gachon.ac.kr

H.-J. Lee · Y.-K. Kim · L. Kim
Department of Psychiatry, Korea University College of Medicine, Seoul, Republic of Korea
e-mail: leehjeong@korea.ac.kr; yongku@korea.edu; leen54@chol.com

Y.-K. Kim (ed.), *Treatment Resistance in Psychiatry*, https://doi.org/10.1007/978-981-10-4358-1_18

polysomnographic findings in major depression are reduced rapid eye movement (REM) sleep latency, reduced slow wave sleep, and disruption of sleep continuity [9, 10]. However, since a decrease in REM sleep latency is also seen in borderline personality disorder, eating disorders, schizophrenia, and alcohol use disorder [11], it is not specific to depression and has not been established as a biomarker for it [12]. A recent study has shown that increased slow wave activities during early sleep after taking ketamine are associated with a favorable response to ketamine [13].

The common sleep and wake problems in patients with psychiatric illness are insomnia, hypnotic use problems, sleep apnea, restless legs syndrome (RLS), sleepiness, hypersomnolence, hypersomnia, irregular circadian sleep-wake cycle, and parasomnia. These problems are either comorbid independent of mental disorders or are caused by the effects of mental disorders, sometimes as a risk factor for mental disorders or as a side effect of psychotropic medications. The problem is that sleep and wake problems make the symptoms of mental illness very complicated and difficult to treat. However, these symptoms and problems are often unrevealed in physician-patient interviews, and in some cases, they are not adequately assessed due to clinicians' lack of understanding of sleep medicine. Therefore, to manage sleep and wake symptoms properly during the treatment of psychiatric disorders, a wider point of view and evaluation are needed.

18.2 Insomnia

Insomnia is a very common symptom that is often experienced in one-third of the population, and one-tenth of people experience chronic insomnia [14]. Insomnia is expected to be more common in psychiatric disorders than in the general population. Conversely, people with insomnia are more likely to have psychological problems, such as depression and anxiety [15]. In clinical practice, insomnia is one of the most common complaints and distressing symptoms. In addition, sleep disturbances can affect the severity and course of psychiatric disorders. According to a previous study, depression patients with sleep problems show treatment resistance, severe depressive symptoms, and suicidality [16].

Insomnia has multiple causes in many psychiatric disorders. Depression and insomnia are known to have a common neurobiology, such as neurotransmitter imbalance, abnormalities in brain activation, and dysregulation of the hypothalamic-pituitary-adrenal axis [10]. In anxiety disorders, insomnia is often associated with generalized anxiety disorder and panic disorder, and insomnia is often accompanied by PTSD. Insomnia symptoms are also very common in bipolar disorder, which is associated with reduced sleep need, delayed sleep phase, and irregular sleep patterns associated with mood episodes [7]. Previous studies have reported that 100% of bipolar disorder patients with depressive episodes and 55% of bipolar disorder patients in inter-episodic periods complain of insomnia [8]. In patients with schizophrenia, insomnia is common in patients with prodromal symptoms, acute psychotic symptoms, and psychotic relapse [17], but insomnia also often occurs in patients with chronic or mild psychotic symptoms due to poor sleep hygiene, negative symptoms, and delayed sleep phases [18–20]. Patients with substance use disorders, such as alcohol use disorder, also frequently complain of insomnia. Alcohol has generally bad effects on sleep. It might slightly reduce the sleep onset latency; however, it suppresses respiration during sleep and ultimately makes the quality of sleep worse. In patients with alcohol use disorder, drinking, discontinuation, and abstinence of alcohol have adverse effects on sleep latency and total sleep time [21]. Patients with severe alcohol use disorder repeatedly sleep and wake up over 24 h with a chaotic sleep cycle during the binge drinking period [22].

Patients with psychiatric disorders often take psychotropic medications. Antidepressants, such as selective serotonin reuptake inhibitors (SSRIs), serotonin-norepinephrine reuptake inhibitors (SNRIs), and norepinephrine-dopamine reuptake inhibitors, might alter the sleep structure, including REM sleep, and sometimes, they have the side effect of insomnia. Psychostimulants, such as methylphenidate and modafinil, can cause insomnia as a side effect, and mood stabilizers, such as lamotrigine, may cause insomnia.

Cognitive behavioral therapy for insomnia (CBT-I) is a very effective and clinically necessary therapy for most other mental disorders as well as primary insomnia. In the case of depression, CBT-I can be applied except for very severe depression. In the case of bipolar disorders, CBT-I is modified because the sleep insufficiency due to strict sleep restriction and stimulus control might induce mood elation or irritability and sometimes trigger manic symptoms [23]. The bipolar disorder-specific modification of CBT-I was developed by integrating interpersonal and social rhythm therapy, chronotherapy, and motivational interviewing, and positive effects have been reported [7]. In recent years, the use of wearable devices and mobile applications in insomnia patients has increased, and interest in them has continued to increase. CBT-I studies using mobile applications and wearable devices have been performed, and the efficacy of these devices has been reported recently [24–27].

Pharmacotherapy is widely used for insomnia when it is difficult to apply CBT-I in clinical settings. The following drugs have been indicated for primary insomnia: benzodiazepine agonists, named Z drugs (zolpidem, zopiclone, eszopiclone, zaleplon), benzodiazepines (quazepam, flurazepam, triazolam, temazepam); doxepin; melatonin receptor agonists (ramelteon); orexin receptor antagonists (suvorexant); and prolonged-release melatonin (Circadin). In psychiatric disorders, not only hypnotics with indications for insomnia but also off-label hypnotic medications with sedative effects are commonly used considering the symptoms that are comorbid with other psychiatric disorders. Typical off-label sedatives include the following: antidepressants, including mirtazapine, trazodone, amitriptyline, imipramine, clomipramine, and agomelatine; antipsychotics, including quetiapine, olanzapine, and chlorpromazine; and anticonvulsants, including gabapentin and pregabalin.

18.3 Hypnotic Abuse Problems

Hypnotics are effective for insomnia in the short term, but they induce shallow sleep, tolerance, and dependency with long-term use. Dependence on benzodiazepines and nonbenzodiazepine $GABA_A$ agonists is already well known, and patients are also aware of this [28–30]. Nonbenzodiazepine $GABA_A$ agonists, such as Z drugs, have been reported to have a low misuse rate in some studies [31], but in the United States, Z drugs are classified as Class IV Drug Enforcement Administration (DEA) restricted agents, which belong to the same group as benzodiazepines [32].

In addition, benzodiazepines, especially long-acting benzodiazepines, inhibit respiration, disrupt sleep quality, and increase the risk of sleep apnea [33]. Occasionally, sleepiness due to benzodiazepines might cause disturbances in the sleep-wake cycle and, ultimately, might cause insomnia at night. These patients should be observed with caution because some of them ask doctors to prescribe more sedative drugs while sleeping during the daytime. We need to pay more attention to patients with substance use disorders, such as alcohol use disorder, regarding the abuse of hypnotics. Sometimes they take sleeping pills, such as benzodiazepine receptor agonists, during the daytime as well as at night [22]. This is thought to be self-medication to minimize daytime physiologic hyperarousal [34]. Doctors should be particularly cautious to prescribe hypnotics in cases of drug use disorders, such as alcohol, because these patients often misuse hypnotics or take alcohol and hypnotics at the same time. This might promote accidents and more serious side effects.

18.4 Sleep Apnea

According to previous studies, many mentally ill patients have sleep apnea, suggesting a high association between mental disorders and sleep apnea. Major depression patients have an increased risk (1.6-fold) for OSA, and those with sleep apnea have an increased risk (1.8-fold) of developing major depression [35]. Treating OSA results in the improvement of depressive symptoms [36].

Attention deficit hyperactivity disorder (ADHD), one of the most common psychiatric disorders in children and adolescents, is also associated with OSA. A recent meta-analysis found a higher apnea-hypopnea index (AHI) in children with ADHD than in healthy children based on polysomnography [37]. There is controversy over the prevalence of sleep-related breathing disorders (SRBDs) in children due to the debate over whether the current AHI criteria are appropriate, but symptoms of SRBD, such as snoring, seem to be common in children with ADHD or ADHD-like behaviors [38]. Approximately 20–66% of children with ADHD have been reported to habitually snore [39–41]. Meanwhile, data from previous studies suggest that treatments such as adenotonsillectomy for SRBD improve ADHD symptoms [42]. Therefore, expert consensus recommends that all children undergoing evaluation for ADHD should be screened for symptoms of SRBD, particularly snoring [43]. If the child snores, then polysomnography is recommended [43]. If the child has AHI >1 on polysomnography, large tonsils, and a small airway, adenotonsillectomy should be considered [43].

Due to the nature of psychotic disorders, the prevalence of OSA among antipsychotic-naïve schizophrenic patients has not been reported. Schizophrenic patients treated with antipsychotics demonstrated a high prevalence rate (17–25%) for sleep-disordered breathing [44–46], although Takahashi et al.'s study did not show a higher SRBD prevalence in schizophrenia than in the control group [45]. In addition to this, more than 46% of schizophrenia patients with suspected sleep disorder had a respiratory disturbance index (RDI) greater than 10, and the mean RDI was 64.8 [47]. The most powerful predictor of OSA was obesity in that study [47]. Although somnolence is a common side effect of antipsychotics, clinician must consider the possibility of comorbid OSA in patients with schizophrenia who show significant somnolence. Therefore, the clinician should evaluate whether patients have OSA symptoms, including snoring, obesity, and weight gain, secondary to antipsychotics [18]. Schizophrenia patients with comorbid OSA can be treated effectively with nasal continuous airway pressure with relatively good compliance and clinical improvement in OSA and schizophrenia [48–50].

Second-generation antipsychotics appear to decrease sleep onset latency and improve sleep efficiency, but they also commonly cause weight gain, which can increase the risk of OSA [10]. Therefore, when antidepressants or antipsychotics with weight gain-inducing potential are prescribed, side effects should be explained to the patient in advance, and attention should be paid to OSA development.

18.5 Restless Legs Syndrome and Periodic Limb Movement During Sleep

Previous literature has reported that 44% of ADHD patients have RLS or RLS symptoms [51]. Recent, less-biased studies have reported an approximately 10–20% RLS prevalence in patients with ADHD [39, 52]. Although the mechanism of the association between the two diseases is unclear, a nigrostriatal deficit may underlie RLS and periodic limb movements during sleep (PLMS) in ADHD [53].

The association between RLS and major depression is not well established [10]. Several studies have shown inconsistent results regarding the association between the two diseases, presumably due to the bias of RLS induced by serotonergic antidepressants [54].

It is unclear how RLS and periodic limb movement disorder (PLMD) are related to schizophrenia because few prevalence studies exist for sleep disorders in antipsychotic-naïve patients [18]. However, our previous study reported that the prevalence of RLS in schizophrenia patients taking antipsychotic medication was 21.4%, twice as common as in normal controls [55]. Because antipsychotics have a dopamine antagonist effect, drug-induced dopamine deficiency appears to cause RLS or PLMS symptoms [55]. In addition, the severity of RLS symptoms is correlated with the severity of psychopathology, suggesting that RLS might play an important role in the deterioration and improvement of symptoms of schizophrenia [55]. Symptoms of RLS are often confused with akathisia. The most important difference is the circadian pattern: RLS symptoms are aggravated at night, but there is no circadian pattern in akathisia symptoms [18]. Previous studies have reported that 13–14% of schizophrenia patients taking first-generation antipsychotics show PLMS in nocturnal polysomnography [44, 56].

The management of RLS/PLMD in psychiatric disorders, such as schizophrenia, depression, and ADHD, includes the elimination of the cause (e.g., stopping the antidepressants or antipsychotics, which might trigger secondary RLS), nonpharmacologic strategies, and, if necessary, pharmacologic strategies. In particulary, the RLS symptoms in psychiatric patients should be assessed for the probability of medication-induced symptoms such as SSRI and antipsychotics should be examined [57, 58]. In this case, adherence to pharmacotherapy deteriorates, and psychiatric disorders often relapse; therefore, ultimately, a reduction or discontinuation/replacement of the medication is necessary for the fundamental solution [59]. Nonpharmacologic strategies include sleep hygiene therapy, physical exercise, and avoiding aggravating factors, such as iron deficiency, pain, caffeine, nicotine, and alcohol [60].

In pharmacotherapy, dopaminergic drugs are used as off-label drugs in children with ADHD [61, 62]; however, there is no established data on their long-term efficacy and tolerability [38]. In cases of low ferritin or iron levels, oral iron supplementation is recommended [63]. In patients with schizophrenia, dopamine agonists, such as ropinirole and pramipexole, may exacerbate psychotic symptoms and should be administered with caution [18].

18.6 Sleepiness and Hypersomnia

In addition to insomnia, hypersomnia is also a common and important symptom in major depression. Depression's atypical features include mood reactivity, weight gain, and hypersomnia symptoms [10]. Approximately 10% of general adults with hypersomnia have major depression [15, 64]. Depressive patients with severe fatigue or hypersomnia may experience an improvement in hypersomnia as well as depressive symptoms when treated with antidepressants, and some patients may benefit from adjunctive use of stimulant medication with antidepressants [10, 65]. Light therapy is also effective for patients with seasonal depression and hypersomnia [10].

Sleepiness and hypersomnia are also common symptoms of bipolar disorder. In particular, bipolar disorder patients with depressive episodes complain of hypersomnia, prolonged time in bed, and excessive sleepiness, and 25% of patients with bipolar disorder complain of hypersomnia in the inter-episode period [66, 67].

First-line treatment medications for psychiatric disorders may also cause sedation [7]. The CATIE study reported significantly prevalent antipsychotic-related somnolence [68]. The rate of somnolence in antipsychotic-treated schizophrenic patients was 24–31% among antipsychotic-treated schizophrenic patients [68]. Sedation can be an adverse reaction due to the direct effect of antipsychotics, sometimes due to negative symptoms or secondary SRBD due to antipsychotic-induced weight gain [18]. Typical low-potency antipsychotic drugs have antihistaminergic and anticholinergic side effects, including sedation [18]. The sedative effect of clozapine, quetiapine, and olanzapine in second-generation antipsychotics is remarkable [18]. If the patient's discomfort or side effects are severe, dose reductions of antipsychotics should be considered to improve patient's quality of life and compliance, even if the medication is needed therapeutically [69]. Quetiapine is often used off-label for insomnia symptoms. The extended release form of quetiapine was originally developed to reduce the side effects of the immediate release form; however, the hangover from quetiapine's extended release form may persist longer through the next morning. In this case, considering the pharmacokinetics of the drug, changing to an immediate release form may be helpful in sleep induction and reducing hangover the next day.

The results of previous studies on modafinil combination therapy to improve antipsychotic-associated sedation or fatigue did not show significantly favorable results compared to a placebo combination [70, 71].

18.7 Disturbances of the Circadian Sleep-Wake Cycle

In bipolar disorder, sleep and circadian rhythms are unstable due to the inadequate and irregular timing of the exposure to light and dark and irregularities in social rhythms. In addition, the clock gene function is also involved in circadian rhythm disturbances [7]. The medication used to treat bipolar disorder also has the effect of delaying or advancing circadian rhythm [72].

Although circadian rhythm abnormalities are common in schizophrenia and there have been many studies on them, the results are largely inconsistent on the proportion of each sleep-wake pattern (e.g., delayed phase, advanced phase, irregular pattern, and free-running pattern) [19, 73–77]. A disturbed pattern of melatonin secretion was reported in both schizophrenic patients with phase-advanced [78] and phase-delayed [79] disease. These inconsistent results may be due to a variety of circumstances, such as the methodological heterogeneity of the studies and environmental/lifestyle factors (sunlight exposure, decreased activity, effective time cues, and lifestyle choices involving preferences for staying awake at night, etc.) [18].

Circadian rhythm abnormalities occur frequently in ADHD patients. The common area of the brain regions identified as a cause of ADHD and circadian rhythm disorder is the locus coeruleus [80]. A clinical study of the melatonin secretion pattern of patients with ADHD shows that delayed sleep phase syndrome is common in that population [81, 82]. According to the recommendations of the expert consensus group, melatonin, light therapy, and chronotherapy can be used for sleep induction difficulties due to delayed sleep phase syndrome [43, 83].

18.8 REM Sleep Behavior Disorder

RBD or RBD-like symptoms frequently occur during pharmacotherapy for psychiatric disorders. In particular, the antidepressants that inhibit REM sleep are closely associated with the RBD occurrence. SSRI, SNRI, and mirtazapine often cause RBD symptoms [84, 85]. Antidepressant-associated RBD symptoms may be caused by a mechanism distinct from synucleinopathy, but others insist that antidepressants tend to unmask RBD symptoms in people with subclinical synucleinopathy [86]. Withdrawal from barbiturates and ethanol is known to trigger RBD symptoms and caffeine abuse, and beta-blockers may also cause RBD [87–90]. If RBD symptoms are suspected, patients and their families should be educated to be cautious of accidents and injuries caused by abnormal behavior during sleep. When the symptoms of RBD are suspected to develop due to medication, it is advisable to reduce the dosage of antidepressants or to switch to other antidepressants (e.g., bupropion) that are less likely to cause RBD symptoms, considering their psychiatric symptoms. Although benzodiazepines, such as clonazepam, may be effective in this case, they are not a fundamental solution for the problem and are likely to cause sleep apnea. In situations where clonazepam is not advisable, 3–15 mg of melatonin can be used [91]. If there is a suspicion of comorbid sleep apnea or if it is necessary to distinguish RBD-like symptoms from other parasomnias or seizures, nocturnal polysomnography should be performed.

Conclusions

Treatment resistance or residual symptoms in many psychiatric disorders are often caused by sleep and wake problems. In long-term treatment situations, sleep-wake disturbances, such as insomnia, become more important problems than the initial chief complaint of psychiatric illness. Sleep and wake problems in major psychiatric disorders, such as depressive disorders, anxiety disorders, bipolar disorders, schizophrenia, and ADHD, impair the quality of life of patients and deteriorate their therapeutic progress. Sleep problems, such as insomnia, sleep apnea, RLS, hypersomnia, hypnotic use and misuse, and circadian disruption, are quite common, and the treatment of psychiatric disorders is jeopardized when they are not properly managed. Occasionally, sleep and wake problems that occur during the treatment of psychiatric illness often require changes in the treatment strategy, including pharmacotherapy. Insomnia, which is the most common sleep-wake symptom, is usually treated effectively with CBT-I, even if it is accompanied by psychiatric illness, but it is better to modify the CBT-I modality for each psychiatric disorder. Weight gain due to psychiatric illness-related or therapeutic drugs is common, and clinicians should always be aware of the possibility of OSA. Patients with psychiatric disorders often do not complain or conceal OSA symptoms themselves; therefore, therapists should be more aggressive in considering the evaluation and management of OSA during pharmacotherapy.

Acknowledgment This research was supported by Basic Science Research Program through the National Research Foundation of Korea (NRF) funded by the Ministry of Education (NRF-2017R1D1A1B03032431).

References

1. Liu X, Buysse DJ, Gentzler AL, Kiss E, Mayer L, Kapornai K, et al. Insomnia and hypersomnia associated with depressive phenomenology and comorbidity in childhood depression. Sleep. 2007;30(1):83–90.
2. Yates WR, Mitchell J, Rush AJ, Trivedi MH, Wisniewski SR, Warden D, et al. Clinical features of depressed outpatients with and without co-occurring general medical conditions in STAR*D. Gen Hosp Psychiatry. 2004;26(6):421–9.
3. Association AP. Diagnostic and statistical manual of mental disorders (DSM-5®). Arlington: American Psychiatric Publishing; 2013.
4. Krystal AD, Stein MB, Szabo ST. Anxiety disorders and posttraumatic stress disorder. In: Principles and practice of sleep medicine. Philadelphia, PA: Elsevier; 2017. p. 1341–51.e5.
5. Johnson EO, Roth T, Breslau N. The association of insomnia with anxiety disorders and depression: exploration of the direction of risk. J Psychiatr Res. 2006;40(8):700–8.
6. Jansson-Frojmark M, Lindblom K. A bidirectional relationship between anxiety and depression, and insomnia? A prospective study in the general population. J Psychosom Res. 2008;64(4):443–9.
7. Harvey AG, Soehner AM, Buysse DJ. Bipolar disorder. In: Principles and practice of sleep medicine. Philadelphia, PA: Elsevier; 2017. p. 1363–9.e4.
8. Harvey AG, Schmidt DA, Scarna A, Semler CN, Goodwin GM. Sleep-related functioning in euthymic patients with bipolar disorder, patients with insomnia and subjects without sleep problems. Am J Psychiatry. 2005;162(1):50–7.
9. Reynolds CF 3rd, Kupfer DJ. Sleep research in affective illness: state of the art circa 1987. Sleep. 1987;10(3):199–215.
10. Minkel JD, Krystal AD, Benca RM. Unipolar major depression. In: Principles and practice of sleep medicine. Philadelphia, PA: Elsevier; 2017. p. 1352–62.e5.
11. Benca RM, Obermeyer WH, Thisted RA, Gillin JC. Sleep and psychiatric disorders. A meta-analysis. Arch Gen Psychiatry. 1992;49(8):651–68; discussion 69–70.
12. Arfken CL, Joseph A, Sandhu GR, Roehrs T, Douglass AB, Boutros NN. The status of sleep abnormalities as a diagnostic test for major depressive disorder. J Affect Disord. 2014;156:36–45.
13. Duncan WC, Sarasso S, Ferrarelli F, Selter J, Riedner BA, Hejazi NS, et al. Concomitant BDNF and sleep slow wave changes indicate ketamine-induced plasticity in major depressive disorder. Int J Neuropsychopharmacol. 2013;16(2):301–11.
14. Ancoli-Israel S, Roth T. Characteristics of insomnia in the United States: results of the 1991 National Sleep Foundation Survey. I. Sleep. 1999;22(Suppl 2):S347–53.
15. Taylor DJ, Lichstein KL, Durrence HH, Reidel BW, Bush AJ. Epidemiology of insomnia, depression, and anxiety. Sleep. 2005;28(11):1457–64.
16. Peterson MJ, Benca RM. Sleep in mood disorders. Sleep Med Clin. 2008;3(2):231–49.
17. Chemerinski E, Ho BC, Flaum M, Arndt S, Fleming F, Andreasen NC. Insomnia as a predictor for symptom worsening following antipsychotic withdrawal in schizophrenia. Compr Psychiatry. 2002;43(5):393–6.
18. Benson KL, Feinberg I. Schizophrenia. In: Principles and practice of sleep medicine. Philadelphia, PA: Elsevier; 2017. p. 1370–9.e5.
19. Wirz-Justice A, Cajochen C, Nussbaum P. A schizophrenic patient with an arrhythmic circadian rest-activity cycle. Psychiatry Res. 1997;73(1–2):83–90.
20. Mansour HA, Wood J, Chowdari KV, Dayal M, Thase ME, Kupfer DJ, et al. Circadian phase variation in bipolar I disorder. Chronobiol Int. 2005;22(3):571–84.
21. Brower KJ. Alcohol's effects on sleep in alcoholics. Alcohol Res Health (The Journal of the National Institute on Alcohol Abuse and Alcoholism). 2001;25(2):110–25.
22. Roehrs T, Roth T. Medication and substance abuse. In: Principles and practice of sleep medicine. Philadelphia, PA: Elsevier; 2017. p. 1380–9.e4.
23. Colombo C, Benedetti F, Barbini B, Campori E, Smeraldi E. Rate of switch from depression into mania after therapeutic sleep deprivation in bipolar depression. Psychiatry Res. 1999;86(3):267–70.
24. Kuhn E, Weiss BJ, Taylor KL, Hoffman JE, Ramsey KM, Manber R, et al. CBT-I coach: a description and

clinician perceptions of a mobile app for cognitive behavioral therapy for insomnia. J Clin Sleep Med. 2016;12(4):597–606.
25. Babson KA, Ramo DE. Mobile app-delivered cognitive behavioral therapy for insomnia: feasibility and initial efficacy among veterans with Cannabis use disorders. JMIR Res Protoc. 2015;4(3):e87.
26. Chen YX, Hung YP, Chen HC. Mobile application-assisted cognitive behavioral therapy for insomnia in an older adult. Telemed J E Health. 2016;22(4):332–4.
27. Kang SG, Kang JM, Cho SJ, Ko KP, Lee YJ, Lee HJ, et al. Cognitive behavioral therapy using a mobile application synchronizable with wearable devices for insomnia treatment: a pilot study. J Clin Sleep Med. 2017;13(4):633–40.
28. Guerlais M, Grall-Bronnec M, Feuillet F, Gerardin M, Jolliet P, Victorri-Vigneau C. Dependence on prescription benzodiazepines and Z-drugs among young to middle-aged patients in France. Subst Use Misuse. 2015;50(3):320–7.
29. Liebrenz M, Gehring MT, Buadze A, Caflisch C. High-dose benzodiazepine dependence: a qualitative study of patients' perception on cessation and withdrawal. BMC Psychiatry. 2015;15:116.
30. Canham SL, Gallo J, Simoni-Wastila L. Perceptions of benzodiazepine dependence among women age 65 and older. J Gerontol Soc Work. 2014;57(8):872–88.
31. Hajak G, Muller WE, Wittchen HU, Pittrow D, Kirch W. Abuse and dependence potential for the non-benzodiazepine hypnotics zolpidem and zopiclone: a review of case reports and epidemiological data. Addiction (Abingdon, England). 2003;98(10):1371–8.
32. Kilduff TS, Mendelson WB. Hypnotic medications: mechanisms of action and pharmacologic effects. In: Principles and practice of sleep medicine. Philadelphia, PA: Elsevier; 2017. p. 424–31.e5.
33. Dolly FR, Block AJ. Effect of flurazepam on sleep-disordered breathing and nocturnal oxygen desaturation in asymptomatic subjects. Am J Med. 1982;73(2):239–43.
34. Roehrs T, Bonahoom A, Pedrosi B, Zorick F, Roth T. Nighttime versus daytime hypnotic self-administration. Psychopharmacology. 2002;161(2):137–42.
35. Peppard PE, Szklo-Coxe M, Hla KM, Young T. Longitudinal association of sleep-related breathing disorder and depression. Arch Intern Med. 2006;166(16):1709–15.
36. Wells RD, Freedland KE, Carney RM, Duntley SP, Stepanski EJ. Adherence, reports of benefits, and depression among patients treated with continuous positive airway pressure. Psychosom Med. 2007;69(5):449–54.
37. Cortese S, Faraone SV, Konofal E, Lecendreux M. Sleep in children with attention-deficit/hyperactivity disorder: meta-analysis of subjective and objective studies. J Am Acad Child Adolesc Psychiatry. 2009;48(9):894–908.
38. Cortese S, Lecendreux M. Sleep disturbances in attention-deficit/hyperactivity disorder. In: Principles and practice of sleep medicine. Philadelphia, PA: Elsevier; 2017. p. 1390–7.e4.
39. Silvestri R, Gagliano A, Arico I, Calarese T, Cedro C, Bruni O, et al. Sleep disorders in children with Attention-Deficit/Hyperactivity Disorder (ADHD) recorded overnight by video-polysomnography. Sleep Med. 2009;10(10):1132–8.
40. Chervin RD, Dillon JE, Bassetti C, Ganoczy DA, Pituch KJ. Symptoms of sleep disorders, inattention, and hyperactivity in children. Sleep. 1997;20(12):1185–92.
41. O'Brien LM, Holbrook CR, Mervis CB, Klaus CJ, Bruner JL, Raffield TJ, et al. Sleep and neurobehavioral characteristics of 5- to 7-year-old children with parentally reported symptoms of attention-deficit/hyperactivity disorder. Pediatrics. 2003;111(3):554–63.
42. Weber SA, Lima Neto AC, Ternes FJ, Montovani JC. Hyperactivity and attention deficit syndrome in obstructive sleep apnea syndrome: is there improvement with surgical management? Braz J Otorhinolaryngol. 2006;72(1):124–9.
43. Cortese S, Brown TE, Corkum P, Gruber R, O'Brien LM, Stein M, et al. Assessment and management of sleep problems in youths with attention-deficit/hyperactivity disorder. J Am Acad Child Adolesc Psychiatry. 2013;52(8):784–96.
44. Benson K, Zarcone V. Sleep abnormalities in schizophrenia and other psychotic disorders. Rev Psychiatry. 1994;13:677–705.
45. Takahashi KI, Shimizu T, Sugita T, Saito Y, Takahashi Y, Hishikawa Y. Prevalence of sleep-related respiratory disorders in 101 schizophrenic inpatients. Psychiatry Clin Neurosci. 1998;52(2):229–31.
46. Waters F, Hanken K, Rock D. Sleep-disordered breathing in schizophrenia: an audit. Schizophr Res. 2013;143(2–3):393–4.
47. Winkelman JW. Schizophrenia, obesity, and obstructive sleep apnea. J Clin Psychiatry. 2001;62(1):8–11.
48. Boufidis S, Kosmidis MH, Bozikas VP, Daskalopoulou-Vlahoyianni E, Pitsavas S, Karavatos A. Treatment outcome of obstructive sleep apnea syndrome in a patient with schizophrenia: case report. Int J Psychiatry Med. 2003;33(3):305–10.
49. Karanti A, Landen M. Treatment refractory psychosis remitted upon treatment with continuous positive airway pressure: a case report. Psychopharmacol Bull. 2007;40(1):113–7.
50. Sugishita K, Yamasue H, Kasai K. Continuous positive airway pressure for obstructive sleep apnea improved negative symptoms in a patient with schizophrenia. Psychiatry Clin Neurosci. 2010;64(6):665.
51. Cortese S, Konofal E, Lecendreux M, Arnulf I, Mouren MC, Darra F, et al. Restless legs syndrome and attention-deficit/hyperactivity disorder: a review of the literature. Sleep. 2005;28(8):1007–13.
52. Zak R, Fisher B, Couvadelli BV, Moss NM, Walters AS. Preliminary study of the prevalence of restless legs syndrome in adults with attention deficit hyperactivity disorder. Percept Mot Skills. 2009;108(3):759–63.

53. Kirov R, Brand S. Sleep problems and their effect in ADHD. Expert Rev Neurother. 2014;14(3):287–99.
54. Ulfberg J, Bjorvatn B, Leissner L, Gyring J, Karlsborg M, Regeur L, et al. Comorbidity in restless legs syndrome among a sample of Swedish adults. Sleep Med. 2007;8(7–8):768–72.
55. Kang SG, Lee HJ, Jung SW, Cho SN, Han C, Kim YK, et al. Characteristics and clinical correlates of restless legs syndrome in schizophrenia. Prog Neuropsychopharmacol Biol Psychiatry. 2007;31(5):1078–83.
56. Ancoli-Israel S, Martin J, Jones DW, Caligiuri M, Patterson T, Harris MJ, et al. Sleep-disordered breathing and periodic limb movements in sleep in older patients with schizophrenia. Biol Psychiatry. 1999;45(11):1426–32.
57. Jagota P, Asawavichienjinda T, Bhidayasiri R. Prevalence of neuroleptic-induced restless legs syndrome in patients taking neuroleptic drugs. J Neurol Sci. 2012;314(1–2):158–60.
58. Rottach KG, Schaner BM, Kirch MH, Zivotofsky AZ, Teufel LM, Gallwitz T, et al. Restless legs syndrome as side effect of second generation antidepressants. J Psychiatr Res. 2008;43(1):70–5.
59. Kang SG, Lee HJ, Kim L. Restless legs syndrome and periodic limb movements during sleep probably associated with olanzapine. J Psychopharmacol (Oxford, England). 2009;23(5):597–601.
60. Allen RP, Montplaisir J, Walters AS, Ferini-Strambi L, Högl B. Restless legs syndrome and periodic limb movements during sleep. In: Principles and practice of sleep medicine. Philadelphia, PA: Elsevier; 2017. p. 923–34.e6.
61. Walters AS, Mandelbaum DE, Lewin DS, Kugler S, England SJ, Miller M. Dopaminergic therapy in children with restless legs/periodic limb movements in sleep and ADHD. Dopaminergic therapy study group. Pediatr Neurol. 2000;22(3):182–6.
62. Konofal E, Arnulf I, Lecendreux M, Mouren MC. Ropinirole in a child with attention-deficit hyperactivity disorder and restless legs syndrome. Pediatr Neurol. 2005;32(5):350–1.
63. Picchietti MA, Picchietti DL. Advances in pediatric restless legs syndrome: iron, genetics, diagnosis and treatment. Sleep Med. 2010;11(7):643–51.
64. Roth T, Jaeger S, Jin R, Kalsekar A, Stang PE, Kessler RC. Sleep problems, comorbid mental disorders, and role functioning in the national comorbidity survey replication. Biol Psychiatry. 2006;60(12):1364–71.
65. Candy M, Jones L, Williams R, Tookman A, King M. Psychostimulants for depression. Cochrane Database Syst Rev 2008;(2):CD006722.
66. Kaplan KA, Gruber J, Eidelman P, Talbot LS, Harvey AG. Hypersomnia in inter-episode bipolar disorder: does it have prognostic significance? J Affect Disord. 2011;132(3):438–44.
67. Kaplan KA, Harvey AG. Hypersomnia across mood disorders: a review and synthesis. Sleep Med Rev. 2009;13(4):275–85.
68. Lieberman JA, Stroup TS, McEvoy JP, Swartz MS, Rosenheck RA, Perkins DO, et al. Effectiveness of antipsychotic drugs in patients with chronic schizophrenia. N Engl J Med. 2005;353(12):1209–23.
69. Kane JM, Sharif ZA. Atypical antipsychotics: sedation versus efficacy. J Clin Psychiatry. 2008;69:18–31.
70. Sevy S, Rosenthal MH, Alvir J, Meyer S, Visweswaraiah H, Gunduz-Bruce H, et al. Double-blind, placebo-controlled study of modafinil for fatigue and cognition in schizophrenia patients treated with psychotropic medications. J Clin Psychiatry. 2005;66(7):839–43.
71. Pierre JM, Peloian JH, Wirshing DA, Wirshing WC, Marder SR. A randomized, double-blind, placebo-controlled trial of modafinil for negative symptoms in schizophrenia. J Clin Psychiatry. 2007;68(5):705–10.
72. Monteleone P, Maj M. The circadian basis of mood disorders: recent developments and treatment implications. Eur Neuropsychopharmacol. 2008;18(10):701–11.
73. Lamont EW, Coutu DL, Cermakian N, Boivin DB. Circadian rhythms and clock genes in psychotic disorders. Isr J Psychiatry Relat Sci. 2010;47(1):27–35.
74. Bersani FS, Iannitelli A, Pacitti F, Bersani G. Sleep and biorhythm disturbances in schizophrenia, mood and anxiety disorders: a review. Riv Psichiatr. 2012;47(5):365–75.
75. Monti JM, BaHammam AS, Pandi-Perumal SR, Bromundt V, Spence DW, Cardinali DP, et al. Sleep and circadian rhythm dysregulation in schizophrenia. Prog Neuropsychopharmacol Biol Psychiatry. 2013;43:209–16.
76. Wirz-Justice A, Haug HJ, Cajochen C. Disturbed circadian rest-activity cycles in schizophrenia patients: an effect of drugs? Schizophr Bull. 2001;27(3):497–502.
77. Wulff K, Dijk DJ, Middleton B, Foster RG, Joyce EM. Sleep and circadian rhythm disruption in schizophrenia. Br J Psychiatry J Ment Sci. 2012;200(4):308–16.
78. Rao ML, Gross G, Strebel B, Halaris A, Huber G, Braunig P, et al. Circadian rhythm of tryptophan, serotonin, melatonin, and pituitary hormones in schizophrenia. Biol Psychiatry. 1994;35(3):151–63.
79. Bromundt V, Koster M, Georgiev-Kill A, Opwis K, Wirz-Justice A, Stoppe G, et al. Sleep-wake cycles and cognitive functioning in schizophrenia. Br J Psychiatry J Ment Sci. 2011;198(4):269–76.
80. Imeraj L, Sonuga-Barke E, Antrop I, Roeyers H, Wiersema R, Bal S, et al. Altered circadian profiles in attention-deficit/hyperactivity disorder: an integrative review and theoretical framework for future studies. Neurosci Biobehav Rev. 2012;36(8):1897–919.
81. Van der Heijden KB, Smits MG, Van Someren EJ, Gunning WB. Idiopathic chronic sleep onset insomnia in attention-deficit/hyperactivity disorder: a circadian rhythm sleep disorder. Chronobiol Int. 2005;22(3):559–70.
82. Van Veen MM, Kooij JJ, Boonstra AM, Gordijn MC, Van Someren EJ. Delayed circadian rhythm in adults with attention-deficit/hyperactivity disorder

and chronic sleep-onset insomnia. Biol Psychiatry. 2010;67(11):1091–6.

83. Rybak YE, McNeely HE, Mackenzie BE, Jain UR, Levitan RD. An open trial of light therapy in adult attention-deficit/hyperactivity disorder. J Clin Psychiatry. 2006;67(10):1527–35.
84. Lee K, Baron K, Soca R, Attarian H. The prevalence and characteristics of REM Sleep without Atonia (RSWA) in patients taking antidepressants. J Clin Sleep Med. 2016;12(3):351–5.
85. Aurora RN, Zak RS, Maganti RK, Auerbach SH, Casey KR, Chowdhuri S, et al. Best practice guide for the treatment of REM sleep behavior disorder (RBD). J Clin Sleep Med. 2010;6(1):85.
86. Silber MH, St. Louis EK, Boeve BF. Rapid eye movement sleep parasomnias. In: Principles and practice of sleep medicine. Philadelphia, PA: Elsevier; 2017. p. 993–1001.e6.
87. Silber M. REM sleep behavior disorder associated with barbiturate withdrawal. Sleep Res. 1996;25:371.
88. Gross MM, Goodenough D, Tobin M, Halpert E, Lepore D, Perlstein A, et al. Sleep disturbances and hallucinations in the acute alcoholic psychoses. J Nerv Ment Dis. 1966;142(6):493–514.
89. Peever J, Luppi PH, Montplaisir J. Breakdown in REM sleep circuitry underlies REM sleep behavior disorder. Trends Neurosci. 2014;37(5):279–88.
90. Ramaligam V, Chen MC, Saper CB, Lu J. Perspectives on the rapid eye movement sleep switch in rapid eye movement sleep behavior disorder. Sleep Med. 2013;14(8):707–13.
91. McCarter SJ, Boswell CL, St Louis EK, Dueffert LG, Slocumb N, Boeve BF, et al. Treatment outcomes in REM sleep behavior disorder. Sleep Med. 2013;14(3):237–42.

Part III

Therapeutic Intervention for Treatment Resistance

Creative, Person-Centered Psychopharmacology for Treatment Resistance in Psychiatry

19

Miro Jakovljevic

19.1 Introduction

Among the leading topics in contemporary psychiatry, treatment resistance is a very hot one, not only from practical clinical perspective but also from research, theoretical, and epistemological points of view. It has always been an important topic in psychiatry, but concerns about increasing costs of psychiatric treatments and high mortality rates have put this topic in hot focus of interest. Despite the introduction of significant number of new mental health medicines since "the decade of the brain," outcomes of mental disorders in our "century of mind" remain poor in both short-term and long-term course of the treatment. Inadequate treatment in psychiatry seems to be more commonly the rule than the exception, and a huge number of patients do not respond in a satisfactory way, in terms of the magnitude of therapeutic response and/or the persistence of the remission [1]. Insufficient treatment response, treatment decrement, and treatment resistance are commonly associated with chronification of many mental disorders. Relationship between relapses, recurrent episodes, and illness chronicity from one side and partial remission, treatment decrement, and treatment resistance/refractoriness from the other side is a very complex one and circular in its nature. Many psychiatric patients suffer from post-episode residual symptoms and have a lower quality of life followed by increased relapse risk and poorer long-term outcomes associated with illness chronification. Major mental disorders are typically chronic disorders with a waxing and waning course and illness progression. Even mental disorders, episodic at the onset, turn chronic with shortening intervals between episodes. It is always important to have in mind that patients who do not achieve a good symptomatic remission and personal recovery after the first or repeated episode of illness have higher probability of relapse or of a new episode of illness, and by extension, of developing treatment decrement or resistance and chronic mental disorder. The high rate of treatment failures, the low effectiveness of mental health medicines, and the rigid and mechanistic pharmaco-centric treatment are currently in contention, both outside and within the field of psychiatry. Some classes of mental health medicines, for example, antidepressants, are wrongly depicted as noneffective, but harmful, and nothing more than "placebos with adverse effects." These negative and wrong views significantly contribute to vilification and condemnation of contemporary technical and impersonal psychopharmacotherapy and to stigmatization and fear of psychiatry. There has been an increasing concern that clinical psychopharmacology has

---

Parts of the chapter were previously published in *Person Centered Psychiatry*, pp. 235–245, Springer 2016.

M. Jakovljevic
Department of Psychiatry, University Hospital Centre Zagreb, Zagreb, Croatia

Y.-K. Kim (ed.), *Treatment Resistance in Psychiatry*, https://doi.org/10.1007/978-981-10-4358-1_19

lost its right way and biological psychiatry its soul, so commonly called "mindless psychiatry."

What causes a good therapeutic outcome and how to prevent or overcome treatment resistance are the fundamental questions from the perspective of transdisciplinary integrative psychiatry (see [2–4]). The challenge for contemporary thinking about treatment resistance in psychiatry arises from the way we understand and treat mental disorders. Treatment outcome is strongly associated with person-centered approach in therapy and the level of resilience (lat. resilare – to rebound), creativity, patient-doctor partnership, and positive therapeutic narratives. In order to increase treatment efficiency, including preventing and overcoming treatment resistance, the author has been trying to develop the concept of creative, person-centered pharmacotherapy [2–5]. The key terms of this concept are the focus on person in treatment instead of blockbuster and stratified medicine approaches, synergistic drug combinations, enhancing resilience and salutogenesis, decreasing general psychopathology or p factor (see [6]), reconstructing disease and therapeutic narratives, and promoting creativity and partnership.

19.2 Reframing Pessimistic Paradigm: Insufficient Treatment Response Is Not Always Treatment Resistance

> The ways in which we define problems often hinder their solutions. Paul Watzlawick (1989)

Our everyday clinical experience confirms Watzlawick's claim that the ways in which we define problems with biases and blunders regularly hinder their solutions. It is also the case with the treatment resistance in psychiatry. Treatment resistance is a metaphor which implies negative and frightening connotations and augments therapeutic pessimism and complicates treatment as well as living of patients with the so-called treatment-resistant mental disorders. For the time being, treatment resistance is unfortunately a badly defined and understood phenomenon with differing conceptualizations, applications, and implications. There are no generally accepted definitions of what defines treatment resistance and refractoriness, as well as treatment nonresponsiveness and ineffectiveness for any of the individual mental disorders. Unfortunately, studies claiming that certain markers could predict treatment response or differentiate treatment-responsive from treatment-resistant mental disorders have not been still replicated (see [7]). Full and clear understanding of neurobiology and psychopathology of major mental disorders has been still elusive. The practice of evidence-biased instead of true evidence-based medicine may significantly contribute to treatment pseudo-resistance. Early differentiation of real treatment resistance from pseudo-resistance and insufficient treatment response is of the great importance because a starting false resistance commonly becomes the real one. The misdiagnosis or rapid labeling of patients as treatment resistant can have very deleterious nocebo effects on treatment outcome. According to the very popular, but not precise definition, treatment resistance "refers to the occurrence of an inadequate response following adequate therapy among patients suffering from a defined psychiatric disorder" [1]. Treatment resistance is a negative and pessimism provoking term which may have double nocebo meaning: that the patient is resisting treatment and that the mental disorder is resistant to treatment. It implies discouraging and disappointing message that remission or recovery is not possible which inhibits patients from continuing treatment long enough or from further searching to get competent treatment. Having in mind this pessimistic connotation, which implies incurability and bad prognosis, it is better to use more neutral terms like insufficient or unsatisfactory treatment response to avoid, among other negativities, the possible nocebo effects on patients. As it is sometimes possible in good clinical practice to achieve favored or even optimal treatment outcome after previous several unsuccessful attempts, several and long treatment failures in fact mean "more-difficult-than-usual treatment." Therefore, instead of treatment resistance, it is better to speak about "for a time being treatment failure," unsatisfactory, or incomplete treatment response and so offering a hope for better treatment success in the future. Learned helplessness and pessimism are essential features of some mental disorders, like depression and anxiety disorders. Optimism is regarded as an indication of positive mental health associated with higher level of subjective well-being. Furthermore, optimism may serve the function to motivate patients in the service of their proactive and cooperative participation and partnership in the treatment. Empathy with positive suggestions, expectations, and optimism are leading to placebo response by many patients, whereas negative suggestions, expectations, and pessimism are commonly followed by nocebo response [8, 9]. It is fundamental for clinicians to create good rapport with patients and balance the need to instill positive thinking and optimism with realistic expectation for desired treatment response and outcome.

19.2.1 Evaluation and General Management of Insufficient Treatment Response and Treatment Failure

Managing patients with previous treatment failures has been challenging, even for the most experienced psychiatrists. Let it be said at the very outset that we do not yet know what are the key processes of therapeutic responses and mechanisms of treatment failures. Treatment resistance is a description of an individual treatment course, and it is not a static but developing phenomenon of several therapeutic failures. As Sigmund Freud noticed in 1912, "the resistance accompanies the treatment step by step." Insufficient therapeutic response and treatment failure can be manifested in various forms (see Table 19.1) and be associated with many diverse factors (see Table 19.2) which should be recognized and eliminated as early as possible. Generally speaking one can differentiate treatment resistance from the illness onset and gradually developed treatment resistance as illness progression in the context of multiple episodes, chronic exposure to medication, or neurochemical sensitization [10].

Treatment failure or negative therapeutic response may be influenced by a myriad of diverse factors: disease, comorbidities, and drug interactions which a patient *has*, what a patients *feels* and how subjectively *suffers*, how a patient is defined or stigmatized by diagnosis, and how the community responds to patient's behavior, who or what of a person a patient *is*, what a patient *does* and how a patient behaves, what a patient *believes in* and tends *to be*, what a patient's

Table 19.1 Diverse form of treatment failures

Absolute or total treatment resistance: nonresponse to adequate treatment, cannot be overcome by manipulating dose or treatment schedule/duration or changing method
Relative treatment resistance: logically inappropriate term for nonresponse to an inadequate treatment
Therapeutic pseudo-resistance: more appropriate term for nonresponse to an inadequate treatment, amenable to treatment corrections
Primary drug resistance: resistance in a patient who has not previously received any mental health medications
Secondary drug resistance: resistance in a patient who was previously treated successfully by mental health medications
Partial treatment resistance: lack of complete remission and full recovery after several appropriate treatment trials
Acquired drug resistance: resistance developed during the treatment due to nonadherence of recommended treatment rules and instructions or due to wrong drug treatments like wrong serial mono-pharmacy or toxic polypharmacy
Therapeutic decrement and progressive treatment resistance: an increasingly more treatment resistance of subsequent episodes of illness and progressive exacerbation or chronification of illness – the so-called "drug tachyphylaxis," reduced neuroplasticity, disturbed plasticity of neuronal receptor regulation, and neurodegenerative mechanisms
Intolerance to medication: an inability to tolerate the adverse effects of a medication at therapeutic or subtherapeutic doses may be related to genetic variations in drug metabolism

Table 19.2 Factors contributing to insufficient or negative therapeutic response and treatment failure (see [11], revised)

Illness-related factors: poor knowing of pathophysiology, unrecognized and undiagnosed psychopathology, unrecognized comorbid medical disorders, comorbid psychiatric disorders (dual disorders), personality/character pathology, and deficiencies in thiamine, vitamin B6, vitamin B12, folates, copper, and zinc
Treatment-related factors: non-adequate treatment, unimodal treatment not covering some important pathological mechanisms, rigid dogmatic treatment approach, the so-called "wait-and-see strategy," inadequate treatment of earlier episodes, and drug therapy as a sole form of treatment with the message to patients: "you don't have to change anything, you just have to take your medication on time and for a long time enough"
Medication-related factors: delayed treatment onset, intolerance to the medication, adverse events and toxic side effects, monotherapy non-covering all important pathological mechanisms, medications with opposite effects, irrational polypharmacy and toxic drug combinations, adverse drug and food interactions
Patient-generated factors: partial adherence or nonadherence to treatment, rapid or slow drug metabolism, pessimism and negative beliefs and expectations, recent psycho-traumatization, reactivation of suppressed psycho-trauma, lack of faith in doctor and treatment, nocebo response, negative meaning response, preoccupation with side effects and negative reactions, negative treatment conditioning, negative therapeutic reaction related to unconscious sense of guilt, self-defeating behavior, strong need to be in charge, pharmacophobia, prejudice, and bad nutritional status
Clinician-related factors: non-adequate communication style; poor fit between type of psychological approach and personality type of patient; nonconscious nocebo induction; lack of optimism; lack of empathy, compassion, and guidance skills; low level of experience and professional knowledge; discomfort with uncertainty; negative countertransference (anger, guilt, dislike, disappointment, helplessness, and powerlessness) and negative emotional reaction to the patient; unsatisfactory self-management; and accusing the patient of being problematic or difficult
Factors associated with doctor-patient relationship: anti-therapeutic relationship, lack of therapeutic alliance, psychiatric care experienced as impersonal, unconcerned and uncaring, lack of rapport, and power games
Patient's family-related factors: stigma, lack of support and care, rejection, high negative emotional expression, and family psychopathology

life story is and *narrative* abou*t* illness and its treatment.

Some general principles for the management of treatment failures may be helpful in overcoming the problem (Table 19.3). First and foremost, clinicians should be rethinking their definition of treatment goals and treatment strategy, always having in mind that the best treatments are those that utilize and integrate multiple modalities at the right time and in good treatment context accepted by patients. For example, rethinking the strategy of long acting injection or depot antipsychotics application could significantly improve treatment response and outcome in patients with schizophrenia.

Despite the evidence-proved advantages offered by long-acting injections of antipsychotics (LAIAs), they are widely underused in many countries all over the world [12, 13]. The LAIAs have long been considered and still are considered as a treatment reserved only for nonadherent and non-compliant patients with frequent relapses or who pose risk for others. Recently, with regard to the schizophrenia staging and critical period concept, the interest of using SG (second generation)-LAIAs in the early stage of schizophrenia has increased [9]. Rethinking schizophrenia as a neurodevelopmental disorder with psychosis and neurodegeneration as a late, potentially preventable stage of illness [14] yields new perspective on SG-LAIAs utilization in early stages of illness aimed to prevent treatment resistance.

Creative, person-centered psychopharmacology is called upon to denounce the metaphor of treatment resistance and to support patients and their families in enhancing their resilience and healthy parts of personalities, thus promoting their positive mental health. At the end of the day, it means to change an inadequate and

Table 19.3 General principles for the management of treatment failure ([11], revised)

Assess factors contributing to treatment failure and formulate and implement a new treatment plan
Ensure accurate diagnosis, including the subtype of mental disorder
Identify patient's strengths and weakness and opportunities and threats (SWOT analysis)
Assess psychiatric and somatic comorbidity
Evaluate psychosocial stressors and enhance social support
Ensure appropriate dose and duration of treatment (e.g., long-acting injectable antipsychotics)
Monitor and treat adverse events
Check and monitor drug concentrations in blood
Evaluate pharmacokinetic parameters
Assess possible undesired drug interactions
Assess drug-induced neurotransmitter dysbalance syndrome, neurotransmitter receptor supersensitivity syndrome (e.g., dopamine supersensitivity psychosis), and drug tachyphylaxis
If applicable assess DHEA/cortisol ratio, thyroid hormones, homocysteine blood level, inflammatory biomarkers like CRP (c-reactive protein), candidate genes ABSB1, FTD7, and WNT2B on antidepressant drug resistance, etc.
Ensure the psycho-education of patient and his or her family
Assess cultural beliefs
Ensure treatment adherence (e.g., LAIAs in schizophrenia and recurrent psychotic disorders) and therapeutic alliance
Ensure integrative and complementary treatment approach
Evaluate and redefine treatment goals and therapeutic narratives
Enhance resilience and placebo response
Integrate treatment from multiple clinicians
Aim for clinical remission, social rehabilitation, and personal recovery

fragmented therapy for a proper and integrative one.

19.3 From Treatment Resistance to Resilience and Positive Mental Health

> Our greatest glory is not in never falling, but in rising every time we fall.
> Confucius

Following the quote of Confucius, resilience may be defined as an ability to rise every time we fall, to bend but not to break, and to adapt well when face to adversity, threats, trauma, disease, or tragedy. The term resilience refers to the process of bouncing back and overcoming adversity, while resiliency means personality traits related to resilience. Resiliency refers to personality traits like adaptability, hardiness, self-directedness, cooperativeness, self-transcendence, and invincibility. With regard to treatment resistance in psychiatry and association between health, resilience, and disease, an essential question arises: Does resilience enhancing help and how in preventing and overcoming treatment resistance in psychiatry? It seems that many major mental disorders may be understood as a limitation of primary resilience [6], while treatment failure or treatment resistance may be associated with limitations of secondary and tertiary resilience. Resilience is a relatively new psychobiological concept which refers to individual's capacity to overcome therapeutic failure and hard-treated mental disorders. The concept of resilience and resiliency promotes positive psychology and positive mental health by increasing individual and collective sense of well-being which may be an important component of favorable treatment outcome [15]. Well-being as "the capacity to live a full and creative life, and the flexibility to deal with life's inevitable challenges" [16] is closely related to resilience.

Research in the psychobiology of resilience, which has epigenetic, neurobiological, psychological, sociocultural, and spiritual underpinnings, could significantly improve our knowledge about where and what the correlates are of treatment failure or resistance and how to prevent and overcome it.

Resilience is a complex, multidimensional, and dynamic process, very important for understanding of salutogenesis and pathogenesis as well as therapeutic and healing mechanisms. *Salutogenesis* (the Latin salus, health; the Greek genesis, origin) is related to healing that is a natural process seen in all forms of life, and it is closely related to resilience. Resilience represents a collection of protective and salutogenic factors that modulate the relationship between a stressful event, adversity or disease, and positive outcomes. It is an indivisible part of mental health and health in general, well-being and quality of life. In psychology, resilience refers to the ability to bounce back from a negative experience (stress, adversity, trauma, threats, tragic) with competent and adaptive functioning [17]. In medicine, resilience refers to one's capability to recover when having an illness or disease. Resilience is considered as a dynamic and modifiable process, gradually developed through the life span, by facing and overcoming of adversary events. In real life resilience manifests itself on continuum that may be present to differing degrees over time across multiple domains of life [17]. Individuals may be resilient in one domain and not in others, or they may be resilient at one spell of time and not at other periods of their lives. Resilience is about the whole person; it includes biological, psychological, social, and spiritual dimension of human existence and enables individuals and communities not only to survive and adapt to challenge but also to be better off and to grow and thrive (posttraumatic growth) in addition to overcoming a specific adversary. *Psychological resilience* is a protective collection of thoughts, actions, and behavior that can be developed and improved by everybody. It consists of intrapersonal (how an individual relates to their own thoughts, feelings, and behaviors) and interpersonal (how an individual relates to others) components. According to hybrid model [18], resilience is related to (1) the one's positive attitude toward restoration and recovery (optimistic thinking, creative faith); (2) the power and confidence to reconstruct, reintegrate, and control one's adversary or disease (coping skills, ability to control relapse prevention and illness, practicing health plan well); and (3) positive mutual interaction with supportive resource (support from institutions and medical experts, from family members, friends, and other people). Resilience may reflect differences in neurobiology, but it also reflects some aspects of personality [19]. Spirituality and religiosity may act as resilience resources to manage adversity like mental illness [20]. Placebo response may be an expression of psychological and spiritual resilience [21].

Resilience depends on individual, family, community, and institutional factors, and it varies over time in different situations. We can speak about primary, secondary, and tertiary resilience. *Primary resilience* is aimed to maintain homeostasis/equilibrium and mental health. The level of primary resilience has been regarded as a protective factor against developing mental disorder, whereas lack of resilience carries a risk for the appearance of mental disorders. It can be described as "bouncing back" and "rebounding after adversary," and as such it is related to the disease prevention. The concept of primary resilience explains why many people do not become ill or do not develop a particular disorder although they are subject to the same kind of adversary events, even after a prolonged period of adversity, with psychological and physical burdens, that cause the disorder in other people [22]. *Secondary resilience* refers to the capability of individuals to cope with illness/disease and successfully recover. It is aimed to regain equilibrium after allostatic load and mental disorder. The capability to achieve clinical, functional/social, and personal recovery implies the presence of secondary resilience. In addition to clinical remission, secondary resilience may lead to a personal growth and developing a meaningful life after the mental illness. On the opposite side, lack of resilience determines onset, course, outcome, distress, and burden of mental illness (see [15]). *Tertiary resilience* enables patients to develop a healthy and productive way to live with their illness, helps them to adapt to limitations in life associated with illness, and has positive and creative life attitudes. Proactive and more efficacious participation of patients with chronic illness and residual symptoms in their medical treatment is also an expression of tertiary resilience.

19.4 Enhancing Resilience: Creative Psychopharmacotherapy May Overcome Treatment Resistance

> It is more important to know what kind of a patient has a disease than what kind of a disease a patient has. William Osler

The model of primary, secondary, and tertiary resilience explains how appropriate resilience-enhancing interventions may help in overcoming the lack of therapeutic response. The level of and pace by which recovery is established is a function of brain resilience, external resources like support, nature of the mental disorder, and chosen drug treatment. However, resiliency as a treatment target has been largely neglected in the field of therapeutics [23], so the lack of favorable treatment outcome may be commonly related to the treatment focus only on symptoms and illness. The route of clinical, functional, and personal recovery lies not only in decreasing illness but also in enhancing resilience and increasing wellness [24]. Full personal recovery does not mean only the absence of symptoms of mental illness but also the presence of resilience and wellness. The concept of resilience enhancing focuses also on strengths and potentials for wellness which are present in patients, not only on their weakness and pathology. Each patient is a unique, responsive, and responsible person, and within every person there is a force that drives them to strive to self-realization, self-understanding and self-transcendence and a sense of cohesion and control over their own life. Resilience is a complex process ranging from surviving to thriving, positive transformation and personal growth. Enhancing patients' resilience by emphasizing their strength and covering up their weakness is an ambitious goal that aims to promote positive mental health in spite of the presence of symptoms [25] and drug treatment failure. Good news is that resilience can be enhanced through learning and training. Resilience training can result in augmented neuroplasticity and balance of neural circuits that modulate reward and motivation, emotion regulation, cognitive reappraisal and executive function, novelty seeking, harm avoidance and fear response, self-directedness, cooperativeness and adaptive social behavior, and self-transcendence. A variety of internal and external events can influence our genes triggering epigenetic reactions, e.g., methylation which turn gene on or turn them off [26]. When a gene is "turned on," it governs the making of gene products, e.g., proteins, and when a gene is "turned off," these products are no longer produced. Genes found to be associated with different aspects of resiliency include the monoamine oxidase A (MAO-A), neuropeptide Y (NPY), brain-derived neurotrophic factor (BDNF), corticotrophin-releasing hormone receptor (CRHR1), oxytocin receptor gene (OXTR), FK-506 binding protein 5 (FKBP5), serotonin-transporter promoter polymorphism (5-HTTLPR), catechol-O-methyltranspherase (COMT), nerve growth factor inducible (NGFI-A), and calcium channel, voltage-dependent, L type, alpha1C subunit (CACNA 1C), apolipoprotein E (ApoE) genes [27–31]. Some authors speak about resilience promoting molecules like DHEA, neuropeptide Y, galanin, serotonin, oxytocin, testosterone, estrogen, HDL and benzodiazepine receptors, and resilience undermining molecules like corticotropin-releasing hormone (CRH) and cortisol [32–34]. The methylation of certain genes, e.g., the glucocorticoid gene promoter, could mediate the long-term effect of adversity (see [6]). It is interesting that low DHEA/cortisol ratio was suggested as useful biological resilience marker in patients with PTSD [32, 34]. According to some studies, resilience may be affected by pharmacological treatments like antidepressants [35].

Antidepressant effects have been reported to be related to reversing hippocampal atrophy by the stimulation of neuronal proliferation and synaptic plasticity as well as that the candidate genes ABCB1, FZD7, and WNT2B can be biomarkers for antidepressant drug resistance [36]. Antidepressants may have resilience-enhancing or saliostatic properties [37] and vice versa; high resilience might contribute to better treatment response in depressed patients [38]. The specific role of resilience in mental disorders like depression, personality disorders, and schizophrenia spectrum disorders is not fully understood; as suggested by literature, it may contribute to the determinism of illness onset, duration, severity, frequency relapses, treatment compliance, and effectiveness [39]. Our growing understanding of the psycho-neurobiology of resilience could have significant implications for predictive, preventive, and person-centered psychopharmacotherapy.

19.4.1 Rethinking Treatment Strategy: Multidimensional and Integrative Therapeutic Approach

> The rational use of multiple medications simultaneously to treat difficult illnesses places psychiatric pharmacotherapy on a par with treatment in other medical specialties. Bernstein (1993) [40]

In the literature one can identify several, mainly empirically supported, recommendations to relieve treatment nonresponse or failure and to prevent developing a real treatment resistance. These recommendations commonly contradict with one another and are changeable as the ever-increasing influx of new information appears and novel therapies are made available. The most popular pharmacological strategies are switching, augmentation, and drug combination from the treatment beginning (see Table 19.4). However, these terms have different meaning for different people which is not good for the scientific image of psychiatry. According to some authors, augmentation is usually defined as the simultaneous administration of the two medications of different classes (e.g., adding antidepressant to antipsychotic drug in patients with schizophrenia), while polypharmacy is defined as the use of two or more medications of the same group such as antipsychotic medications (see [41]). Polypharmacy (lat. multiple drugs) refers to the concurrent use of multiple medications by a patient for the same illness or different illnesses in the case of comorbidity. It usually implies a negative connotation of too many medications which is a wrong apprehension. Within the concept of creative psychopharmacotherapy, creative drug combinations mean as many medications as needed, each for a specific target of illness, to obtain optimal therapeutic response and personal recovery. Medications which become not-needed or un-tolerable over time are discontinued.

In the case of treatment failure, first and foremost, clinicians should be rethinking their treatment philosophy and strategy. The best treatments are those that utilize and integrate multiple complementary modalities aimed to clear defined therapeutic goals addressing all presenting important syndromes. The concept of creative, person-centered narrative psychopharmacotherapy gives a hope for overcoming treatment nonresponse and failure (Table 19.5).

The concept of creative psychopharmacotherapy offers an overarching theoretical framework that permits the integration of different levels of explanation from neuroscience, clinical psychopharmacology, psychodynamics, evolutionary psychobiology, and positive psychology in order to predict and prevent or identify and resolve treatment resistance. It represents an art and practice of the learning organization (see [43]) in the frame of transdisciplinary, integrative, narrative, person-centered, and neuroscience-based psychiatry [5, 2, 3, 11]. Each therapy is a learning process which involves systemic thinking, creative mental model, personal mastery, therapeutic vision, and therapeutic dialogue (see [43]). The more complicated the treatment case is, the more art and learning with the patient are needed for a successful therapeutic outcome. Creative psychopharmacotherapy is much more than pre-

Table 19.4 Management strategies for overcoming insufficient treatment response ([11], modified)

Pharmacological strategies
Increasing the dosage of medication to the maximal recommended dose
Switching strategies: stopping the medication to which the patient is not responding and prescribing another medicine, usually from an another group of the same class
Augmentation strategies: adding another agent to an ongoing medication that has been insufficient in order to augment or maximize its effectiveness
Adjunctive, adjuvant, or add-on therapy: another treatment used with or added to the primary treatment with an ancillary role in treating an illness (in addition to drugs also horticultural, art, music, recreation therapy)
Neoadjuvant therapy: in contrast to adjuvant therapy, it is applied before the application of the main therapy
Supplementations (brain-healthy diet, vitamins, omega-3 fatty acids, amino-acids, S-adenosyl-L- methionine (SAM-e), dehydroepiandrosterone (DHEA), Saint John's wort, *Ginkgo biloba*, etc.)
Combination strategies (COMBOs): adding another compound very soon or starting with two or more compounds of the same or different class with a well-established efficacy as a single agent for the treatment of the mental disorder
Off-label indication drugs: ketamine, oxytocin, memantine, armodafinil, thyroid hormones, riluzole, minocycline, COX-2 inhibitors, etc.
Non-pharmacological strategies
Electroconvulsive therapy (ECT): better term is electroneuromodulatory therapy
Vagus nerve stimulation
Repetitive transcranial magnetic stimulation (rTMS)
Cognitive enhancement therapy based on the brain neuroplasticity model
Psychotherapy and psychosocial treatments, assertive community treatment
Psycho-education and cooperation with family and social skills training
Individual resiliency training
The health belief dialogue and improving treatment adherence and proactivity
Psychological strategies: respecting the patient, being nonjudgmental, careful active listening, validating feelings and behaviors, supportive and understanding attitude, framing a clear treatment strategy and contract, enhancing motivation for change (motivational enhancement therapy)
Creating favorable therapeutic context
Partnership-based guidance of the patient and building a stable therapeutic alliance
Increasing placebo and decreasing nocebo responses
Creating positive treatment narrative: narrative psychopharmacology
Psychodynamic pharmacotherapy
Life coaching strategies
Enhancing resilience and resiliency: cognitive restructuring and improving coping strategies
Promoting patients' creativity
Improving illness self-management skills and coping with persistent symptoms
Supporting patients to achieve personal goals
Complementary medicine: therapeutic disciplines that are used together with conventional medicine as add-on therapy
Acupuncture, homeopathy, spiritual healing, yoga, tai chi, etc.
Integrated strategies
-Use of mental health medications together with other modes of treatment like psychotherapy, family therapy, narrative therapy, risk management strategies, complementary, and alternative medicine
Creative, person-centered narrative psychopharmacotherapy

scribing mental health medicines in rational manner and careful control of their use. It is a relational, contextual, multimodal, personalized, and individualized application of the creative thinking and systemic information processing strategy. Creative psychopharmacotherapy includes not only creative and rational use of mental health medicines and their combinations but it is also about creating favorable treatment context, reconstructing narratives that fuel mental

Table 19.5 Creative person-centered narrative psychopharmacotherapy ([11, 42] revised)

1. Not only to decrease illness but also to increase wellness enhancing salutogenesis and resilience, resetting self-awareness, self-esteem, self-motivation, self-affirmation, hedonic capacity, and positive thinking
2. Evidence-based practice and practice-based evidence, value- and narrative-based practice, pluralistic, personal and respective of individuality, and personal life stories
3. Individualistic and more humanistic (postmodern science)
4. In addition to rational thinking based on lateral and systems thinking and imagination and inductive logic
5. Self-determination of patients is promoted; patients are more proactive subjects and participants and the stars of treatment; alliance is much more than compliance
6. Partnership between doctors and patients and their families, not paternalism
Patients and their families have also access to the information. Doctors and patients together know what's the best, shared decisions; patients are best experts on their life
7. Focus on self-actualization, positive health and quality of life, and strengths and advantages; increase wellness
8. Therapeutic goals drive treatment. In addition to clinical remission, personal recovery is valued; drug treatment is rooted in creative and systematic thinking in addition to treatment guidelines
9. Responsible benefit-risk ratio evaluation, personal growth
10. "Poly-therapy as soon as needed" strategy
11. More optimistic concepts, terms like insufficient or incomplete treatment response, lack of treatment response
12. Treatment goals of therapeutic journey: acute phase – clinical remission, stabilizing phase – social recovery, stable or final phase – personal recovery
13. Psychopharmacotherapy closely joined with psychotherapy

health problems, resilience enhancing, and fostering patients' creativity and personal mastery. It is an alternative to dogmatic, rigid, and authoritarian application of official treatment guidelines and marketing-based practice.

19.4.2 Tailoring the Best Drug Combinations as Soon as Possible for Specific Mental Disorders on Individual Basis

> Good clinicians practice rational poly-pharmacy, and those who do it expertly are leaders in their field. Doran [44]

Dr. Jonathan Cole (1925–2009) coined the term creative psychopharmacology in 1992 referring to "the rational use of multiple medications simultaneously to treat difficult illnesses" (according [40]). Rational and safe combinations of multiple medications are usually recommended to achieve clinical improvement when simpler regimens have failed [40, 44]. Drug treatment guidelines mainly promote a next decision-making procedure: (1) single drug treatment of the first choice; (2) switching, if there is no treatment response; and (3) augmentation or drug combinations (COMBOs), if treatment fails again. Although many of the evidence support "COMBOs as soon as needed" strategy (see [45, 46]), international consensus treatment guidelines for all major mental disorders strongly recommend single drug of choice as the first-line treatment in spite of the fact that many psychiatric patients do not recover after their initial monotherapy trial. The so-called treatment pseudo-resistance may be commonly a result of this treatment strategy. The use of a single mental health medication is always the simplest and safest, but very often not the most effective or sufficient treatment [44]. Approximately half of depressed patients, for example, show an insufficient response to monotherapy, and every fifth patient has chronic depression despite multiple interventions. In general, creative COMBOs with an additive, synergistic, and therapeutic effect between two and more medicines make the overall treatment benefit greater than that achieved by either of the medications alone. Patients with panic disorder, for example, respond better and sooner to the COMBO of an SSRI antidepressant and a high potent benzodiazepine than to either of the medications alone. When panic attacks disappear soon, the benzodiazepine is excluded, while

Table 19.6 Some examples of some synergistic drug combinations

Antipsychotics:
Risperidone or paliperidone in the morning or during the day + clozapine or olanzapine or quetiapine in the evening
Aripiprazole in the morning + clozapine or olanzapine or quetiapine in the evening
Haloperidol or fluphenazine + clozapine or olanzapine or quetiapine
Paliperidone long-acting injection every 4 weeks or every 3 months + clozapine or olanzapine or quetiapine in the evening
Aripiprazole long-acting injection every 4 weeks + clozapine or olanzapine or quetiapine in the evening
Antidepressants
Escitalopram or sertraline or fluoxetine or paroxetine in the morning + trazodone or mirtazapine in the evening
Escitalopram or sertraline or fluoxetine or paroxetine in the morning + maprotiline in the evening
Reboxetine in the morning + trazodone or mirtazapine in the evening
Escitalopram or sertraline or fluoxetine or paroxetine in the morning + agomelatine in the evening
Escitalopram or sertraline or fluoxetine or paroxetine in the morning + olanzapine or quetiapine in small doses in the evening
Mood stabilizers
Lithium carb + valproate
Lithium carb + lamotrigine
Lithium carb or valproate or lamotrigine + olanzapine long-acting injection or paliperidone long-acting injection or aripiprazole long-acting injection
Anxiolytic drugs
Alprazolam or klonazepam + escitalopram or fluvoxamine or paroxetine or sertraline or fluoxetine
Buspirone + alprazolam or klonazepam or diazepam, etc.

maintenance treatment is continued with the antidepressant. Individual antipsychotics are not effective in treating the entire range of symptoms in schizophrenia as well as antidepressants in monotherapy which do not cover all the aspects of psychopathology in depression. It is quite rational to treat depressed patients with two or more antidepressants simultaneously if they have different mechanisms of action and synergistic therapeutic effects, e.g., stimulating one in the morning and sedating one in the evening (see Table 19.6). It is similar with combinations of mood stabilizers, antipsychotics, etc. Many bipolar patients simply cannot be stabilized with one mood stabilizer alone but improve considerably or achieve a full recovery when treated with a combination of mood stabilizers from different drug families. A common example of monotherapy ineffectiveness may be seen in bipolar depressed patients, when patients on a mood stabilizer alone have breakthrough depressions but when on an antidepressant alone have lack of response, manic overstimulation, or erratic, unpredictable response [44]. Rational combination of two or more mental health medicines may help patients to be mood stable and free from depression. Comorbidity increases risk of treatment failure, and because of that it is also an important reason supporting the rationale of polypharmacy. For example, patients with comorbid depression and anxiety disorder, like panic disorder, treated with antidepressant alone, may become overstimulated or respond only partially, while treated with a high potent benzodiazepine alone may have breakthrough depressive symptoms or breakthrough panic attacks (see [44]). Combination of these two classes of drugs together (COMBOs) may eliminate both depression and panic attacks.

As mental disorders contribute enormously to psychological, social, and economic suffering of patients and their families, the achievement of complete remission as soon as possible is a very important goal of creative psychopharmacotherapy. Rapid remission and complete recovery, what is the best prevention of treatment failures and resistance, can be achieved in majority cases only with rational drug combinations and creative polypharmacy. Creative and rational polypharmacy means multiple drug treatment with “only as many drugs as necessary, each for a

Table 19.7 Some interesting evidence-based and practice-based COMBOs according to Stephen Stahl [45, 46]

Combos for unipolar depression
Triple-action combo: SSRI/SNRI+NDRI
California rocket fuel: SNRI + mirtazapine
Arousal combos: SNRI + stimulant or modafinil
Lithium combo: 1st line agent + lithium
Thyroid combo: 1st line agent + T3/T4
Serotonin 1A combo: 1st line agent + buspirone (?pindolol)
Insomnia anxiety combo: 1st line agent + eszopiclone/zolpidem or benzodiazepine
Serotonin 2A combo: 1st line agent + SARI + mirtazapine + SDA/DPA
Dopaminergic combo: NDRI/NRI + stimulant + modafinil + DA agonist (e.g., pramipexole)
Heroic combo: high-dose SNRI/SSRI + alfa2 antagonist + NDRI/NRI + stimulant
Bipolar combos
Atypical + lithium (evidence-based)
Atypical + valproate (evidence-based)
Li-Vo: lithium + valproate (practice-based)
La-Vo: lamotrigine + valproate (practice-based – caution)
La-Li: lamotrigine + lithium (practice-based)
La-Li-Vo: lamotrigine + lithium + valproate (practice-based – caution)
Lami-quel: lamotrigine + quetiapine (practice-based)
Boston bipolar brew: any combo but antidepressant
California careful cocktail: any combo + antidepressant
Tennessee mood shine: atypical + antidepressant
Walt Disney's combo: any combo containing ziprasidone
California sunshine: ziprasidone + lithium + transdermal selegiline or ziprasidone + lithium + venlafaxine
Schizophrenia combos
The second-line treatment of positive symptoms: clozapine or conventional AP + SDA or DPA
The third-line treatment: first line AP + mood stabilizer

AP antipsychotic, *DPA* dopamine partial agonist, *NDRA* noradrenalin dopamine reuptake inhibitor, *NRI* noradrenaline reuptake inhibitor, *SDA* serotonin dopamine antagonist, *SNRI* serotonin noradrenaline reuptake inhibitor, *SSRI* selective serotonin reuptake inhibitor

specific target symptom, each evaluated individually for efficacy and side effects and adjusted optimally, with the elimination of each one that is no longer necessary" [47]. Creative COMBOs provide synergistic benefits and mitigate or eliminate adverse effects by using lower doses of each medication and targeting complementary physiological (compensatory) mechanisms.

General strategy "monotherapy before polytherapy" is one of the significant causes of treatment resistance or better to say pseudo-resistance. It is evident that finding the right medication for an individual in serial mono-pharmacy approach is not so easy. Many patients usually try several different medicines before finding the right one. In addition, we are now confronted with the fact that mental disorders are the result of abnormalities in the complex interactions between several neurotransmitter and psychobiological systems rather than in the abnormalities of any only one simple system. In clinical practice it is very difficult to achieve a full remission or recovery with drug monotherapy, so polypharmacy of mental health medicines should be rather a rule than an exception.

In general, creative COMBOs (see Tables 19.6 and 19.7) with an additive, synergistic therapeutic effect between two and more medicines, make the overall treatment benefit greater than that achieved by either of the medications alone. Rapid remission and complete recovery can be achieved in a majority of cases only with rational drug combinations and creative polypharmacy.

19.4.3 Creating Favorable Therapeutic Relationship/Context

Unfavorable treatment context contributes very often to the lack of desirable therapeutic response and treatment resistance as consequence. In addition to the optimal treatment regime in terms of drug selection, dosage and duration, creating specific favorable treatment context for each patient individually is crucial for obtaining treatment success. The term context refers to the particular setting, such as time, place, and people present, which gives meaning to all events and activities during treatment. The fact is that in addition to the physical world, we also live in the world of ideas, symbols, stories, and meanings. The patient's beliefs concerning the origin of symptoms and mental health medicines action may contribute positively (placebo) or negatively (nocebo) to drug treatment response and treatment adherence. In addition to their pharmacodynamic mechanisms, mental health medications work also on account of meanings, expectations, and relationships related to the context of treatment. Hence, treatment effectiveness depends on (1) what psychiatrists and patients believe how medications work, (2) quality of a physician-patient relationship including rapport (mutual trust and respect) and patient's confidence in the psychiatry as a whole, (3) characteristics of the treatment (color, shape, smell, taste and name of medications, method and place of application, etc.), (4) communication and emotional expressiveness within the patient's family, and (5) respect for patients' human rights. Always we should have in mind that "pharmakon," which means both "remedy" and "poison," is closely related to "pharmakos," which means "scapegoat," and to "pharmakeus," "magician" or "sorcerer" (see [48]). Positive beliefs and good human relations may be "ariston pharmakon," "most effective remedy," whereas negative and wrong beliefs and bad human relations may be scapegoating.

The creation of favorable therapeutic context is significantly associated with proactive participation of patients and their commitment to treatment. The purpose of person-centered pharmacotherapy is to empower the patients to control their disease, to improve resilience and obtain full personal recovery, and to regain control over their life. However, taking medications only is often not enough for full treatment success. Pharmacotherapy as a sole form of treatment may carry the wrong message that patients don't have to change their lifestyle and don't have to learn any new skill; they just have to take their medication on time because the only problem is in brain chemistry. Pharmacotherapy is one essential external support, alongside a whole range of other type of resilience-promoting supports, skills, and strengths. As previously mentioned the goals of medication treatment are not only to decrease illness and prevent relapse but also to help patients learn new ways of thinking, emotional response, and behavior to get more love, freedom, power, joy, and sense of life. Learning in this context does not mean getting more information but expanding the ability to produce the results truly wanted. Improving personal mastery, involving self-care and self-management of patients, goes beyond competence and skills; it means living life from a creative as opposed to reactive viewpoint [43]. Creative collaboration with patients and their families includes building the shared treatment goals as well as the pictures of their future that foster their genuine commitment and enrollment more than simple compliance. Alliance is of much more value than compliance. A shared vision is the first step in allowing people who mistrusted each other to begin to work together [43]. Motivational interviewing with matching, pacing, and leading techniques is an essential step in establishing a creative treatment context because it helps the patients to articulate personally meaningful goals while taking medications may facilitate achieving their goals. Being able to set and pursue personal goals provide much of the motivation for better cooperation and active participation in treatment. As patients develop more personal mastery over their symptoms, they become able to better master over their lives and to realize their own vision of recovery. Creating and fostering treatment context of hope, meaning, personal responsibility, and commitment can significantly contribute to overall positive response to pharmacotherapy, but in the other way round, drug treatment can contribute to creation and fostering hope, meaning, personal responsibility, spirit of optimism, and commitment. Hope, which includes perceived external resources, perceived internal resources and positive expectations, is recognized as the starting point for treatment success and personal recovery. Hope is not hype or only wishful thinking so that the treatment context of hope refers to creating appropriate ways for overcoming treatment failures and achieving positive treatment goals. Incenting hope makes patients invest energy and activities toward treatment goals and personal recovery. Personal recovery involves a journey from disengagement to engagement and from surviving to living and growing; it has many routes, and each patient's journey is unique with taking back control over one's own life and finding hope for a better future (see [49].

19.4.4 Deconstructing the Therapeutic Narratives: Person-Centered Narratives of Therapeutic Benefit

> The good physician will treat the disease,
> but the great physician will treat the patient.
> William Osler

Treatment resistance may be associated with diverse iatrogenic hopeless nocebo tales within losing life scripts or destructive unconscious life scenarios. Lack of hope in positive treatment outcome is both demoralizing for patients and contributing to their pessimistic self-fulfilling prophecies as well as influencing negatively on psychiatrists and their devotion to the patients well-being [13]. Repeated treatment failures can reflect the negative ways on how patients define and explain their mental disorder (lifelong lasting, uncurable), how they are defined by diagnosis (stigmatization), and how community responds to them (secondary gain) as well as how they imagine their treatment and future life (situating in a nowhere-land or in a losing game). Narrative psychiatry is predicated on the conceptualization of human beings as narrators who live their lives in relationships and connect and cooperate with one another through the stories they create, tell, and live. Human beings are immersed in narrative; the stories they tell about themselves not only describe themselves but also shape their lives [50]; telling and listening stories, they recognize themselves in the stories of others, and others in their stories. One's ability to create, live, and tell a coherent, hopeful, and self-actualizing story of his or her life is a fundamental component of mental health and well-being. Creative person-centered psychopharmacotherapy is based on a deep and empathic understanding of the patients' as persons with unique individual life stories, and therapy involves their re-authoring and retelling the stories of their lives in a creative and hopeful way. Patients simply have a fundamental need for narrative because human life itself is structured narratively and narratives are strongly associated with personal understandings, purpose, and meaning, in health as well as in illness.

All therapies from psychopharmacologic ones to all kinds of psychotherapies involve a therapeutic narrative and start with therapist listening to the patient's story and then helping him to recognize a new perspective on the problem and gain new coping and resilience skills [51]. Mental health medications have diverse physical and neurochemical as well as rhetorical and symbolical effects, both of which are responsible for treatment outcome. In addition to their diverse pharmacodynamic mechanisms, they work also on account of meanings, expectations, and relationships which may modify neurobiological effects of medications. Treatment failure may be related to the inconvenient drugs biological effects as well as to the negative meanings the patient ascribes to the medicine and its effects. Deconstructing narratives that fuel mental health problems and treatment failures is essential whenever desired treatment goals are not obtained. Through illness narratives patients form their own explanations about the causes of their illnesses, in a useful or harmful way. Deconstructing hopeless and harmful into hopeful and useful narratives may help in overcoming treatment failure. Therapeutic narrative refers to explanations on how mental health medications work. These explanations are different during acute, stabilizing, and maintenance phase of treatment. Treatment failure may be related to an inappropriate narrative in specific situations. The restitution narrative presumes the illness to be cured or overcome so that the patient becomes the same or healthy again. While restitution story "yesterday I was healthy, today I am sick, but tomorrow I'll be healthy again" may work for some illness experience, it can be problematic in the context of some other mental disorders for which cure, or return to previous health as it was once, may not be forthcoming [52]. So, patients with severe major mental disorders need alternative narrative resources to preserve or reinstate sense of self, meaning, identity, hope, well-being, and mental health. In chaos narrative, the illness destroys the life of the patient. The quest narrative is characterized by the patient's search for meaning and the idea that something can be learned or gained from the illness experience [52]. The recovery narratives involve the four component process: recognizing the problem, transforming the self through recovery narratives, reconciling with the system, and reaching out to others. Establishing a personal relationship with the patient should help the patient to find a new self as a person with a mental disorder who can recover from that disorder with a new perspective on life. The main focus is on the person, not on the symptoms and problems. This approach allows the patient to reconnect with his or her true healthy self. Finding a new, true self is associated with a re-authoring life story, personal growth, self-actualization, and reaching one's full potential. Person-centered psychopharmacotherapy supports hope, self-actualization, and self-directed growth focused on patients' strengths and resources. Narrative psychopharmacology combines the resources of re-authoring conversations and mental health medications. The purpose of psychopharmacotherapy is to empower the patients' to control their disease, to change losing into winning life story, and to regain control over their life to get more love, freedom, power, joy, and sense of life [9, 11, 49, 53]. Psychopharmacotherapy is one essential external support, alongside a whole range of other types of transformation and resilience-promoting supports, skills, and strengths.

19.4.5 Enhancing Placebo and Eliminating Nocebo Responses

> The doctor-patient relationship is critical to the placebo effect. Irwing Kirsch

Placebo (Latin, I shall please) and nocebo (Latin, I shall harm) phenomena are a part of every treatment procedure and thus require careful approach by all clinicians [21]. These phenomena of positive "pleasing" and negative "harming" response of patients to any kind of treatment have potential to powerfully improve or worsen mental and/or somatic symptoms and can significantly modify the overall treatment outcome. However, they have been usually viewed in pharmacology through reductionist lenses. Some treatment failures may be predicated and predicted on nocebo response. As causal factors of some mental disorders are linked to adverse life experiences and negative beliefs, views, and expectations, they can be described in some way as nocebo responses to stressful and important life events. Many psychiatric patients are characteristically engaged in a negative view of themselves, in a negative view of the world, and in a negative view of their future and prone to pharmacophobia, negative self-fulfilling prophecy, or nocebo response. For proper understanding of placebo and nocebo phenomena in pharmacology, it is of great importance to be familiar with quite a number of explanatory models which can be identified in scientific literature (Table 19.8). The creative use the potential of these mechanisms to master strategies on how to manage these phenomena to increase the quality of clinical practice [54, 55] may help in preventing and overcoming treatment failures. Goal-oriented utilization of placebo responses may

Table 19.8 Explanatory models of placebo and nocebo effects and responses [8, 21, 56–61] modified

The individual, personality differences model: placebo and nocebo responsiveness may be related to the certain types of personalities so that one can speak about placebo reactors and nocebo reactors (placebo-prone and nocebo-prone personality). Factors such as dispositional optimism, hypnotic suggestibility, somatic focus, empathy, neuroticism, altruism, social desirability, dopamine-related traits, fear of pain, locus of ego-resilience, anxiety, pessimism, pain catastrophizing, harm avoidance, and persistence have been linked to placebo and nocebo effects
The interpersonal dynamics model: placebo and nocebo responsiveness should be understood in terms of the complex dynamics of the physician-patient relationship. Some physicians are themselves powerful placebos: central components in all healer-patient relationships such as hope, trust, caring, empathy, and compassion play an important role in placebo response
The perceptual filtering model: placebo and nocebo responsiveness can be explained in terms of patients' positive or negative perceptual filtering and misattribution. Patients with placebo response are typically motivated to get better and to please their physicians, and in doing so they tend to foreground beneficial changes. In addition, they frequently filter out negative changes and outcomes
The neurobiological model: placebo and nocebo responsiveness can be understood in neurobiological terms as the activation of the different psychophysiological and neurotransmitters systems. For example, placebo and nocebo phenomena are related to the opposite responses of dopaminergic and endogenous opioid neurotransmissions in various brain areas, as well as of the brain reward – punishment system; oxytocin increases trust and placebo response by binding to its receptors in amygdala
The conditioning model: placebo and nocebo responsiveness can be explained in terms of classical conditioning theory because they resembles to a positive or negative conditioned stimulus. They can be related to nonconscious associative learning processes and priming effects
The meaning making model: placebo and nocebo responsiveness can be understood in terms of cultural practices of positive and negative meaning making. Placebo is positive, and nocebo is negative meaning response
The logic of expectation model: placebo and nocebo responsiveness can be explained in terms of a logic of expectation in which cultural conceptions of the effectiveness of medications, or imagined expectations, can override their pharmacological action. Patients' knowledge about and expectations of a treatment may affect the treatment outcome
The narrative pharmacology model: the patient's beliefs and stories concerning the origin of symptoms and medicines action may contribute positively (placebo) or negatively (nocebo) to drug treatment response
The resilience model: beliefs, actions, and behavior may have salutogenic or pathogenic effects. Resilience is a protective collection of thoughts, actions, and behavior that can be developed and improved by everybody. Thus, placebo effect can be understood as a form of resilience activating or enhancing by treatment
The multidimensional integrative model includes all of the above models based on transdisciplinary systemic approach

contribute to overall drug treatment effectiveness and while having in mind and preventing nocebo responses may provide a useful possibility to reduce adversary events and prevent treatment failures. It seems that psychiatric patients with good treatment response are likely to possess a common biological, psychological, and/or spiritual resilience component that largely controls recovery from mental disorders. Some authors, for example, suggest "a common resilience mechanism underlying antidepressant drug response" because "once triggered recovery appears to follow a pattern similar to the course observed with placebo, despite marked pharmacologic differences of triggers" [56]. This antidepressant resilience mechanism can be activated by diverse procedures like medications, talking psychotherapies, music therapy, dancing therapy, psychodrama, etc.

The placebo and nocebo phenomena represent a very good model for our better understanding of the role of treatment context and how the words, thoughts, meanings, images, beliefs, anticipations, and expectancies act on our brain and mind producing positive or negative health effects [62]. Placebo and nocebo might be considered as the personal responses to any kind of treatment; they are universal phenomena in human communication and so very important from the perspective of the person-centered medicine. Patients are always subjects who give sense and respond more or less actively to meanings that disease, illness, and treatment have for them and their physicians. While the physician is an expert with specialized knowledge about drug treatments, the patient is the expert on his or her life and the best judge of the treatment outcome. Patients always bring into treatment unique characteristics related to their sensibility, vulnerability, resilience, narration, and potential for personal growth as well as proneness to placebo or nocebo responsiveness. Disease has to be treated, illness has to be healed, and the needs of the suffering person have to be met and satisfied. There are many placebo-inducing psychological interventions which involve creating and fostering hope, meaning, personal responsibility, spirit of optimism, and commitment. Patients just need to learn specific skills of positive psychology: how to have more positive thinking and emotions, more novelty seeking and engagement, more gratitude, love, and sense of life, more accomplishment, and better human relations (see [63]). Properly choice of drug treatment can contribute to the creation and fostering hope, meaning, and personal commitment. Hope is an important part of an effective coping or treatment strategy which involves a positive perspective of future, the expectation of achieving a favorable outcome, and an inner power that helps one to overcome treatment failure.

19.4.6 Individual Resilience and Creativity Enhancing Training

> The great thing, than, in all education, is to make our nervous system our ally instead our enemy.
> William James: The Principals of Psychology, 1892

Treatment failures may appear due to diminished secondary or tertiary resilience and lack of creativity, on both clinician's and patient's side. Creativity and resilience are qualities that exist more or less in all people, and they are strongly related to each other. Resilience is in a way an ability to learn from failure, whereas therapy in psychiatry is also a complex learning process in which patients learn new dimensions of themselves and their lives. Creativity involves new perspective improvement and creation, it asserts life, frees human spirit, and helps to overcome both mental disorders and somatic diseases [4]. Everyday creativity is an ability to cope effectively with life problems and adversaries and find new solutions. In this spirit the creative, person-centered psychopharmacotherapy may be defined as an art and practice of learning organization [11, 42, 43] aimed to increase resilience, foster creativity, and help patients to reset their own selves. The patient is a person, a body-mind-spirit unit, capable of resilience which involves self-regulation, self-healing, and salutogenesis or health maintenance (see [64]). The idea of fostering resilience and creativity of patients who experienced treatment failure is an issue of growing interest. The concept of resilience and creativity explains us why one person differs from another, and what makes each of patients the person they are. Resilience of each individual is based on intrinsic and extrinsic protective factors promoting strength and compensating for weakness of patients as well as maximizing opportunities and protecting against threats. Extrinsic factors operate indirectly modifying exposure to, or the impact of, adverse events or illness, while intrinsic protective factors are the accumulated physiological, psychological, social, and spiritual capital that patients can mobilize [65]. Resilience can be both built and maintained through life coaching the proactive efforts of patients using self-help resources [66]. Enhancing resilience involves the protective and salutogenic processes aimed to (1) reduce the impact of risks; (2) reduce the negative chain reactions that follow adversities; (3) establish and maintain positive mindset, self-esteem, and self-efficacy; (4) create opportunities to revert the damaging effects and change circulus viciosus into circulus virtuosus; and (5) help finding new meaning and constructing new pathways in the face of adversity (see [67]). Adversities and failures are inevitable in life, and it is very important to recognize and learn the lessons they offer. Resiliency known as "the hard-resilient style" appears as (1) a strong sense of commitment and self-esteem, a belief that individual can control or influence outcomes; (2) an open-minded and exploring approach to living, a sense of challenge and novelty seeking; (3) a strong future orientation and optimism, living at the present and learning from the past; and (4) a sense of humor and joy [33].

All treatments in general may be roughly divided into creativity-promoting and creativity-killing ones. Creativity promoting means resilience enhancing. Psychopharmacotherapy may preserve, foster, or damage patients' creativity in ways that significantly influence their resilience, quality of life, and personal recovery. Many psychiatric patients commonly discontinue medication due to complaints of creativity blocking and cognitive impairments caused by drug treatment [68]. The programs of individual resiliency and creativity training focus on positive mental health and individual improvement and recovery goals, improving illness management skills, making progress toward a meaningful life, and finding new pathways [4, 69]. Treatment failure may be associated in a circular way with despair, helplessness, meaninglessness, isolation, resentment, and sorrow, while favorable treatment outcome is associated with a state of resilience which involves love (attachment, connecting, belonging, communion), personal mastery (power, inner peace, learning, achievement, control), freedom (choice, independence, autonomy), happiness (gratitude, joy, fun, play, pleasure, enjoyment), and purpose (meaning, sense of life, personal life's mission). Person-centered creative psychopharmacotherapy has included varied combinations of resilience-enhancing and creativity-fostering interventions in addition to psychopharmacologic treatment. Resilience-enhancing and creativity-fostering techniques on a therapeutic journey of healing and transformation enable patients with a mental disorder to live a meaningful life in their community while striving to achieve their own potential of self-actualization. It helps them to live a satisfying, hopeful, and contributing life even with the limitations caused by illness. Resilience-enhancing training is aimed to improve functional expression of character dimensions: self-directedness, cooperativeness, and self-transcendence (see [64, 70]). According to Cloninger et al. [70], "the synergistic quality of all three character dimensions" represents "creativity and the healthy personality configuration, called the creative character profile." Resilience is not about just to survive but also to thrive. Improving self-directedness involves promoting disposition attributes of the patient such as personal mastery and healthy lifestyle, growth and learning, physical condition and robustness, vitality, optimism, positive cognitive reappraisal, and affiliative behavior. It means also cultivating a positive mindset and living life from a creative and proactive as opposed to passive and reactive viewpoint. Interestingly enough research showed that nonresponders to antidepressant medication scored low in self-directedness, both before and after treatment, in comparison with responders who had scored normally after treatment [71]. A high capacity for cooperativeness is one of the pillars of resilience. Improving cooperativeness refers to learning successful communication skills and assertiveness as well as to practicing positive mutual interaction and forming attachments and bonds with supportive resources. Being kind, empathic, and compassionate and working in the service of others enhances physical, mental, social, and spiritual well-being and improves different aspects of mental health and health in general. Mindful meditation and contemplation effectively increase the total well-being of previously treatment-resistant patients too. Improving self-transcendence is related to existential personal journey and transcendent relationship with an entity that is beyond physical, psychological, or social dimensions of life. Self-transcendence means growing in spirituality and awareness of right purpose and meaning life beyond limitations of mental disorders and material possessions.

At the end of the day, creative, person-centered psychopharmacotherapy may be represented as a therapeutic journey of evolving therapeutic challenges and treatment goals by enhancing secondary and tertiary resilience and creativity that promotes the flourishing of healthy, happy, and virtuous life and thus changes treatment resistance into treatment response. With regard to achieving successful treatment outcome, the motto is "better late than never, but never late is better."

Conclusions

Despite a huge progress in clinical psychopharmacology, the treatment outcome for many psychiatric patients has remained not good enough. Much remains to be improved in psychiatry to prevent and overcome treatment failures and increase treatment effectiveness. The time is ripe for psychiatry to find its transdisciplinary integrative soul and increase treatment effectiveness. Creative, person-centered narrative psychopharmacotherapy as multimodal resilience-enhancing concept may significantly contribute to better treatment effectiveness and efficiency in current psychiatry.

References

1. Riva Posse P, Nemeroff CB. The problem of treatment resistant psychiatric disorders. In: Nemeroff CB, editor. Management of treatment-resistant major psychiatric disorders. USA: Oxford University Press; 2012. p. 1–21.
2. Jakovljevic M. How to increase treatment effectiveness and efficiency in psychiatry: creative psychopharmacotherapy – Part 1: definition, fundamental principles and higher effectiveness polypharmacy. Psychiatr Danub. 2013a;25:269–73.
3. Jakovljevic M. How to increase treatment effectiveness and efficiency in psychiatry: creative psychopharmacotherapy – Part 2: creating favorable treatment context and fostering patients' creativity. Psychiatr Danub. 2013b;25:274–9.
4. Jakovljevic M. Creativity, mental disorders and their treatment: recovery-oriented psychopharmacotherapy. Psychiatr Danub. 2013c;25:311–5.
5. Jakovljević M. The creative psychopharmacotherapy and personalized medicine: the art and practice of the learning organization. Psychiatr Danub. 2010;22:309–12.
6. Fonagy P, Luyten P, Allison E, Campbell C. What we have changed our minds about: Part 1. Borderline personality disorder as a limitation of resilience. Borderline Personal Disord Emot Dysregulation. 2017;4:11. https://doi.org/10.1186/s40479-017-0061-9.
7. Gillespie AL, Samanaite R, Mill J, Egerton A, MacCabe JH. Is treatment-resistant schizophrenia categorically distinct from treatment responsive schizophrenia? A systemic review. BMC Psychiatry. 2017;17:12.
8. Jakovljevic M. The placebo-nocebo response: controversies and challenges from clinical and research perspective. Eur Neuropsychopharmacol. 2014a;24:333–41.
9. Jakovljević M. The placebo-nocebo response in patients with depression: do we need to reconsider our treatment approach and clinical trial designs? Psychiatr Danub. 2014b;26:92–5.
10. Demjaha A, Lappin JM, Stahl D, Patel MX, MacCabei JH, Howes OD, et al. Antipsychotic treatment resistance in first-episode psychosis: prevalence, subtypes and predictors. Psychol Med. 2017;47:1981–9.
11. Jakovljevic M. Person-centered psychopharmacotherapy: what is it? – Each patient is a unique, responsive and responsible subject. Psychiatr Danub. 2015;27(suppl 1):s28–33.
12. Jakovljevic M. Long-acting injectable (depot) antipsychotics and changing treatment philosophy: possible contribution to integrative care and personal recovery of schizophrenia. Psychiatr Danub. 2014c;26:304–7.
13. Bressan RA, Grohs GEM, Matos G, Shergil S. Hope or hype in the treatment of schizohrenia – what's the role of the physician. Br J Psychiatry. 2018;212:1–3.
14. Insel TR. Rethinking schizophrenia. Nature. 2010;468:187–93.
15. Shrivastava A, De Sousa A, Sonavane S, Shah N. Resilience improves neurocognition and treatment outcomes in schizophrenia: a hypothesis. Open J Psychiatry. 2016;6:173–87.
16. Nabi A, Khan I. Resilience as predictor of mental well-being among cardiovascular disorder. Int J Indian Psychol. 2017;4:182–90.
17. Southwick SM, Charney DS. Resilience – the science of mastering life's greatest challenges. New York: Cambridge University Press; 2013.
18. Shin SJ, Yung DY, Hwang EA. Concept analysis of resilience in patients with cardiovascular diseases. J Korean Acad Nurs. 2009;39:788–95. https://doi.org/10.4040/jkan.2009.39.6.788.
19. Clarke J, Nicholson J. Resilience – bounce back from whatever life throws at you. Great Britain: Crimson Publishing; 2010.
20. Reutter KK, Bigatti SM. Religiosity and spirituality as resilience resources: moderation, mediation, or moderated mediation? J Sci Study Relig. 2014;53:56–72.
21. Jakovljevic M. Placebo and nocebo phenomena from the perspective of evidence based and person centered medicine. Hosp Pharmacol Int Multidiscip J. 2017;4:512–20.
22. Kalisch R, Mueller MB, Tuescher O. A conceptual framework for the neurobiological study of resilience. Behav Brain Sci. 2015;62:1–79.
23. Davidson JRT, Payne VM, Connor KM, Foa EB, Rothbaum BO, Hertzberg MA, et al. Trauma, resilience and saliostasis: effects of treatment in post-traumatic stress disorder. Int Clin Psychopharmacol. 2005;20:43–8.
24. Jakovljevic M. Contemporary psychopharmacotherapy in the context of brave new psychiatry, well-

being therapy and life coaching. Psychiatr Danub. 2007;19:195–201.
25. Bolos A. Considerations on assisted resilience and individualized therapy in bipolar affective disorder, with a clinical case exemplification. Clujul Med. 2015;88:462–7.
26. Jakovljević M, Borovecki F. Epigenetics, resilience, comorbidity and treatment outcome. Psychiatr Danub. 2018;30. (In press).
27. Feder A, Nestler EJ, Charney DS. Psychobiology and molecular genetics of resilience. Nat Rev Neurosci. 2009;10:446–57.
28. Dudley KJ, Li X, Kobor MS, Kippin TE, Bredy TW. Epigenetic mechanisms mediating vulnerability and resilience to psychiatric disorders. Neurosci Biobehav Rev. 2011;35:1544–51.
29. Wu G, Feder A, Cohen H, Kim JJ, Calderon S, Charney DS, et al. Understanding resilience. Front Behav Neurosci. 2013;7:10.
30. Moore RC, Eyler LT, Mills PJ, O'Hara RM, Wachmann K, Lavretsky H. Biology of positive psychiatry. In: Jeste DV, Palmer BW, editors. Positive psychiatry – a clinical handbook. Washington, DC: American Psychiatric Publishing; 2015. p. 261–83.
31. James LM, Engdahl BE, Georgopoulous AP. Apolipoprotein E: the resilience gene. Exp Brain Res. 2017;235:1853–9.
32. Yehuda R, Brand SR, Golier JA, Yang RK. Clinical correlates of DHEA associated with post-traumatic stress disorder. Acta Psychiatr Scand. 2006;114:187–93.
33. Bartone PT, Spinosa T, Robb J, Pastel RH. Hardy-resilient style is associated with high density lipoprotein levels. Presented at the Association of Military surgeons of the United States annual meeting, San Antonio, Texas, 11 November, 2008.
34. van Zuiden M, Haverkort SO, Tan Z, Daams J, Lok A, Olf M. DHEA and DHEA-S levels in posttraumatic stress disorder: a meta-analytic review. Psychoneuroendocrinology. 2017;84:76–82.
35. Binder E, Karim M, Paya Cano JL, Fernandes C, Aitchison KJ, Mathe AA, et al. Antidepressants and the resilience to early-life stress in inbred mouse strains. Pharmacogenet Genomics. 2011;21:779–89.
36. Breitfeld J, Scholl C, Steffens M, Laje G, Stingl JC. Gene expression and proliferation for antidepressant treatment resistance. Transl Psychiatry. 2017;7(3):e1061.
37. Davidson J, Baldwin DS, Stein D, Pederson R, Ahmed S, Musgnung J, et al. Effects of venlafaxine extended release on resilience in posttraumatic stress disorder: an item analysis of the Conor-Davidson Resilience Scale. Int Clin Psychopharmacol. 2008;23:299–303.
38. Min JA, Lee NB, Lee CU, Lee C, Chae JH. Low trait anxiety, high resilience, and their interaction as possible predictors for treatment response in patients with depression. J Affect Disord. 2012;137:61–9.
39. Camera P, Molino C, Girardi L, Gattoni E, Feggi A, Gramaglia C, et al. The role of resilience and coping strategies in different psychiatric diseases: a comparison among schizophrenic spectrum, depression and personality disorders. Evid Based Psychiatr Care. 2016;2:123–6.
40. Bernstein JG. Creative psychopharmacology: medication-intolerant and refractory patients. In: Bernstein JG, editor. Drug treatment in psychiatry. 3rd ed. St. Louis: Mosby; 1995. p. 522–45.
41. Jasovic Gasic M. Is treatment resistance in psychiatric disorders a trap for polypharmacy. Psychiatr Danub. 2015;27:308–13.
42. Jakovljevic M, Abou-Salex MT. Person centered psychopharmacotherapy. In: Mezzich JE, Botbol M, Christodoulou GN, Cloninger CR, Salloum IM, editors. Person centered psychiatry. Switzerland: Springer, International Publishing AG; 2016. p. 235–45.
43. Senge PM. The fifth discipline – the art and practice of the learning organisation. London: Random House; 2006.
44. Doran CM. Prescribing mental health medication – the practitioner's guide. New York: Routledge; 2003.
45. Stahl SM. Stahl's essential psychopharmacology – neuroscientific basis and practical applications. 4th ed. New York: Cambridge University Press; 2013.
46. Stahl SM. Stahl's essential psychopharmacology – neuroscientific basis and practical applications. 3rd ed. New York: Cambridge University Press; 2008.
47. Joseph S. Symptom-focused psychiatric drug therapy for managed care. New York: The Haworth Medical Press; 1997.
48. Pakman M. A systemic frame for mental health practices. In: Prosky PS, Keith DV, editors. Family therapy as an alternative to medication – an appraisal of Pharmaland. New York: Brunner – Routhledge; 2003. p. 93–110.
49. Slade M. Personal recovery and mental illness – a guide for mental health professionals. New York: Cambridge University Press; 2011.
50. Lewis B. Narrative and psychiatry. Curr Opin Psychiatry. 2011b;24:489–94.
51. Hamkins SE. The art of narrative psychiatry. USA: Oxford University Press; 2014.
52. Frank A. The wounded story teller: body, illness and ethics. Chicago: University of Chicago Press; 1995.
53. Rufener C, Depp CA, Gawronska MK, Saks ER. Recovery in mental illness. In: Jeste DV, Palmer BW, editors. Positive psychiatry – a clinical handbook. Washington, DC: American Psychiatric Publishing; 2015. p. 91–110.
54. Kamperman L, Nestoriuc Y, Shedden-Mora MC. Physicians' beliefs about placebo and nocebo effects in antidepressants – an online survey among German practitioners. PLoS One. 12(5):e0178719. https://doi.org/10.1371/journal,pone.0178719.
55. Chavarria V, Vian J, Pereira C, Data-Franco, Fernandes BS, Merck M, et al. The placebo and nocebo phenomena: their clinical management and impact on treatment outcomes. Clin Ther. 2017;39:477–86.
56. Stassen HH, Angst J, Hell D, Sharfetter C, Szegedi A. Is there a common resilience mechanism underlying antidepressant drug response? Evidence from 2848 patients. J Clin Psychiatry. 2007;68:1195–205.

57. Jopling DA. Talking cures and placebo effects. Oxford: Oxford University Press; 2008.
58. Jaksic N, Aukst-Margetic B, Jakovljevic M. Does personality play a relevant role in the placebo effect? Psychiatr Danub. 2013;25:17–23.
59. Benedetti F. Placebo effects. 2nd ed. Oxford: Oxford University Press; 2014.
60. Planes S, Villier C, Mallaret M. The nocebo effect of drugs. Pharmacol Res Perspect. 2016;4(2):e00208.
61. Corsi N, Colloca L. Placebo and nocebo effects: the advantage of measuring expectations and psychological factors. Front Psychol Published online. 2017;8:308.
62. Benedetti F, Armanzio M. The placebo response: how words and rituals change the patient's brain. Patient Educ Couns. 2011;84:413–9.
63. Seligman MEP. Flourish – a visionary new understanding of happiness and well-being. New York: Free Press; 2012.
64. Cloninger CR, Cloninger KM, Mezzich JE. Holistic framework for ill health and positive health. In: Mezzich JE, Botbol M, Christodoulou GN, Cloninger CR, Salloum IM, editors. Person centered psychiatry. Springer: International Publishing AG Switzerland; 2016. p. 47–59.
65. Hatch S, Huppert FA, Abbott R, Croudace T, Ploubidis G, Wadsworth M, Richards M, Kuh D. A life course approach to well-being. In: Haworth J, Hart G, editors. Well-being – individual, community and social perspective. London: Palgrave Macmillan; 2012.
66. Trivedi RB, Bosworth HB, Jackson GL. Resilience in chronic illness. In: Resnick B, Gwyther LP, Roberto KA, editors. Resilience in aging – concepts, research, and outcomes. Switzerland: Springer, International Publishing AG; 2011. p. 181–97.
67. Lima de Moura Cal SF, Glustak ME, Mittermayer Bareto S. Psychological resilience and immunity. Innovative Immunology. 2015. www.austinpublishinggroup.com/ebooks.
68. Flaherty AW. Brain illness and creativity: mechanisms and treatment risks. Can J Psychiatr. 2011;56:132–43.
69. Meyer PS, Gottlieb JD, Penn D, Mueser K, Gingerich S. Individual resiliency training: an early intervention approach to enhance well-being in people with first-episode psychosis. Psychiatr Ann. 2015;45:554–60.
70. Cloninger CR. Feeling good: the science of well-being. New York: Oxford University Press; 2004.
71. Wikipedia. Self-directedness. 2018. https://en.m.wikipedia.org.

A Psychodynamic Approach to Treatment Resistance

20

Elizabeth Weinberg, Erin Seery, and Eric M. Plakun

20.1 Introduction

In the past 50 years, psychiatry has hailed the development of numerous treatments for psychiatric illness, only to discover the problem of "treatment resistance"—the failure of many patients to benefit from evidence-based treatments. As authors in this volume and others have noted, the problem of treatment resistance affects a significant proportion of psychiatric patients [1–3]. The severity of the problem is underlined by the troubling growth of advocacy for the use of assisted suicide as an option for patients struggling with treatment-resistant psychiatric illness [4]. New treatments, strategies, and algorithms for treatment resistance proliferate. Meanwhile, although some treatments such as clozapine for psychosis or ECT for depression offer substantial advantages for some severely ill patients, often new strategies have failed to offer striking benefits.

There is evidence that patients with "treatment resistance" share some characteristics, such as higher incidence of personality disorders [5], histories of trauma [6], and other social adversity [7]. Part of the difficulty in understanding treatment resistance may lie in the reality that pharmacologic treatment trials usually use exclusion criteria, such as psychiatric or substance use disorder comorbidity and suicide risk, such that results may not fully apply to real-life patient populations [8]. Some causes of treatment resistance relate to the approach of the prescriber, including improper diagnosis or misunderstanding treatment needs. A psychodynamic approach to psychiatry, including but not limited to psychodynamic psychotherapy (PDT), argues that to treat patients effectively, we must make the "overall diagnosis" [9] and treat the whole person, not psychiatric symptoms alone.

Plakun [10] has noted the pressures that drive psychiatrists to spend less time and effort seeking to understand their patients. Resource limitations in the forms of reduced inpatient and outpatient mental health services and low reimbursement from third-party payers, the proliferation and increased availability of psychiatric medications, and a cultural shift away from interest in psychodynamic thought all have led to reduced focus on conducting comprehensive biopsychosocial assessment. As Plakun [10] notes in his experience as a senior psychiatrist, supervisor, and board examiner, the result can be the genesis of psychiatrists who see patients in terms of symptom checklists and who assess psychiatric pathology but do not know how to make contact with the person who is suffering.

In 2010, Insel and co-authors [11] noted that DSM and ICD diagnoses, while important, have

E. Weinberg (✉) · E. Seery · E. M. Plakun
The Austen Riggs Center, Stockbridge, MA, USA
e-mail: Elizabeth.Weinberg@austenriggs.net; Seery@musc.edu; Eric.Plakun@AustenRiggs.Net

Y.-K. Kim (ed.), *Treatment Resistance in Psychiatry*, https://doi.org/10.1007/978-981-10-4358-1_20

not led to adequate improvements in treatment or understanding of illness. "The boundaries of these categories have not been predictive of treatment response. And, perhaps most important, these categories, based upon presenting signs and symptoms, may not capture fundamental underlying mechanisms of dysfunction [11]." While this statement was made to advocate for increased focus on basic neuroscience, it is also the case that focusing on neuroscience has not resulted in interventions that consistently predict treatment response. Moreover, neuroscience has not yet explained in a satisfactory manner the mechanisms underlying psychiatric illness or the resistance of illness to treatment. As Insel later said in an interview with *Wired* magazine [12], "I spent 13 years at NIMH really pushing on the neuroscience and genetics of mental disorders.... I don't think we moved the needle in reducing suicide, reducing hospitalizations, improving recovery for the tens of millions of people who have mental illness." A psychodynamic approach offers a significant opportunity to reframe the problem of treatment-resistant psychiatric conditions.

The psychodynamic approach takes as its starting point the experience of the individual patient and seeks to understand the meaning of the patient's illness. This approach does not by any means reject the findings of neuroscience or biological intervention but accepts these findings in the context of awareness that the human brain changes in response to life experience and to medical manipulation, that our brains and our minds are constantly responding to and accommodating more environmental and biological factors than we possibly can identify, and that awareness of neurology does not diminish the central importance of lived experience. While this approach acknowledges the contributions of other fields, such as neurobiology and cognitive science, the integrative nature of psychodynamic thought offers new possibilities for treatment. Moreover, there is increasing evidence that psychodynamic treatments can be as effective in the treatment of mental illness as other evidence-based treatments, challenging the dominance of biological and cognitive-behavioral interventions [13, 14].

Despite the increasing importance of "patient-centered medicine" in primary care [15], there has been relatively less focus on patient-centered care in psychiatry. The term "patient-centered medicine" derives from the work of Michael and Enid Balint, [16] who were both psychoanalysts and who worked with primary care physicians to integrate psychotherapy into ordinary medical care. Patient-centered medicine has been judged to be a priority central to the development of high-quality medical care by the Institute of Medicine [17]. Central features of patient-centered care, as described by Mead and Bower [18], include practice grounded in the biopsychosocial perspective, awareness of the "patient-as-person" and the "doctor-as-person," attention to the therapeutic alliance, and a stance in which power and responsibility are shared. It is an irony of current psychiatric practice that it has been slow to embrace this approach, even as it becomes increasingly valued by general medicine. Enid and Michael Balint emphasized the importance of assessing psychological and social factors as well as the use of psychotherapy in the treatment of "fat envelope patients," [19] that is, the treatment-resistant patients with very large charts. The comprehensive biopsychosocial, alliance-based approach of psychodynamic psychiatry is consistent with patient-centered practice, allows for the assessment of psychosocial complexity and adversity, and supports a treatment approach appropriate for work with complex, treatment-resistant patients.

The effort to define mental illness as a brain disorder or a medical illness "like any other" in part was intended to reduce stigma [20, 21] but in fact has either not affected or has increased rejection of those with mental illness [21, 22]. Assuming that mental illness is entirely due to genetics or immutable biological deficits can contribute to the sense that the patient has no capacity to learn or to change. Rather than taking sides in a "nature versus nurture" debate, an informed perspective favors investigating the complex interplay between genetic and environmental influences. In this context, a psychodynamic approach includes the use of appropriate biological interventions—while attending to their meaning.

Psychodynamic principles apply to psychodynamic psychotherapy (PDT) but also apply to psychodynamically informed psychopharmacologic treatment and general psychiatric practice. Blagys and Hilsenroth [23], reviewing the comparative psychotherapy literature, determined seven areas of focus that characterize psychodynamic treatment, including patients' emotional states; exploration of resistance and avoidance; identification of recurrent patterns in thoughts, feelings, and relationships; exploration of experiences from the patient's past; interpersonal experiences; the therapeutic relationship; and conscious and unconscious dreams and fantasies. Plakun [24] has proposed a set of principles to guide psychodynamic interventions for treatment-resistant patients, including attention to the patient's affect states, to recurrent themes, and to transference and countertransference in the therapeutic relationship. In addition, Plakun recommends that the clinician addresses diagnostic comorbidity, consciously integrates the use of medication and therapy, anticipates and makes use of treatment enactments to aid in understanding, and continuously negotiates and maintains the treatment alliance. Finally, Mintz and Belnap [25] have contributed six technical principles for the psychodynamically informed psychopharmacologic treatment of patients who experience treatment resistance. These are: (1) avoid a mind-body split, (2) seek to know the patient, (3) be aware of ambivalence about the loss of symptoms, (4) address specific resistances to medications, (5) be aware of inappropriate uses of medications, and (6) anticipate and address enactments that arise in relation to prescribing.

20.2 The Mind-Body Problem and Psychodynamic Psychiatry

It is widely accepted that Cartesian dualism does not accurately describe the relationship between the body and the mind [26]. Since mind and body cannot be disentangled, an effective understanding of mental illness cannot be based in biological observations alone. Nevertheless, psychiatry risks losing sight of the patient as an individual, focusing on brain and biology. An exclusive focus on the biology of the brain omits much of what we know about the mind: that psychological stress can influence medical health, that psychological interventions such as biofeedback and meditation can influence physical symptoms, and that psychological experience is part of a complex brain-body system that involves all aspects of human physiology.

An exclusively biological approach to treatment resistance in psychiatry is characterized by the following "false assumptions" described by Plakun [27].

- "Treatment resistance" is a characteristic of an underlying biological disorder affecting psychiatric function.
- Psychiatric conditions are adequately understood illnesses with indicated treatments that can be expected to work for most affected patients.
- Treatment resistance is a feature of the patient and the psychiatric condition and does not reflect the limits of the treater, the treatment approach, or the larger psychosocial environment.
- Effective treatments for psychiatric conditions should be based on placebo-controlled treatment trials for carefully selected patients with a single disorder and are usually biological interventions.
- The treatment of psychiatric illness should be focused on amelioration of symptoms.

In treating illness as a purely biological phenomenon, ignoring its consequences for the patient's sense of self, we miss what illness means to the individual. When a patient's distress becomes radically located in the body, the body may then become a container for disavowed, negative views of the self. This location of negative self-concepts in the body then may contribute to attacks on the body in the form of self-destructive and suicidal behavior. Psychiatric illness can represent stigma and can identify the patient as different from others, conferring meanings such as isolation, inferiority, defectiveness, or even a special, elevated status. The illness of the patient itself may carry meaning that otherwise may be lost, such as a narrative of trauma or loss. Finally, even treatment failures carry meaning. When treatment fails the patient, this may be experienced as one more rejection or abandonment by an uncaring world. Conversely, a patient's active resistance to treatment may signify unwillingness to submit to an authority who has not earned the patient's trust, and stubborn symptoms such as pain may articulate an emotional truth that otherwise would be forgotten. The point here is not a simplistic argument that unacknowledged dynamics cause mental illness. Rather, a psychodynamic approach posits a more complex interaction of meaning and distress, of mind and body, in which a multitude of physical and experiential factors join to create a unique narrative that must be engaged in order to achieve the most effective treatment approach.

Mintz and Flynn [28] note patient characteristics that impact treatment response to medications. Factors predicting response or non-response to medication can include attachment style, defensive style, neuroticism, locus of control, expectations of treatment, ambivalence about medications, readiness to change, and treatment preference. Thase et al. [29] address the importance of attention to psychosocial factors in the psychopharmacological treatment of treatment-resistant depression. Noting that as much as 75% of the effectiveness of an initial antidepressant trial may be due to "nonspecific elements" of treatment, such as the placebo response and the experience of interpersonal contact, these authors argue that a strong therapeutic alliance is necessary to maximize the likelihood of response to any kind of treatment. Patient adherence, the presence or absence of social support, and underlying personality traits such as neuroticism all can affect the likelihood of treatment success. Similarly, McKay et al. [30] found that the outcome of treatment both for placebo and active drug was mediated by the alliance with the person prescribing it. Patients with a positive therapeutic alliance had a more robust response. Psychological and relationship factors are neglected in the current emphasis on biological aspects of treatment, perhaps contributing to the likelihood of treatment resistance.

20.3 Psychodynamic and Other Psychotherapies

Cognitive-behavioral therapy (CBT), designed to be measurable and usable in a short, defined time frame, has been studied much more than psychodynamic and other therapies. Nevertheless, arguing that meaningful, "bona fide" therapies share effective common factors, Wampold and coauthors [31] argue for the "dodo effect." All contestants (i.e., psychotherapies) have won, and "all must have prizes." Plakun, Sudak, and Goldberg [32] have argued that teaching of psychotherapy could be conceptualized according to the "Y" model, in which effective psychotherapies share characteristics in common, such as the use of empathy and development of a treatment alliance, but diverge, having significant differences one from the other.

While CBT has been most studied, psychodynamic therapy (PDT) has a smaller but significant evidence base supporting its use [33]. Leichsenring et al. reviewed evidence for effectiveness of psychodynamic psychotherapy for a broad range of psychiatric diagnoses, using rigorously defined PDT, and found that psychodynamic psychotherapy was superior to control conditions and as efficacious as established treatments [34]. A Cochrane Review of 33 studies of short-term psychodynamic psychotherapy used in a range of psychiatric conditions [35] showed that the psychodynamic psychotherapies studied were generally superior to treatment as usual. Steinert and colleagues conducted a systematic analysis of the equivalence of PDT as compared to established treatments, chiefly CBT or medication trials, controlling for researcher allegiance, and found equivalence [13].

The NICE guidelines for treatment of depression [36] note that CBT has a strong evidence base, but is not effective for all patients. Some patients may benefit from some of the common elements shared by psychotherapies, such as interpersonal support, understanding, and identification and experience of challenging emotional states, and find these most accessible in a psychodynamic context. Others may benefit preferentially from elements specific to psychodynamic psychotherapy such as the focus on developmental experiences, on the therapy relationship, or on the meaning of recurrent themes in the patient's life [37].

Apart from the clinical benefits of PDT, the psychodynamic approach offers conceptual advantages. The psychodynamic approach privileges meaning, the value of historical understanding, and the uniqueness of the individual. These concepts may benefit any practitioner, whether applying a psychodynamic, a behavioral, or a biological treatment. Psychodynamic thinking often is caricatured in academic literature as rigid, unscientific, or dated. As Blatt et al. [38] have pointed out, such accusations appear impervious to the growing literature that applies scientific methods to the study of psychoanalytic concepts and treatments. Markowitz et al. [39] note the self-reinforcing nature of the dominance of CBT, which creates a situation in which CBT has replaced the hegemony in American psychiatry previously enjoyed by psychoanalysis. Abbas et al. [40] describe the frequent bias in the depiction of psychodynamic psychotherapy. PDT often is depicted in an inaccurate, exaggerated manner that contributes to its marginalization, and evidence of the effectiveness of PDT frequently is overlooked in reviews and treatment guidelines.

Motivated by the intractable nature of treatment resistance and the need for new approaches, researchers have sought to rectify the lack of research regarding the effectiveness of psychodynamic psychotherapy. Leichsenring et al. [41] carried out a meta-analysis of studies from 1970 to 2004 examining the effectiveness of short-term psychodynamic psychotherapy with a design that was carefully selected for adequately conducted psychotherapy, finding large effect sizes not significantly different from other therapies. Leichsenring and Rabung [42] conducted a meta-analysis of research published between 1960 and 1988 addressing the effectiveness of long-term psychodynamic psychotherapy, finding that outcomes were superior in patients receiving long-term psychodynamic psychotherapies compared to those treated with shorter therapies and that this was particularly true for patients with complex mental disorders.

20.4 Psychodynamic Approaches to Psychiatric Disorders: The Evidence Base

While some studies address treatment resistance across a range of psychiatric disorders, most research is disorder-specific, particularly focusing on mood, psychotic, and anxiety disorders. Since most research addresses specific conditions, research focused on specific disorders must be included in a full review of approaches to treatment resistance. Nevertheless, it is likely that organizing research by psychiatric condition to some extent misses the mark. Increasingly, there is evidence that psychiatric diagnoses may not be clearly distinguished one from the other. Rather, different psychiatric conditions may represent varying presentations of overlapping pathologies that emerge as the result of complex interactions between genetic and environmental influences. Kessler et al. [43], for example, found in the WHO World Mental Health Surveys that childhood adversity was strongly related to the lifetime occurrence of psychiatric disorders, but there was no specificity in the relationship between adversities and disorders. Caspi et al. [44], in analyzing longitudinal data from a sample of over 1000 subjects found that psychopathology was best modeled using a single factor, the "p-factor," indicating the presence and severity of psychopathology, as opposed to discrete diagnoses or multiple factors. These findings have been replicated by Martel and Lehey in examining the symptoms of young children and their families [45, 46].

Reviewing the literature on treatment resistance addressing specific diagnoses leads to several general observations. First, in almost all treatment resistance research, accepted definitions refer to lack of response to biological therapies, and recommendations focus on medication. As noted by Thase et al. [29], psychotherapy is not created or funded by profit-oriented corporations, and cannot compete with the corporate interests and funding that ensures that medication marketing is supported by research evidence as soon as it becomes available. For this reason, it is not likely that psychotherapies can achieve the same evidence base as medication yet may be essential in achieving clinical response for treatment-resistant patients. In particular, patients with histories of early adversity respond better to psychotherapy than to medications, though the combination is superior to either alone [47]. Second, although there is evidence that trauma and childhood adversity can contribute to mood, anxiety, psychotic, personality disorders, and general psychopathology, not enough research addresses the consequences of trauma and adversity in the lives of affected patients. Third, scientific study in this field appears oriented toward addressing treatment response organized by diagnosis, not common themes in psychopathology or in treatment, despite growing awareness of the overlapping psychopathology of psychiatric disorders.

20.5 Treatment Resistance and Mood Disorders

Treatment resistance has been most studied in depressive disorders. Numerous authors [14, 48–50] have noted the cost to society of treatment-resistant depression. Definitions of treatment-resistant depression vary, but a commonly used definition is the failure of the patient's depressive illness to remit after two adequate trials of different antidepressants [51]. Treatment recommendations for resistant depression rarely include psychotherapy [52, 53]. In characterizing current approaches to treatment-resistant depression, Jenkins and Goldner [54] reviewed research articles related to treatment-resistant depression in adults from 2005 to 2010. Eighty-one percent of the papers studied fell within a biological paradigm, with 3% judged to be within a psychological paradigm.

Efforts to describe patients with treatment-resistant depression have yielded a picture of a complex population, more likely to suffer from personality pathology and trauma than treatment-responsive patients. Kaplan and Klinetor [55] studied outpatients treated for major depressive disorder, and found that non-responders differed from responders in being significantly more functionally impaired, more likely to have comorbid anxiety diagnoses, more likely to show personality pathology, and were more likely to show evidence of chronic post-traumatic stress disorder. Moreover, childhood trauma in one study appeared to moderate preferential response to psychotherapy [47]. In this study, CBASP (cognitive-behavioral analysis system of psychotherapy) was developed specifically to attend to the difficulties of depressed patients, with a focus on understanding and addressing interpersonal relationships. Such studies suggest that an approach to treatment-resistant depression should include awareness of psychological and syndromal complexity, as well as sensitivity to the prevalence and experience of trauma.

Numerous studies have linked depression to psychological stress [56]. Bryant and co-authors [57] found that the degree of depression experienced after a disaster was related to the extent of social connectedness of the affected individual, suggesting that stress effects can be mitigated by interpersonal connections. Caspi et al. [58] found evidence of a direct interaction between the presence of a genetic polymorphism of the serotonin transporter promoter gene and stress in the etiology of depression. While there has been controversy about this significant finding, it now has been replicated repeatedly and converges with newer findings regarding effects of stress on the amygdala that are linked to the serotonin transporter polymorphism [59]. Such data suggest a complex interplay between psychological stress, gene-environment interactions, and the presence or absence of social networks.

Increasing evidence demonstrates effectiveness of short-term psychodynamic psychotherapy (STPP) for depression. Town et al. [60] found STPP to be superior to treatment as usual in a treatment-resistant sample. Driesen and co-authors

[61] found that among patients recruited from a Dutch outpatient clinic, a trial of STPP was non-inferior to CBT. Gibbons et al. [62] also found non-inferiority for STPP as compared to CBT. It is possible that the effectiveness of psychotherapy in the treatment of depression rests on "common factors" of effective psychotherapy [63], such as the development of an alliance within the treatment relationship and the experience of hope linked to shared goals, rather than to the name given to the psychotherapy. So far, research has not clarified the usefulness and effectiveness of specifically psychodynamic versus behavioral interventions.

Given the complex nature of treatment-resistant depression, longer-term treatment may be indicated. This hypothesis was tested in the Tavistock Adult Depression Study [14], which followed patients receiving weekly long-term psychodynamic psychotherapy (LTPP) for 18 months, as compared to patients receiving standard treatment according to British NHS recommendations. Both groups had access to medication treatment, and the treatment-as-usual group received more non-psychodynamic psychotherapy interventions, such as CBT. Although both groups had similar rates of remission at the end of the treatment phase, differences between the groups widened significantly at 24, 30, and 42 months, with 30% of the psychodynamic treatment group as opposed to 4% of the control group achieving partial remission.

Less is known about treatment resistance in bipolar disorder than in depression, especially potential benefits of psychotherapy. Nevertheless, Miklowitz [64] and Miklowitz and co-authors [65] have noted superiority of intensive psychotherapeutic interventions compared to less intensive interventions, such as intermittent "collaborative care" visits in the treatment of bipolar disorder. Bipolar disorder generally is conceptualized as a "brain disorder," yet trials of aggressive medical intervention yield limited results. In one comparison between ECT and algorithm-assisted treatment for patients with treatment-resistant bipolar disorder, results did not distinguish the two groups and were modest at roughly 30% remission [66]. In one study, patients with treatment-resistant bipolar depression were found to have a number of distinguishing characteristics that included premorbid personality and social stress, factors likely to be useful targets for psychotherapy [67].

Mood disorders, although considered psychiatric illnesses, also involve the same emotions that are part of ordinary life. The neurovegetative symptoms of depression can be understood at least in part as physiologic reactions to intense, sustained emotional distress. Evidence-based therapies for mood disorders, including CBT, interpersonal therapy (IPT), and STPP, have common goals of helping patients to recognize and tolerate awareness of emotional and interpersonal problems. Each of these techniques has significant advantages, and each is likely not to suit every patient. A full biopsychosocial assessment, including a psychodynamic formulation, can help the clinician to understand what feelings, conflicts, and needs contribute to the perpetuation of unresolved sadness and emotional instability.

20.6 Treatment Resistance and Psychosis

Since the introduction of antipsychotic medications in the 1950s, psychotic disorders have been reconceptualized as biomedical disorders. Even more than in the case of depression, published criteria for treatment resistance in psychosis exclusively rely on medication trials [68]. The success of antipsychotic medications catalyzed a movement toward biological explanations for psychosis. Hallucinations, delusions, disorganized behavior, and paranoia are the most prominent symptoms of psychosis. Medications have helped countless patients to contain these symptoms well enough to avoid prolonged hospitalization and limit the disruptive effects of illness on their lives.

Despite our growing understanding of the biology of psychotic disorders, psychosis remains difficult to treat. There is a growing literature base on treatment-resistant psychotic disorders. At the time of this writing, there are over 1900 references for treatment-resistant schizophrenia on PubMed [69]. In seeking an explanation for treatment resistance, it is possible that at least part of the responsibility lies in currently predominant treatment approaches. Within the United States, pharmacotherapy has been the primary mode of treatment for psychosis. Despite the advances in medication development, not all patients respond to medications, medications do not treat all symptoms equally, and even for those whom medications are effective, nonadherence is a common cause of relapse in psychotic illness [70]. Current studies indicate that for roughly 40% of patients, medications alone are partially to minimally effective [71].

Treatment that addresses psychosis as only a medical illness, disconnected from relationships and meaning, both eclipses the patient's experience of psychosis and contributes to the further isolation and stigmatization of the patient. To understand problems with medication adherence, it is necessary to understand patients' concerns. Reasons for poor adherence can include side effects, reluctance to accept a diagnostic label, and even a need to protect the symptoms that the patient may value. The psychotic patient may be isolated by having perplexing symptoms but also may feel more powerful through being different and presenting mysterious difficulties. Hallucinations can be a source of comfort and company and sometimes may actually be felt to provide useful information. Particularly following trauma, paranoia may be experienced as a helpful reminder to be vigilant. Delusions may confer otherwise elusive feelings of grandeur and power. In understanding the perceived value of psychosis, we may consider Don Quixote, whose madness expressed nobility and revealed nuances of meaning.

The use of coercion further complicates treatment of psychosis. Hospital systems institute involuntary medication protocols for acute stabilization of psychosis, and outpatient community psychiatry clinics can request court orders for involuntary treatment. In 2017, the FDA approved Abilify MyCite as the first psychiatric medication with an ingestible digital sensor to record medication adherence [72]. Although ensuring adherence with treatment, such interventions circumvent negotiation of the therapeutic alliance. While involuntary medication may have a place in treatment when there are acute safety concerns and other resources are limited or not adequate, it also has consequences for treatment effectiveness and the treatment alliance [28, 29]. In understanding "treatment resistance," we may wish to consider the reasonable resistance of a patient who feels disrespected or whose concerns have not been heard.

Although in the last 60 years schizophrenia and related psychoses have been seen through a biomedical lens, we have yet to identify specific sets of genes that cause psychosis. Instead, studies have demonstrated correlations between specific chromosomal areas and single nucleotide polymorphisms (SNPs) which confer vulnerability to development of psychoses [73]. What we call schizophrenia is more likely a heterogeneous group of related disorders that each has their own course and prognosis and responds differently to pharmacological and psychotherapeutic interventions [74]. In recent decades, there has emerged a rich and provocative body of evidence demonstrating links between psychosis and environmental stress. Increased risks of psychosis have been related to life in urban environments, social fragmentation [75], and immigrant status, as well as to childhood trauma and early adversity [76]. Selten and Cantor-Graae [77] have proposed that social defeat is linked to schizophrenia, mediated by increased dopaminergic sensitivity. This literature challenges a reductionist view by demonstrating the complex interweaving between biological and psychosocial development.

In 1998, the Agency for Healthcare Policy and the National Institute of Mental Health funded the Schizophrenia Patient Outcomes Research Team (PORT) report [78]. This report reviewed available scientific literature in order to determine the most efficacious evidence-based treatments for schizophrenia with the aim of unifying standards of care. The initial report provided substantial recommendations for pharmacotherapy but understated the value of psychosocial treatments. In particular, the report recommended against the use of psychodynamic individual or group psychotherapy. This recommendation was based on the limited evidence available and concerns about the potential for regression and development of psychotic transferences [78]. The report recommended therapies focused on behavioral and cognitive skills training as well as supportive interventions, despite a similar lack of scientific study and despite lack of evidence of regression using contemporary models of PDT.

It is by now a truism that "absence of evidence of effectiveness is not evidence of absence [of effectiveness]" [79]. Research in psychodynamic treatment of psychosis is a developing field, yet the psychodynamic approach offers value to patients and treaters. Taking a patient-centered approach, psychotic patients are people first, who have ordinary concerns such as navigating relationships and finding meaning in work. The psychotic patient must adapt to having a disabling illness that can complicate meeting developmental, emotional, and interpersonal goals. There is increasing evidence that psychosocial interventions are important to maximize treatment response and recovery from psychosis. In one survey of patients with serious mental illness, three quarters felt psychotherapy had brought positive change to their lives. Most preferred a combination of psychotherapy and medications, but psychotherapy was valued more than medications [80].

Rather than focusing on symptom reduction, some treatments have shifted toward a more patient-centered approach with a framework of recovery and emphasis on individualized care [81–85]. Several recent studies have found that intensive treatment with integration of many modalities, including psychotherapy, can reduce morbidity associated with chronic psychosis. The PORT report was further updated in 2003 and 2009 with greater emphasis on the importance of psychosocial treatments [81, 82]. Recommendations included assertive community treatment, supported employment, life skills training, family-based services, treatment of comorbid substance use, and group or individual CBT [82]. In addition, the 2003 report recommended that psychotherapy should include the development of a shared understanding of the illness between patient and therapist and recognized that lacking a full range of offerings deprives patients of optimal treatment [81]. Although the report recommended CBT, studies of actual CBT interventions effective in treatment of psychosis overlap with core psychodynamic principles. They include emphasis on collaborative understanding of the development and experience of symptoms, examining the antecedents of psychotic symptoms, and generating a shared case formulation [86].

In 2008, the National Institute of Mental Health launched the Recovery After an Initial Schizophrenia Episode (RAISE) project with 17 sites and over 400 patients [83]. The RAISE project examined the important components of treatment for patients with first episode psychosis. As recommended in the revised PORT report, the treatment integrated psychotherapy, medication management, family education, case management, and employment and education support, although still with emphasis on psychopharmacology [83].

The need-adapted (NA) approach to treatment [84, 87] and open dialogue (OD) [85, 86] interventions developed in Scandinavia highlight essential elements in addressing treatment resistance in psychotic conditions. NA was developed from studies of schizophrenic patients in Finland with a goal of developing a comprehensive and therapeutically oriented approach to psychosis that could be applied to community mental health treatment [87]. NA emphasizes individualized and flexible treatment to meet "the real and changing needs" of patients and family members [84]. OD is a type of need-adapted approach developed to focus on acute psychosis and crisis intervention [85]. The dialogue between patients, staff, and family is "open," with no treatment decisions made without the patient [85, 86].

Both NA and OD are community, family, and team oriented, with all staff, including doctors, psychologists, nurses, and social workers, given extensive training in family and individual therapies including PDT and CBT [87]. In one review of the effectiveness of these approaches, patients in the treatment group had fewer days in the hospital, were less likely to be living on a disability pension, were more likely to be free from psychotic symptoms on follow-up, and required less psychiatric medication [85, 88]. NA and OD approaches empower patients to make their own treatment decisions, attend to the meaning of their experiences, individualize the use of medications, and strengthen networks of relationships. Psychotherapeutic interventions are primary with medication use kept to a minimum, always in collaboration with the patient.

With growing evidence of the importance of psychosocial interventions in psychosis, acknowledgement of the heterogeneity of psychotic illness, and the movement toward patient-centered care, there has been more interest in the use of psychodynamic therapy. Supportive psychodynamic psychotherapy (SPP) was developed and manualized for use with psychotic patients [89]. SPP employs a modified psychodynamic approach aimed at reducing regression and vulnerability to overwhelming affect. As in NA and OD approaches, SPP is grounded in a belief that psychotic experiences hold meaning and that treatment of psychosis is best approached through genuine respect for the patient's experience [89].

The Danish Schizophrenia Project, a multisite prospective longitudinal study of first-episode psychosis, compared treatment as usual (TAU) with SPP in addition to TAU [90]. TAU consisted of psychoeducational programs, groups, and individual meetings with nurses, psychologists, and social workers as well as medication assessment. The study followed 269 patients over 2 years and found that the SPP group improved significantly with moderate to strong effect sizes in social function, positive and negative symptoms, as well as reduced general psychopathology when compared to TAU [90]. In SPP, the therapist attends to issues of mistrust, difficulties in communication, and the patient's degree of awareness of his or her illness. SPP not only builds trust and enhances adherence but also can reduce pathological vigilance and increase capacities for metacognition [89]. In later sessions, the therapist addresses disavowed aspects of reality as well as defenses such as denial, projection, projective identification, splitting, and attacks on linking [91]. Finally, the therapist makes use of the treatment relationship to assist the patient in developing the ability to manage daily reality and to enhance interpersonal skills [89].

20.6.1 Treatment Resistance and Anxiety Disorders, Eating Disorders, and Trauma

While the bulk of research investigating treatment resistance in specific disorders has addressed mood and psychotic disorders, disorders discussed in this section are characterized by being highly heterogeneous, subject to treatment resistance, and generally acknowledged to be best treated by psychotherapeutic interventions. CBT continues as the most recognized therapy, despite evidence of effectiveness of other modalities. Given the complexity of these disorders, their comorbidity with histories of trauma and personality disorders and limited treatment response to medications and CBT, psychodynamic approaches are valuable both in offering frameworks for a patient-centered, biopsychosocial formulation and also in providing treatment alternatives. Although these disorders are diagnostically distinct from mood disorders and psychoses, as already discussed in this paper, treatment-resistant disorders are characterized by diagnostic overlap and comorbidity [27, 44, 55]. Observations made in the preceding section regarding contributions of personality disorders, trauma, and social adversity in most cases apply to these disorders as well.

Although medications frequently are used in treatment of anxiety disorders, there is at present no consensus regarding underlying neurobiological mechanisms. Moreover, psychological therapies have been highly successful and may be considered treatments of choice for anxiety disorders. As in other disorders, CBT has been the most studied. In particular, techniques of desensitization, exposure, and cognitive restructuring have been important tools in the treatment of anxiety disorders. Nevertheless, as Bystritsky notes [92] in a comprehensive review of interventions for treatment-resistant anxiety disorders, narrowly defined behavioral approaches may have limited benefit, particularly for more complex, treatment-resistant patients. Anxiety disorders are often chronic and comorbid with mood and personality disorders, suggesting a need for complex treatment strategies that go beyond isolated symptom targets.

A psychodynamic approach includes attending to the developmental context, the meanings of anxiety to the patient, and the nature of interpersonal interactions and transactions relating to anxiety. A useful concept drawn from psychoanalytic theory is that of "signal anxiety," which suggests that anxiety is a signal of potential psychological danger. The task of encountering and mastering this anxiety becomes a building block for psychological structure in the developing child [93]. Plakun notes, "In psychodynamic thinking, signal anxiety is seen as a symptom of a deeper problem rather than necessarily as a specific focus of clinical attention, just as the dashboard "check engine" warning light in a motor vehicle is a warning to deal with some hidden but discoverable danger, not a warning to turn off the light [94]."

Specific psychodynamic psychotherapies have been designed to target anxiety disorders. Leichsenring et al. [95] found short-term PDT and CBT to be similarly effective for treatment of generalized anxiety disorder, while Leichsenring et al. [30] found short-term PDT and CBT to be equally effective in both short- and long-term follow-up in treatment of social anxiety. Shear et al. [96] have noted psychodynamic themes commonly identified in patients with panic disorder, and Milrod and co-authors [97] studied a form of manualized psychodynamic psychotherapy for panic disorder based on core psychodynamic concepts and found this therapy to be more effective than a relaxation training treatment condition. Given these promising findings, a trial of PDT could be considered in patients who have not benefited adequately from other modalities and may be a first-line approach for patients who highly value psychological understanding.

PTSD stands alone among diagnoses associated with serious mental illness in that by definition its etiology involves the psychological experience of traumatic stress. Numerous medications have been studied in the treatment of PTSD, and some sources emphasize the role of medications in treatment-resistant PTSD [98]. Nevertheless, the United States Department of Veterans' Affairs in their most recent guidelines [99] have recommended individual trauma-focused psychotherapies as the treatments of choice. The Cochrane Review [100] of psychological interventions for PTSD described psychodynamic psychotherapies as insufficiently studied but also noted that research in this area overall was affected by methodologic problems and bias and that non-exposure-based therapies may have an advantage over exposure-based therapy in patient dropout. A randomized controlled trial of prolonged exposure treatment versus time-limited PDT found both treatments to be effective but prolonged exposure significantly more effective [101]. Notably, however, the PDT condition was used as an "active control," and researchers are known experts in CBT. It is likely the allegiance of the authors was not equally balanced for the two conditions. Moreover, the PDT condition involved an unusual condition in that therapists explicitly did not ask about or explore the subject of trauma with patients, a limitation that violates basic tenets of PDT.

Newer research suggests CBT-based therapies are not the only effective therapies for PTSD. One study used nonrandom assignments to assign patients either to CBT or PDT [102] based on individual patient characteristics. Both treatments were equally effective. Noting that exposure therapy has disadvantages in being "grueling," and often unacceptable to patients, Markowitz et al. [103] randomly assigned patients to IPT, prolonged exposure, or relaxation training. Findings were that IPT was non-inferior to prolonged exposure and both significantly more effective than relaxation training.

Response rates often are poor in treatment of eating disorders [104]. Eating disorders often are ego-syntonic, and eating-disordered patients frequently directly resist treatment [105]. While medications have been studied in the treatment of eating disorders, primary established treatments are nutritional and psychotherapeutic. As in other disorders, CBT has been the most studied but may have disadvantages for subgroups of patients. Psychodynamic psychotherapies offer an important alternative, and psychodynamic concepts may be useful to clinicians working in any modality in clarifying the meanings and purposes of eating disorder symptoms.

Halmi [104] notes that patients with anorexia nervosa share characteristic developmental experiences, including histories of difficulty with developmental transitions, fears of autonomy, and difficulties developing social effectiveness. Zipfel et al. [106] found that PDT, CBT, and "optimized" treatment as usual, consisting of psychotherapy in combination with medical care, were similarly effective with respect to weight gain in the treatment of anorexia nervosa, with somewhat quicker results shown by CBT and somewhat greater results shown by PDT 1 year after treatment. McIntosh et al. [107] reported that nonspecific supportive psychotherapy, when performed by trained therapists, was superior to either IPT or CBT, performed by the same therapists, demonstrating that nonspecific factors of psychotherapy likely were more important than specific interventions and that CBT in particular may have had disadvantages in focusing on performance correction of thought patterns and skill acquisition in a group of patients already high in perfectionistic characteristics.

Cognitive-behavioral treatments have shown greater success in treatment of bulimia nervosa. Poulsen et al. [108] showed marked superiority for CBT compared to PDT, but Stefini et al. [109] found comparable results from PDT and CBT in treatment of bulimia nervosa. Fairburn et al. [110] showed that in their sample, IPT and CBT had similar results, suggesting that a direct focus on eating-related behavior and thoughts was not necessary for effective treatment, while a simple behavioral therapy had an extremely high attrition rate, suggesting that an exclusive focus on eating-disordered behavior alone is likely to be unacceptable to many patients.

Conclusion

Despite expanding knowledge in biological psychiatry in recent decades, patients and practitioners continue to struggle to find effective ways to address treatment-resistant psychiatric disorders. Treatments may fail when narrowly conceived psychiatric diagnoses and biologically focused interventions do not adequately address the full context for the patient's distress. Treatment has its best chance to succeed when it acknowledges comorbidity, the influence of personality, and relevant events in the patient's life, and attends to the relationship between the patient and clinician. Psychodynamic approaches have value in work with the treatment-resistant patient both in (1) providing a person-centered, biopsychosocial perspective that avoids reductionism and includes awareness of the complex effects of the treatment relationship and (2) contributing psychotherapies that provide an alternative to symptom-focused treatments such as CBT. Despite resistance to recognizing evidence-based psychodynamic treatments, increasingly treatment research demonstrates that: 1) psychotherapy is an effective treatment for many patients, and is the most effective treatment for some patients, such as trauma survivors; (2) recommendations against psychodynamic psychotherapy in the past have not been based on high-quality trials; (3) when psychodynamic psychotherapy is studied appropriately, research shows it is as efficacious as other evidence-based treatments; and (4) effective psychotherapies share important characteristics, such as attention to affect, to the treatment relationship, and to recurrent problematic patterns in the patient's thinking and behavior.

References

1. Mathew SJ. Review of treatment resistant depression: a roadmap for effective care. J Psychiatr Pract. 2012;18(5):388–9.
2. Posse PR, Nemeroff CB. The problem of treatment-resistant psychiatric disorders. In: Nemeroff CB, editor. Management of treatment-resistant major psychiatric disorders. Oxford, New York: Oxford University Press; 2012. p. 3–21.
3. Plakun EM, editor. Treatment resistance and patient authority: the Austen Riggs reader. 1st ed. New York: W.W. Norton & Co; 2011. 305 p

4. Schuklenk U, van de Vathorst S. Treatment-resistant major depressive disorder and assisted dying. J Med Ethics. 2015;41(8):577–83.
5. Souery D, Oswald P, Massat I, Bailer U, Bollen J, Demyttenaere K, et al. Clinical factors associated with treatment resistance in major depressive disorder: results from a European multicenter study. J Clin Psychiatry. 2007;68:1062–70.
6. Kaplan M, Klinetob N. Childhood emotional trauma and chronic posttraumatic stress disorder in adult outpatients with treatment-resistant depression. J Nerv Ment Dis. 2000;188(9):596–601.
7. Hassan AN, De Luca V. The effect of lifetime adversities on resistance to antipsychotic treatment in schizophrenia patients. Schizophr Res. 2015;161(2–3):496–500.
8. Zimmerman M, Mattia JI, Posternak MA. Are subjects in pharmacological treatment trials of depression representative of patients in routine clinical practice? Am J Psychiatry. 2002;159(3):469–73.
9. Balint E. A study of the doctor-patient relationship using randomly selected cases. J Coll Gen Pract. 1967;13(2):163–73.
10. Plakun EM. Finding psychodynamic psychiatry's lost generation. J Am Acad Psychoanal Dyn Psychiatry. 2006;34(1):135–50.
11. Insel T, Cuthbert B, Garvey M, Heinssen R, Pine DS, Quinn K, et al. Research domain criteria (RDoC): toward a new classification framework for research on mental disorders. Am J Psychiatry. 2010;167(7):748–51.
12. Rogers A. Star neuroscientist Tom Insel leaves the Google-spawned verily for… a Startup? WIRED. 2017.
13. Steinert C, Munder T, Rabung S, Hoyer J, Leichsenring F. Psychodynamic therapy: as efficacious as other empirically supported treatments? A meta-analysis testing equivalence of outcomes. Am J Psychiatry. 2017;174(10):943–53.
14. Fonagy P, Rost F, Carlyle J-A, Mcpherson S, Thomas R, Pasco Fearon RM, et al. Pragmatic randomized controlled trial of long-term psychoanalytic psychotherapy for treatment-resistant depression: the Tavistock Adult Depression Study (TADS). World Psychiatry. 2015;14:312–21.
15. Bardes CL. Defining "patient-centered medicine.". N Engl J Med. 2012;366(9):782–3.
16. Balint E. The possibilities of patient-centered medicine. J R Coll Gen Pract. 1969;17(82):269–76.
17. Institute of Medicine (US) Committee on Quality of Health Care in America. Crossing the quality chasm: a new health system for the 21st century. Washington, DC: National Academies Press (US); 2001. [cited 2017 Oct 27]. Available from https://www.ncbi.nlm.nih.gov/books/NBK222271/.
18. Mead N, Bower P. Patient-centredness: a conceptual framework and review of the empirical literature. Soc Sci Med. 2000;51(7):1087–110.
19. Balint M. The doctor, his patient and the illness. London: Pitman Medical Publishing Co; 1964.
20. Stigma SM. Stigma. Adv Psychiatr Treat. 2002;8(5):317–25.
21. Pescosolido BA, Martin JK, Long JS, Medina TR, Phelan JC, Link BG. "A disease like any other"? A decade of change in public reactions to schizophrenia, depression, and alcohol dependence. Am J Psychiatry. 2010;167:1321–30.
22. Schnittker J. An uncertain revolution: why the rise of a genetic model of mental illness has not increased tolerance. Soc Sci Med. 2008;67(9):1370–81.
23. Blagys MD, Hilsenroth MJ. Distinctive feature of short-term psychodynamic-interpersonal psychotherapy: a review of the comparative psychotherapy process literature. Clin Psychol Sci Pract. 2000;7(2):167–88.
24. Plakun EM. Treatment refractory mood disorders: a psychodynamic perspective. J Psychiatr Pract. 2003;9(3):209–18.
25. Mintz D, Belnap BA. View from Riggs: treatment resistance and patient authority—III. What is psychodynamic psychopharmacology? An approach to pharmacologic treatment resistance. J Am Acad Psychoanal Dyn Psychiatry. 2016;34(4):581–601.
26. Kendler KS. Toward a philosophical structure for psychiatry. Am J Psychiatry. 2005;162(3):433–40.
27. Plakun EM. Psychotherapy and psychosocial treatment: recent advances and future directions. Psychiatr Clin North Am. 2015;38(3):405–18.
28. Mintz DL, Flynn DF. How (not what) to prescribe: nonpharmacologic aspects of psychopharmacology. Psychiatr Clin North Am. 2012;35(1):143–63.
29. Thase ME, Friedman ES, Howland RH. Management of treatment-resistant depression: psychotherapeutic perspectives. J Clin Psychiatry. 2001;62(SUPPL. 18):18–24.
30. McKay KM, Imel ZE, Wampold BE. Psychiatrist effects in the psychopharmacological treatment of depression. J Affect Disord. 2006;92(2–3):287–90.
31. Wampold BE, Mondin GW, Moody M, Stich F, Benson K, Ahn H. A meta-analysis of outcome studies comparing bona fide psychotherapies: empirically, "all must have prizes.". Psychol Bull. 1997;122(3):203–15.
32. Plakun EM, Sudak DM, Goldberg D. The Y model: an integrated, evidence-based approach to teaching psychotherapy competencies. J Psychiatr Pract. 2009;15(1):5–11.
33. Fonagy P. The effectiveness of psychodynamic psychotherapy: an update. World Psychiatry. 2015;14:137–50.
34. Leichsenring F, Luyten P, Hilsenroth MJ, Abbass A, Barber JP, Keefe JR, et al. Psychodynamic therapy meets evidence-based medicine: a systematic review using updated criteria. Lancet Psychiatry. 2015;2(7):648–60.
35. Abbass AA, Kisely SR, Town JM, Leichsenring F, Driessen E, De Maat S, et al. Short-term psychodynamic psychotherapies for common mental disorders. Cochrane Database Syst Rev. 2014;7:CD004687.

36. National Collaborating Centre for Mental Health (UK). Depression: the treatment and management of depression in adults (Updated Edition) [Internet]. Leicester: British Psychological Society; 2010 [cited 2017 Dec 21]. (National Institute for Health and Clinical Excellence: Guidance). Available from: http://www.ncbi.nlm.nih.gov/books/NBK63748/.
37. Shedler J. The efficacy of psychodynamic psychotherapy. Am Psychol. 2010;65(2):98–109.
38. Blatt SJ, Corveleyn J, Luyten P. Minding the gap between positivism and hermeneutics in psychoanalytic research. J Am Psychoanal Assoc. 2006;54(2):571–610.
39. Markowitz JC, Lipsitz J, Milrod BL. Critical review of outcome research on interpersonal psychotherapy for anxiety disorders. Depress Anxiety. 2014;31:316–25.
40. Abbass A, Luyten P, Steinert C, Leichsenring F. Bias toward psychodynamic therapy: framing the problem and working toward a solution. J Psychiatr Pract. 2017;23(5):361–5.
41. Leichsenring F, Rabung S, Leibing E. The efficacy of short-term psychodynamic psychotherapy in specific psychiatric disorders: a meta-analysis. Arch Gen Psychiatry. 2004;61(12):1208–16.
42. Leichsenring F, Rabung S. Effectiveness of long-term psychodynamic psychotherapy: a meta-analysis. JAMA. 2008;300(13):1551–65.
43. Kessler RC, McLaughlin KA, Green JG, Gruber MJ, Sampson NA, Zaslavsky AM, et al. Childhood adversities and adult psychopathology in the WHO world mental health surveys. Br J Psychiatry. 2010;197(5):378–85.
44. Caspi A, Houts RM, Belsky DW, Goldman-Mellor SJ, Harrington H, Israel S, et al. The p factor: one general psychopathology factor in the structure of psychiatric disorders? Clin Psychol Sci. 2014;2(2):119–37.
45. Martel MM, Pan PM, Hoffmann MS, Gadelha A, do Rosário MC, Mari JJ, et al. A general psychopathology factor (P factor) in children: structural model analysis and external validation through familial risk and child global executive function. Abnorm Psychol. 2017;126(1):137–48.
46. Lahey BB, Rathouz PJ, Keenan K, Stepp SD, Loeber R, Hipwell AE. Criterion validity of the general factor of psychopathology in a prospective study of girls. J Child Psychol Psychiatry. 2015;56(4):415–22.
47. Nemeroff CB, Heim CM, Thase ME, Klein DN, Rush AJ, Schatzberg AF, et al. Differential responses to psychotherapy versus pharmacotherapy in patients with chronic forms of major depression and childhood trauma. Proc Natl Acad Sci. 2003;100(24):14293–6.
48. Thase ME. New approaches to managing difficult-to-treat depressions. J Clin Psychiatry. 2003;64:3–4.
49. Rush AJ, Trivedi MH, Wisniewski SR, Nierenberg AA, Stewart JW, Warden D, et al. Acute and longer-term outcomes in depressed outpatients requiring one or several treatment steps: a STAR*D report. Am J Psychiatry. 2006;163(11):1905–17.
50. Emslie GJ, Mayes T, Porta G, Vitiello B, Clarke G, Wagner KD, et al. Treatment of resistant depression in adolescents (TORDIA): week 24 outcomes. Am J Psychiatry. 2010;167(7):782–91.
51. Greden J, Riba M, McInnis M. Treatment resistant depression: a roadmap for effective care. 1st ed. Arlington: American Psychiatric Publishing; 2011. p. 193–212.
52. Crismon ML, Trivedi M, Pigott TA, Rush AJ, Hirschfeld RMA, Kahn DA, et al. The Texas medication algorithm project: report of the Texas consensus conference panel on medication treatment of major depressive disorder. J Clin Psychiatry. 1999;60(3):142–56.
53. Association AP. Practice guideline for the treatment of patients with major depressive disorder (revision). Am J Psychiatry. 2000;157:1.
54. Jenkins E, Goldner EM. Approaches to understanding and addressing treatment-resistant depression: a scoping review. Depress Res Treat. 2012;2012:469680.
55. Kaplan MJ, Klinetor NA. Childhood emotional trauma and chronic posttraumatic stress disorder in adult outpatients with treatment-resistant depression. J Nerv Ment Dis. 2000;188(9):596–601.
56. Flynn H, Himle J. Psychotherapy strategies for treatment resistant depression. In: Greden J, Riba M, McInnis M, editors. Treatment resistant depression: a roadmap for effective care. Arlington: American Psychiatric Publishing; 2011. p. 193–212.
57. Bryant RA, Gallagher HC, Gibbs L, Pattison P, MacDougall C, Harms L, et al. Mental health and social networks after disaster. Am J Psychiatry. 2017;174(3):277–85.
58. Caspi A. Influence of life stress on depression: moderation by a polymorphism in the 5-HTT gene. Science. 2003;301(5631):386–959.
59. Caspi A, Hariri AR, Holmes A, Uher R, Moffitt TE. Genetic sensitivity to the environment: the case of the serotonin transporter gene and its implications for studying complex diseases and traits. Am J Psychiatry. 2010;167(5):509–27.
60. Town JM, Abbass A, Stride C, Bernier D. A randomised controlled trial of intensive short-term dynamic psychotherapy for treatment resistant depression: the Halifax Depression Study. J Affect Disord. 2017;214:15–25.
61. Driessen E, Van HL, Don FJ, Peen J, Kool S, Westra D, et al. The efficacy of cognitive-behavioral therapy and psychodynamic therapy in the outpatient treatment of major depression: a randomized clinical trial. Am J Psychiatry. 2013;170(9):1041–50.
62. Gibbons MB, Gallop R, Thompson D, Luther D, Crits-Christoph K, Jacobs J, et al. Comparative effectiveness of cognitive therapy and dynamic psychotherapy for major depressive disorder in a community mental health setting: a random-

ized clinical noninferiority trial. JAMA Psychiat. 2016;73(9):904–11.
63. Wampold BE. How important are the common factors in psychotherapy? An update. World Psychiatry. 2015;14(3):270–7.
64. Miklowitz DJ. Adjunctive psychotherapy for bipolar disorder: state of the evidence. Am J Psychiatry. 2008;165:1408–19.
65. Miklowitz DJ, Otto MW, Frank E, Reilly-Harrington NA, Kogan JN, Sachs GS, et al. Intensive psychosocial intervention enhances functioning in patients with bipolar depression: results from a 9-month randomized controlled trial. Am J Psychiatry. 2007;164(9):1340–7.
66. Schoeyen HK, Kessler U, Andreassen OA, Auestad BH, Bergsholm P, Malt UF, et al. Treatment-resistant bipolar depression: a randomized controlled trial of electroconvulsive therapy versus algorithm-based pharmacological treatment. Am J Psychiatry. 2015;172(1):41–51.
67. Parker GB, Graham RK. Clinical characteristics associated with treatment-resistant bipolar disorder. J Nerv Ment Dis. 2017;205(3):188–91.
68. Howes OD, McCutcheon R, Agid O, de Bartolomeis A, van Beveren NJ, Birnbaum ML, et al. Treatment-resistant schizophrenia: treatment response and resistance in psychosis (TRRIP) working group consensus guidelines on diagnosis and terminology. Am J Psychiatry. 2017;174(3):216–29.
69. Search performed 12/24/17, with keywords "treatment," "resistant," and "schizophrenia." https://www.ncbi.nlm.nih.gov/pubmed/.
70. Lacro JP, Dunn LB, Dolder CR, Leckband SG, Jeste DV. Prevalence of and risk factors for medication nonadherence in patients with schizophrenia. J Clin Psychiatry. 2002;63(10):892–909.
71. Kane JM. Treatment-resistant schizophrenic patients. J Clin Psychiatry. 1996;57(suppl 9):35–40.
72. U.S. Food and Drug Administration. FDA approves pill with sensor that digitally tracks if patients have ingested their medication [Internet]. 2017 Nov 13 [updated 2017 Nov 14; cited 2017 Dec 7]. Available from: https://www.fda.gov/NewsEvents/Newsroom/PressAnnouncements/ucm584933.htm.
73. Harrison PJ. Recent genetic findings in schizophrenia and their therapeutic relevance. J Psychopharmacol. 2014;29(2):85–96.
74. Alanen YCBO. Towards a more humanistic psychiatry: development of need-adapted treatment of schizophrenia group psychoses. Psychosis. 2009;1(2):156–66.
75. Veling W, Susser E, van Os J, Mackenbach JP, Selten J-P, Hoek HW. Ethnic density of neighborhoods and incidence of psychotic disorders among immigrants. Am J Psychiatry. 2008;165(1):66–73.
76. Varese F, Smeets F, Drukker M, Lieverse R, Lataster T, Viechtbauer W, et al. Childhood adversities increase the risk of psychosis: a meta-analysis of patient-control, prospective- and cross-sectional cohort studies. Schizophr Bull. 2012;38(4):661–71.
77. Selten J-P, Cantor-Graae E. Social defeat: risk factor for schizophrenia? Br J Psychiatry. 2005;187:101–2.
78. Lehman AF, Steinwachs DM. Translating research into practice: the schizophrenia patient outcomes research team (PORT) treatment recommendations. Schizophr Bull. 1998;24(1):1–10.
79. Altman DG, Bland JM. Absence of evidence is not evidence of absence. Br Med J. 1995;311(7003):485.
80. Coursey RD, Keller AB, Farrel EW. Individual psychotherapy and persons with serious mental illness: the clients' perspective. Schizophr Bull. 1995;21(2):283–301.
81. Lehman AF, Kreyenbuhl J, Buchanan RW, Dickerson FB, Dixon LB, Qoldberg R, et al. The schizophrenia patient outcomes research team (PORT): updated treatment recommendations 2003 Schizophrenia Bulletin. Schizophr Bull. 2004;30(2):193–217.
82. Dixon LB, Dickerson F, Bellack AS, Bennett M, Dickinson D, Goldberg RW, et al. The 2009 schizophrenia PORT psychosocial treatment recommendations and summary statements. Schizophr Bull. 2010;36(1):48–70.
83. Azrin ST, Goldstein AB, Heinssen RK. Early intervention for psychosis: the recovery after an initial schizophrenia episode project. Psychiatr Ann. 2015;45(11):548–53.
84. Alanen YO, Lehtinen K, Räkköläinen V, Aaltonen J. Need-adapted treatment of new schizophrenic patients: experiences and results of the Turku project. Acta Psychiatr Scand. 1991;83(5):363–72.
85. Seikkula J, Alakare B, Aaltonen J. The comprehensive open-dialogue approach in Western Lapland: II. Long-term stability of acute psychosis outcomes in advanced community care. Psychosis. 2011;3(3):192–204.
86. Sensky T, Turkington D, Kingdon D, Scott JL, Scott J, Siddle R, et al. A randomized controlled trial of cognitive-behavioral therapy for persistent symptoms in schizophrenia resistant to medication. Arch Gen Psychiatry. 2000;57(2):165–72.
87. Alanen YO. Towards a more humanistic psychiatry: development of need-adapted treatment of schizophrenia group psychoses. Psychosis. 2009;1(2):156–66.
88. Gromer J. Need-adapted and open-dialogue treatments: empirically supported psychosocial interventions for schizophrenia and other psychotic disorders. Ethical Hum Psychol Psychiatry. 2012;14(3):162–77.
89. Rosenbaum B, Martindale B, Summers A. Supportive psychodynamic psychotherapy for psychosis. Adv Psychiatr Treat. 2013;19(4):310–8.
90. Rosenbaum B, Harder S, Knudsen P, Køster A, Lindhardt A, Lajer M, et al. Supportive psychodynamic psychotherapy versus treatment as usual for first-episode psychosis: two-year outcome. Psychiatry: Interpersonal Biol Process. 2012;75(4):331–41.
91. Martindale B, Summers A. The psychodynamics of psychosis. Adv Psychiatr Treat. 2013;19(2):124–31.

92. Bystritsky A. Treatment-resistant anxiety disorders. Mol Psychiatry. 2006;11(9):805–14.
93. Tolpin M. On the beginnings of a cohesive self: an application of the concept of transmuting internalization to the study of the transitional object and signal anxiety. Psychoanal Study Child. 197(26):316–52.
94. Plakun EM. Psychoanalytic treatment of anxiety disorders, obsessive-compulsive and trauma-related disorders. In: Kaplan & Sadock's comprehensive textbook of psychiatry. 10th ed. Philadelphia: Walters Kluwer; 2017. p. 2666–72.
95. Leichsenring F, Salzer S, Jaeger U, Kachele H, Kreische R, Leweke F, et al. Short-term psychodynamic psychotherapy and cognitive-behavioral therapy in generalized anxiety disorder: a randomized, controlled trial. Am J Psychiatry. 2009;166(8):875–81.
96. Shear MK, Cooper AM, Klerman GL, Busch FN, Shapiro T. A psychodynamic model of panic disorder. Am J Psychiatry. 1993;150:859–66.
97. Milrod B, Leon AC, Busch F, Rudden M, Schwalberg M, Clarkin JF, et al. A randomized controlled clinical trial of psychoanalytic psychotherapy for panic disorder. Am J Psychiatry. 2007;164(2):265–72.
98. Stein DJ, Louw K-A. Management of treatment-resistant post-traumatic stress disorder. In: Nemeroff CB, editor. Management of treatmentresistant major psychiatric disorders. Oxford, New York: Oxford University Press; 2012.
99. Management of Post-Traumatic Stress Working Group. Management of posttraumatic stress disorder and acute stress reaction 2017 – VA/DoD Clinical Practice Guidelines. [cited 2017 Dec 18]. Available from: https://www.healthquality.va.gov/guidelines/MH/ptsd/.
100. Bisson JI, Roberts NP, Andrew M, Cooper R, Lewis C. Psychological therapies for chronic post-traumatic stress disorder (PTSD) in adults. In: The Cochrane Collaboration, editor. Cochrane database of systematic reviews. Chichester: Wiley; 2013 [cited 2017 Dec 18]. Available from. https://doi.org/10.1002/14651858.CD003388.pub4.
101. Gilboa-Schechtman E, Foa E, Shafran N, et al. Prolonged exposure vs dynamic therapy for adolescent PTSD: a pilot randomized controlled trial. J Am Acad Child Adolesc Psychiatry. 2010;49(10):1034–42.
102. Levi O, Bar-Haim Y, Kreiss Y, Fruchter E. Cognitive-behavioural therapy and psychodynamic psychotherapy in the treatment of combat-related post-traumatic stress disorder: a comparative effectiveness study. Clin Psychol Psychother. 2016;23(4):298–307.
103. Markowitz JC, Petkova E, Neria Y, Van Meter PE, Zhao Y, Hembree E, et al. Is exposure necessary? A randomized clinical trial of interpersonal psychotherapy for PTSD. Am J Psychiatry. 2015;172(5):430–40.
104. Halmi KA. Perplexities of treatment resistance in eating disorders. BMC Psychiatry. 2013;13(1):292.
105. Fassino S, Abbate-Daga G. Resistance to treatment in eating disorders: a critical challenge. BMC Psychiatry. 2013;13(1):282.
106. Zipfel S, Wild B, Groß G, Friederich H-C, Teufel M, Schellberg D, et al. Focal psychodynamic therapy, cognitive behaviour therapy, and optimised treatment as usual in outpatients with anorexia nervosa (ANTOP study): randomised controlled trial. Lancet. 2013;383:127–37.
107. McIntosh VVW, Jordan J, Carter F a, Luty SE, McKenzie JM, Bulik CM, et al. Three psychotherapies for anorexia nervosa: a randomized, controlled trial. Am J Psychiatry. 2005;162(4):741–7.
108. Poulsen S, Lunn S, Daniel SIF, Folke S, Mathiesen BB, Katznelson H, et al. A randomized controlled trial of psychoanalytic psychotherapy or cognitive-behavioral therapy for bulimia nervosa. Am J Psychiatry. 2014;171(1):109–16.
109. Stefini A, Salzer S, Reich G, Horn H, Winkelmann K, Bents H, et al. Cognitive-behavioral and psychodynamic therapy in female adolescents with bulimia nervosa: a randomized controlled trial. J Am Acad Child Adolesc Psychiatry. 2017;56(4):329–35.
110. Fairburn CG, Jones R, Peveler RC, Hope RA, O'Connor M. Psychotherapy and bulimia nervosa. Longer-term effects of interpersonal psychotherapy, behavior therapy, and cognitive behavior therapy. Arch Gen Psychiatry. 1993;50:419–28.

Cognitive Behavioral Therapy and Behavioral Activation Therapy for Treatment-Resistant Depression: Traditional and Digital Therapy Perspectives

21

Jennifer Apolinário-Hagen, Lara Fritsche, Liesemarie Albers, and Christel Salewski

21.1 Introduction

According to the WHO World Mental Health (WMH) Surveys [1], mood disorders, including unipolar depression, have high lifetime prevalence worldwide, for instance, with up to 21.4% of the population in the United States. Insofar, depression is a global burden and one of the primary causes of chronic disease and disability with respect to mental diseases [1, 2]. Major depressive disorder (MDD) is characterized by depressed or nervous mood, negative thoughts, and loss of interest or pleasure in everyday activities. These symptoms have to be present for at least 2 weeks and yield significant psychological strain and reduced psychosocial, work-related, or physical functioning [3].

J. Apolinário-Hagen (✉)
Department of Health Psychology, University of Hagen, Hagen, Germany

Department of Health Psychology, University of Hagen, Institute for Psychology, Hagen, Germany
e-mail: jennifer.apolinario-hagen@fernuni-hagen.de

L. Fritsche · L. Albers · C. Salewski
Department of Health Psychology, University of Hagen, Hagen, Germany
e-mail: lara.fritsche@fernuni-hagen.de; liesemarie.albers@fernuni-hagen.de; Christel.Salewski@fernuni-hagen.de

Treatment as usual (TAU) for MDD includes pharmacotherapy. Yet, treatment resistance is a significant issue for the treatment of MDD [4]. Definitions of treatment-resistant depression (TRD) vary in the literature. Commonly, TRD is defined as non-response to pharmacotherapy for depressive disorders. It is estimated that about one-third of depressed patients are non-responders [5]. Hence, TRD is a complex issue for health-care providers requiring integrated therapy approaches and various treatment options for patients [5]. In clinical practice, 50–60% of patients suffering from depression do not respond adequately to antidepressant treatment [6]. If depression is untreated or inappropriately treated, it can be an enormous burden for individuals and societies and produce both direct and indirect costs [7]. Therefore, it is important to understand which well-established psychological treatments work for whom and which delivery mode is appropriate.

Different psychotherapeutic approaches are proven to be effective in the treatment of depression, with comparable benefits across therapeutic strategies [8]. Behavioral and cognitive therapies are suggested as complement or alternative treatment options for TRD, for example, cognitive behavioral therapy (CBT) and behavioral activation (BA) [9]. Meta-analyses of randomized controlled trials (RCTs) showed that both CBT and

Y.-K. Kim (ed.), *Treatment Resistance in Psychiatry*, https://doi.org/10.1007/978-981-10-4358-1_21

BA are effective and efficient stand-alone treatment options for MDD in traditional face-to-face health care [10, 11]. However, treatment gaps in mental health care exist. More treatment spots are needed for large-scale provision of psychological treatment options [12]. To overcome barriers for face-to-face mental health services for depression, the Internet is proposed as a delivery mode for evidence-based digital interventions. Internet-based CBT (ICBT) is suggested to be an efficient format for self-help and treatment of various mental health problems [13]. Internet interventions for depression can be delivered via computer, tablet, or smartphone. In recent years, numerous mobile health applications (mHealth apps), which could provide convenience and easily accessible support for persons suffering from depression, are available through app stores [14]. However, the evidence base for mHealth apps is still scarce, and progress is hard to evaluate for patients and health-care providers [15]. Due to these innovations, health professionals need to provide advice regarding the effectiveness and usefulness of Internet-based self-help programs, ICBT, and mHealth apps for depression. Thus, it is important for health professionals to know about the latest advances in evidence-based psychological treatments.

This chapter summarizes evidence for the effectiveness of different delivery modes of CBT and BA in order to derive recommendations for the traditional and digital psychological therapy of TRD, especially in light of persistent treatment gaps in mental health care.

21.2 Cognitive Therapy and Behavioral Activation for Depression: Theoretical Underpinnings, Approaches, and Key Components of Therapy Programs

CBT is one of the most popular and most researched psychological treatments for depression [16]. It is a client-centered second-wave psychological treatment which suggests that cognitive factors play a major role in the development and maintenance of psychological disorders [17]. Beck's cognitive model of depression [18] constitutes a theoretical foundation for CBT. The model suggests three core mechanisms that are characteristic for depression: Typically, patients engage in negatively biased information processing. Additionally, they develop negative cognitive schemas. Finally, the negative cognitive triad describes patients' negative cognitions about the self, the world, and the future. Generally, negative cognitions, behavior, and emotions maintain each other [19]. The goal of CBT is to unlearn these cognitive patterns and, thereby, to break the cycle of cognitions, emotions, and behavior [20, 21]. In CBT it is assumed that these thoughts are automatic but not unconscious. This implies that patients can be made aware of these maladaptive cognitions and alter them. The task of the therapist is to actively guide the patient through therapy [22]. Techniques that are applied are both cognitive and behavioral with a stronger emphasis placed on cognitive components. Behavioral techniques, which are commonly implemented, are activity planning, assessment of pleasure and mastery activities, gradual goal setting, cognitive rehearsal, and role playing [23]. Usually, these techniques are applied early in the therapeutic process in order to restore minimum functioning and to subsequently change cognitions [24]. Common cognitive techniques are explaining the treatment rationale, cognitive reattribution, assessment of dysfunctional thoughts, and self-monitoring. It is essential that the patient develops a solid understanding of the relation between cognitions and emotions as well as the nature of maladaptive cognitions. This enables the patient to recognize and assess maladaptive automatic cognitions and to self-observe in what type of situations these commonly occur. The key to cognitive reattribution is the search for alternative explanations [23]. CBT can be delivered in individual format, in group format, or in guided self-help format. Duration of treatment can vary from a single session up to 25 sessions [11].

BA originated from a component analysis of CBT, which suggested that behavioral components alone are as effective as cognitive and behavioral components combined to treat acute depression [25] as well as to prevent relapse [26]. The authors consequently suggested that it is not a necessary condition to address cognitions explicitly during treatment. They argued that addressing maladaptive behavior suffices and serves as a mechanism to change cognitions as well [25]. Consequently, BA as a treatment based on the behavioral components of Beck's CBT manual emerged [27]. BA gained attention as a more parsimonious and more efficient way to treat depression that increases reinforcing experiences by activating the client. Benefits of BA include that it is simpler to conduct than CBT and that it does not require extensive training of mental health staff. Therefore, widespread dissemination can be achieved more easily [28].

Behavioral explanations for depression were already proposed 25 years before BA was introduced as a treatment. For example, Ferster [29] assumed that a lack of reinforcement plays a major role in the maintenance of depression. Moreover, he emphasized a strong tendency toward avoidance and escape behaviors to be characteristic of depression. Additionally, Lewinsohn [30] introduced a behavioral treatment for depression where he aimed to increase reinforcing experiences by aiding the client to engage in pleasurable experiences. Comparable to Ferster's [29] explanation of depression, a key premise of BA is that avoidance behaviors are typical for emotional disorders, such as depression. On the one hand, this avoidance pattern may downregulate emotion intensity in the short term. On the other hand, it decreases opportunities for the experience of positive emotions resulting from pleasurable activities long term. In contrast to these previous approaches, BA nowadays does not only target classes of behaviors that are assumed to be pleasurable. Rather any behavior that is potentially beneficial for the client's healthy functioning or mood is targeted [27]. Jacobson and colleagues [27] provide a brief overview over the typical course of treatment in BA. First, they emphasize the importance of establishing a good therapeutic relationship as well as explaining the treatment rationale. Secondly, treatment goals, usually several short-term and fewer long-term goals, are set in collaboration between the practitioner and the client. Higher emphasis is set on short-term goals in order to maintain BA. Usually the goals that are addressed first are those that are concerned with avoidance behavior in order to enable reinforcing experiences. BA treatment usually consists of up to 25 weekly sessions. Brief behavioral activation treatment of depression (BATD), which is a shorter version of BA, usually constitutes 12 weekly sessions [31].

Commonly BA utilizes a variety of techniques. A review by Kanter and colleagues identified the most common ones [32]. These include activity monitoring, activity scheduling, assessment of goals and values, as well as contingency management. Activity monitoring does not only serve to identify behaviors that should be targeted; it also serves to demonstrate the association between mood and behavior to the client. Activity scheduling is a common feature among interventions. Formerly, its purpose was to increase scheduling of pleasant activities. However, focus nowadays has shifted toward scheduling functional activities even if they are not instantly rewarding. The purpose of contingency management is to balance the immediate reinforcement of previously engaged behavior with the long-term benefit of the goal behavior. Contingency management typically has lower priority in treatment than activity scheduling. Some BA interventions also include skills training, verbal training, and relaxation training. Few interventions contain components explicitly directed at avoidance behavior.

21.3 Evidence Base for Face-to-Face CBT and BA

Systematic reviews and meta-analyses yield increasing support for the effectiveness of CBT and BA as stand-alone or complement psychological treatments for MDD in face-to-face care. For instance, a review of 16 meta-analyses by Butler and colleagues [33] showed that CBT is effective for various mental disorders, including unipolar depression, achieving large effect sizes. A recent meta-analysis by Cujpers and colleagues [11] also confirmed the effectiveness of traditional CBT in reducing the symptoms of MDD compared to a waiting-list control condition with large effect sizes. However, effect sizes were small to moderate for CBT compared to TAU or placebo. Cujpers and colleagues [11] criticized the mostly low study quality and publication bias. Another meta-analysis of 16 RCTs on the effectiveness of CBT as monotherapy of chronic depression and dysthymia [34] demonstrated significant but small effects of CBT compared to control conditions and smaller effects compared to antidepressant pharmacotherapy. A meta-analysis [35] on 32 RCTs targeting depressive disorders that combined CBT and pharmacotherapy yielded enhanced therapeutic effects.

Several predictors and mediators for the effectiveness of CBT are discussed. For instance, pretreatment patient predictors of negative outcome or poor response to cognitive therapy for depression involve higher symptom severity scores, number of previous episodes and chronicity, younger age at onset of disease, as well as dysfunctional attitudes and beliefs about depression [36]. Moreover, some patients do not respond to pharmacotherapy; especially adolescents are non-responders. According to a review by Hamill-Skoch and colleagues [37], adolescents suffering from TRD benefit most from a switch in medication combined with appropriately dosed CBT, especially if CBT includes the components social skills training and problem-solving training. However, they also note that more large-scale research is needed to assess moderators of the effectiveness of CBT for adolescents. Additionally, as a review of meta-analyses on CBT has demonstrated [17], there is a lack of meta-analytic studies of CBT with other subgroups, such as ethnic minorities and low-income populations.

Like CBT, BA is an effective psychological approach for the treatment of MDD in face-to-face settings. For instance, a meta-analysis by Cujpers and colleagues [9] including 16 RCTs showed that BA, activity scheduling in particular, and CBT have comparable effectiveness; both had large effect sizes in the treatment of depression. This meta-analysis [9] further revealed no significant difference between activity scheduling and cognitive therapy in long-term effectiveness at the follow-up assessments that ranged between few weeks up to 24 months. Mazzucchelli and colleagues [38] included 34 RCTs in their meta-analysis and review on BA for depressed adults. Most studies met the criteria for moderate quality. Overall, BA was identified as effective in the treatment of depression. They also found no differences in the effectiveness of BA and cognitive therapy. Conversely, the authors [38] also noted that more research is needed to determine whether simpler BA interventions are as effective as more complex BA therapy approaches. Another meta-analysis by Ekers and colleagues [39] including 26 RCTs also confirmed the effectiveness of BA for depression compared to control conditions. However, the authors [39] criticized the low study quality and brief follow-up periods of the BA studies for depression.

Overall, both CBT and BA appear to be attractive alternatives or supplements for the medication of TRD. If a patient is not responsive to medication, health-care providers should consider adding CBT to the treatment. Alternatively, they can consider BA as a simpler approach. Nonetheless, several barriers for using face-to-face mental health services exist, for example, treatment gaps in health care [12]. Apart from structural barriers, an individual barrier to seek professional face-to-face help is that many persons suffering from mild to moderate mental health problems prefer self-help programs [40]. Another individual barrier for depressed persons to seek face-to-face help is stigmatization. Internet interventions have the potential to reduce this burden as they grant more anonymity [41]. Thus, promoting early utilization of professional help and increasing access to evidence-based interventions could be achieved by the provision of Internet-based and smartphone app-delivered mental health interventions for persons with TRD.

21.4 Internet-Based CBT and Mobile Health CBT/BA Apps for Depression as Innovative Strategy

Internet interventions for depression are proposed to reduce treatment gaps [41]. Generally, the Internet provides additional possibilities for the large-scale dissemination of evidence-based psychological interventions [42, 43]. Further potential advantages of standardized and highly structured Internet interventions, such as ICBT, include cost-effectiveness and reduced efforts for therapist [44].

Most of the evidence-based Internet interventions for depression follow the structure and principles of CBT [45]. Such digital interventions involve various Internet-delivered treatment formats with varying degrees of human support, ranging from unguided to therapist-guided self-help interventions, and videoconferencing psychotherapy (VCP). Unguided ICBT programs are characterized as structured computerized programs that are designed for specific psychological problems and provided without personalized support. Most ICBT programs for depression provide at least minimal professional support, including scheduled therapist assistance through weekly text-based personalized feedback about the individual progress of the self-help modules [45]. In contrast to highly standardized ICBT programs, VCP. can use flexible therapeutic strategies [46]. Similar to guided ICBT, VCP has the potential to improve access to psychotherapy regardless of geographical and temporal limitations [46]. Conversely, VCP sessions require the simultaneous presence of a licensed psychotherapist and the patient. However, in VCP. as with face-to-face therapies in clinical practice, deviations from treatment manuals are probable; highly structured Internet intervention for depression can rather guarantee an evidence-based procedure in contrast to face-to-face therapies [41]. Various evidence-based ICBT programs are available, such as the self-help program "MoodGYM" (free-to-use) from Australia or "Beating the Blues" (pay-to-use) from England [47]. Another example for a commercial ICBT program for the adjunctive or self-help treatment of mild to moderate depression is "deprexis" from Germany that aims to support patients to bridge waiting time for traditional psychotherapy [48]. Both, an unguided self-help and a therapist-guided version of deprexis, are available for computers, tablets, and smartphones. This nine-module ICBT program combines different evidence-based components, such as cognitive restructuring, BA elements, relaxation exercises, acceptance- and mindfulness-based lessons, as well as social skill training [48]. Deprexis is shown to be effective and has high acceptance rates in RCTs [49].

Benefits of mHealth apps for TRD include convenient public access through app stores and use in everyday life via smartphones [14]. Apps provide the opportunity for ecological momentary assessment (EMA) as well as activity monitoring and tracking [15]. A systematic review of depression apps [50] identified 243 eligible apps from app stores. The main purposes of these apps were providing therapeutic treatment (33.7%, $n = 82$), psychoeducation (32.1%, $n = 78$), medical assessment (16.9%, $n = 41$), symptom management (8.2%, $n = 20$), and supportive resources (1.6%, $n = 4$). As functions, some apps included an e-book (20.6%, $n = 50$), audio therapy (16.9%, $n = 41$), or screening (16.9%, $n = 41$). The majority of these reviewed depression apps used a dynamic user interface (72.4%, $n = 176$) and text as the main type of media (51.9%, $n = 126$) [50].

Examples of the most downloaded CBT/BA apps are "Mood Tools – Depression Aid" (most usable) and "Depression CBT Self-Help Guide" (most theory based, Textbox 1) [14]. Another example is the commercially available "Moodivate" app for iOS [51]. Moodivate is a mobile app adaptation of BATD with usually five to ten sessions to be utilized in primary care. This app aims to help depressed persons to identify, schedule, and reengage with positive, non-depressed activities. BATD, as it is delivered via the Moodivate app, includes four treatment components: (1) psychoeducation regarding the BATD model; (2) identification of life areas, values, and related activities; (3) daily monitoring and activity planning; and (4) contacts with respect to the identification of supportive individuals [51].

Textbox 1: App "Depression CBT Self-Help Guide (Author: Excel at Life)

Commercial market (cost)	Popularity	(Adherence with) core ingredients[a]	(Adherence with) usability heuristics[a]	Privacy policy and safety[a]
Google play (0€)	Average satisfaction rating: 4.2/5 stars	CBT (75%):	Use (62%):	Privacy:
https://play.google.com/store/apps/details?id=com.excelatlife.depression&hl=de	1373 reviews	Depression education	Match between system and real world	
✓	100,000–500,000 downloads	Model explanation	User control and freedom	(This app, other apps by the author, and homepage)
		Depression rating	Error prevention	Type of information collected
		Monitoring cognitions	Documentation and help (recognize, diagnose, and recover from errors)	Rationale for collection
		Cognitive techniques	Flexibility and efficiency	Sharing of information
		Behavioral techniques	Visibility of system status	User control
		Monitoring behaviors	Consistency and standards	Safety
		Conceptualization	Recognition rather recall	✗
		BA (25%):	Aesthetic and minimalist design	
		Depression education		
		Depression rating		

[a]Data on the usability assessment was obtained from Huguet et al. [14]

21.5 Evidence Base for Internet-Based CBT and Mobile CBT/BA Apps for Depression

Over the past two decades, a growing evidence base clearly indicated the helpfulness of ICBT in the treatment of mild to moderate forms of depression [13, 52] For instance, a systematic review (40 studies) and meta-analysis (19 RCTs) by Richards and Richardson [53] demonstrated the effectiveness of ICBT for depression treatment. Another systematic review by Arnberg and colleagues [54] showed short-term efficacy of ICBT (versus waiting-list control condition) for adults suffering from mild to moderate depression. As a meta-analysis [55] of 3876 depressed adults revealed, self-help ICBT was effective compared to control condition, especially for patients who did not want to have personal therapeutic contact. Moreover, the online self-help interventions for depression MoodGYM and Beating the Blues are shown to be effective when added to TAU (up to the 12-month follow-up) in a pragmatic RCT with 239 patients, though the benefits of using both, self-help interventions and TAU, including cost-effectiveness were marginal [47]. This is in line with a previous meta-review [56] that showed the effectiveness of ICBT for depression but also questioned the cost-effectiveness of such combined interventions (blended treatment). A meta-analysis by Twomey and O'Reilly [57] identified support for the effectiveness of the freely available self-help ICBT program MoodGYM for depression in adults by comparing 11 studies. Several confounding factors restricted the conclusions, including publication bias. Furthermore, high attrition rates up to 90% were found. Regarding different delivery modes, a systematic review [46] revealed that VCP is also a feasible treatment option that has been used in various therapeutic settings and several populations. In addition, results indicated that VCP was generally associated with good participant satisfaction and similar clinical outcomes to face-to-face psychotherapy. Despite an increasing number of publications on VCP, it should be noted that large-scale clinical trials are still necessary for assessing its effectiveness [46].

Furthermore, there is research evidence that therapeutic support in ICBT programs is associated with improved outcomes in the treatment of depression [53, 58]. For instance, a review by Schröder and colleagues [45] concluded that stand-alone self-help Internet interventions yielded small to medium effects in reducing the symptoms of depression, whereas therapist-guided Internet interventions resulted in medium to large effects. In line with this, a systematic review and meta-analysis by Andersson and colleagues [13] provided preliminary evidence that therapist-guided ICBT is effective comparable to face-to-face CBT. However, the evidence base regarding direct comparisons (two studies) is too small to derive conclusions on the equivalence of ICBT and face-to-face CBT. Different factors could influence the effectiveness and acceptability of ICBT. For instance, data from a large cohort study ($N = 1738$) of adult outpatients [59] identified that the perceived credibility of an ICBT treatment for depression was a strong predictor for treatment response. The authors [59] concluded that assessing patients' expectations and beliefs about the treatment could be a useful tool for clinicians to decide which patient might benefit from ICBT for depression.

Like ICBT programs for the treatment of depression, mHealth apps improve the access to evidence-based treatments for depression. BA apps potentially provide another way to ease the implementation of behavior changes in daily life by better matching the habits and preferences especially of younger adults than traditional face-to-face interventions [14, 15]. A review by Donker and colleagues [15] on eight mental health apps, with three apps targeting depression ("Mobilyze," "mobiletype," and "Get Happy Program") within four studies, demonstrated overall positive results. Whereas the apps Mobilyze using EMA [60] and the CBT Get Happy Program [61] yielded significant improvements in depressive symptoms, the app mobiletype using EMA tested within two RCTs against active control groups with adolescents showed no improvements concerning depression [62, 63]. Another systematic review by Huguet and colleagues [14] identified 12 evidence-based

CBT/BA apps for depression. Overall, the authors postulated lack of effective studies as well as scarce usage of the core components of both CBT and BA models. Furthermore, utility and usability of these apps were found to be questionable or variable. Explicit privacy or safety policies were found to be rarely included in CBT/BA apps for depression [14]. This is in line with another review by Bakker and colleagues [64]. The authors concluded that current evidence for the effectiveness and application of user-centered design features of many mental health apps is still lacking [64]. For this purpose, qualitative research on user perspectives and experiences appears to be a necessary step. Concerning the user experience with BA, Ly and colleagues [65] conducted in-depth interviews with 12 selected participants that received guided smartphone-delivered BA treatment for depression that has been shown to be effective in previous research [66]. Their analyses revealed three important areas for individual experience: commitment, expectations, and motivation. For instance, motivational factors varied, but most participants found the reminder function, mobility of the BA therapy app, and feedback from a therapist motivating [65].

21.6 Uptake of and Adherence to Digital CBT/BA Interventions for Depression

Currently, the promotion of the uptake and implementation of Internet interventions for depression into routine care remain a challenge in several countries, despite promising results on the effectiveness and acceptability from clinical studies [41]. In clinical trials ($n = 5$), a systematic review and meta-analysis by Andrews and colleagues [67] identified evidence for both the effectiveness and acceptability of ICBT, including good adherence and satisfaction ratings. According to a meta-analysis of individual participant data [55], adherence to self-help ICBT program improved clinical outcomes. Regarding the dissemination of ICBT in primary care, Hedman and colleagues [52] performed a cohort study examining all patients ($N = 1203$) who had received therapist-guided ICBT for the treatment of depression between 2007 and 2013 in a routine care setting (at an outpatient psychiatric clinic). Results showed significant improvements at the posttreatment that were maintained at 6-month follow-up. Conversely, the attrition rate was assessed as high at 6-month follow-up [52].

Another important question regarding the adherence to ICBT for depression is whether face-to-face and digital therapies achieve comparable adherence rates in routine care settings. A systematic review [13], for instance, found no significant differences in terms of attrition rates between therapist-guided ICBT and face-to-face CBT for different mental health problems (two studies targeting depression). Generally, it should be considered that studies on direct comparisons between the attrition and non-completer rates of therapist-guided ICBT and traditional face-to-face CBT in primary care are quite rare. A systematic review [68] identified 24 studies published between 2000 and 2013 that described 26 treatment conditions (14 face-to-face CBT, 12 guided ICBT) targeting depressed adults. None of the studies compared guided ICBT and face-to-face CBT in a single trial. Face-to-face CBT interventions involved more sessions: while face-to-face CBT therapies ranged from 12 to 28 sessions, guided ICBT interventions contained 5 to 9 sessions. On average, participants in face-to-face CBT completed 83.9% of the treatment program. This rate did not differ significantly from participants in guided ICBT (80.8%). However, the percentage of completers was significantly higher in face-to-face CBT intervention studies (84.7%) than in guided ICBT (65.1%). In addition, this review showed that non-completers of face-to-face CBT completed on average significantly less (24.5%) of the treatment compared to guided ICBT (42.1%) [68].

Concerning the acceptability of ICBT for depression, a systematic review by Rost and colleagues [69] including 29 studies demonstrated that most of the studies reported very high (8 studies) or high (17 studies) level of acceptance. However, the operationalization of user acceptance was heterogeneous across included studies.

Another review by Donker and colleagues [44] has also demonstrated that mHealth apps were associated with good ratings of acceptability, perceived usefulness, and utility. Nonetheless, the number of included apps was very low (eight papers investigating five evidence-based apps for different mental health problems). In contrast to the high acceptability ratings reported in RCTs [44, 69], the uptake of ICBT in public health can be demanding. The slow dissemination and implementation of Internet interventions in primary care in different countries worldwide could be due to the poor acceptability of digital treatment services in the general population [70, 71] and among patients as well as health professionals [72]. Various barriers and facilitators for the dissemination and implementation of Internet interventions in primary care are discussed, such as determinants of their acceptability [72], which can be, in the case of low acceptance, the result of poor awareness or knowledge about digital interventions for common mental health problems [70]. Acceptance-facilitating interventions (AFI) represent a potential way to increase the acceptability of ICBT by providing appropriate information for potential service users. Research on the effectiveness of AFI resulted in promising results regarding the improvement of the acceptability of Internet interventions in clinical practice. For instance, a RCT in primary care [73] demonstrated that AFI using a brief psychoeducational video was effective in improving the acceptance of an Internet intervention among patients with depression.

21.7 Implications of Digital CBT/BA Depression Interventions for Research and Practice

Considering the overall positive research evidence on the effectiveness and acceptability of different delivery modes of CBT and BA, it can be concluded that patients and therapists can choose between different but comparably helpful adjunctive and stand-alone psychological treatments of TRD. Since meta-analyses [9, 38] have shown that face-to-face CBT and BA are comparably effective in reducing symptoms of depression, BA interventions appear especially attractive for clinicians, because they are easy to learn for professionals [28]. Also, BA interventions could reach more patients with TRD due to their simplicity and lower demands for the cognitive functioning of patients compared to CBT [8]. Nonetheless, more research is required to determine whether simpler types or variants of BA are as effective as more complex interventions [38]. Furthermore, predictors of individual treatment response to face-to-face therapies for depression should be considered and investigated in more detail across different populations and settings within public health [17]. Digital delivery modes of CBT and BA represent an additional strategy for the self-help or adjunctive treatment of TRD. Taken together, research suggests that digital mental health interventions hold great promise to improve the access to evidence-based treatments and reduce treatment gaps in traditional health care in the future [45, 74]. Among the digital treatment options for depression, the strongest evidence base exists for therapist-guided ICBT programs. Guided ICBT programs have demonstrated to be effective in the treatment of mood disorders, achieving comparable effects to traditional face-to-face CBT [13]. To make use of the best of both worlds, the advantages of traditional and digital treatments in routine care and blended treatments, a combination of both traditional and digital interventions, could be a suitable, well-accepted strategy for the psychological treatment of depression [75].

Apart from these positive findings indicating the helpfulness of digital treatments for mild to moderate forms of depression, several uncertainties remained, especially with respect to the efficient dissemination of such interventions for patients with TRD in clinical practice. This includes, for instance, the questionable transferability of interpersonal therapeutic principles from traditional to digital treatments with respect to clinical outcomes and adherence. While it can be concluded that at least some degree of professional guidance in ICBT seems to be important to achieve clinical outcomes comparable to face-to-face CBT [13], other aspects regarding the quality of therapeutic relationships and of perceived individual support are less clear for ICBT, for example, the role of the therapeutic relationship between patient and therapist, respectively; the therapeutic working alliance that is an important component of traditional face-to-face psychotherapy, in ICBT, can be classified as unclear due to the limited amount of studies available targeting this outcome. However, there is also evidence that the therapeutic relationship or working alliance can be evaluated as different as or less relevant for the effectiveness of the therapy than in face-to-face therapies, as a narrative review suggested [76]. According to another systematic review [77] on the therapeutic working alliance in Internet therapies, the results of the 11 included studies indicated that the therapeutic working alliance was assessed positively, but the authors mentioned numerous limitations of the included studies, such as the small number of eligible studies, the heterogeneous operationalization of the measured constructs, and the highly selective sample in terms of selection bias. For example, most participants were recruited online via social media websites and familiar with the Internet, which could promote positive evaluations of therapeutic interactions in Internet interventions [77]. Concerning the transferability of these findings to real-world primary care, a limitation for the external validity is especially the use of such selective samples with persons that are well educated and have access to and an affinity for new media. Keeping in mind that Internet interventions are supposed to close treatment gaps, a broader range of patient populations should be considered in view of social inequalities in terms of the so-called digital divide that can turn out as a significant drawback of the large-scale implementation of ICBT into primary care [78]. Additionally, data security concerns of users and clinicians are potential obstacles for developers and providers of digital mental health interventions [74]. In countries where the implementation of electronic (e-)health services into health care is at an early stage, low knowledge about Internet interventions for depression and rather skeptical opinions are other significant barriers for the utilization of such services [75]. To improve the awareness and the acceptability of digital treatment services for mental health problems, such as TRD, educating the public and health professionals via information campaigns [70, 71] and patients with depression in primary care via AFI [73] appear to be suitable strategies. Further research and practice should therefore develop and assess psychoeducational material provided using different media formats for different stakeholder groups.

To better understand the specific conditions for an effective dissemination of ICBT programs and BA apps for the treatment of depression, future studies should explore differences regarding the delivery modes of psychological treatments in real-world public health settings. For instance, there is an overall scarcity of RCTs comparing face-to-face CBT and ICBT for depression that should be addressed in future research [13]. Open questions further include, for instance, the clarification of the cost-effectiveness of ICBT programs in mental health care [44, 54]. Furthermore, it should also be considered that many evidence-based, Internet-based, or app-delivered psychological interventions are presently inaccessible for the public [42]. Therefore, it can be hard to decide for help-seeking laypersons whether a freely accessible digital service is useful. Despite the growing public demand, it should be noted that the helpfulness of most BA apps remains unclear at present [14, 15]. There is a deficiency of appropriate CBT and BA apps for depression from both a clinical and legal perspective [14]. Generally, regarding the development of evidence-based mHealth apps for depression, more rigorous research is needed [15]. In addition, a limitation for clinical practice is that mobile apps for depression appear to be only suitable for mild or moderate forms of depression [79]. Besides a lack of experimental validation, Bakker and colleagues [64] identified a low application of design principles for many of the available apps. Evidence-based guidelines that have been developed for other self-help interventions, like for mHealth apps to promote physical activity, can be rarely found among mental health apps [64]. Finally, because only very few evidence-based mHealth apps for depression are available, the public should be educated on how to identify helpful apps [15].

Conclusions

In this chapter, we evaluated the evidence base for the effectiveness of both traditional face-to-face and digital Internet-based CBT as well as CBT/BA apps for TRD. Research evidence indicates that both face-to-face and Internet-based CBT and BA programs are effective in reducing the symptoms of depression. ICBT and BA programs have the potential of closing present treatment gaps for milder forms of depression and spare therapeutic resources. However, the evidence base for individual predictors of CBT and BA outcomes, such as the role of different delivery modes, appears insufficient for definitive recommendations, especially for Internet-based or smartphone-delivered therapy of TRD in primary care. Concerning the effective implementation of Internet interventions for depression, some questions, concerning specific predictors, individual drivers, and barriers of their uptake, also remain open that need to be addressed in future research and practice. Nonetheless, health professionals should be informed about recent advances in the psychological therapy of TRD, including Internet-based and smartphone-delivered interventions, to counsel their patients or clients about both traditional and digital treatments and help them in finding an appropriate and accessible treatment option that best matches their individual needs and preferences.

References

1. Kessler RC, Aguilar-Gaxiola S, Alonso J, Chatterji S, Lee S, Ormel J, et al. The global burden of mental disorders: an update from the WHO World Mental Health (WMH) surveys. Epidemiol Psychiatr Sci. 2009;18:23–33.
2. World Health Organization. Depression and other common mental disorders: Global health estimates. Geneva; 2017.
3. American Psychiatric Association: diagnostic and statistical manual of mental disorders. 5th ed. Arlington: American Psychiatric Publishing; 2013.
4. Hetrick SE, Cox GR, Merry SN. Treatment-resistant depression in adolescents: is the addition of cognitive behavioral therapy of benefit? Psychol Res Behav Manag. 2011;4:97.
5. Al-Harbi KS. Treatment-resistant depression: therapeutic trends, challenges, and future directions. Patient Prefer Adherence. 2012;6:369.
6. Fava M. Diagnosis and definition of treatment-resistant depression. Biol Psychiatry. 2003;53:649–59.
7. Lépine J-P, Briley M. The increasing burden of depression. Neuropsychiatr Dis Treat. 2011;7:3.
8. Barth J, Munder T, Gerger H, Nüesch E, Trelle S, Znoj H, et al. Comparative efficacy of seven psychotherapeutic interventions for patients with depression: a network meta-analysis. PLoS Med. 2013;10:e1001454.
9. Cuijpers P, van Straten A, Warmerdam L. Behavioral activation treatments of depression: a meta-analysis. Clin Psychol Rev. 2007;27:318–26.
10. Cuijpers P, Dekker JJ, Hollon SD, Andersson G. Adding psychotherapy to pharmacotherapy in the treatment of depressive disorders in adults: a meta-analysis. J Clin Psychiatry. 2009;70:1219–29.
11. Cuijpers P, Cristea IA, Karyotaki E, Reijnders M, Huibers MJH. How effective are cognitive behavior therapies for major depression and anxiety disorders? A meta-analytic update of the evidence. World Psychiatry. 2016;15:245–58.
12. Patel V, Maj M, Flisher AJ, Silva MJ, Koschorke M, Prince M, et al. Reducing the treatment gap for mental disorders: a WPA survey. World Psychiatry. 2010;9:169–76.
13. Andersson G, Cuijpers P, Carlbring P, Riper H, Hedman E. Guided internet-based vs. face-to-face cognitive behavior therapy for psychiatric and somatic disorders: a systematic review and meta-analysis. World Psychiatry. 2014;13:288–95.
14. Huguet A, Rao S, McGrath PJ, Wozney L, Wheaton M, Conrod J, et al. A systematic review of cognitive behavioral therapy and behavioral activation apps for depression. PLoS One. 2016;11:e0154248.
15. Donker T, Petrie K, Proudfoot J, Clarke J, Birch M-R, Christensen H. Smartphones for smarter delivery of mental health programs: a systematic review. J Med Internet Res. 2013;15:e247.
16. McMain S, Newman MG, Segal ZV, DeRubeis RJ. Cognitive behavioral therapy: current status and future research directions. Psychother Res. 2015;25:321–9.
17. Hofmann SG, Asnaani A, Vonk IJJ, Sawyer AT, Fang A. The efficacy of cognitive behavioral therapy: a review of meta-analyses. Cognit Ther Res. 2012;36:427–40.
18. Beck AT. Thinking and depression: I. Idiosyncratic content and cognitive distortions. Arch Gen Psychiatry. 1963;9:324–33.
19. Beck AT. Cognitive therapy and the emotional disorders. New York, NY, USA, Penguin; 1979.
20. Beck AT. Thinking and depression: II. Theory and therapy. Arch Gen Psychiatry. 1964;10:561–71.

21. Beck AT. Cognitive therapy: nature and relation to behavior therapy. Behav Ther. 1970;1:184–200.
22. Beck AT, Rush AJ, Shaw BF, Emery G. Cognitive therapy of depression. Chichester: Wiley; 1980.
23. Beck AT, Rush AJ, Shaw BF, Emery G. Kognitive Therapie der Depression. 5th ed. Weinheim: Beltz; 2017.
24. Rupke SJ, Blecke D, Renfrow M. Cognitive therapy for depression. Am Fam Physician. 2006;73:83–6.
25. Jacobson NS, Dobson KS, Truax PA, Addis ME, Koerner K, Gollan JK, et al. A component analysis of cognitive-behavioral treatment for depression. J Consult Clin Psychol. 1996;64:295–304.
26. Gortner ET, Gollan JK, Dobson KS, Jacobson NS. Cognitive-behavioral treatment for depression: relapse prevention. J Consult Clin Psychol. 1998;66:377.
27. Jacobson NS, Martell CR, Dimidjian S. Behavioral activation treatment for depression: returning to contextual roots. Clin Psychol. 2001;8:255–70.
28. Ekers DM, Dawson MS, Bailey E. Dissemination of behavioural activation for depression to mental health nurses: training evaluation and benchmarked clinical outcomes. J Psychiatr Ment Health Nurs. 2013;20:186–92.
29. Ferster CB. A functional analysis of depression. Am Psychol. 1973;28:857–70.
30. Lewinsohn PM, Graf M. Pleasant activities and depression. J Consult Clin Psychol. 1973;41:261.
31. Lejuez CW, Hopko DR, Acierno R, Daughters SB, Pagoto SL. Ten year revision of the brief behavioral activation treatment for depression: revised treatment manual. BMO. 2011;35:111–61.
32. Kanter JW, Manos RC, Bowe WM, Baruch DE, Busch AM, Rusch LC. What is behavioral activation?: a review of the empirical literature. Clin Psychol Rev. 2010;30:608–20.
33. Butler AC, Chapman JE, Forman EM, Beck AT. The empirical status of cognitive-behavioral therapy: a review of meta-analyses. Clin Psychol Rev. 2006;26:17–31.
34. Cuijpers P, van Straten A, Schuurmans J, van Oppen P, Hollon SD, Andersson G. Psychotherapy for chronic major depression and dysthymia: a meta-analysis. Clin Psychol Rev. 2010;30:51–62.
35. Cuijpers P, Sijbrandij M, Koole SL, Andersson G, Beekman AT, Reynolds CF. Adding psychotherapy to antidepressant medication in depression and anxiety disorders: a meta-analysis. World Psychiatry. 2014;13:56–67.
36. Hamilton KE, Dobson KS. Cognitive therapy of depression: pretreatment patient predictors of outcome. Clin Psychol Rev. 2002;22:875–93.
37. Hamill-Skoch S, Hicks P, Prieto-Hicks X. The use of cognitive behavioral therapy in the treatment of resistant depression in adolescents. Adolesc Health Med Ther. 2012;3:95.
38. Mazzucchelli T, Kane R, Rees C. Behavioral activation treatments for depression in adults: a meta-analysis and review. Clin Psychol. 2009;16:383–411.
39. Ekers D, Webster L, van Straten A, Cuijpers P, Richards D, Gilbody S. Behavioural activation for depression; an update of meta-analysis of effectiveness and sub group analysis. PLoS One. 2014;9:e100100.
40. Andrade LH, Alonso J, Mneimneh Z, Wells JE, Al-Hamzawi A, Borges G, et al. Barriers to mental health treatment: results from the WHO World Mental Health surveys. Psychol Med. 2014;44:1303–17.
41. Schröder J, Berger T, Westermann S, Klein JP, Moritz S. Internet interventions for depression: new developments. Dialogues Clin Neurosci. 2016;18:203.
42. Kvillemo P, Brandberg Y, Bränström R. Feasibility and outcomes of an internet-based mindfulness training program: a pilot randomized controlled trial. JMIR Ment Health. 2016;3:e33.
43. Spijkerman MP, Pots WT, Bohlmeijer ET. Effectiveness of online mindfulness-based interventions in improving mental health: a review and meta-analysis of randomised controlled trials. Clin Psychol Rev. 2016;45:102–14.
44. Donker T, Blankers M, Hedman E, Ljótsson B, Petrie K, Christensen H. Economic evaluations of internet interventions for mental health: a systematic review. Psychol Med. 2015;45:3357–76.
45. Schröder J, Sautier L, Kriston L, Berger T, Meyer B, Späth C, et al. Development of a questionnaire measuring attitudes towards psychological online interventions-the APOI. J Affect Disord. 2015;187:136–41.
46. Backhaus A, Agha Z, Maglione ML, Repp A, Ross B, Zuest D, et al. Videoconferencing psychotherapy: a systematic review. Psychol Serv. 2012;9:111.
47. Littlewood E, Duarte A, Hewitt C, Knowles S, Palmer S, Walker S, et al. A randomised controlled trial of computerised cognitive behaviour therapy for the treatment of depression in primary care: the Randomised Evaluation of the Effectiveness and Acceptability of Computerised Therapy (REEACT) trial. Health Technol Assess. 2015;19:1.
48. Meyer B, Berger T, Caspar F, Beevers GC, Andersson G, Weiss M. Effectiveness of a novel integrative online treatment for depression (Deprexis): randomized controlled trial. J Med Internet Res. 2009;11:e15.
49. Krieger T, Meyer B, Sude K, Urech A, Maercker A, Berger T. Evaluating an e-mental health program ("deprexis") as adjunctive treatment tool in psychotherapy for depression: design of a pragmatic randomized controlled trial. BMC Psychiatry. 2014;14:285.
50. Shen N, Levitan M-J, Johnson A, Bender JL, Hamilton-Page M, Jadad AAR, et al. Finding a depression app: a review and content analysis of the depression app marketplace. JMIR Mhealth Uhealth. 2015;3:e16.
51. Dahne J, Lejuez CW, Kustanowitz J, Felton JW, Diaz VA, Player MS, et al. Moodivate: a self-help behavioral activation mobile app for utilization in primary care—development and clinical considerations. Int J Psychiatry Med. 2017;52:160–75.
52. Hedman E, Ljótsson B, Kaldo V, Hesser H, El Alaoui S, Kraepelien M, et al. Effectiveness of internet-based cognitive behaviour therapy for depression in routine psychiatric care. J Affect Disord. 2014;155:49–58.

53. Richards D, Richardson T. Computer-based psychological treatments for depression: a systematic review and meta-analysis. Clin Psychol Rev. 2012;32:329–42.
54. Arnberg FK, Linton SJ, Hultcrantz M, Heintz E, Jonsson U. Internet-delivered psychological treatments for mood and anxiety disorders: a systematic review of their efficacy, safety, and cost-effectiveness. PLoS One. 2014;9:e98118.
55. Karyotaki E, Riper H, Twisk J, Hoogendoorn A, Kleiboer A, Mira A, et al. Efficacy of self-guided internet-based cognitive behavioral therapy in the treatment of depressive symptoms: a meta-analysis of individual participant data. JAMA Psychiatry. 2017;74:351–9.
56. Foroushani PS, Schneider J, Assareh N. Meta-review of the effectiveness of computerised CBT in treating depression. BMC Psychiatry. 2011;11:131.
57. Twomey C, O'Reilly G. Effectiveness of a freely available computerised cognitive behavioural therapy programme (MoodGYM) for depression: meta-analysis. Aust N Z J Psychiatry. 2017;51:260–9.
58. Johansson R, Andersson G. Internet-based psychological treatments for depression. Expert Rev Neurother. 2012;12:861–970.
59. El Alaoui S, Ljótsson B, Hedman E, Svanborg C, Kaldo V, Lindefors N. Predicting outcome in internet-based cognitive behaviour therapy for major depression: a large cohort study of adult patients in routine psychiatric care. PLoS One. 2016;11:e0161191.
60. Burns MN, Begale M, Duffecy J, Gergle D, Karr CJ, Giangrande E, et al. Harnessing context sensing to develop a mobile intervention for depression. J Med Internet Res. 2011;13:e55.
61. Watts S, Mackenzie A, Thomas C, Griskaitis A, Mewton L, Williams A, et al. CBT for depression: a pilot RCT comparing mobile phone vs. computer. BMC Psychiatry. 2013;13:49.
62. Kauer SD, Reid SC, Crooke AHD, Khor A, Hearps SJC, Jorm AF, et al. Self-monitoring using mobile phones in the early stages of adolescent depression: Randomized controlled trial. J Med Internet Res. 2012;14:e67.
63. Reid SC, Kauer SD, Hearps SJC, Crooke AHD, Khor AS, Sanci LA, et al. A mobile phone application for the assessment and management of youth mental health problems in primary care: a randomised controlled trial. BMC Fam Pract. 2011;12:131.
64. Bakker D, Kazantzis N, Rickwood D, Rickard N. Mental health smartphone apps: Review and evidence-based recommendations for future developments. JMIR Ment Health. 2016;3:e7.
65. Ly KH, Janni E, Wrede R, Sedem M, Donker T, Carlbring P, et al. Experiences of a guided smartphone-based behavioral activation therapy for depression: a qualitative study. Internet Interv. 2015;2:60–8.
66. Ly KH, Topooco N, Cederlund H, Wallin A, Bergström J, Molander O, et al. Smartphone-supported versus full behavioural activation for depression: a randomised controlled trial. PLoS One. 2015;10:e0126559.
67. Andrews G, Cuijpers P, Craske MG, McEvoy P, Titov N. Computer therapy for the anxiety and depressive disorders is effective, acceptable and practical health care: a meta-analysis. PLoS One. 2010;5:e13196.
68. van Ballegooijen W, Cuijpers P, van Straten A, Karyotaki E, Andersson G, Smit JH, et al. Adherence to internet-based and face-to-face cognitive behavioural therapy for depression: a meta-analysis. PLoS One. 2014;9:e100674.
69. Rost T, Stein J, Löbner M, Kersting A, Luck-Sikorski C, Riedel-Heller SG. User acceptance of computerized cognitive behavioral therapy for depression: systematic review. J Med Internet Res. 2017;19:e309.
70. Apolinário-Hagen J, Kemper J, Stürmer C. Public acceptability of E-mental health treatment services for psychological problems: a scoping review. JMIR Ment Health. 2017;4:e10.
71. Musiat P, Goldstone P, Tarrier N. Understanding the acceptability of e-mental health-attitudes and expectations towards computerised self-help treatments for mental health problems. BMC Psychiatry. 2014;14:109.
72. Hennemann S, Beutel ME, Zwerenz R. Drivers and barriers to acceptance of web-based aftercare of patients in inpatient routine care: a cross-sectional survey. J Med Internet Res. 2016;18:e337.
73. Ebert DD, Berking M, Cuijpers P, Lehr D, Pörtner M, Baumeister H. Increasing the acceptance of internet-based mental health interventions in primary care patients with depressive symptoms. A randomized controlled trial. J Affect Disord. 2015;176:9–17.
74. Lal S, Adair CE. E-mental health: a rapid review of the literature. Psychiatr Serv. 2014;65:24–32.
75. Topooco N, Riper H, Araya R, Berking M, Brunn M, Chevreul K, et al. Attitudes towards digital treatment for depression: a European stakeholder survey. Internet Interv. 2017;8:1–9. https://doi.org/10.1016/j.invent.2017.01.001.
76. Berger T. The therapeutic alliance in internet interventions: a narrative review and suggestions for future research. Psychother Res. 2017;27:511–24.
77. Sucala M, Schnur JB, Constantino MJ, Miller SJ, Brackman EH, Montgomery GH. The therapeutic relationship in e-therapy for mental health: a systematic review. J Med Internet Res. 2012;14:e110.
78. Apolinario-Hagen JA, Tasseit S. Access to psychotherapy in the era of web 2.0-new media, old inequalities?/Zugang zur Psychotherapie in der Ära des Web 2.0-Neue Medien, Alte Ungleichheiten? Int J Health Prof. 2015;2:119–29.
79. Arean PA, Hallgren KA, Jordan JT, Gazzaley A, Atkins DC, Heagerty PJ, et al. The use and effectiveness of mobile apps for depression: results from a fully remote clinical trial. J Med Internet Res. 2016;18:e330.

22 Novel Neurostimulation Therapeutic Approaches for Treatment-Resistant Psychiatric Disorders

Ralph J. Koek, Janine Roach, Nicholas Athanasiou, and Arkady Korotinsky

Abbreviations

BD	Bipolar disorder
BDI	Beck depression inventory [1]
CAPS	Clinician administered posttraumatic stress disorder rating scale [2]
CBT	Cognitive-behavioral therapy
CGI	Clinical global impressions [3]
DLPFC	Dorsolateral prefrontal cortex
HDRS	Hamilton depression rating scale [4]
MADRS	Montgomery-Asberg depression rating scale [5]
NAc	Nucleus accumbens
OCD	Obsessive-compulsive disorder
OFC	Orbitofrontal cortex
PTSD	Post-traumatic stress disorder
SCG	Subgenual cingulate gyrus
SZP	Schizophrenia
TRD	Treatment-resistant depression
vALIC	Ventral anterior limb of the internal capsule
VC/VS	Ventral internal capsule/ventral striatum

22.1 Overview of Neuromodulatory Strategies

22.1.1 Electroconvulsive Therapy (ECT)

Electroconvulsive therapy (ECT) (Fig. 22.1) is recognized in many parts of the world as one of the most effective somatic treatments in

R. J. Koek (✉)
Mood Disorders Clinic, Sepulveda Amublatory Care Center, VA Greater Los Angeles Healthcare System, Los Angeles, CA, USA

Department of Psychiatry and Biobehavioral Sciences, David Geffen School of Medicine at UCLA, Los Angeles, CA, USA
e-mail: rkoek@ucla.edu

J. Roach
Mood Disorders Clinic, Sepulveda Amublatory Care Center, VA Greater Los Angeles Healthcare System, Los Angeles, CA, USA

Department of Psychiatry and Biobehavioral Sciences, David Geffen School of Medicine at UCLA, Los Angeles, CA, USA

Department of Psychiatry, Olive View-UCLA Medical Center, Sylmar, CA, USA
e-mail: JRoach@dhs.lacounty.gov

N. Athanasiou · A. Korotinsky
Mood Disorders Clinic, Sepulveda Amublatory Care Center, VA Greater Los Angeles Healthcare System, Los Angeles, CA, USA

Department of Psychiatry and Biobehavioral Sciences, David Geffen School of Medicine at UCLA, Los Angeles, CA, USA
e-mail: nathanas@ucla.edu; Arkady.Korotinsky@va.gov

Y.-K. Kim (ed.), *Treatment Resistance in Psychiatry*, https://doi.org/10.1007/978-981-10-4358-1_22

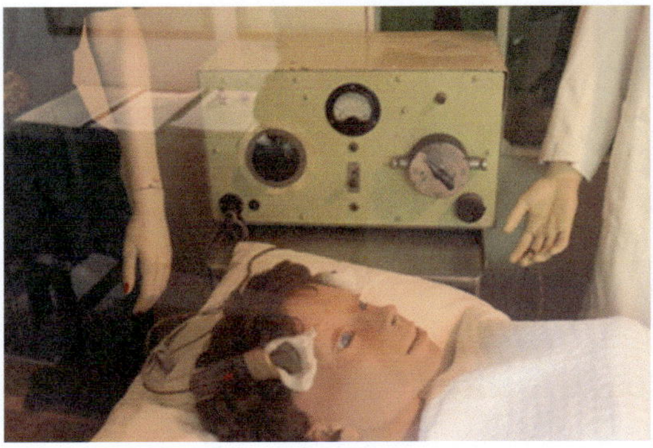

Fig. 22.1 Electroconvulsive therapy (ECT). (https://upload.wikimedia.org/wikipedia/commons/2/21/ECT_machine_03.JPG)

psychiatry. It has been used for severe and treatment-resistant mental illnesses, including psychosis, mania, catatonia, and depression [6, 7].

An ECT treatment *session* involves the application of electrical current to the skull, to produce a generalized seizure discernible on an electroencephalogram. The number of treatment sessions in an ECT *course* varies by diagnosis/symptom cluster and is guided by individual patient response. An *index course* consists of a series of typically twice or thrice weekly treatments sufficient to produce maximal improvement for an acute illness episode. Continuation and maintenance ECT consists of less frequent treatments delivered over months to years to prevent relapse and recurrence, respectively. During the procedure, stimulating electrodes are placed either on one (unilateral ECT, usually right, to reduce cognitive side effects: RUL ECT) or both (bilateral ECT/BL ECT) sides of the patient's head; a seizure is induced by applying a brief electrical pulse. In modern (modified) ECT, the patient is under anesthesia, and neuromuscular blockade is given to prevent muscular contractions (convulsions) [8, 9]. Since 1976 the US Food and Drug Administration has categorized ECT. devices as class III (high risk), although this classification is currently under review for some specific indications.

22.1.2 Transcranial Magnetic Stimulation (TMS)

The mechanism of TMS (Fig. 22.2) is based on the laws of electromagnetic induction. An electrical coil placed above the head generates an electrical current which induces a magnetic field able to penetrate the brain. The magnetic field subsequently induces electrical activity in the cortical neurons below (about 2–3 cm) which are thought to exert therapeutic benefit through neurotransmitter modulation. Initial trials demonstrated that stimulation of neurons in the DLPFC exerted therapeutic benefits in depression and different parameters are important to consider for treatment protocols. Location of the coil can affect different brain regions (DLPFC, SMA, OFC, etc.) and can impact different psychiatric illness (MDD, OCD, schizophrenia, etc.). Stimulus intensity (usually 90–130% of resting motor threshold) should be considered when balancing therapeutic benefits and adverse effects (seizure, headaches, etc.), and the frequency of stimulation can generally be considered stimulatory between 10 and 20 Hz (high frequency) or inhibitory between 1 and 5 Hz (low frequency). The total number of pulses delivered per session is determined by the frequency of stimulation, the length of time for each pulse train, and the total number

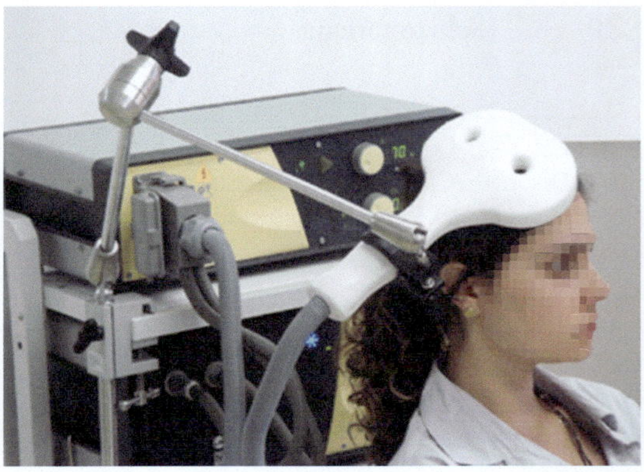

Fig. 22.2 Transcranial magnetic stimulation (TMS). (TMS: https://commons.wikimedia.org/wiki/File:Neuro-ms.png. Page ID 39754391)

of trains delivered. At the time of this publication, rTMS has an indication by the US Food and Drug Administration for treatment of MDD in patients who have failed antidepressant treatment. Other uses remain experimental [10, 11].

22.1.3 Transcranial Direct Current Stimulation (TDCS)

Transcranial direct current stimulation (tDCS) (Fig. 22.3) is a noninvasive neuromodulatory technique, which places two electrodes against the scalp with a headband. A weak current is delivered through the skull; the anodal stimulation brings neuronal membranes toward depolarization, whereas the cathodal stimulation shifts toward hyperpolarization [12]. Action potentials are not reached because of subthreshold stimulation. Electrodes are placed to stimulate or inhibit areas implicated in the psychiatric disorder being treated. TDCS is currently cleared by the FDA for treatment-resistant depression, has received CE mark approval in the EU for depression, and is used off-label for a number of other disorders. Most protocols involve a 1–2 mA current throughout a 20–30 min session, 5 days per week [13]. The most common side effects are redness, itching and tingling at the electrode site, and headache [14].

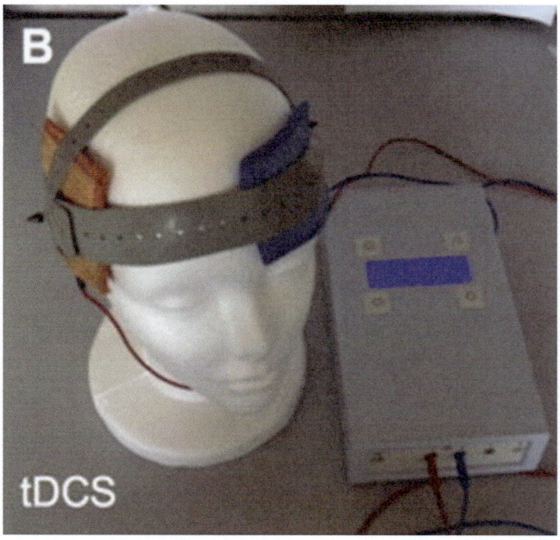

Fig. 22.3 Transcranial direct current stimulation (tDCS). (Open access under the CC BY-NC-ND license (http__creativecommons.org_licenses_by-nc-nd_4.0_).jpg)

22.1.3.1 Trigeminal Nerve Stimulation (TNS)

Trigeminal nerve stimulation (TNS) (Fig. 22.4) is another noninvasive technique where electrodes are placed on the forehead to stimulate the V1 branches of the trigeminal nerve, most commonly at 120 Hz, 250 μs pulse width for 30 s on/30 s off. Stimulation of the trigeminal nerve is thought to carry information to structures in the brainstem which then connect to forebrain structures. Side effects include mild discomfort at the electrode site as well as headache [15]. TNS has received EU CE certification as adjunctive treatment of MDD, though has not received FDA approval in the USA (http://www.medscape.com/viewarticle/770512).

22.1.4 Vagus Nerve Stimulation (VNS) and Transcutaneous Vagus Nerve Stimulation (tVNS)

VNS (Fig. 22.5) stimulates the vagus nerve intermittently at a low frequency; the proposed mecha-

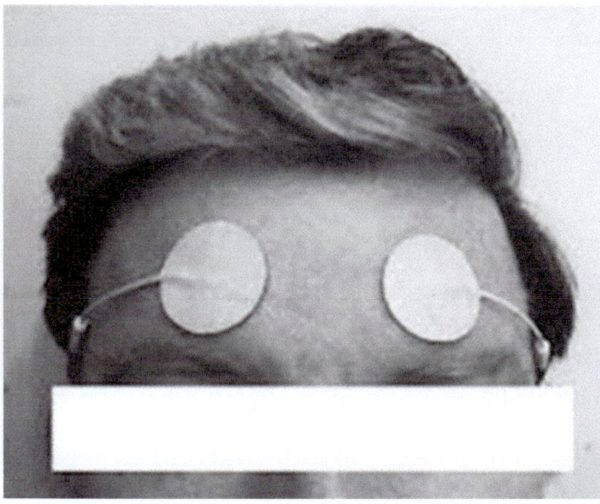

Fig. 22.4 Trigeminal nerve stimulation (TNS). (Reprinted from Ref. 15, with permission from Elsevier)

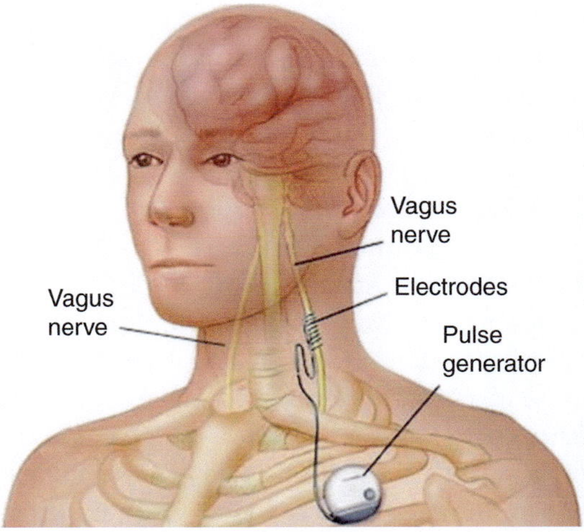

Fig. 22.5 Vagus nerve stimulation (VNS) https://vimeo.com/leehealth (labeled "for reuse")

nism of action is that stimulation of vagal afferent fibers activates the nucleus tractus solitarius in the brainstem, in turn stimulating the prefrontal cortex and medial temporal regions [16, 17]. Wire electrodes are wrapped around the vagus nerve in the neck and connected to a pulse generator surgically implanted in the chest wall. The device is implanted on the left, as there are more cardiac efferent fibers on the right. Side effects are most commonly voice changes, pharyngitis, and cough, although headache, nausea, vomiting, and dyspepsia are also seen [16]. VNS is currently FDA approved for the treatment of severe, recurrent unipolar and bipolar depression [18]. More recently, transcutaneous or noninvasive VNS (tVNS) (Fig. 22.6) is being tested for psychiatric disorders. In this method, instead of wrapping a wire around the vagus nerve, the nerve is stimulated transcutaneously through

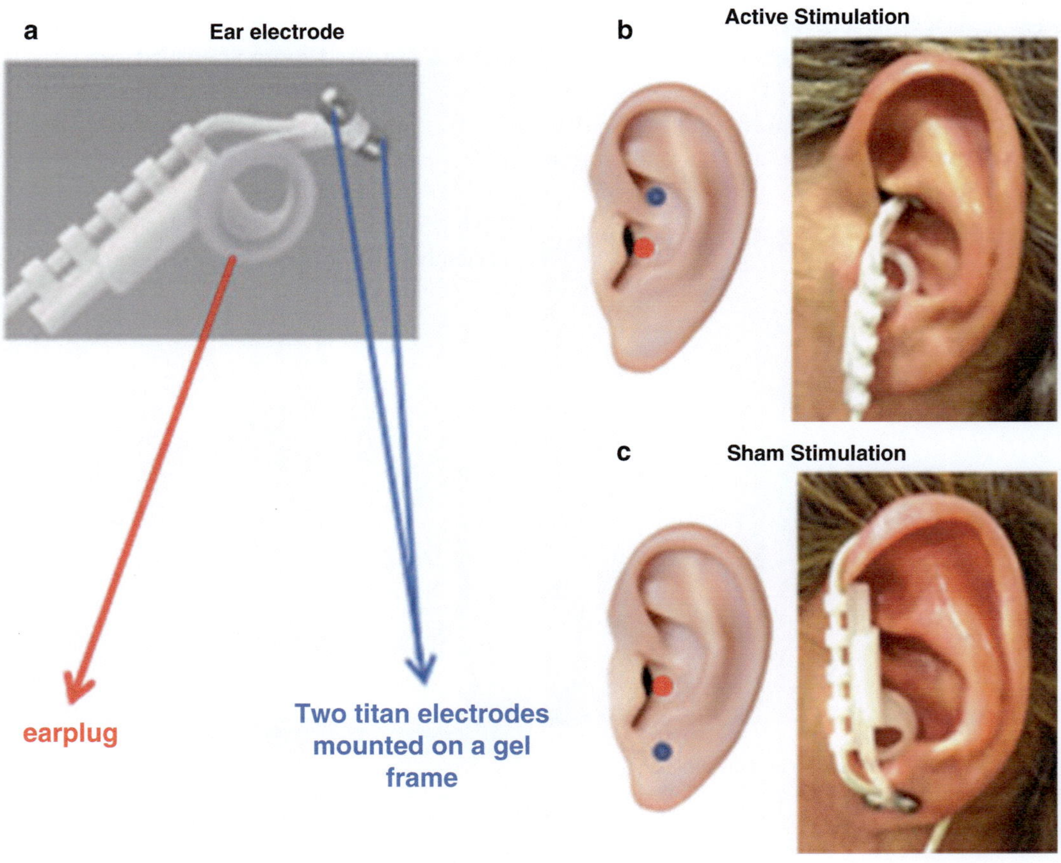

Fig. 22.6 Transcutaneous vagus nerve stimulation (tVNS). (Reprinted with permission from Elsevier)

the auricular branch of the vagus nerve in the outer ear. This device is battery powered and appears like a headset, with electrodes placed in both ears [19]. At this time tVNS is not FDA approved for any psychiatric conditions.

22.1.5 Deep Brain Stimulation (DBS)

DBS (Fig. 22.7) involves surgical implantation of typically 1.3 mm diameter platinum-iridium electrodes (Fig. 22.8) bilaterally into a gray or white matter target determined optimal for a given condition by functional neuroimaging (see Dr. S-H Lee's chapter in Section I and individual chapters in Section II). Within the target structure, four stimulating contacts allow precise stimulation of subregions. After implantation, wires

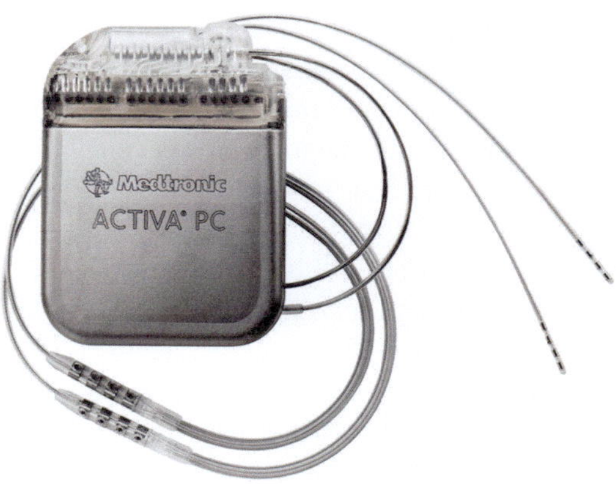

Fig. 22.8 Deep brain stimulation (DBS) example of pulse generator and stimulating electrodes. (Used with permission of Medtronic, Inc.: 7000 Central Avenue NE, RCE240 | Minneapolis, Minnesota, 55,432 | USA)

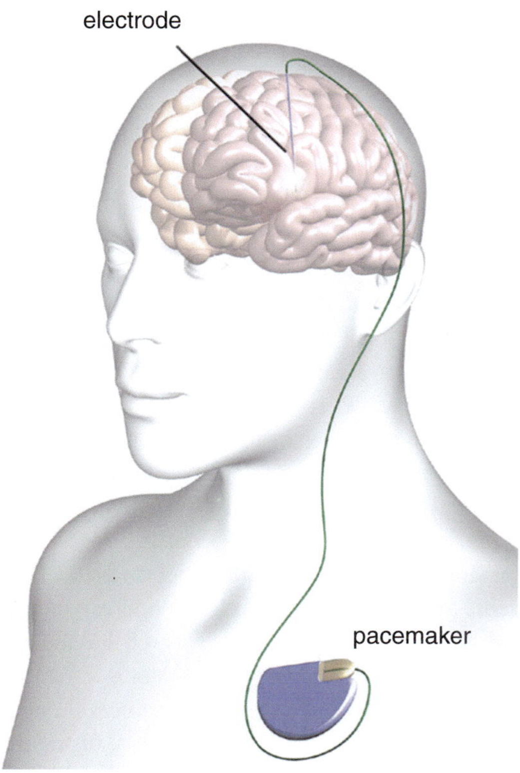

Fig. 22.7 Deep brain stimulation (DBS) schematic depiction. (Shamir R, Noecker A, McIntyre C [CC BY 3.0 (http://creativecommons.org/licenses/by/3.0)], via Wikimedia. Commons: https://commons.wikimedia.org/wiki/File%3ATypical_deep_brain_stimulation_setup.jpg)

are buried under the scalp, connecting the stimulating electrodes to a pulse generator implanted subcutaneously below the clavicle (Figs. 22.7 and 22.8). A hand-held wireless programmer allows adjustment of stimulus pulse width (in microseconds), frequency in hertz, and intensity in volts or milliamperes. Drs. Nejensohn and Dega discuss additional stimulation variables, along with new technological developments to optimize desired effects on brain circuitry, in more detail in a later chapter. In most of the clinical research described below, high-frequency (e.g., 130 Hz) stimulation is used to *reduce* hyperactivity in a target structure, which creates a reversible, "functional lesioning" effect—although neurophysiologic mechanisms are complex and incompletely understood.

Deep brain stimulation (DBS) is distinct from other forms of neuromodulation in several ways. First, it is the most invasive treatment, and thus patients referred are usually the most clearly refractory to standard treatments. In the USA, DBS is FDA approved only under a Humanitarian Device Exemption for treatment-refractory OCD. Thus, all other uses are experimental and "off-label." Inclusion of patients who have well-documented refractoriness to standard treatments makes positive outcomes with DBS more remarkable, particularly if they are long term and associated with improvement of functioning. The second distinction of DBS compared to other forms of neuromodulation is its fidelity in terms of the brain target. This makes DBS a particularly valuable tool for better understanding the specifics of brain-behavior relationships via integrating DBS with functional neuroimaging and, in the future, with simultaneous micro-recording. A third distinction of DBS is shared with VNS, i.e., it can be a continuous, adjustable, "maintenance" (once efficacy is established) intervention. This is valuable because our most treatment-refractory patients are almost always long suffering, with symptoms that vary in severity and quality over time.

22.2 Clinical Application of Neuromodulation in Treatment-Resistant Psychiatric Disorders

22.2.1 Addiction

In addiction, the DLPFC plays an important role in craving, and inhibitory control [20] abnormalities in reward circuitry are also prominent. Neuromodulation has targeted the DLPFC for cravings [21], and high-frequency L DLPFC rTMS has shown benefit for cravings in cigarette smokers, although results have been inconsistent [22]. Similarly, five sham-controlled trials of L DLPFC tDCS have shown reduced cravings in cigarette smokers [23–27], although at least two others have not [28, 29]. Hayashi et al. combined fMRI and low-frequency TMS (LF-rTMS) to inactivate the left DLPFC and were able to decrease cravings during cue-induced exposure to cigarettes but also, importantly, demonstrate the role of the DLPFC in modulating the medial OFC when assigning value to the anticipated drug [30]. Notably, tDCS over the DLPFC has been associated with reduction of drug craving in alcohol [31, 32], cocaine [33], and cannabis [34] users. In addition, some investigations have found worsening of actual drug use [34, 35] despite acutely reduced craving, and one sham-controlled RCT of tDCS in methamphetamine users found reduced craving at rest but increased craving in association with cues [36]. In terms of actual reduction in substance use in patients unresponsive to standard intervention with neuromodulatory intervention, case reports describe substantial, even long-term abstinence with DBS targeting the nucleus accumbens—a key structure in the reward circuit—in alcohol [37, 38], opioid [39–41], and cocaine [42] addiction. Based on the compulsivity inherent in addiction, the subthalamic nucleus (STN) is currently being targeted with DBS (NCT02892851).

22.2.2 Bipolar Disorder

22.2.2.1 ECT

A randomized controlled trial (RTC) conducted in Norway assigned a total of 73 bipolar depressed patients to receive either ECT or algorithm-based pharmacological treatment. A linear mixed-effect modeling analysis found that ECT was significantly more effective than algorithm-based pharmacological treatment for both symptom reduction and treatment response (73.9% versus 35%). [43] The remission rate did not differ (34.8% versus 30.0%), highlighting the degree of treatment resistance in this population. Perugi et al. (2017) published a meta-analysis of ECT in drug-resistant bipolar depression, mania, and mixed state and with catatonia [44]. The study sample included 522 total patients with bipolar depression, evaluated prior to and after an index ECT course. Responders and nonresponders were compared in subsamples of depressed and mixed patients. Descriptive analyses were reported for patients with mania and with catatonic features. After the ECT course, 344 (68.8%) patients were considered responders (final CGI-I score ≤ 2) and 156 (31.2%) nonresponders. Response rates were, respectively, 68.1% for BD depression, 72.9% for mixed state, 75% for mania, and 80.8% for catatonic features. Length of current episode and global severity of the illness were the only statistically significant predictors of nonresponse, a finding consistently seen in most treatment-resistant disorders. ECT was found to be an effective and safe treatment for all phases of severe and drug-resistant BD. Positive response was observed in approximately two-thirds of the cases and in 80% of catatonic patients. It is also worth noting that in this review the risk of ECT-induced mania was virtually absent and mood destabilization very unlikely, often significant concerns with other available treatments. The ECT was well tolerated, with only 22 out of 522 patients excluded for adverse effects of withdrawal of consent for ECT. In general, ECT treatment of bipolar mania has not been rigorously evaluated, and thus most national/professional guidelines do not recommend or include mania as an indication for ECT treatment.

22.2.2.2 rTMS

As rTMS began showing positive outcomes for treatment-resistant depression, researchers have been looking for new applications in bipolar mania and bipolar depression. Grisaru et al. found benefit of right-sided in comparison to left-sided prefrontal HF-rTMS in reducing manic symptoms in patients who met criteria for mania while on pharmacotherapy [45]. However, a sham-controlled study of right-sided HF-rTMS could not demonstrate benefit in a similar population [46]. Others have shown benefit of TMS as an add-on to standard pharmacotherapy [47, 48].

Although there is notable efficacy for rTMS in TRD, the evidence is mixed in regard to bipolar depression. Initially, Dolberg et al. found that rTMS for 2 weeks was superior to sham in 20 patients with various symptom duration and treatments (including ECT) [49], while a subsequent trial found that rTMS over the DLPFC was no more efficacious than sham, but the study did find the risk for inducing mania to be minimal [50]. More recently, a controlled trial of sequential bilateral rTMS in patients with treatment-resistant bipolar depression who received both HF-rTMS applied to the left DLPFC followed by LF-rTMS applied to the right did not show benefit over sham [51]. However, a naturalistic study of 150 unipolar and 50 bipolar depressed patients who failed multiple antidepressants found similar efficacy in response and remission rates between the two groups when given bilateral sequential rTMS or LF-rTMS to the right DLPFC. The study lacked a sham group for comparison. Further studies will be needed to better understand a future role for TMS in the treatment of both bipolar mania and depression [52].

22.2.2.3 tDCS

Most tDCS studies for depression include both unipolar and bipolar depression, as criteria include major depressive episode but do not specify primary diagnosis. A meta-analysis of tDCS in bipolar depression including 7 studies with 46 patients showed significant decrease in depression, with 6 total affective switches [53]. In a case report, tDCS was used in a patient who presented with acute mania while taking lithium, olanzapine, and sertraline. The patient received a 5-day course of tDCS in combination with clozapine and oxcarbazepine, and after the 3rd day, there was a reduction in manic symptoms and inappropriate behaviors. Seventy-two hours after completing tDCS, symptoms reappeared and did not improve until approximately 12 days later, presumably when medications took effect [54].

22.2.2.4 VNS

Vagal nerve stimulation has not been studied as extensively in bipolar disorder as treatment-resistant depression. In a 2-year open-label study, the response rates of unipolar TRD and bipolar TRD were 32% vs 34%, suggesting that the difference in response rate to VNS in these two illnesses is not significant [55]. There is a case report of a patient with bipolar disorder who had 9 years of remission after 20 months of adjunct VNS whose battery in the device died, and there was considerable time in getting replacement. The patient subsequently had recurrences of manic, depressed, and mixed episodes until 17 months after reinitiation of VNS therapy [56]. Rapid cycling bipolar disorder is often treatment resistant, and these patients tend to be excluded from studies, though one study included nine outpatients with rapid cycling bipolar disorder who were assessed after 40 weeks of open-label adjunct VNS. Over 1 year there was a 38% reduction in total illness (combination of depression and mania symptoms) with significant reductions in HDRS, MADRS, and CGI, though not mania scores [57].

22.2.2.5 DBS

To date, no study utilizing DBS specifically for bipolar disorder has been published [58], although in trials of DBS for TRD, both improvements in bipolar depression [59–61] and development of hypomania [60] have been seen. Hypomania has been reported as a rapidly reversible side effect of DBS in Parkinson's disease and OCD. ClinicalTrials.gov shows several ongoing studies in TR bipolar disorder (NCT01372722, NCT01973478, NCT01476527, NCT01372722, NCT01973478) so the next few years may reveal valuable data.

22.2.3 Depression (TRD)

22.2.3.1 ECT

For prospectively defined TRD, it is worth noting that RCTs are few and often small. The literature is complicated by varying definitions of treatment resistance, various subtypes of depression, and different modalities of ECT administered (RUL vs BL ECT, brief pulse ECT) and treatment number (a course of 6–12 sessions over 2–4 weeks has been found to result in remission in 55–86% of major depression patients in general [62], but this hasn't been compared for TRD versus non-TRD). In one frequently referenced RCT, Folkerts et al. (1997) randomized 39 patients with TRD, defined as ≥ two failed antidepressant trials from different classes (mean 4.9), to either paroxetine mean dose 44 mg ($n = 18$) or RUL ECT ($n = 21$). After 6 weeks, during which the ECT group received six treatments over 14 days (7.1 on average), the authors found a 59% HDRS score reduction with ECT compared to 29% for paroxetine ($P < 0.001$ paired t-test). In the ECT group, 71% of subjects fulfilled the response criteria (at least a 50% decrease in total HDRS score). In this study, ECT was superior to paroxetine in medication-resistant major depression in both degree and speed of response [63]. It is worth noting that patients who had psychotic symptoms or pronounced suicidal tendencies were excluded from this study. This limits generalizability to clinical populations, which is surprising given that suicidal tendencies and psychotic depression (in addition to medication-refractoriness and catatonic features) are widely regarded as particular indications for ECT in depression.

An important clinical consideration in the discussion of ECT for TRD is the role of concomitant antidepressant treatment. There are understandably not only questions about which treatment is responsible for antidepressant effect but also concerns about possible worsening of side effects, including cognitive effects. In a 2015 meta-analysis, Song et al. attempted to answer this question [64]. The review included a total of 17 studies, 13 regarding ECT plus antidepressant versus antidepressant alone and 4 concerning ECT versus antidepressant alone, comprising a total of 1098 patients. The head-to-head comparison suggested that response rate can be improved in the ECT plus antidepressant (RR, 1.82; 95% CI, 1.55–2.14) and ECT alone group (RR, 2.24, 95% CI, 1.51–3.33) compared with antidepressant alone, respectively; adverse complications including memory deterioration and somatization were not significantly increased except incidence of memory deterioration in ECT plus antidepressant in the 4th week after treatment (RR, 0.09, 95% CI, 0.02–0.49). An indirect comparison meta-analysis showed no significant differences in response rate and memory deterioration between ECT plus antidepressant and ECT alone. However, ECT plus antidepressant increased the incidence of memory deterioration relative to ECT alone. These authors [64] concluded that ECT plus antidepressant should not be preferentially recommended for TRD relative to ECT alone.

In addition to its established place as an effective treatment for severe, psychotic, or catatonic depression, ECT offers other potential benefits for severe treatment-resistant mood disorders. The rapid onset of its beneficial effects is a key advantage of ECT over pharmacotherapy and psychotherapy, which may take 1–3 weeks or longer to achieve clinically significant response. ECT can be particularly important in clinical situations where severity of symptoms, functional disability, catatonia, and acute suicidal ideation are present and require a rapid clinical intervention. Finally, some evidence supports the specific anti-suicidal effect of ECT. Data from the first phase of an ongoing, collaborative, multicenter study suggested profound short-term benefit in patients with suicidal ideation who received ECT. One hundred thirty-one patients (representing 29.5% of the entire study group) reported suicidal thoughts and acts (either active suicidal thoughts or a suicidal event during current episode, a 3 or 4 on the Hamilton depression scale) at baseline. Scores decreased to 0 after 1 week (three ECT sessions) in 38.2% of the patients, after 2 weeks (six ECT sessions) in 61.1%, and in 80.9% at the end of the course of treatment. The resolution of suicidal thoughts further improved with increased number of ECT sessions [65]. Another study [66] noted more rapid improvement in depression and expressed suicidal intent in a group of 30 patients receiving ECT compared with a control group receiving pharmacotherapy. The ECT group received between five and ten bilateral treatments administered at three times/week. Outcome was assessed with the 24-item Brief Psychiatric Rating Scale (BPRS) before and after the ECT course. There were significant advantages for ECT on BPRS depression and suicide item scores. Finally, an RCT ($N = 73$) found that ECT reduced depressive symptoms and suicidal ideation scores on both the HDRS and BDI more rapidly and effectively than rTMS [67].

22.2.3.2 rTMS

TMS is an effective treatment for major depressive disorder in patients who have not responded to pharmacotherapy [10]. In 2008, the US Food and Drug Administration approved TMS for treatment of MDD based on a double-blind multisite study of 301 patients who failed 1–4 antidepressants [68], and subsequently a study sponsored by the National Institutes of Mental Health found fourfold greater remission rates with active HF-rTMS targeting the left DLPFC when compared to sham [69]. Since those trials, more than 15 meta-analyses and reviews have been published demonstrating the efficacy of TMS in depression, and the Clinical TMS Society provides a thorough review and recommendations for clinical use [10].

It has been shown that there is likely a dose effect with a higher total number of pulses delivered resulting in a better antidepressant effect [70]. Several studies have found that rTMS can have benefits past the initial treatment phase and with better durability in patients who show more robust response to acute TMS. Mantovani et al. (2012) found that 58% of acute rTMS responders maintained benefits up to 3 months afterward with or without medication; of those who did relapse, the average time was 7 weeks [71]. Other studies have found relapse rates as low as 10% at 6 months with pharmacotherapy maintenance only, and one-third at 1 year with pharmacotherapy or TMS reintroduction as needed [72]. These promising results suggest further consideration of TMS as a maintenance treatment for TRD. Fitzgerald et al. used clustered maintenance, consisting of five sessions over 2 days, monthly, to delay relapse until a mean of 10 months [73], while Richieri et al. found benefits of TMS maintenance using a tapering frequency of weekly, biweekly, and then monthly over 18 weeks [74]. However, a recent study where patients who responded to acute TMS treatment were placed on monthly maintenance TMS for 1 year without medications did not show a statistically significant benefit [75].

The left DLPFC is most often targeted in depression, but it is worth noting that rTMS likely affects other regions that may help explain response to treatment. In the future, other targets and possibly depression subgroups will likely guide treatment. Recently, Drysdale et al. published a study in which they calculated resting state-functional MRI connectivity in limbic and frontostriatal networks to develop four neurophysiological subtypes ("biotypes") of depression [76]. They then evaluated response to HF-rTMS of the dorsomedial PFC and found that a certain biotype (type 1) showed the highest response rate (83%). Even more remarkably, their method distinguished responders from nonresponders with up to 90% accuracy. Such advances in rTMS for TRD may improve applicability of this modality to other treatment-resistant psychiatric illness.

22.2.3.3 tDCS

There are numerous open-label as well as placebo-controlled trials of tDCS in depression [13, 77]. Ferrucci studied a cohort of 14 severe treatment-resistant patients who were hospitalized for major depression and high risk of suicide and referred for ECT. After ten tDCS sessions over 5 days, BDI and HDRS scores improved by 30% in this very difficult to treat population [78]. Thus far, three sham-controlled RCTs studied the effect of tDCS in TRD, defined as failing at least two trials of antidepressants in different classes [79–81]. All three trials failed to demonstrate significant improvement with active compared to sham tDCS. Study size ranged from 22 to 24 subjects who received between 10 and 15 sessions.

22.2.3.4 TNS

There is one open pilot study of TNS in depressed patients who failed to respond to at least two antidepressants at therapeutic dose for 6 weeks. After 8 weeks, subjects showed a significant decrease in the severity of symptoms and improvement in quality of life [15].

22.2.3.5 VNS

Vagal nerve stimulation for chronic TRD has been examined in a number of open-label and naturalistic studies, most demonstrating a benefit in depression over 12 months [82–84]. Long-term sham-controlled trials may be difficult and unethical because of the invasive nature of VNS. One study compared VNS + treatment as usual (TAU) with TAU. After 12 months, the VNS group showed a response rate of 27%, compared with 13% for TAU [85].

A recent 5-year observational study of 795 patients who had failed at least four treatments, including ECT, for either unipolar or bipolar depression compared VNS+ TAU with TAU. The group with VNS showed a 67.6% response rate (vs. 40.9% TAU) and a 43.3% remission rate (vs. 25.7% TAU) at some point during the 5-year follow-up period [86].

22.2.3.6 DBS

Given that TRD is associated with a high rate of relapse after initial improvement despite maintenance treatment [87], long-term use with ongoing adjustability is a potential advantage of DBS (as well as VNS). The subgenual cingulate gyrus (SCG) was the target of the first DBS study in TRD [88]. At 6 months, four out of six initial patients showed a response [88], and at study completion, substantial symptomatic and functional improvements in most of 20 subjects were seen up to 6 years [89]. A meta-analysis of four open-label SCG DBS trials from three different groups found a 1-year pooled response rate of 40% and remission rate of 26% [90], which compares favorably with TAU response and remission rates of 11.6% and 3.6% [91], respectively, in such severely refractory patients. Case reports and open-label investigations have found benefit with DBS in other brain targets, including the VC/VS, NAc, inferior thalamic peduncle, and habenular nucleus, with 6–12 month pre-post comparisons demonstrating no deterioration on extensive neurocognitive assessment batteries [92]. Substantial functional improvements, perhaps a more meaningful benefit than depressive symptom ratings per se for such long-suffering individuals, have been found with long-term SCG, VC/VS, or vALIC DBS for TRD [93].

While long-term, parallel group sham-controlled RCTs are unethical, a sham-controlled phase within a long-term trial, allowing all subjects implanted to eventually receive active stimulation, can control for nonspecific effects in an ethically justifiable way. In one study, a sham phase was dropped from the study when the first three subjects rapidly deteriorated [94]. Another pilot study of five subjects showed relatively greater benefit during active compared with sham SCG stimulation [95]. Notably, however, a large (planned $N = 75$) industry-sponsored RCT of SCG DBS was halted based on an early futility analysis showing a 17% likelihood of finding active > sham DBS at study completion [96]. The two published sham-controlled RCTs of DBS for TRD both included ~30 patients. In one study [97] targeting the VC/VS, improvements were low and similar over 4 months (3/15 active and

2/14 sham patients responded (p = 0.53)). Notably in this study, the randomization phase occurred after a few days of programming optimization. The second RCT involved 25 subjects and was positive [98]. These investigators targeted the nearby vALIC, but compared 4 months active to sham stimulation in the 16/25 subjects who had improved after up to 12 months of initial, open-label programming adjustment.

The optimal site of stimulation is not yet clear. Schlaepfer and colleagues in Germany have targeted the superolateral branch of the medial forebrain bundle (slMFB) based on its involvement in the reward system and the potential benefit for anhedonia [99]. Rapid benefit (within a week) was seen in six out of seven initial patients, four of whom were in remission at 3–8 months [99]. At 1 year, six out of eight patients were responders and four out of eight were remitters, with substantial improvements during most of 4 years of stimulation in seven out of eight subjects [100]. Results from additional subjects and a sham phase are anticipated in this ongoing multiphase study, which has been independently replicated in a ten-patient sham-controlled pilot study [101]. Epidural plate electrode stimulation of simultaneously the frontal pole and DLPFC was safe and effective in five patients with TRD [102]. Both RCTs [97, 98] in TRD found no neurocognitive differences between sham and active stimulation [103, 104], although better cognitive outcomes were seen on some measures in responders, compared with nonresponders in one study [104]. Ongoing trials include another sham-controlled SCG investigation (NCT00367003), R vs L SCG (NCT01898429), and a study with simultaneous recording of local field potentials—the "Brain Radio" (NCT01984710) and bilateral habenula DBS (NCT03254017).

22.2.4 OCD

Neuromodulation has targeted a number of brain areas to treat OCD, with varying success. A 2014 review article found a positive response in 60% of case reports/series when using ECT to treat OCD, though the level of treatment resistance is unclear [105]. Initial experiments showed application of HF-rTMS to the DLFPC to be helpful [106, 107], although some subsequent reviews suggested overall lack of benefit for HF-rTMS to the DLPFC [108, 109]. Some research has found improvement with LF-rTMS to the supplemental motor area (SMA) and OFC [109]. The most recent meta-analysis found clear advantage for active vs. sham rTMS that was not influenced by study heterogeneity [110]. In patients with OCD who had failed multiple medication trials as well as CBT, VNS showed statistically significant improvement in symptoms in three of seven patients over 4 years [111]. Multiple case reports and open-label studies suggest that tDCS targeting the OFC, DLPFC, and SMA leads to reduction in OCD symptoms in some patients who have failed at least two SSRIs and CBT. [112–116] The only RCT to date involving tDCS and OCD showed significant reduction in symptoms when electrodes were placed to decrease cortex excitability and blood flow to the pre-SMA, an area thought to be hyperactive in patients with OCD [117]. A meta-analysis of DBS studies targeting limbic structures including the VC/VS, NAc, STN, ALIC, and inferior thalamic peduncle (ITP) found a decrease in symptoms regardless of target in patients who have failed at least three medication trials and CBT [118]. Other studies have shown improvement of quality of life and long-term benefit in active vs. sham studies [119–122], leading the FDA to approve Medtronic's Reclaim® device, targeting the vALIC, under a Humanitarian Device Exemption for severe, non-hoarding OCD patients who have failed ≥3 medication trials and intensive CBT. Benefit has been shown with DBS targeting the BNST, MFB, and thalamus as well [123–125].

22.2.5 Panic and Other Anxiety Disorders

There are limited data regarding neuromodulation and anxiety disorders. One patient with generalized anxiety disorder who had failed four trials of pharmacotherapy reported a 93%

decrease in symptoms after ten sessions of TNS, which was maintained for 1 month [126]. One patient with panic disorder showed greater than 50% reduction in anxiety symptoms with VNS which was maintained over the 1-year study period [111]. Kuhn et al. (2007) found no efficacy in a single patient receiving NAc DBS for treatment-refractory panic disorder [37], though studies of vALIC DBS for OCD have found improvements in anxiety ratings [121].

22.2.6 PTSD

The most clinical data in treatment-refractory PTSD comes from rTMS studies, with three meta-analyses documenting benefit [127–129]. Karsen et al. (2014) found pooled effect size for PTSD symptoms of 2.67 (0.73–3.78, Hedges g) in one meta-analysis of three RCTs, while Berlim et al. found a pooled effect size 1.65 for clinician-rated response in another three-study meta-analysis [130]. While the left DLPFC is the primary target for TRD, there is evidence that targeting the right DLPFC may be more effective in PTSD, with no clear advantage of high- versus low-frequency stimulation [127, 128, 130]. With ECT, there was one open trial of 6 B-ECT in 20 patients with severe, chronic, extensively antidepressant, and CBT refractory PTSD. An intent-to-treat analysis showed statistically and clinically significant improvement, with a mean 34.4% CAPS total score reduction and a response rate of 70% (CAPS reduction of ≥30% from baseline). There were no remitters (CAPS endpoint <20) and three dropouts [131]. Notably, CAPS improvement was independent of both baseline depression severity and improvement in depression with ECT. An open study of 12 patients with comorbid PTSD and MDD who failed to respond to an adequate trial of one antidepressant underwent 8 weeks of TNS adjunctive to their current treatment. Study subjects showed a significant decrease in symptoms of both depression and PTSD [132].

Neuroimaging findings in treatment-refractory PTSD suggest an inadequate vmPFC inhibition of an over-reactive amygdala, preventing extinction learning. To date, one tDCS study based on this hypothesis in 28 veterans found greater effect on skin conductance reactivity during extinction consolidation than during extinction learning, in a 2-day Pavlovian fear conditioning paradigm [133]. With DBS, only one case report has been published, a 48-year-old man with extremely severe combat PTSD (baseline CAPS, 119) who obtained a 38% improvement after 8 months of bilateral DBS targeting the basolateral nucleus of the amygdala (BLn) [134]. Clinical and electrophysiologic safety was demonstrated at 1 year [135].

22.2.7 Schizophrenia

Several neuromodulatory techniques have been used in both positive and negative symptoms of treatment-resistant schizophrenia, though it is difficult to define treatment-resistant negative symptoms as there is currently no recognized effective treatment.

22.2.7.1 Positive Symptoms

A meta-analysis of ECT augmentation of clozapine in schizophrenia found positive symptom treatment response in 66% of 192 patients treated in an RCT ($N = 39$), 4 open-label studies ($N = 32$), as well as chart reviews and case series [136]. More sessions (11–15, mean 11.3) are often required in schizophrenia than for other clinical indications [136–138]. ECT also has a critical role in the treatment of catatonia [139], where fewer sessions than in TRD may be required, and in malignant/lethal catatonia, where its emergency application may be indicated [140]. It is believed that the left temporoparietal cortex (TPC) participates in generation of auditory hallucinations (AH). Low-frequency rTMS to reduce neural excitability in the TPC has been recommended after studies noted improvement in severity of AH when targeting this region, though little benefit is seen for other positive symptoms and effects appear to diminish after about 4 weeks [110, 141–144]. An RCT of tVNS in treatment-resistant schizophrenia found no significant difference between the active vs. sham groups in improving positive or negative symptoms [145]. When using tDCS for the treatment of positive symptoms, the anode was placed on the left DLPFC (hypoactive area) and the cathode on the L temporoparietal (hyperactive) area [146]. Of five sham-controlled RCTs exploring treatment of positive symptoms in patients who failed to respond to two or more antipsychotics, three demonstrated a reduction in AH [147–149], and two did not [150, 151]. TNS was used for a patient with olfactory hallucinations refractory to treatment with two antipsychotics; the patient reported complete remission of olfactory hallucinations after ten sessions [152]. The earliest efforts to use DBS for psychiatric illness were carried out by Heath and colleagues, beginning in the mid-1950s, for "schizophrenia" [153]. Unfortunately, methodologic limitations made the results of their trials in over 20 patients difficult to apply to today's understanding of either DBS or schizophrenia [154]. A 2016 report described marked improvement in treatment-refractory positive symptoms over a 10-month period after NAc DBS [155] in a 27-year-old woman enrolled in an ongoing study comparing NAc to PFC DBS (NCT02377505). Additional ongoing trials include a comparison of NAc vs SCG and DBS of the substantia nigra pars reticulata (NCT02361554).

22.2.7.2 Negative Symptoms

Negative symptoms of schizophrenia are hypothesized to arise from prefrontal dysfunction and hypoactivity of the DLPFC. There are several meta-analyses demonstrating efficacy of HF-TMS and even an expert consensus determination of "probably effective" (level B) [110, 156]. However, a more recent large-scale, multicenter trial of 175 patients failed to demonstrate efficacy of HF-rTMS to the DLPFC when compared to sham TMS [157], though it is worth considering that the effects of TMS on negative symptoms could be delayed for as long as 8 weeks, while most studies measure response in shorter time intervals [158]. An open pilot study of both bilateral and unilateral tDCS did not show any benefit for either positive or negative symptoms in patients who had failed at least two antipsychotics [150]; however, one double-blind sham-controlled trial showed a significant decrease in negative symptoms of schizophrenia after ten sessions of dTCS [14], and another study showed a decrease in negative but not positive symptoms with left DLPFC stimulation [159]. A case report of patient who had tried four different antipsychotics including clozapine underwent ten sessions of TNS and showed improvement in negative symptoms [160].

22.3 Adverse Effects

In neuromodulation, an important general consideration is discerning whether a given event is attributable to the device and its application/implantation, the stimulation from the device, or the psychiatric condition being treated [161]. Additional cost-benefit analysis considerations affecting the clinical applicability of neuromodulation in treatment-refractory conditions include (1) limited FDA approvals (as of December 2017, only rTMS and VNS for TRD and DBS for TR-OCD under HDE); (2) device cost, availability, and standardization; and (3) availability of professionals qualified in utilization of the device, including long-term monitoring and management in the case of VNS and DBS.

22.3.1 ECT

The most frequent immediate adverse effects of ECT with modern techniques include, but are not limited to, headache, nausea, and vomiting [8]. Many of the side effects of ECT are related to the risk of anesthesia used for the ECT procedures. Serious medical complications are rare, even in patients with severe cardiovascular risk factors. The most common adverse effect of ECT is acute cognitive impairment lasting from few minutes to few days [162] or amnesia [163]. The two types of ECT-related memory loss are anterograde and retrograde amnesia. Marked hippocampal plasticity triggered by ECT has been implicated as a potential mechanism [164]. The incidence of these and other adverse effects of ECT have been reduced with improved modern ECT/anesthesia techniques.

22.3.2 rTMS

TMS does not require anesthesia or seizure induction, as is the case with ECT, and it is a noninvasive brain stimulation therapy that does not pose risks of surgical complications such as VNS or DBS. The risk of seizure induction from TMS is relatively small with less than 1% in the general population, and these have been self-limited, occurring during treatment sessions [10]. More commonly, patients may complain of headache (28%) or localized pain (38%), but these rarely cause patients to discontinue treatment and can oftentimes resolve within the first few weeks [10, 165].

22.3.3 tDCS

Transcranial direct current stimulation has some risks, the most significant being affective switches at an incidence of 3.2% [166], as well as burning at site and tingling under the electrodes. The cost of the devices is relatively low, running at approximately $100 USD, and they can be purchased online without a prescription. Studies of tDCS show considerable heterogeneity in study parameters including concomitant medications, psychotherapy, session length (10–35 min), number of sessions (1–20), and electrode size, placement, and current strength [12]. A relatively low risk-benefit ratio is noted in tDCS studies, but these heterogeneities require further sham-controlled RCTs and long-term data before firm conclusions can be drawn.

22.3.4 TNS

Trigeminal nerve stimulation has few associated side effects, the most prominent are headache, irritation at the stimulation site, and mild discomfort during stimulation. Thus far there have been no documented treatment-related affective switches [166]. The TNS studies have limited data for treatment-resistant psychiatric illnesses; almost all data derive from case reports or small open-label studies.

22.3.5 VNS

Vagal nerve stimulation is an invasive procedure, and it runs the risk of complications of surgery (e.g., infection, bleeding), as well as cost estimated at approximately $25,000 USD, and the common adverse effects of hoarseness, dyspnea, nausea, and pain. Like with tDCS, heterogeneity in study design makes systematic adverse effect risk difficult to estimate: lack of sham-controlled data beyond 10 weeks, limited sample size, variations in stimulus parameters, and widely varying durations of follow-up [167].

22.3.6 DBS

A very recent review found serious hardware complications in 11.75% of 8983 patients in 96 studies of DBS for neurologic and psychiatric indications combined [168]. In TRD studies, rates of attempted and completed suicide are high, although this can attributed to the condition as much as to the treatment [61, 64].

Some psychiatric side effects may result directly from stimulation, since they are quickly reversible upon change in stimulation parameters, e.g., hypomania in depression or OCD, anxiety and panic with striatal DBS for OCD, and impulsivity with NAc DBS in OCD [92, 161].

Besides its invasiveness, DBS has other important limitations. Patients eligible for research protocols are severely ill despite multiple therapeutic interventions, and the relatively high risk of suicide and other poor outcomes must be carefully considered. The risk of hopelessness—which must be explicitly and carefully addressed before DBS—is significant. Thus, a healthy treatment alliance and carefully considered long-term therapeutic framework are critical. Finally, DBS is expensive at outset, time intensive, and requires long-term commitment by a multidisciplinary team of experts as well as patients and their families.

22.4 Conclusions and Future Directions

22.4.1 ECT

At present time, ECT is arguably the most recognized, widely available internationally, and studied/reviewed neuromodulation technique. However, there remain several important questions, issues, and limitations to this treatment modality. Efforts continue to improve and minimize the adverse effects of the ECT and its associated anesthesia procedures, in particular to reduce the cognitive adverse events of ECT. Several questions also remain about the long-term impact of ECT treatment, not only about its adverse long-term effects, but also the need for ongoing maintenance of ECT after an acute ECT course, given the known high and often rapid relapse rates after acute ECT treatment discontinuation. Treatment protocols, access to initial index and subsequent maintenance ECT, and exploration of the role of other neuromodulating technologies like rTMS in maintenance after ECT gains should be explored. Finally, although ECT in clinical practice is still often reserved for the most severe and refractory cases, given evidence of its safety vs. effectiveness profile in all phases and for various severity of the illness warrant further research of ECTs use more broadly. In particular, ECT research and clinician education should focus on the possible rapid onset of benefits from ECT treatment that suggest it should be considered earlier in the illness course and for more patients, versus the current standard of ECT being the "last line therapy" in many treatment settings.

22.4.2 rTMS

Over the past decade, significant progress has been made in the use of TMS for the treatment of TR-MDD, and recent clinical trials continue to show efficacy of this modality [11]. Given its relatively low side effect profile [68] and the increasing awareness of its efficacy, more patients are choosing TMS as an alternative to more traditional treatments of depression; however, there is still much to be learned. Although there is a generally accepted range for certain treatment parameters, including stimulus intensity, frequency, and number of pulses delivered, further understanding of treatment protocols is necessary for improving outcomes. Newer TMS machine designs, including deep TMS, are also showing benefit [10]. A few studies referenced above show the potential of TMS as a maintenance treatment in TR-MDD which is important for any treatment modality of chronic illness [71, 74, 75], and recent studies combining neuroimaging are showing the potential power of predicting subgroups that may best respond to TMS [76]. Although the use of TMS in other treatment-resistant psychiatric illness is still considered experimental, it is likely we will see similar progress as was made with TR-MDD. As has been shown in OCD, schizophrenia, and substance use disorders, determining the optimal stimulus location is a significant first step. This combined with multiple treatment parameters leaves us with many variables to optimize. The important consideration is recognizing that TMS is a noninvasive neurostimulation technique that allows us to target specific brain regions believed to contribute to severe, psychiatric illness.

22.4.3 tDCS

There are numerous sham-controlled RCTs examining tDCS in a number of refractory psychiatric conditions, with mixed results. Unfortunately, there is little research involving long-term maintenance of illness after response to treatment or the long-term effects of this modality. The vast majority of studies measure response immediately after treatment, and some measure response after 4 weeks. Few studies have looked at the persistence of improvement over time, though one case study used quarterly booster treatments with tDCS for schizophrenia and maintained a positive response over 1 year [169]. Studies of tDCS are often small and underpowered, and results are inconsistent across studies. Protocols also vary the location of stimulation, number of sessions, and amount of current; optimizing these aspects of tDCS research will be necessary to clarify the potential of this modality for treatment-resistant patients.

22.4.4 TNS

There is a paucity of data regarding maintenance treatments for trigeminal nerve stimulation and long-term safety. There are a limited number of studies utilizing TNS, the majority of which involve about 2–4 weeks of treatment followed by 1-month follow-up. Trigeminal nerve stimulation has shown some promise in the treatment of major depression, PTSD, and psychosis; however, there are limited data and no RCTs in treatment-refractory patients. Given the noninvasive nature of this technique, further investigation is warranted.

22.4.5 VNS

Observational studies suggest that VNS requires long-term and continuous treatment in order to maintain improvement. Naturalistic studies lasting 5 years have shown benefit of VNS over treatment as usual [86]. At this time, optimal protocol for long-term maintenance remains to be determined. There are limitations in the current data, because of the inability to directly compare sham treatment vs. control. Thus far, the data for the sham vs. control groups compare data for use of the device for 10 weeks prior to its activation to data after the device is activated; however, studies suggest that VNS may require more time to show benefit and may be better for maintenance than acute episodes. Given the positive results in highly treatment-resistant populations, this modality should continue to be explored.

22.4.6 DBS

DBS in psychiatry remains in its early stages, and several unanswered questions emerge from the literature. First, the technology, in combination with modern neuroimaging, allows highly precise targeting of neuromodulation with ongoing adjustment. However, in psychiatry there are limitations in specificity among disorders and lack of individual patient utility of neuroimaging findings. In addition, the optimal approach to a sham phase, optimal site of stimulation, and optimal combination(s) of other stimulation variables remain far from established and require ongoing research, with innovative methodologies [170]. Second, a series of targets have been used for several different conditions, and several different targets have shown equal efficacy in the same condition. Future research may require targeting and stimulation parameters focused on symptom domains within conditions [59, 171]. There are reports of safe use of two sets of bilateral DBS electrodes for distinct symptom targets in the same patient [102, 172, 173]. Further, targeting of specific symptom domains *across* categorical diagnoses, as in NIMH Research Domain Criteria (RDoC) approach [174], is likely to be fruitful. Examples include ongoing studies of ventral striatal DBS on reward motivation (NCT01590862) and impulsivity (NCT01506206) in patients with *either* TRD or OCD. Third, while gray matter structures are most often targeted with DBS, some neuroimaging investigations have found adjacent white matter pathways to be the active site of therapeutic stimulation effects [175, 176]. Tractography approaches to identifying optimal projection targets of white matter stimulation are frontier areas of DBS research [100, 177], NCT03244852. Investigators in China are studying the use of electrodes capable of independently stimulating adjacent gray and white matter targets (NCT02590445). Interestingly, in the MFB, retrograde effects in the ventral tegmental area, with secondary effects on projections to forebrain reward centers, may mediate anti-hedonic effects of DBS [99]. Neuroimaging advances will remain an ongoing complement to the intricate merger of psychiatry, neurosurgery, neuropsychology, and neurophysiology that allows DBS to provide hope for some of our most daunting sufferers.

References

1. Beck AT, Ward CH, Mendelson M, Mock J, Erbaugh J. An inventory for measuring depression. Arch Gen Psychiatry. 1961;4:561–71.
2. Blake DD, Weathers FW, Nagy LM, Kaloupek DG, Gusman FD, Charney DS, et al. The development of a clinician-administered PTSD scale. J Trauma Stress. 1995;8:75–90.
3. Guy W, editor. ECDEU assessment manual for psychopharmacology. Rockville: US Department of Heath, Education, and Welfare Public Health Service Alcohol, Drug Abuse, and Mental Health Administration; 1976.
4. Hamilton M. A rating scale for depression. J Neurol Neurosurg Psychiatry. 1960;23:56–62.
5. Montgomery SA, Asberg M. A new depression scale designed to be sensitive to change. Br J Psychiatry. 1979;134:382–9.
6. American Psychiatric Association. Practice guidelines for the treatment of patients with major depressive disorder. 3rd ed. Am J Psychiatry. 2010;167(Suppl):S1–S152.
7. Payne NA, Prudic J. Electroconvulsive therapy: Part I. A perspective on the evolution and current practice of ECT. J Psychiatr Pract. 2009;15:346–68.
8. Baghai TC, Möller H-J. Electroconvulsive therapy and its different indications. Dialogues Clin Neurosci. 2008;10:105–17.
9. Frankel F. The use of ECT therapy in suicidal patients. Am J Psychother. 1984;38:384.
10. Perera T, George MS, Grammer G, Janicak PG, Pascual-Leone A, Wirecki TS. The clinical TMS society consensus review and treatment recommendations for TMS therapy for major depressive disorder. Brain Stimul. 2016;9:336–46.
11. Lefaucheur J-P, André-Obadia N, Antal A, Ayache SS, Baeken C, Benninger DH, et al. Evidence-based guidelines on the therapeutic use of repetitive transcranial magnetic stimulation (rTMS). Clin Neurophysiol. 2014;125:2150–206.
12. Kekic M, Boysen E, Campbell I, Schmidt U. A systematic review of the clinical efficacy of transcranial direct current stimulation (tDCS) in psychiatric disorders. J Psychiatr Res. 2016;74:70–86.
13. Fregni F, Boggio P, Nitsche M, Marcolin M, Rigonatti S, Pascual-Leone A. Treatment of major depression with transcranial direct current stimulation. Bipolar Disord. 2006;8:203–4.
14. Palm U, Keeser D, Hasan A, Kupka MJ, Blautzik J, Sarubin N, et al. Prefrontal transcranial direct current stimulation for treatment of schizophrenia with predominant negative symptoms: a double-blind, sham-controlled proof-of-concept study. Schizophr Bull. 2016;42:1253–61.
15. Cook I, Schrader L, DeGiorgio C, Miller P, Maremont E, Leuchter A. Trigeminal nerve stimulation in major depressive disorder: acute outcomes in an open pilot study. Epilepsy Behav. 2013;28:221–6.
16. Shah A, Carreno F, Frazer A. Therapeutic modalities for treatment resistant depression: focus on vagal nerve stimulation and ketamine. Clin Psychopharmacol Neurosci. 2014;12:83–93.
17. Mu Q, Bohning D, Nahas Z, Walker J, Anderson B, George M. Acute vagus nerve stimulation using different pulse widths produces varying brain effects. Biol Psychiatry. 2004;55:816–25.
18. O'Reardon J, Cristancho P, Peshek A. Vagus nerve stimulation (VNS) and treatment of depression: to the brainstem and beyond. Psychiatry (Edgmont). 2006;3:54–63.
19. Hein E, Nowak M, Kiess O, Biermann T, Bayerlein K, Kornhuber J, et al. Auricular transcutaneous electrical nerve stimulation in depressed patients: a randomized controlled pilot study. J Neural Transm. 2013;120:821–7.
20. Koob GF, Volkow ND. Neurocircuitry of addiction. Neuropsychopharmacology. 2010;35:217–38.
21. Rachid F. Neurostimulation techniques in the treatment of nicotine dependence: a review. Am J Addict. 2016;25:436–51.
22. Amiaz R, Levy D, Vainiger D, Grunhaus L, Zangen A. Repeated high-frequency transcranial magnetic stimulation over the dorsolateral prefrontal cortex reduces cigarette craving and consumption. Addiction. 2009;104:653–60.
23. Meng Z, Liu C, Yu C, et al. Transcranial direct current stimulation of the frontal-parietal-temporal area attenuates smoking behavior. J Psychiatr Res. 2014;54:19–25.
24. Falcone M, Bernardo L, Ashare RL, et al. Transcranial direct current brain stimulation increases ability to resist smoking. Brain Stimul. 2016;9:191–6.
25. Fregni F, Liguori P, Fecteau S, et al. Cortical stimulation of the prefrontal cortex with transcranial direct current stimulation reduces cue provoked smoking craving: a randomized, sham-controlled study. J Clin Psychiatry. 2008;69:32–40.
26. Boggio PS, Liguori P, Sultani N, et al. Cumulative priming effects of cortical stimulation on smoking cue-induced craving. Neurosci Lett. 2009;463:82e6.

27. Fecteau S, Agosta S, Hone-Blanchet A, et al. Modulation of smoking and decision-making behaviors with transcranial direct current stimulation in tobacco smokers: a preliminary study. Drug Alcohol Depend. 2014;140:78–84.
28. Smith RC, Boules S, Mattiuz S, et al. Effects of transcranial direct current stimulation (tDCS) on cognition, symptoms, and smoking in schizophrenia: a randomized controlled study. Schizophr Res. 2015;168:260–6.
29. Xu J, Fregni F, Brody AL, et al. Transcranial direct current stimulation reduces negative affect but not cigarette craving in overnight abstinent smokers. Front Psychol. 2013; https://doi.org/10.3389/fpsyt.2013.00112.
30. Hayashi T, Ko JH, Strafella AP, Dagher A. Dorsolateral prefrontal and orbitofrontal cortex interactions during self-control of cigarette craving. Proc Natl Acad Sci U S A. 2013;110:4422–7.
31. Boggio PS, Sultani N, Fecteau S, Merabet L, Mecca T, Pascual-Leone A, et al. Prefrontal cortex modulation using transcranial DC stimulation reduces alcohol craving: a double-blind, sham controlled study. Drug Alcohol Depend. 2008;92:55–60.
32. den Uyl T, Gladwin T, Wiers R. Transcranial direct current stimulation, implicit alcohol associations and craving. Biol Psychiatry. 2015;105:37–42.
33. Batista E, Klauss J, Fregni F, Nitsche M, Nakamura-Palacios E. A randomized placebo-controlled trial of targeted prefrontal cortex modulation with bilateral tDCS in patients with crack cocaine dependence. Int J Neuropsychopharmacol. 2015; https://doi.org/10.1093/ijnp/pyv066.
34. Boggio P, Zaghi S, Villani A, Frecteau S, Pascal-Leone A, Fregni F. Modulation of risk-taking in marijuana users by transcranial direct current stimulation of the dorsolateral prefrontal cortex. Drug Alcohol Depend. 2010;112:220–5.
35. da Silva MC, Conti CL, Klauss J, et al. Behavioral effects of transcranial direct current stimulation (tDCS) induced dorsolateral prefrontal cortex plasticity in alcohol dependence. J Physiol-Paris. 2013;107:493–502.
36. Shahbabaie A, Golesokhi M, Zamanian B, Ebrahimpoor M, Keshvari F, Nejati V, et al. State dependent effect of transcranial direct current stimulation (tDCS) on methamphetamine craving. Int J Neuropsychopharmacol. 2014;10:1591–8.
37. Kuhn J, Lenartz D, Huff W, Lee SH, Koulousakis A, Klosterkoetter J, et al. Remission of alcohol dependency following deep brain stimulation of the nucleus accumbens: valuable therapeutic implications? J Neurol Neurosurg Psychiatry. 2007;78:1152–3.
38. Müller UJ, Sturm V, Voges J, Heinze HJ, Galazky I, Büntjen L, et al. Nucleus accumbens deep brain stimulation for alcohol addiction – safety and clinical long-term results of a pilot trial. Pharmacopsychiatry. 2016;49:170–3.
39. Kuhn J, Möller M, Treppmann JF, Bartsch C, Lenartz D, Gruendler TO, et al. Deep brain stimulation of the nucleus accumbens and its usefulness in severe opioid addiction. Mol Psychiatry. 2014;19:145–6.
40. Valencia-Alfonso CE, Luigjes J, Smolders R, Cohen MX, Levar N, Mazaheri A, et al. Effective deep brain stimulation in heroin addiction: a case report with complementary intracranial electroencephalogram. Biol Psychiatry. 2012;71:e35–7.
41. Zhou H, Xu J, Jiang J. Deep brain stimulation of nucleus accumbens on heroin-seeking behaviors: a case report. Biol Psychiatry. 2011;69:e41–2.
42. Gonçalves-Ferreira A, do Couto FS, Rainha Campos A, Lucas Neto LP, Gonçalves-Ferreira D, Teixeira J. Deep brain stimulation for refractory cocaine dependence. Biol Psychiatry. 2016;79:e87–9.
43. Schoeyen HK, Kessler U, Andreassen OA, Auestad BH, Bergsholm P, Malt UF, et al. Treatment-resistant bipolar depression: a randomized controlled trial of electroconvulsive therapy versus algorithm-based pharmacological treatment. Am J Psychiatry. 2015;172(1):41–51.
44. Perugi G, Medda P, Toni C, Mariani MG, Socci C, Mauri M. The role of electroconvulsive therapy (ECT) in bipolar disorder: effectiveness in 522 patients with bipolar depression, mixed-state, mania and catatonic features. Curr Neuropharmacol. 2017;15:359–71.
45. Grisaru N, Chudakov B, Yaroslavsky Y, Belmaker RH. Transcranial magnetic stimulation in mania: a controlled study. Am J Psychiatry. 1998;155:1608–10.
46. Kaptsan A, Yaroslavsky Y, Applebaum J, Belmaker RH, Grisaru N. Right prefrontal TMS versus sham treatment of mania: a controlled study. Bipolar Disord. 2003;5:36–9.
47. Michael N, Erfurth A. Treatment of bipolar mania with right prefrontal rapid transcranial magnetic stimulation. J Affect Disord. 2004;78:253–7.
48. Praharaj SK, Ram D, Arora M. Efficacy of high frequency (rapid) suprathreshold repetitive transcranial magnetic stimulation of right prefrontal cortex in bipolar mania: a randomized sham controlled study. J Affect Disord. 2009;117:146–50.
49. Dolberg OT, Dannon PN, Schreiber S, Grunhaus L. Transcranial magnetic stimulation in patients with bipolar depression: a double blind, controlled study. Bipolar Disord. 2002;4(Suppl 1):94–5.
50. Nahas Z, Kozel FA, Li X, Anderson B, George MS. Left prefrontal transcranial magnetic stimulation (TMS) treatment of depression in bipolar affective disorder: a pilot study of acute safety and efficacy. Bipolar Disord. 2003;5:40–7.
51. Fitzgerald PB, Hoy KE, Elliot D, McQueen S, Wambeek LE, Daskalakis ZJ. A negative double-blind controlled trial of sequential bilateral rTMS in the treatment of bipolar depression. J Affect Disord. 2016;198:158–62.
52. Carnell BL, Clarke P, Gill S, Galletly CA. How effective is repetitive transcranial magnetic stimulation for bipolar depression? J Affect Disord. 2017;209:270–2.

53. Dondé C, Amad A, Nieto I, Brunoni AR, Neufeld NH, Bellivier F, et al. Transcranial direct-current stimulation (tDCS) for bipolar depression: a systematic review and meta-analysis. Prog Neuro-Psychopharmacol Biol Psychiatry. 2017; 78:123–31.
54. Schestatsky P, Janovik N, Lobato MI, Belmonte-de-Abreu P, Schestatsky S, Shiozawa P, et al. Rapid therapeutic response to anodal tDCS of right dorsolateral prefrontal cortex in acute mania. Brain Stimul. 2013;6:701–3.
55. Nierenberg A, Alpert J, Gardner-Schuster S, Mischoulon D. Vagus nerve stimulation: 2 year outcomes for bipolar vs. unipolar treatment resistant depression. Biol Psychiatry. 2008;64:455–60.
56. Pardo JV. Adjunctive vagus nerve stimulation for treatment-resistant bipolar disorder: managing device failure or the end of battery life. BMJ Case Rep. 2016;2016:bcr2015213949.
57. Marangell LB, Suppes T, Zboyan HA, Prashad SJ, Fischer G, Snow D, et al. A 1-year pilot study of vagus nerve stimulation in treatment-resistant rapid-cycling bipolar disorder. J Clin Psychiatry. 2008;69:183–9.
58. Gippert SM, Switala C, Bewernick BH, Kayser S, Brauer A, Coenen VA, et al. Deep brain stimulation for bipolar disorder—review and outlook. CNS Spectr. 2017;22:254–7.
59. Holzheimer PE, Kelley ME, Gross RE, et al. Subcallosal cingulate deep brain stimulation for treatment-resistant unipolar and bipolar depression. Arch Gen Psychiatry. 2012;69(2):150–8.
60. Malone DA Jr, Dougherty DD, Rezai AR, et al. Deep brain stimulation of the ventral capsule/ventral striatum for treatment resistant depression. Biol Psychiatry. 2009;65(4):267–75.
61. Schlaepfer TE, Bewernick BH, Kayser S, Mädler B, Coenen VA. Rapid effects of deep brain stimulation for treatment-resistant major depression. Biol Psychiatry. 2013;73(12):1204–12.
62. Fink M, Kellner CH, McCall WV. The role of ECT in suicide prevention. J ECT. 2014;30:5–9.
63. Folkerts HW, Michael N, Tölle R, Schonauer K, Mücke S, Schulze-Mönking H. Electroconvulsive therapy vs. paroxetine in treatment-resistant depression—a randomized study. Acta Psychiatr Scand. 1997;96:334–42.
64. Song GM, Tian X, Shuai T, Yi LJ, Zeng Z, Liu S, et al. Treatment of adults with treatment-resistant depression: electroconvulsive therapy plus antidepressant or electroconvulsive therapy alone? Evidence from an indirect comparison meta-analysis. Medicine. 2015;94(26):e1052.
65. Kellner CH, Fink M, Knapp R, Petrides G, Husain M, Rummans T, et al. Relief of expressed suicidal intent by ECT: a consortium for research in ECT study. Am J Psychiatry. 2005;162:977–82.
66. Patel M, Patel S, Hardy DW, Benzies BJ, Tare V. Should electroconvulsive therapy be an early consideration for suicidal patients? J ECT. 2006;22:113–5.
67. Keshtkar M, Ghanizadeh A, Firoozabadi A. Repetitive transcranial magnetic stimulation versus electroconvulsive therapy for the treatment of major depressive disorder, a randomized controlled clinical trial. J ECT. 2011;27:310–4.
68. O'Reardon JP, Solvason HB, Janicak PG, Sampson S, Isenberg KE, Nahas Z, et al. Efficacy and safety of transcranial magnetic stimulation in the acute treatment of major depression: a multisite randomized controlled trial. Biol Psychiatry. 2007;62:1208–16.
69. George MS, Lisanby SH, Avery D, McDonald WM, Durkalski V, Pavlicova M, et al. Daily left prefrontal transcranial magnetic stimulation therapy for major depressive disorder: a sham-controlled randomized trial. Arch Gen Psychiatry. 2010;67:507–16.
70. Gershon AA, Dannon PN, Grunhaus L. Transcranial magnetic stimulation in the treatment of depression. Am J Psychiatry. 2003;160:835–45.
71. Mantovani A, Pavlicova M, Avery D, Nahas Z, McDonald WM, Wajdik CD, et al. Long-term efficacy of repeated daily prefrontal transcranial magnetic stimulation (TMS) in treatment-resistant depression. Depress Anxiety. 2012;29:883–90.
72. Janicak PG, Nahas Z, Lisanby SH, Solvason HB, Sampson SM, McDonald WM, et al. Durability of clinical benefit with transcranial magnetic stimulation (TMS) in the treatment of pharmacoresistant major depression: assessment of relapse during a 6-month, multisite, open-label study. Brain Stimul. 2010;3:187–99.
73. Fitzgerald PB, Grace N, Hoy KE, Bailey M, Daskalakis ZJ. An open label trial of clustered maintenance rTMS for patients with refractory depression. Brain Stimul. 2013;6:292–7.
74. Richieri R, Guedj E, Michel P, Loundou A, Auquier P, Lançon C, et al. Maintenance transcranial magnetic stimulation reduces depression relapse: a propensity-adjusted analysis. J Affect Disord. 2013;151:129–35.
75. Philip NS, Dunner DL, Dowd SM, Aaronson ST, Brock DG, Carpenter LL, et al. Can medication free, treatment-resistant, depressed patients who initially respond to TMS be maintained off medications? A prospective, 12-month multisite randomized pilot study. Brain Stimul. 2016;9:251–7.
76. Drysdale AT, Grosenick L, Downar J, Dunlop K, Mansouri F, Meng Y, et al. Resting-state connectivity biomarkers define neurophysiological subtypes of depression. Nat Med. 2016;23:28–38.
77. Palm U, Hasan A, Strube W, Padberg F. tDCS for the treatment of depression: a comprehensive review. Eur Arch Psychiatry Clin Neurosci. 2016;266:681–94.
78. Ferrucci R, Bortolomasi M, Vergari M, Tadini L, Salvoro B, Giacopuzzi M, et al. Transcranial direct current stimulation in severe, drug-resistant major depression. J Affect Disord. 2009;118(1–3):215–9.
79. Palm U, Schiller C, Fintescu Z, Obermeier M, Keeser D, Reisinger E, et al. Transcranial direct current stimulation in treatment resistant depression: a randomized double-blind, placebo-controlled study. Brain Stimul. 2012;5(3):242–51.

80. Blumberger DM, Tran LC, Fitzgerald PB, Hoy KE, Daskalakis ZJ. A randomized double-blind sham-controlled study of transcranial direct current stimulation for treatment-resistant major depression. Front Psychiatry. 2012;3:74.
81. Bennabi D, Nicolier M, Monnin J, Tio G, Pazart L, Vandel P, et al. Pilot study of feasibility of the effect of treatment with tDCS in patients suffering from treatment-resistant depression treated with escitalopram. Clin Neurophysiol. 2015; 126(6):1185–9.
82. Cristancho P, Cristancho MA, Baltuch GH, Thase ME, O'Reardon JP. Effectiveness and safety of vagus nerve stimulation for severe treatment-resistant major depression in clinical practice after FDA approval: outcomes at 1 year. J Clin Psychiatry. 2011;72:1376–82.
83. Christmas D, Steele JD, Tolomeo S, Eljamel MS, Matthews K. Vagus nerve stimulation for chronic major depressive disorder: 12-month outcomes in highly treatment-refractory patients. J Affect Disord. 2013;150:1221–5.
84. Eljamel S. Vagus nerve stimulation for major depressive episodes. Prog Neurol Surg. 2015;29:53–63.
85. George MS, Rush AJ, Marangell LB, Sackeim HA, Brannan SK, Davis SM, et al. A one-year comparison of vagus nerve stimulation with treatment as usual for treatment-resistant depression. Biol Psychiatry. 2005;58:364–73.
86. Aaronson ST, Sears P, Ruvuna F, Bunker M, Conway CR, Dougherty DD, et al. A 5-year observational study of patients with treatment-resistant depression treated with vagus nerve stimulation or treatment as usual: comparison of response, remission, and suicidality. Am J Psychiatry. 2017;174:640–8.
87. Fekadu A, Wooderson SC, Markopoulo K, Donaldson C, Papadopoulos A, Cleare AJ. What happens to patients with treatment-resistant depression? A systematic review of medium to long term outcome studies. J Affect Disord. 2009;116:4–11.
88. Mayberg HS, Lozano AM, Voon V, McNeely HE, Seminowicz D, Hamani C, et al. Deep brain stimulation for treatment-resistant depression. Neuron. 2005;45:651–60.
89. Kennedy SH, Giacobbe P, Rizvi SJ, Placenza FM, Nishikawa Y, Mayberg HS, et al. Deep brain stimulation for treatment-resistant depression: follow-up after 3 to 6 years. Am J Psychiatry. 2011;168:502–10.
90. Berlim MT, McGirr A, Van den Eynde F, Fleck MP, Giacobbe P. Effectiveness and acceptability of deep brain stimulation (DBS) of the subgenual cingulate cortex for treatment-resistant depression: a systematic review and exploratory meta-analysis. J Affect Disord. 2014;159:31–8.
91. Dunner DL, Rush AJ, Russell JM, Burke M, Woodard S, Wingard P, et al. Prospective, long-term, multicenter study of the naturalistic outcomes of patients with treatment-resistant depression. J Clin Psychiatry. 2006;67:688–95.
92. Graat I, Figee M, Denys D. The application of deep brain stimulation in the treatment of psychiatric disorders. Int Rev Psychiatry. 2017;29:178–90.
93. Saleh C, Hasler G. Deep brain stimulation for psychiatric disorders: is there an impact on social functioning? Surg Neurol Int. 2017;8:134.
94. Holzheimer PE, Kelley ME, Gross RE, Filkowski MM, Garlow SJ, Barrocas A, et al. Subcallosal cingulate deep brain stimulation for treatment-resistant unipolar and bipolar depression. Arch Gen Psychiatry. 2012;69:150–8.
95. Puigdemont D, Portella M, Pérez-Egea R, Molet J, Gironell A, de Diego-Adeliño J, et al. A randomized double-blind crossover trial of deep brain stimulation of the subcallosal cingulate gyrus in patients with treatment-resistant depression: a pilot study of relapse prevention. J Psychiatry Neurosci. 2015;40:224–31.
96. Morishita T, Fayad SM, Higuchi MA, Nestor KA, Foote KD. Deep brain stimulation for treatment-resistant depression: systematic review of clinical outcomes. Neurotherapeutics. 2014;11:475–84.
97. Dougherty DD, Rezai AR, Carpenter LL, et al. A randomized sham-controlled trial of deep brain stimulation of the ventral capsule/ventral striatum for chronic treatment-resistant depression. Biol Psychiatry. 2015;78:240–8.
98. Bergfeld IO, Mantione M, Hoogendoorn ML, Ruhé HG, Notten P, van Laarhoven J, et al. Deep brain stimulation of the ventral anterior limb of the internal capsule for treatment-resistant depression: a randomized clinical trial. JAMA Psychiat. 2016;73:456–64.
99. Schlaepfer TE, Bewernick BH, Kayser S, Hurlemann R, Coenen VA. Deep brain stimulation of the human reward system for major depression—rationale, outcomes and outlook. Neuropsychopharmacology. 2014;39:1303–14.
100. Bewernick BH, Kayser S, Gippert SM, Switala C, Coenen VA, Schlaepfer TE. Deep brain stimulation to the medial forebrain bundle for depression- long-term outcomes and a novel data analysis strategy. Brain Stimul. 2017;10:664–71.
101. Fenoy AJ, Schulz P, Selvaraj S, Burrows C, Spiker D, Cao B, et al. Deep brain stimulation of the medial forebrain bundle: distinctive responses in resistant depression. J Affect Disord. 2016;203:143–51.
102. Williams NR, Short EB, Hopkins T, Bentzley BS, Sahlem GL, Pannu J, et al. Five-year follow-up of bilateral epidural prefrontal cortical stimulation for treatment-resistant depression. Brain Stimul. 2016;9:897–904.
103. Kubu CS, Brelje T, Butters MA, Deckersbach T, Malloy P, Moberg P, et al. Cognitive outcome after ventral capsule/ventral striatum stimulation for treatment-resistant major depression. J Neurol Neurosurg Psychiatry. 2017;88:262–5.
104. Bergfeld IO, Mantione M, Hoogendoorn MLC, Ruhe HG, Horst F, Notten P, et al. Impact of deep

brain stimulation of the ventral anterior limb of the internal capsule on cognition in depression. Psychol Med. 2017;47:1647–58.
105. Fontenelle LF, Coutinho ES, Lins-Martins NM, Fitzgerald PB, Fujiwara H, Yücel M. Electroconvulsive therapy for obsessive-compulsive disorder: a systematic review. J Clin Psychiatry. 2015;76:949–57.
106. Greenberg BD, George MS, Martin JD, Benjamin J, Schlaepfer TE, Altemus M, et al. Effect of prefrontal repetitive transcranial magnetic stimulation in obsessive-compulsive disorder: a preliminary study. Am J Psychiatry. 1997;154:867–9.
107. Mantovani A, Lisanby SH, Pieraccini F, Ulivelli M, Castrogiovanni P, Rossi S. Repetitive transcranial magnetic stimulation (rTMS) in the treatment of obsessive-compulsive disorder (OCD) and Tourette's syndrome (TS). Int J Neuropsychopharmacol. 2006;9:95–100.
108. Jaafari N, Rachid F, Rotge J-Y, Polosan M, El-Hage W, Belin D, et al. Safety and efficacy of repetitive transcranial magnetic stimulation in the treatment of obsessive-compulsive disorder: a review. World J Biol Psychiatry. 2012;13:164–77.
109. Berlim MT, Neufeld NH, Van den Eynde F. Repetitive transcranial magnetic stimulation (rTMS) for obsessive-compulsive disorder (OCD): an exploratory meta-analysis of randomized and sham-controlled trials. J Psychiatr Res. 2013;47:999–1006.
110. Trevizol AP, Shiozawa P, Cook IA, Sato IA, Kaku CB, Guimarães FB, et al. Transcranial magnetic stimulation for obsessive-compulsive disorder: an updated systematic review and meta-analysis. J ECT. 2016;32:262–6.
111. George MS, Ward HE, Ninan PT, Pollack M, Nahas Z, Anderson B, et al. A pilot study of vagus nerve stimulation (VNS) for treatment-resistant anxiety disorders. Brain Stimul. 2008;1:112–21.
112. Silva RM, Brunoni AR, Miguel EC, Shavitt RG. Transcranial direct current stimulation for treatment-resistant obsessive-compulsive disorder: report on two cases and proposal for a randomized, sham-controlled trial. Sao Paulo Med J. 2016;134:446–50.
113. Palm U, Leitner B, Kirsch B, Behler N, Kumpf U, Wulf L, et al. Prefrontal tDCS and sertraline in obsessive compulsive disorder: a case report and review of the literature. Neurocase. 2017;23:173–7.
114. Narayanaswamy JC, Jose D, Chhabra H, Agarwal SM, Shrinivasa B, Hegde A, et al. Successful application of add-on transcranial direct current stimulation (tDCS) for treatment of SSRI resistant OCD. Brain Stimul. 2015;8:655–7.
115. Mondino M, Haesebaert F, Poulet E, Saoud M, Brunelin J. Efficacy of cathodal transcranial direct current stimulation over the left orbitofrontal cortex in a patient with treatment-resistant obsessive-compulsive disorder. J ECT. 2015;31:271–2.
116. Bation R, Poulet E, Haesebaert F, Saoud M, Brunelin J. Transcranial direct current stimulation in treatment-resistant obsessive-compulsive disorder: an open-label pilot study. Prog Neuro-Psychopharmacol Biol Psychiatry. 2016;4(65):153–7.
117. D'Urso G, Brunoni AR, Mazzaferro MP, Anastasia A, de Bartolomeis A, Mantovani A. Transcranial direct current stimulation for obsessive-compulsive disorder: a randomized, controlled, partial crossover trial. Depress Anxiety. 2016;33:1132–40.
118. Alonso P, Cuadras D, Gabriëls L, Denys D, Goodman W, Greenberg BD, et al. Deep brain stimulation for obsessive-compulsive disorder: a meta-analysis of treatment outcome and predictors of response. PLoS One. 2015;10:e0133591.
119. Huff W, Lenartz D, Schormann M, Lee SH, Kuhn J, Koulousakis A, et al. Unilateral deep brain stimulation of the nucleus accumbens in patients with treatment-resistant obsessive-compulsive disorder: outcomes after one year. Clin Neurol Neurosurg. 2010;112:137–43.
120. Okun MS, Mann G, Foote KD, Shapira NA, Bowers D, Springer U, et al. Deep brain stimulation in the internal capsule and nucleus accumbens region: responses observed during active and sham programming. J Neurol Neurosurg Psychiatry. 2007;78:310–4.
121. Goodman WK, Foote KD, Greenberg BD, Ricciuti N, Bauer R, Ward H, et al. Deep brain stimulation for intractable obsessive compulsive disorder: pilot study using a blinded, staggered-onset design. Biol Psychiatry. 2010;67:535–42.
122. Fayad SM, Guzick AG, Reid AM, Mason DM, Bertone A, Foote KD, et al. Six-nine year follow-up of deep brain stimulation for obsessive-compulsive disorder. PLoS One. 2016;11:e0167875.
123. Islam L, Franzini A, Messina G, Scarone S, Gambini O. Deep brain stimulation of the nucleus accumbens and bed nucleus of stria terminalis for obsessive-compulsive disorder: a case series. World Neurosurg. 2015;83:657–63.
124. Coenen VA, Schlaepfer TE, Goll P, Reinacher PC, Voderholzer U, Tebartz van Elst L, et al. The medial forebrain bundle as a target for deep brain stimulation for obsessive-compulsive disorder. CNS Spectr. 2017;22:282–9.
125. Maarouf M, Neudorfer C, El Majdoub F, Lenartz D, Kuhn J, Sturm V. Deep brain stimulation of medial dorsal and ventral anterior nucleus of the thalamus in OCD: a retrospective case series. PLoS One. 2016;11:e0160750.
126. Trevizol AP, Shiozawa P, Sato IA, Calfat EL, Alberto RL, Cook IA, et al. Trigeminal nerve stimulation (TNS) for generalized anxiety disorder: a case study. Brain Stimul. 2015;8:659–60.
127. Karsen EF, Watts BV, Holtzheimer PE. Review of the effectiveness of transcranial magnetic stimulation for post-traumatic stress disorder. Brain Stimul. 2014;7:151–7.

128. Clark C, Cole J, Winter C, Williams K, Grammer G. A review of transcranial magnetic stimulation as a treatment for post-traumatic stress disorder. Curr Psychiatry Rep. 2015;17:83.
129. Philip NS, Barredo J, van't Wout-Frank M, Tyrka AR, Price LH, Carpenter LL. Network mechanisms of clinical response to transcranial magnetic stimulation in posttraumatic stress disorder and major depressive disorder. Biol Psychiatry. 2018;83:263–72.
130. Berlim MT, Van Den Eynde F. Repetitive transcranial magnetic stimulation over the dorsolateral prefrontal cortex for treating posttraumatic stress disorder: an exploratory meta-analysis of randomized, double-blind and sham-controlled trials. Can J Psychiatr. 2014;59:487–96.
131. Margoob MA, Ali Z, Andrade C. Efficacy of ECT in chronic, severe, antidepressant-and CBT-refractory PTSD: an open, prospective study. Brain Stimul. 2010;3:28–35.
132. Cook IA, Abrams M, Leuchter AF. Trigeminal nerve stimulation for comorbid posttraumatic stress disorder and major depressive disorder. Neuromodulation. 2016;19:299–305.
133. Van't Wout M, Longo SM, Reddy MK, Philip NS, Bowker MT, Greenberg BD. Transcranial direct current stimulation may modulate extinction memory in posttraumatic stress disorder. Brain Behav. 2017;7(5):e00681.
134. Langevin JP, Koek RJ, Schwartz HN, Chen JW, Sultzer DL, Mandelkern MA, et al. Deep brain stimulation of the basolateral amygdala for treatment-refractory posttraumatic stress disorder. Biol Psychiatry. 2016;79:e82–4.
135. Langevin JP, Chen JW, Koek RJ, Sultzer DL, Mandelkern MA, Schwartz HN, et al. Deep brain stimulation of the basolateral amygdala: targeting technique and electrodiagnostic findings. Brain Sci. 2016;6(3):28.
136. Lally J, Tully J, Robertson D, Stubbs B, Goghran F, MacCabe JH. Augmentation of clozapine with electroconvulsive therapy in treatment resistant schizophrenia: a systematic review and meta-analysis. Schizophr Res. 2016;171:215–24.
137. Charlson F, Siskind D, Doi SAR, McCallum E, Broome A, Lie DC. ECT efficacy and treatment course: a systematic review and meta-analysis of twice vs thrice weekly schedules. J Affect Disord. 2012;138:1–8.
138. Waite J, Easton A. The ECT handbook. 3rd ed. The Royal College of Psychiatrists' Special Committee on ECT. London: Royal College of Psychiatrists; 2013.
139. Unal A, Altindag A, Demir B, Aksoy I. The use of lorazepam and electroconvulsive therapy in the treatment of catatonia: treatment characteristics and outcomes in 60 patients. J ECT. 2017;33:290–3.
140. Bulteau S, Laforgue EJ, Chimot L, Dumont R, Loutrel O, Etcheverrigaray F, et al. Management of emergency electroconvulsive therapy in the intensive care unit for lifethreatening psychiatric conditions: a case series. J ECT. 2018;34:55–9.
141. Buchanan RW, Kreyenbuhl J, Kelly DL, Noel JM, Boggs DL, Fischer BA, et al. The 2009 schizophrenia PORT psychopharmacological treatment recommendations and summary statements. Schizophr Bull. 2010;36:71–93.
142. Hoffman RE, Hawkins KA, Gueorguieva R, Boutros NN, Rachid F, Carroll K, et al. Transcranial magnetic stimulation of left temporoparietal cortex and medication-resistant auditory hallucinations. Arch Gen Psychiatry. 2003;60:49–56.
143. Freitas C, Fregni F, Pascual-Leone A. Meta-analysis of the effects of repetitive transcranial magnetic stimulation (rTMS) on negative and positive symptoms in schizophrenia. Schizophr Res. 2009;108:11–24.
144. Slotema CW, Blom JD, van Lutterveld R, Hoek HW, Sommer IEC. Review of the efficacy of transcranial magnetic stimulation for auditory verbal hallucinations. Biol Psychiatry. 2014;76:101–10.
145. Hasan A, Wolff-Menzler C, Pfeiffer S, Falkai P, Weidinger E, Jobst A, et al. Transcutaneous noninvasive vagus nerve stimulation (tVNS) in the treatment of schizophrenia: a bicentric randomized controlled pilot study. Eur Arch Psychiatr Clin Neurosci. 2015;265:589–600.
146. Lefaucheur J-P, Antal A, Ayache SS, Benninger DH, Brunelin J, Cogiamanian F, et al. Evidence-based guidelines on the therapeutic use of transcranial direct current stimulation (tDCS). Clin Neurophysiol. 2017;128:56–92.
147. Brunelin J, Mondino M, Gassab L, Haesebaert F, Gaha L, Suaud-Chagny M-F, et al. Examining transcranial direct-current stimulation (tDCS) as a treatment for hallucinations in schizophrenia. Am J Psychiatry. 2012;169:719–24.
148. Mondino M, Haesebaert F, Poulet E, Suaud-Chagny M-F, Brunelin J. Fronto-temporal transcranial Direct Current Stimulation (tDCS) reduces source-monitoring deficits and auditory hallucinations in patients with schizophrenia. Schizophr Res. 2015;161:515–6.
149. Mondino M, Poulet E, Suaud-Chagny M-F, Brunelin J. Anodal tDCS targeting the left temporo-parietal junction disrupts verbal reality-monitoring. Neuropsychologia. 2016;89:478–84.
150. Fitzgerald PB, McQueen S, Daskalakis ZJ, Hoy KE. A negative pilot study of daily bimodal transcranial direct current stimulation in schizophrenia. Brain Stimul. 2014;7:813–6.
151. Fröhlich F, Burrello TN, Mellin JM, Cordle AL, Lustenberger CM, Gilmore JH, et al. Exploratory study of once-daily transcranial direct current stimulation (tDCS) as a treatment for auditory hallucinations in schizophrenia. Eur Psychiatry. 2016;33:54–60.
152. Gomes JS, Akiba H, Dias ÁM, Soares A, Taiar I, Gadelha AA, et al. Trigeminal nerve stimulation for olfactory hallucinations in schizophrenia: case study. Schizophr Res. 2016;176:203–5.

153. Heath RG, Russell MD, Monroe R, Mickle WA. Stimulation of the amygdaloid nucleus in a schizophrenic patient. Am J Psychiatry. 1955;111:862–3.
154. O'Neal CM, Baker CM, Glenn CA, Connor AK, Sughrue ME, Robert G. Heath: a controversial figure in the history of deep brain stimulation. Neurosurg Focus. 2017; https://doi.org/10.3171/2017.6.FOCUS17252.
155. Salgado-Lopez L, Pomarol-Clotet E, Roldán A, Rodríguez R, Molet J, Sarró S, et al. Letter to the editor: deep brain stimulation for schizophrenia. J Neurosurg. 2016;125:229–30.
156. Shi C, Yu X, Cheung EFC, Shum DHK, Chan RCK. Revisiting the therapeutic effect of rTMS on negative symptoms in schizophrenia: a meta-analysis. Psychiatry Res. 2014;215:505–13.
157. Wobrock T, Guse B, Cordes J, Wölwer W, Winterer G, Gaebel W, et al. Left prefrontal high-frequency repetitive transcranial magnetic stimulation for the treatment of schizophrenia with predominant negative symptoms: a sham-controlled, randomized multicenter trial. Biol Psychiatry. 2015;77:979–88.
158. Li Z, Yin M, Lyu X-L, Zhang L-L, Du X-D, GC-L H. Delayed effect of repetitive transcranial magnetic stimulation (rTMS) on negative symptoms of schizophrenia: findings from a randomized controlled trial. Psychiatry Res. 2016;240:333–5.
159. Gomes J, Shiozawa P, Dias A, Akiba H, Tevizol A, Bikson M, et al. Left dorsolateral prefrontal cortex anodal tDCS effects on negative symptoms in schizophrenia. Brain Stimul. 2015;8:974–91.
160. Shiozawa P, Fasanella NA, Marinho C, Taiar I, Soares A, Calderoni DM, et al. Trigeminal nerve stimulation (TNS) for treating negative symptoms in schizophrenia: a case study. Schizophr Res. 2017;184:139–40.
161. Buhmann C, Huckhagel T, Engel K, Gulberti A, Hidding U, Poetter-Nerger M, et al. Adverse events in deep brain stimulation: a retrospective long-term analysis of neurological, psychiatric and other occurrences. PLoS One. 2017;12:e0178984.
162. Semkovska M, McLoughlin DM. Objective cognitive performance associated with electroconvulsive therapy for depression. A systematic review and meta-analysis. Biol Psychiatry. 2010;68:568–77.
163. Fraser LM, O'Carroll RE, Ebmeier KP. The effect of electroconvulsive therapy on autobiographical memory: a systematic review. J ECT. 2008;24:10–7.
164. Chang AD, Vaidya PV, Retzbach EP, Chung SJ, Kim U, Baselice K, et al. Narp mediates antidepressant-like effects of electroconvulsive seizures. Neuropsychopharmacology. 2018;43:1088–98.
165. Rossi S, Hallett M, Rossini PM, Pascual-Leone A, Safety of TMS Consensus Group. Safety, ethical considerations, and application guidelines for the use of transcranial magnetic stimulation in clinical practice and research. Clin Neurophysiol. 2009;120:2008–39.
166. Shiozawa P, Cordeiro Q, Cho HJ, Trevizol AP, Brietzke E. A critical review of trials of transcranial direct current stimulation and trigeminal nerve stimulation for depression: the issue of treatment-emergent mania. Trends Psychiatry Psychother. 2017;39:48–53.
167. Cimpianu C, Strube W, Falkai P, Palm U, Hasan A. Vagus nerve stimulation in psychiatry: a systematic review of the available evidence. J Neural Transm. 2017;124:145–58.
168. Jitkritsadakul O, Bhidayasiri R, Suneil K, Kalia SK, Hodaie M, Lozano AM, et al. Systematic review of hardware-related complications of deep brain stimulation: do new indications pose an increased risk? Brain Stim. 2017;10:967–76.
169. Shivakumar V, Chhabra H, Subbanna M, Agarwal S, Bose A, Kalmady S, et al. Effect of tDCS on auditory hallucinations in schizophrenia: influence of catechol-O-methyltransferase (COMT) Val158Met polymorphism. Asian J Psychiatr. 2015;16:75–7.
170. Fins JJ, Kubu CS, Mayberg HS, Merkel R, Nuttin B, Schlaepfer TE. Being open minded about neuromodulation trials: finding success in our "failures". Brain Stimul. 2017;10:181–6.
171. Volpini M, Giacobbe P, Cosgrove GC, Levitt A, Lozano AM, Lipsman N. The history and future of ablative neurosurgery for major depressive disorder. Stereotact Funct Neurosurg. 2017;95:216–28.
172. Israel M, Steiger H, Kolivakis T, McGregor L, Sadikot AF. Deep brain stimulation in the subgenual cingulate cortex for an intractable eating disorder. Biol Psychiatry. 2010;67:e53–4.
173. Blomstedt P, Naesström M, Bodlund O. Deep brain stimulation in the bed nucleus of the stria terminalis and medial forebrain bundle in a patient with major depressive disorder and anorexia nervosa. Clin Case Rep. 2017;5:679–84.
174. Kozak MJ, Cuthbert BN. The NIMH research domain criteria initiative: background, issues, and pragmatics. Psychophysiology. 2016;53:286–97.
175. van den Munckhof P, Bosch DA, Mantione MH, Figee M, Denys DA, Schuurman PR. Active stimulation site of nucleus accumbens deep brain stimulation in obsessive-compulsive disorder is localized in the ventral internal capsule. Acta Neurochir Suppl. 2013;117:53–9.
176. Riva-Posse P, Choi KS, Holtzheimer PE, McIntyre CC, Gross RE, Chaturvedi A, et al. Defining critical white matter pathways mediating successful subcallosal cingulate deep brain stimulation for treatment-resistant depression. Biol Psychiatry. 2014;76:963–9.
177. Riva-Posse P, Choi KS, Holtzheimer PE, Crowell AL, Garlow SJ, Rajendra JK, et al. A connectomic approach for subcallosal cingulate deep brain stimulation surgery: prospective targeting in treatment-resistant depression. Mol Psychiatry. 2018;23:843–9.

When Clozapine Fails: Augmentation Strategies in the Management of Clozapine-Resistant Schizophrenia

23

Domenico De Berardis, Michele Fornaro, Annalisa Anastasia, Federica Vellante, Alessandro Valchera, Marilde Cavuto, Giampaolo Perna, Marco Di Nicola, Gianluca Serafini, Alessandro Carano, Maurizio Pompili, Laura Orsolini, Carmine Tomasetti, Gabriella Di Emidio, Giovanni Martinotti, and Massimo Di Giannantonio

D. De Berardis (✉)
National Health Service, Department of Mental Health, Psychiatric Service of Diagnosis and Treatment, Hospital "G. Mazzini", Teramo, Italy

Department of Neuroscience, Imaging and Clinical Science, University "G. D'Annunzio", Chieti, Italy
e-mail: domenico.deberardis@aslteramo.it

M. Fornaro
Polyedra Research Group, Teramo, Italy

Department of Neuroscience, Reproductive Science and Odontostomatology, School of Medicine 'Federico II' Naples, Naples, Italy

A. Anastasia
Department of Neuroscience, Reproductive Science and Odontostomatology, School of Medicine 'Federico II' Naples, Naples, Italy

F. Vellante · M. Di Giannantonio
Department of Neuroscience, Imaging and Clinical Science, University "G. D'Annunzio", Chieti, Italy
e-mail: digiannantonio@unich.it

A. Valchera
Polyedra Research Group, Teramo, Italy

Villa S. Giuseppe Hospital, Hermanas Hospitalarias, Ascoli Piceno, Italy

M. Cavuto
Department of Theory, Analysis, Composition and Direction, Music Conservatory "L. Canepa", Sassari, Italy

G. Perna
Department of Clinical Neurosciences, Hermanas Hospitalarias, FoRiPsi, Villa San Benedetto Menni, Como, Italy

Department of Psychiatry and Neuropsychology, University of Maastricht, Maastricht, The Netherlands

Department of Psychiatry and Behavioral Sciences, Leonard Miller School of Medicine, University of Miami, Coral Gables, FL, USA

M. Di Nicola
Institute of Psychiatry and Psychology, Catholic University of Sacred Heart, Rome, Italy

G. Serafini
Department of Neuroscience, Rehabilitation, Ophthalmology, Genetics, Maternal and Child Health, Section of Psychiatry, University of Genoa, Genoa, Italy
e-mail: gianluca.serafini@unige.it

Y.-K. Kim (ed.), *Treatment Resistance in Psychiatry*, https://doi.org/10.1007/978-981-10-4358-1_23

A. Carano
NHS, Department of Mental Health, Psychiatric Service of Diagnosis and Treatment, Hospital "Madonna Del Soccorso", San Benedetto del Tronto, Italy

M. Pompili
Department of Neurosciences, Mental Health and Sensory Organs, Suicide Prevention Center, Sant'Andrea Hospital, Sapienza University of Rome, Rome, Italy
e-mail: maurizio.pompili@uniroma1.it

L. Orsolini
Polyedra Research Group, Teramo, Italy

Psychopharmacology, Drug Misuse and Novel Psychoactive Substances Research Unit, School of Life and Medical Sciences, College Lane Campus, University of Hertfordshire, Hatfield, Herts, UK

C. Tomasetti
NHS, Department of Mental Health, Psychiatric Service of Diagnosis and Treatment, Hospital of Giulianova, Teramo, Italy
e-mail: carmine.tomasetti@aslteramo.it

G. Di Emidio
NHS, Department of Mental Health, Psychiatric Service of Diagnosis and Treatment, Mental Health Center of Giulianova, Teramo, Italy
e-mail: gabriella.diemidio@aslteramo.it

G. Martinotti
Department of Neuroscience, Imaging and Clinical Science, University "G. D'Annunzio", Chieti, Italy

Psychopharmacology, Drug Misuse and Novel Psychoactive Substances Research Unit, School of Life and Medical Sciences, College Lane Campus, University of Hertfordshire, Hatfield, Herts, UK

23.1 Introduction

Schizophrenia is a chronic and debilitating illness affecting about 0.5% of the population [1–3]. Schizophrenia comprises positive, negative, cognitive, and affective symptoms [2, 4]. It is known that, considering the complex symptom profile and the numerous theories on its etiopathogenesis [3, 5], the complete remission or recovery of symptoms is relatively rare in schizophrenia and the treatment resistance remains one of the most important challenges in psychiatry [6].

Antipsychotics are the mainstay of the pharmacological treatment of such burdensome condition, although documented that roughly 20% up to 60% of the patients with schizophrenia do not respond sufficiently to conventional treatments [7–9].

Clozapine, a dibenzodiazepine compound developed in 1961, is a multireceptorial atypical antipsychotic approved for the treatment of resistant schizophrenia (TRS) [10]. It has been demonstrated that clozapine is more effective than any other first (FGA)- or second-generation (SGA) antipsychotic in the treatment of TRS [11–13]. It has been estimated that almost two-thirds of patients who do not respond adequately to treatment with FGAs or other SGAs may respond adequately to treatment with clozapine [14]. Undoubtedly, despite its adverse effects that may be particularly bothersome or even potentially life-threatening for some poorly compliant and/or oversensitive patients, clozapine is a very effective drug in everyday clinical practice, and many of those in its receipt actually tolerating it would experience remarkable symptom relief, often protracted over the time allowing overall satisfactory quality of life [15, 16].

However, despite the superior efficacy of clozapine over alternative antipsychotics in the management of schizophrenia corroborated by everyday clinical practice, a remarkable number of patients fails to achieve satisfactory response, even when cases of "pseudo-resistance" are excluded (i.e., for those patients with poor treatment adherence, heavy smokers, and/or caffeine users without dosage adjustment) [6, 17, 18]. It has been estimated that around 40–70% of patients with ascertained TRS receiving clozapine may have an incomplete remission and are referred to as "ultra-resistant" or "refractory" [19–21] (see Table 23.1). Clozapine-resistant schizophrenia represents a challenge for the clinician and a misfortune for the patients, and several strategies

Table 23.1 Criteria for clozapine-resistant schizophrenia

Clinical characteristics	Clinical evaluation
Clozapine-refractory schizophrenia	No less than 8-week clozapine treatment with serum levels ≥350 μg/L
	No improvement or failure to improve by at least 20% in total Brief Psychiatric Rating Scale score
Persistence of positive symptoms	Item score ≥4 on at least two of four positive symptom items on the Brief Psychiatric Rating Scale
Actual presence of at least moderately severe disorder	Total Brief Psychiatric Rating Scale score≥45
	Score of ≥4 on the Clinical Global Impression Scale
Persistence of disorder and low functioning	Lack of a stable period of a satisfactory social and/or occupational functioning within the last 5 years regardless of clozapine treatment
	Global assessment of functioning scale score ≥40

Modified from Mouaffak et al. [19]

have been proposed to overcome this problem, yet, to date, it remains high-bar goal [22–24].

The aim of this chapter was to provide an overview of the managing strategies of clozapine-resistant schizophrenia with a particular focus on augmentation strategies aimed to improve efficacy on schizophrenia symptoms.

23.2 Clozapine Augmentation with Antipsychotics

23.2.1 Second-Generation Antipsychotics (SGAs)

23.2.1.1 Amisulpride

Amisulpride is a SGA promoting dopaminergic neurotransmission blocking presynaptic dopamine D2/D3 autoreceptors when administered at low doses; the converse is true when amisulpride is administered at higher doses when postsynaptic D2/D3 blockade occurs [25]. Several studies have been conducted so far, aiming at investigating whether amisulpride may be beneficial for patients with clozapine-resistant schizophrenia, and, overall, the majority of them have shown encouraging positive results [26, 27].

Assion et al. [28] showed that the augmentation with amisulpride improved the global outcome of patients suffering from chronic schizophrenia and tended to be a helpful treatment option in cases of partial or non-responsiveness to clozapine. Hotham et al. [29] found that amisulpride augmentation of clozapine in patients with schizophrenia and a history of violence led to a clinical improvement and reduced aggression and violence, thus showing anti-aggressive properties. It has been also suggested that the augmentation with amisulpride may reduce the sialorrhea often seen in patients treated with clozapine, thus improving their quality of life [30–32].

However, this combination is not void from potential risks. It has been observed that often this combined treatment may lead to high rates of relevant side effects including bradykinesia, akathisia, tremor, and an increase of prolactin serum levels, and therefore patients should be accurately monitored [28].

To sum-up, the amisulpride add-on to clozapine may be a useful strategy especially in violent patients, but the development of adverse effects should be taken into account.

23.2.1.2 Aripiprazole

One of the most used strategies in clozapine-resistant schizophrenia is to augment with aripiprazole, a 5HT2 antagonist and dopamine D2 partial agonist featuring 5-HT1A partial agonist [33, 34]. It has been suggested and is often seen in clinical practice that aripiprazole add-on to clozapine may improve metabolic adverse effects that often may appear with clozapine treatment [35, 36]. However, relatively few studies have investigated the effect of the aripiprazole augmentation on disease symptoms, and results were controversial.

Some earlier studies have demonstrated that, despite its favorable effects on metabolic parameters, aripiprazole augmentation may only slightly improve the symptoms of schizophrenia on Brief Psychiatric Rating Scale (BPRS) and Positive and Negative Syndrome Scale (PANSS) [37–39]. In a multicenter, naturalistic, randomized, superiority study, Cipriani et al. [40]

compared clinical efficacy and tolerability of haloperidol versus aripiprazole as combination treatment with clozapine in patients with resistant schizophrenia. The investigators found that the augmentation with aripiprazole offered no substantial benefit over haloperidol in terms of efficacy profile.

However, other studies have demonstrated an efficacy of aripiprazole-clozapine combination in treatment-resistant schizophrenia [41–44]. De Risio et al. [45] demonstrated a statistically significant improvement in psychopathology and functional outcome measures from baseline to endpoint (6 weeks) after augmentation with aripiprazole. As well, Muscatello et al. [46] showed that the aripiprazole add-on to clozapine resulted in a valuable effect on both positive and general psychopathological symptoms in a sample of TRS subjects. Moreover, a recent meta-analysis conducted on selected studies evaluating aripiprazole-clozapine combination in TRS has suggested that aripiprazole augmentation of clozapine would minimize the cardiometabolic risk and may be effective in attenuating psychotic symptoms but may cause agitation and akathisia. Furthermore, aripiprazole augmentation would be somewhat beneficial in reducing negative symptoms [47].

In conclusion, balancing the results of the studies, it seems that aripiprazole add-on to clozapine may be useful in some patients, especially in those who experienced metabolic symptoms. However, more larger studies are required to confirm such results.

23.2.1.3 Risperidone

The augmentation with risperidone may have a rationale considering the high affinity of this drug for D2 receptor compared with the lower affinity of clozapine on such receptors [48, 49]. Thus, this combination may be beneficial especially when positive symptoms are not recovered by clozapine [50, 51]. A critical review published in 2006 [52] points out that lower risperidone dosages and a longer duration of the augmentation would be associated with a better outcome, although some adverse effects such as extrapyramidal symptoms, akathisia, sedation, and sialorrhea may occur.

However, in a double-blind placebo-controlled parallel-group trial of a fixed dose of 4 mg/day of risperidone added for 6 weeks in 24 outpatients with schizophrenia partially responders to clozapine, Freudenreich et al. found that patients who received risperidone showed a nonsignificant decrease in PANSS total score although the disorganized thought subscale improved significantly. Moreover, Akdede et al. [53] found that adjunctive treatment with risperidone for 6 weeks in patients with schizophrenia who had received sustained treatment with clozapine did not significantly improve cognitive function. In a short-term study (8 weeks of daily augmentation with 3 mg of risperidone or with placebo), the addition of risperidone to clozapine did not result in improved symptoms in patients with severe schizophrenia, whereas a small decline in the verbal working-memory index was observed in the risperidone group [54]. These negative results were confirmed in another double-blind, placebo-controlled, randomized clinical trial (RCT) in partially responsive people with schizophrenia treated with clozapine [55]. In addition, another trial yielded negative results [56].

On the other hand, in a head-to-head trial (risperidone vs ziprasidone augmentation of clozapine), the augmentation with both drugs resulted in significant psychopathological improvement even if the side effects differed between the treatment groups (with prominent hyperprolactinemia, extrapyramidal symptoms, and weight gain in the risperidone group) [57]. These findings confirmed those previous positive ones of Raskin et al. [49]. Moreover, it has been suggested that also long-acting risperidone may be beneficial in some patients when added to clozapine [58].

In conclusion, risperidone augmentation of clozapine is controversial even if some patients may have benefits especially when positive symptoms are poorly controlled by clozapine alone. However, the adverse effects may be very burdensome and potentially threatening.

23.2.1.4 Ziprasidone

Ziprasidone is a SGA with a combined serotonin and dopamine receptor antagonist and a relatively favorable metabolic adverse effect profile (even if may induce QT prolongation).

In some open studies and case reports, positive results were attained in clozapine augmentation with ziprasidone, alongside with weight loss [59, 60].

Two studies compared ziprasidone and risperidone as clozapine augmentation strategies, and both drugs were shown to have comparable clinical efficacy but different side effect profiles [57, 61]. In fact, subjects with ziprasidone had an increased risk of QTc interval prolongation. However, all these studies had limitations due to the small sample size, the short observation time, and the absence of a placebo group.

Recently, Muscatello et al. [62] conducted a 16-week double-blind RCT to evaluate the efficacy of ziprasidone add-on clinical symptoms and cognitive functioning in 40 schizophrenic patients with residual symptoms refractory to clozapine monotherapy at the highest tolerated dosage. They found that ziprasidone added to clozapine was effective on negative and cognitive symptoms improving semantic fluency in treated patients. The effect on QTc was minimal but statistically significant.

In conclusion, the efficacy of ziprasidone augmentation of clozapine is encouraging and may be proposed as a helpful treatment in schizophrenia, mainly for those patients who partially respond to clozapine monotherapy and have a lower risk of QTc prolongation. However, the action of ziprasidone on QTc must be always considered also in patients who don't take clozapine [63].

23.2.1.5 Other SGAs

Overall speaking, the olanzapine/clozapine combination should be avoided due to high risk of developing severe weight gain and metabolic syndrome, even if it may be somewhat beneficial on clinical symptoms [64, 65].

The augmentation with the SGA sertindole was not superior to placebo and caused a significant worsening of positive symptoms in some subjects, and minor, yet significant, QTc prolongation thus is not recommended [66].

Some encouraging data are available concerning the combination of clozapine with paliperidone, but the majority are case reports, and therefore further controlled studies are needed [67–69].

23.2.2 First-Generation Antipsychotics (FGAs)

The augmentation with FGAs was proposed in earlier studies mostly because SGAs weren't yet available [70, 71].

There are some data on haloperidol augmentation in order to achieve improvement mainly on positive symptoms, but the effect wasn't significant, whereas adverse effects were prominent [40, 71]. Other data are available concerning pimozide, a FGA with potent D2 inhibition properties [72]. However the results were controversial with studies that demonstrated an overall good efficacy on positive symptoms [73] and others that reported negative findings [74, 75]. However, the incidence of adverse effects with pimozide/clozapine combination was remarkable and included QT prolongation and parkinsonism.

In conclusion, clozapine augmentation with FGAs isn't recommended due to a relative lack of efficacy and higher risk of adverse effects.

23.3 Clozapine Augmentation with Antidepressants

23.3.1 Selective Serotonin Reuptake Inhibitors (SSRIs)

The combination with antidepressants and especially the selective serotonin reuptake inhibitors (SSRIs) may have a rationale when depressive or negative symptoms are prominent and poorly controlled by clozapine. Similarly, this combination may be useful in the presence of relevant anxiety and obsessive-compulsive symptoms despite clozapine treatment. However, the SSRIs/clozapine combination should take into account the pharmacokinetics of such agents in order to avoid dangerous interactions.

The most studied SSRI in combination with clozapine was fluvoxamine. Fluvoxamine is an inhibitor of almost all cytochromes (CYP) and, in particular, CYP1A2 and therefore may increase the serum levels of clozapine proportionally to the administered dose of fluvoxamine. Thus, in the case of coadministration, a clozapine serum level monitoring or a dose reduction is recommended. However, in everyday clinical practice, this combination is often discouraged and avoided, even if it has been demonstrated that fluvoxamine seems effective on global symptomatology in patients who did not achieve a good response with clozapine and/or experienced weight gain [76, 77].

On the other hand, Wigard et al. [78], following the suggestions of a previous study [79], proposed that even if adding fluvoxamine to clozapine may produce a dangerous rise of clozapine serum concentrations, this can also be used to prescribe a lower number of clozapine pills improving treatment adherence, but assuming that a regular control of clozapine serum concentrations is compulsory.

Recently, Lu et al. [80] conducted a 12-week double-blind RCT to evaluate the effects of fluvoxamine on metabolic parameters and psychopathology in 85 clozapine-treated patients with schizophrenia and found that treatment with adjunctive fluvoxamine with clozapine reduced weight gain and metabolic abnormalities in patients with schizophrenia, without sacrificing the clinical effect when compared with clozapine monotherapy. Moreover, they did not observe differences in the plasma clozapine level between the two groups with the monotherapy group showing higher levels of norclozapine and clozapine N-oxide than the combined group. The beneficial effects on metabolic parameters may be due to the fact that fluvoxamine decreases plasma levels of norclozapine, a toxic metabolite of clozapine, which has been reported to contribute to weight gain, hyperglycemia, and serum lipid alterations in clozapine-treated patients [76, 81, 82].

The results of a recent meta-analysis, on the clinical potentials of adjunctive fluvoxamine to clozapine treatment [83], suggested that adjunctive fluvoxamine should be considered in patients not responding optimally to clozapine when it is difficult to achieve plasma levels above 350–420 ng/mL. This may not only reduce the number of ingested tablets needed but also prolong the clozapine half-life ensuring more stable plasma levels. However, clozapine serum level monitoring is mandatory to avoid dangerous and toxic raises in clozapine levels as it is a substrate of CYP1A2, whereas fluvoxamine is one of the most potent inhibitors of the isoenzyme CYP1A2 [84].

It has been demonstrated that fluoxetine add-on increased clozapine serum levels but without substantial clinical effects [85–87]. On the other hand, sertraline has showed to improve clozapine treatment, mainly concerning negative and obsessive symptoms without affecting clozapine plasma levels, but data are limited [88, 89]. The data on citalopram or escitalopram add-on to clozapine is, to date, inconsistent [90, 91].

23.3.2 Noradrenergic and Specific Serotoninergic Antidepressant (NaSSA)

The only available NaSSA is mirtazapine that acts by antagonizing the adrenergic alpha2-autoreceptors and alpha2-heteroreceptors as well as by blocking 5-HT2 and 5-HT3 receptors [92, 93]. Thus, mirtazapine enhances the release of noradrenaline and 5-HT1A-mediated serotonergic transmission [94].

The interest for mirtazapine as adjunctive therapy for clozapine rose due to the potential benefits on negative and cognitive symptoms without affecting clozapine serum levels [95]. In an 8-week double-blind RCT of 30 mg adjunctive mirtazapine to clozapine therapy, Zoccali et al. [96] demonstrated a significant reduction of negative symptoms as measured by the Scale for the Assessment of Negative Symptoms (SANS) in the mirtazapine group with a significant improvement on the SANS subscales avolition/apathy and anhedonia/asociality. Concerning adverse effects, weight gain and drowsiness were reported in few patients in the mirtazapine group. In an 8-week open-label trial, Delle Chiaie et al. [97] reported that mirtazapine add-on to clozapine induced a significant improvement in cognitive performance, as measured by the Repeatable Battery for the Assessment of Neuropsychological Status (RBANS), independently of negative and depressive symptoms. However, no other studies are available concerning this combination.

Moreover, the possibility of adverse metabolic effects should be considered due to the high propensity of both mirtazapine and clozapine to cause weight gain [98, 99], and therefore caution is recommended when mirtazapine is added to clozapine.

23.3.3 Other Antidepressants

Concerning serotonin and norepinephrine reuptake inhibitors (SNRIs), no data concerning clinical efficacy as add-on therapy are available for venlafaxine, even if it seems to not influence clozapine serum levels at least at low-to-moderate doses [100]. In a 16-week double-blind RCT of duloxetine augmentation in a sample of 33 patients with TRS receiving clozapine, Mico et al. [101] found that duloxetine augmentation showed a beneficial effect on the negative and general psychopathological symptomatology although without significant effects on executive cognitive functions and was well tolerated.

Only one study concerning the melatonergic antidepressant agomelatine is, to date, available. Bruno et al. conducted a 16-week, open-label, uncontrolled pilot trial evaluating the augmentation of partial responders to clozapine with agomelatine and found a promising effect of agomelatine on clinical and cognitive symptoms with a good tolerability.

The add-on with older antidepressants such as tricyclics has been suggested [102, 103], but data are very limited and cardiac and cholinergic adverse effects should be considered. The addition of amitriptyline seems to be beneficial in clozapine-induced sialorrhea [104].

23.3.4 Conclusions

Adding the SSRI fluvoxamine to ongoing clozapine treatment may be useful in some clinical conditions, especially in patients with negative or depressive symptoms or difficulty in achieving sufficiently high plasma levels for an adequate response. However, critical raises in clozapine serum levels may happen and need a careful monitoring or a clozapine dose reduction when coadministered with fluvoxamine. However, generally, the best rationale for a combined clozapine-SSRIs therapy may be the presence of moderate-to-severe depressive or obsessive symptoms that are not controlled or even worsened by clozapine, but, even if in the clinical practice this combination is relatively common [23], more longitudinal tolerability studies are definitely needed.

Some promising data are present for mirtazapine which seems to have a limited but beneficial effect on negative and cognitive symptoms, but the risk of additive metabolic adverse effects should be taken into account.

Too few data are available concerning other antidepressants in combination with clozapine to allow a definite conclusion.

23.4 Clozapine Augmentation with Mood Stabilizers or Anticonvulsants

23.4.1 Lithium

The lithium add-on to clozapine may have a rationale when administered to severe and treatment-resistant patients with schizoaffective disorder or bipolar disorder (wherein the latter clozapine has an established clinical efficacy [105–107]) or in the case of clozapine-treated patients with a still high risk of suicide despite the known anti-suicidal effect of clozapine [108, 109]. However, surprisingly, only few studies have evaluated this association in clozapine-resistant patients, whereas the majority has pointed out the beneficial effects of lithium in clozapine-induced neutropenia [110, 111].

In a retrospective study, Kelly et al. [112] evaluated adjunctive divalproex or lithium in TRS patients taking clozapine compared to clozapine monotherapy and observed that the 6-month general symptomatology was similarly improved in all treatment groups, but a significantly greater improvement occurred in the first month for those on divalproex or lithium than clozapine alone. However, in patients treated with lithium, several adverse effects were reported such as weight gain and increased glycemia. Small et al. [113] in a mixed sample of patients with TRS and treatment-resistant schizoaffective disorder (SD) showed that SD subjects improved with lithium concerning the overall outcome, the Positive and Negative Syndrome Scale (PANSS) total and negative subscales, and the cognitive measures, whereas schizophrenic patients did not. Authors concluded that, for TRS patients, lithium add-on did not improve but increased the risk of a possible lithium toxicity.

In conclusion, the available evidences concerning lithium add-on provide only support for the utility of lithium in preventing or managing clozapine-related neutropenia, but its effect on symptoms is somewhat limited and further studies are needed.

23.4.2 Valproic Acid

Valproic acid add-on to the ongoing clozapine therapy is mainly used to treat or avoid, in a preventive way in at risk subjects, clozapine-related seizures [114, 115].

Besides the addition as anticonvulsant, valproic acid also may play a significant role in the treatment of some symptoms in TRS [116]. Valproic acid is commonly used for individuals with schizophrenia with violent episodes, because it is reported to decrease aggression and hostility [117, 118]. However, the addition of valproate has been reported to increase the plasma or serum levels of clozapine [119, 120] through an inhibiting effect on the CYP1A2- or CYP3A4-mediated conversion of clozapine to norclozapine, but this interaction is unlikely to be clinically significant [120].

Concerning add-on therapy to clozapine, Kando et al. [121] found that the combination of clozapine and valproate was efficacious and well tolerated in 55 patients with affective and psychotic disorders without severe adverse effects. In the abovementioned (see Sect. 23.4.1) retrospective study, Kelly et al. [112] showed that the addition of divalproex was significantly more effective in reducing global symptoms (especially hostility and anxiety) in the first month of add-on treatment when compared to clozapine monotherapy and to previous clozapine treatment.

However, it has been reported that the combination of clozapine and valproate may be associated to increased risk of several severe adverse effects such as neutropenia [122, 123], myocarditis, and pericarditis [16, 124, 125]. Therefore, if not used for controlling the risk of clozapine-related seizures, this combination should be possibly avoided and used only when the clinical benefits overcome the risk of harmful effects.

23.4.3 Topiramate

The topiramate does not affect the plasma levels of clozapine [126] and has been proposed as an effective add-on to clozapine especially in patients who experienced weight gain [127, 128] and to prevent or treat seizures [129].

Hahn et al. [130] carried out a 12-week naturalistic, open study to evaluate the potential benefits of topiramate in clozapine-treated patients with a suboptimal clinical response. They found that topiramate augmentation caused a 14% improvement in total BPRS score together with a reduction in body weight. Topiramate was well tolerated and the most common side effect was paraesthesia. In a 24-week RCT, Muscatello et al. [131] aimed to explore the efficacy and tolerability of topiramate add-on pharmacotherapy on clinical symptomatology and cognitive functioning in a sample of TRS patients receiving clozapine. They reported that topiramate appeared to be poor effective for reducing clinical symptomatology in schizophrenic patients who have had an incomplete clinical response to clozapine. However, the patients included in the topiramate groups showed a slight worsening of performances on cognitive tasks.

Therefore, on the basis of the current evidence, topiramate add-on cannot be recommended for controlling symptomatology of clozapine-resistant schizophrenia, even if maybe cautiously used to reduce weight and prevent seizures.

23.4.4 Lamotrigine

The use of lamotrigine as add-on therapy to clozapine has been proposed in several studies besides its antiepileptic effect [132]. It has been suggested that lamotrigine add-on may reduce alcohol consumption in TRS patients taking clozapine [133].

The comprehensive meta-analysis of Tiihonen et al. concerning lamotrigine add-on [134] included 5 trials with overall 161 patients. They found that lamotrigine was superior to placebo augmentation in both the primary (total symptom score from the PANSS or BPRS rating scales) and secondary outcome measures (positive and negative symptoms score from the PANSS or BPRS rating scales). The results of Tiihonen et al. [134] pointed out that about 20 to 30% of clozapine-resistant patients may achieve clinically significant benefits from lamotrigine augmentation. On the other hand, in a 12-week prospective study, Vayisoglu et al. [135] did not reported any benefit of augmentation of clozapine with lamotrigine in TRS patients with partial response.

However, all considered, overall evidences for lamotrigine as add-on therapy to clozapine are favorable, even if further studies may be useful. A slow lamotrigine titration is recommended, and the careful monitoring for potential severe adverse effects (i.e., rash and agranulocytosis) is required [136–138].

23.5 Clozapine Augmentation with Drug Treatments for Alzheimer's Disease

23.5.1 Acetylcholinesterase Inhibitors (AChEIs)

The rationale for using drug treatments for Alzheimer's disease in addition to clozapine is mainly to address cognitive symptoms associated with schizophrenia and often poorly improved by clozapine.

The AChEI donepezil has been tried in combination with clozapine with encouraging results [139]. However, Stryjer et al. [140], in an 18-week double-blind crossover study, found no significant differences in the total positive and negative symptom scale scores when donepezil add-on was compared with placebo, even if three patients improved in the total PANSS scores during the donepezil treatment phase. Only one case series is available for galantamine with a positive effect as a cognitive enhancer [141].

Therefore, the data concerning donepezil and galantamine add-on are too few to make a definite conclusion.

23.5.2 Memantine

The memantine has shown positive results on residual negative and cognitive symptoms of schizophrenia when added to stable antipsychotic regimen in patients with schizophrenia even if they are not treatment-resistant [142].

The memantine add-on to clozapine has been evaluated in several trials and, to date, the data are very encouraging [143, 144]. In a RCT on 21 patients, de Lucena et al. [145] randomized subjects to receive either 20 mg/day memantine or placebo in addition to clozapine for 12 weeks and found a significant improvement with memantine on the total BPRS score (and its positive and negative subscales), the Clinical Global Impression (CGI) score, and the Mini Mental State Examination (MMSE) score when compared with placebo. No significant changes in extrapyramidal symptoms were observed.

Veerman et al. [146] randomized clozapine-treated patients to 12 weeks of double-blind adjunctive treatment with memantine or placebo and found that, if compared with placebo, memantine improved a composite memory score comprising verbal recognition memory and paired associates learning task scores on the Cambridge Neuropsychological Test Automated Battery (CANTAB) and PANSS negative subscale score. In addition, adverse effects were rare and mild and transient. In 2017, the same group conducted an open-label 1-year extension of the previous trial [147] and found that, in the 1-year extension phase, the favorable effect of adjunctive memantine on memory was persistent, and a further improvement of negative, positive, and overall symptoms in patients with clozapine-treated TRS was observed. The memantine was well tolerated without severe adverse effects.

In conclusion, the overall evaluation of published data is very encouraging. The effect of memantine in clozapine-resistant patients seems to improve both cognitive and positive/negative symptoms without evidence of severe adverse effect. Thus, this strategy may be recommended at least in some clozapine-resistant patients, even if further studies would be useful to confirm adjunctive memantine as the first strategy of choice in such cases.

23.6 Other Augmentation Strategies

Due to the "black hole" of clozapine-resistant management strategies, several nonpsychiatric drugs or other bioactive compounds were tried to find a possible way to cope with this serious condition [148–151]. This trial aimed not only to overcome treatment refractoriness but also to improve the physical health of clozapine-treated patients [24, 152].

Some encouraging data come from the omega-3 fatty acid add-on that have demonstrated to improve some anthropometric indices (such as weight, body mass index [BMI], wrist and waist circumference) in patients with schizophrenia who were taking clozapine pharmacotherapy [153]. Peet and Horrobin [154] conducted a 12-week placebo-controlled dose-ranging exploratory study (1, 2, and 4 g/day of ethyl-eicosapentaenoate [E-EPA]) on 115 patients with persistent symptoms of schizophrenia, receiving either clozapine (31 patients), SGAs (48 patients), or FGAs (36 patients). In the clozapine group only, a post hoc analysis showed a clinically important and significant effect on all PANSS subscales, which was most pronounced at an E-EPA dosage of 2 g/day. Moreover, omega-3 fatty acids may be useful in patients taking clozapine who have elevated serum triglyceride levels [155]. However, in a 12-week study, Emsley et al. [156] found no significant changes in positive, negative, or overall symptoms of schizophrenia in patients taking clozapine after treatment with E-EPA 3 g/day. Moreover, Fenton et al. [157] found similar results confirming the negative results.

There are several evidences that minocycline, a tetracycline antibiotic that has anti-inflammatory and neuroprotective properties, may play a role in schizophrenia as inflammation has been suggested as one of the potential mechanisms leading to pharmacoresistance [151, 158–160]. Adjunctive minocycline has been successfully employed in patients with persistent schizophrenia symptoms despite clozapine treatment [150, 161]. In a 10-week, double-blind RCT, Kelly et al. [162] randomized 52 patients with persistent symptoms to receive adjunct minocycline (100 mg twice daily) or placebo to clozapine. They found that significant improvements with minocycline were seen in working memory, avolition, and anxiety/depressive symptoms in such patients. However, it is possible that minocycline effects may be mediated by an increase in clozapine levels [163].

Further augmentation strategies have involved other glutamatergic agents than memantine (such as glycine, D-cycloserine, D-serine, and ampakine). Several double-blind, placebo-controlled trials have evaluated glycine add-on to clozapine alone or together with other antipsychotics, but the results about its effectiveness on positive and negative symptoms were inconsistent and generally negative [164–166].

Recently, some preliminary data suggested that the extract of *Ginkgo biloba* was found useful for enhancing the effect of clozapine on negative symptoms in patients with treatment-resistant schizophrenia [167].

23.7 Adjunctive Electroconvulsive Therapy (ECT)

ECT is one of the oldest treatments in psychiatry, which has luckily survived till today and is considered to be very useful in patients with several severe psychiatric disorders including schizophrenia [168, 169]. Many studies have shown that ECT may be effective in patients with TRS [170, 171].

Moreover, there are several earlier reports that suggested an important positive effect of adjunctive ECT in patients with partial or non-response to clozapine [172–175].

More recently, a renewed interest has grown up from the results of several trials and reviews that have further investigated the effect of adjunctive ECT to clozapine [176–179]. Kho et al. [180] observed a remission in eight patients with adjunctive ECT treatment. After remission of symptoms, five subjects experienced a relapse, and three of the five subjects who relapsed had a second effective ECT course and did not experience further relapses with maintenance ECT and clozapine. No adverse effects were reported. Masoudzadeh et al. [181] assigned 18 TRS patients to three identical groups: one group was given clozapine, another group was treated with ECT, and the last group was treated with the clozapine-ECT combination. They found that the clozapine-ECT combination was superior to single therapies with a fast response to combination treatment and a higher improvement in both positive and negative symptoms. There were no significant adverse effects with clozapine-ECT combination. In a randomized single-blind 8-week study by Petrides et al. [182], patients with clozapine-resistant schizophrenia were assigned to treatment as usual (clozapine group) or a course of bilateral ECT plus clozapine (ECT plus clozapine group). Authors found that the 50% of the ECT plus clozapine patients met the response criterion (≥40% reduction in symptoms based on BPRS scores, a CGI-severity rating <3, and a CGI-improvement rating ≤2), whereas none of the patients in the clozapine group met it. In the crossover phase, response was 47%, and ECT combination was well tolerated. Kim et al. [183] confirmed these positive observations in a sample of seven patients with a significant reduction on PANSS total score. As well, other reports were positive [184–186].

In conclusion, combination treatment with clozapine and ECT was safe and effective in clozapine-resistant patients without severe adverse effects. It should be always considered, where available, for the treatment of clozapine-resistant patients.

Conclusions

When clozapine fails there are several strategies that can be employed [152]. However, such strategies are mostly empirical and should be considered on a case-by-case basis for those individuals who haven't achieved a good response and/or experienced some clozapine-related adverse effects [20, 187]. It should be noted that the majority of the studies that have evaluated augmentation strategies are mostly case report, case series, and open trials with a relative few number of patients and several biases [24, 188]. There are too few available RCTs that may allow to define a precise guideline on what to do in the unluckily case of clozapine resistance [21, 188]. Nevertheless, given the devastating effect of the clozapine-refractory schizophrenia and the pervasive consequences on patients as well as caregivers quality of life and functioning, even a modest response to a particular augmenting agent may be clinically significant for each subject [189].

Some augmentations may be more useful to manage clozapine adverse effects such as metabolic adverse effects and seizures (i.e., aripiprazole, valproate, and topiramate add-on), to address pharmacokinetics and pseudo-resistant problems (i.e., fluvoxamine add-on), or to target specific symptoms (such as depressive symptoms with antidepressant add-on).

However, some strategies seem more promising than others on some symptom domains (i.e., memantine augmentation on cognitive symptoms) or may be effective to improve positive and negative symptoms (i.e., lamotrigine, mirtazapine, and ECT add-on), but further larger studies are undoubtedly needed.

As a concluding remark, we underline that, while augmenting, the adverse effect profile of each augmenting agent must be carefully considered, and, in case of intolerability or inefficacy, the clozapine monotherapy should be promptly restored. We are absolutely aware that clozapine-refractory schizophrenia is a great challenge and a real troublesome condition, but we fully agree with Jain et al. [19] when they wrote "…the progressive nature of schizophrenia needs to be kept in mind while setting goals for functional recovery as unrealistic expectations may do more harm than good…"

References

1. Simeone JC, Ward AJ, Rotella P, Collins J, Windisch R. An evaluation of variation in published estimates of schizophrenia prevalence from 1990 horizontal line 2013: a systematic literature review. BMC Psychiatry. 2015;15:193.
2. Galderisi S, Rucci P, Kirkpatrick B, Mucci A, Gibertoni D, Rocca P, et al. Interplay among psychopathologic variables, personal resources, context-related factors, and real-life functioning in individuals with schizophrenia: a network analysis. JAMA Psychiat. 2018;75:396–404.
3. Ebisch SJ, Mantini D, Northoff G, Salone A, De Berardis D, Ferri F, et al. Altered brain long-range functional interactions underlying the link between aberrant self-experience and self-other relationship in first-episode schizophrenia. Schizophr Bull. 2014;40(5):1072–82.
4. Marasco V, De Berardis D, Serroni N, Campanella D, Acciavatti T, Caltabiano M, et al. Alexithymia and suicide risk among patients with schizophrenia: preliminary findings of a cross-sectional study. Riv Psichiatr. 2011;46(1):31–7.
5. Ebisch SJ, Salone A, Ferri F, De Berardis D, Romani GL, Ferro FM, et al. Out of touch with reality? Social perception in first-episode schizophrenia. Soc Cogn Affect Neurosci. 2013;8(4):394–403.
6. Iasevoli F, Giordano S, Balletta R, Latte G, Formato MV, Prinzivalli E, et al. Treatment resistant schizophrenia is associated with the worst community functioning among severely-ill highly-disabling psychiatric conditions and is the most relevant predictor of poorer achievements in functional milestones. Prog Neuro-Psychopharmacol Biol Psychiatry. 2016;65:34–48.
7. Howes OD, McCutcheon R, Agid O, de Bartolomeis A, van Beveren NJ, Birnbaum ML, et al. Treatment-resistant schizophrenia: treatment response and resistance in psychosis (TRRIP) working group consensus guidelines on diagnosis and terminology. Am J Psychiatry. 2017;174(3):216–29.
8. Orsolini L, Tomasetti C, Valchera A, Vecchiotti R, Matarazzo I, Vellante F, et al. An update of safety of clinically used atypical antipsychotics. Expert Opin Drug Saf. 2016;15(10):1329–47.
9. De Berardis D, Marini S, Carano A, Lang AP, Cavuto M, Piersanti M, et al. Efficacy and safety of long acting injectable atypical antipsychotics: a review. Curr Clin Pharmacol. 2013;8(3):256–64.
10. Warnez S, Alessi-Severini S. Clozapine: a review of clinical practice guidelines and prescribing trends. BMC Psychiatry. 2014;14:102.
11. Kane J, Honigfeld G, Singer J, Meltzer H. Clozapine for the treatment-resistant schizophrenic. A double-blind comparison with chlorpromazine. Arch Gen Psychiatry. 1988;45(9):789–96.
12. Siskind D, McCartney L, Goldschlager R, Kisely S. Clozapine v. first- and second-generation antipsychotics in treatment-refractory schizophrenia: systematic review and meta-analysis. Br J Psychiatry. 2016;209(5):385–92.
13. De Berardis D, Serroni N, Campanella D, Olivieri L, Marini S, Moschetta FS, et al. Safety and efficacy of combined clozapine-azathioprine treatment in a case of resistant schizophrenia associated with Behcet's disease: a 2-year follow-up. Gen Hosp Psychiatry. 2013;35(2):213.e9–11.
14. Essali A, Al-Haj Haasan N, Li C, Rathbone J. Clozapine versus typical neuroleptic medication for schizophrenia. Cochrane Database Syst Rev. 2009;21(1):CD000059.
15. Nucifora FC Jr, Mihaljevic M, Lee BJ, Sawa A. Clozapine as a model for antipsychotic development. Neurotherapeutics. 2017;14(3):750–61.
16. De Berardis D, Serroni N, Campanella D, Olivieri L, Ferri F, Carano A, et al. Update on the adverse effects of clozapine: focus on myocarditis. Curr Drug Saf. 2012;7(1):55–62.
17. Williams L, Newton G, Roberts K, Finlayson S, Brabbins C. Clozapine-resistant schizophrenia: a positive approach. Br J Psychiatry. 2002;181:184–7.
18. Dratcu L, Grandison A, McKay G, Bamidele A, Vasudevan V. Clozapine-resistant psychosis, smoking, and caffeine: managing the neglected effects of substances that our patients consume every day. Am J Ther. 2007;14(3):314–8.
19. Jain M, Karia S, De Sousa A. Clozapine-resistant schizophrenia: strategies for the busy clinician. Ind J Priv Psychiatry. 2017;11(2):17–23.
20. Li YY, Zhang YS, Wang J, Li KQ, Wang HY. Optimal treatment strategies of clozapine for refractory schizophrenia. Zhongguo Yi Xue Ke Xue Yuan Xue Bao. 2016;38(6):666–78.
21. Mouaffak F, Tranulis C, Gourevitch R, Poirier MF, Douki S, Olie JP, et al. Augmentation strategies of clozapine with antipsychotics in the treatment of ultraresistant schizophrenia. Clin Neuropharmacol. 2006;29(1):28–33.
22. Remington G, Saha A, Chong SA, Shammi C. Augmenting strategies in clozapine-resistant schizophrenia. CNS Drugs. 2006;20(2):171.
23. Kudva G, Gupta D. Strategies in clozapine-resistant schizophrenia: a literature review. J Ment Health Hum Behav. 2016;21(1):6–15.
24. Vayisoglu S, Anil YE. Augmentation strategies in patients with schizophrenia who show partial response to clozapine treatment. Turk Psikiyatri Derg. 2014;25(3):201–11.
25. Komossa K, Rummel-Kluge C, Hunger H, Schmid F, Schwarz S, Silveira da Mota Neto JI, et al. Amisulpride versus other atypical antipsychotics for schizophrenia. Cochrane Database Syst Rev. 2010;1:CD006624.

26. Tufan AE, Yalug I. Clozapine augmented with amisulpride in 3 cases of treatment-resistant early- and very early-onset schizophrenia. J Clin Psychopharmacol. 2013;33(4):572–4.
27. Zink M, Knopf U, Henn FA, Thome J. Combination of clozapine and amisulpride in treatment-resistant schizophrenia – case reports and review of the literature. Pharmacopsychiatry. 2004;37(1):26–31.
28. Assion HJ, Reinbold H, Lemanski S, Basilowski M, Juckel G. Amisulpride augmentation in patients with schizophrenia partially responsive or unresponsive to clozapine. A randomized, double-blind, placebo-controlled trial. Pharmacopsychiatry. 2008;41(1):24–8.
29. Hotham JE, Simpson PJ, Brooman-White RS, Basu A, Ross CC, Humphreys SA, et al. Augmentation of clozapine with amisulpride: an effective therapeutic strategy for violent treatment-resistant schizophrenia patients in a UK high-security hospital. CNS Spectr. 2014;19(5):403–10.
30. Kreinin A, Miodownik C, Sokolik S, Shestakova D, Libov I, Bergman J, et al. Amisulpride versus moclobemide in treatment of clozapinein-duced hypersalivation. World J Biol Psychiatry. 2011;12(8):620–6.
31. Kreinin A, Novitski D, Weizman A. Amisulpride treatment of clozapine-induced hypersalivation in schizophrenia patients: a randomized, double-blind, placebo-controlled cross-over study. Int Clin Psychopharmacol. 2006;21(2):99–103.
32. Croissant B, Hermann D, Olbrich R. Reduction of side effects by combining clozapine with amisulpride: case report and short review of clozapine-induced hypersalivation-a case report. Pharmacopsychiatry. 2005;38(1):38–9.
33. De Berardis D, Fornaro M, Serroni N, Marini S, Piersanti M, Cavuto M, et al. Treatment of antipsychotic-induced hyperprolactinemia: an update on the role of the dopaminergic receptors D2 partial agonist aripiprazole. Recent Pat Endocr Metab Immune Drug Discov. 2014;8(1):30–7.
34. Martinotti G, Orsolini L, Fornaro M, Vecchiotti R, De Berardis D, Iasevoli F, et al. Aripiprazole for relapse prevention and craving in alcohol use disorder: current evidence and future perspectives. Expert Opin Investig Drugs. 2016;25(6):719–28.
35. de Bartolomeis A, Tomasetti C, Iasevoli F. Update on the mechanism of action of aripiprazole: translational insights into antipsychotic strategies beyond dopamine receptor antagonism. CNS Drugs. 2015;29(9):773–99.
36. Sepede G, Di Iorio G, Spano MC, Lorusso M, Sarchione F, Santacroce R, et al. A case of resistant schizophrenia successfully treated with clozapine/long-acting injectable aripiprazole combination. Clin Neuropharmacol. 2016;39(6): 322–4.
37. Chang JS, Ahn YM, Park HJ, Lee KY, Kim SH, Kang UG, et al. Aripiprazole augmentation in clozapine-treated patients with refractory schizophrenia: an 8-week, randomized, double-blind, placebo-controlled trial. J Clin Psychiatry. 2008;69(5):720–31.
38. Fleischhacker WW, Heikkinen ME, Olie JP, Landsberg W, Dewaele P, McQuade RD, et al. Effects of adjunctive treatment with aripiprazole on body weight and clinical efficacy in schizophrenia patients treated with clozapine: a randomized, double-blind, placebo-controlled trial. Int J Neuropsychopharmacol. 2010;13(8):1115–25.
39. Henderson DC, Kunkel L, Nguyen DD, Borba CP, Daley TB, Louie PM, et al. An exploratory open-label trial of aripiprazole as an adjuvant to clozapine therapy in chronic schizophrenia. Acta Psychiatr Scand. 2006;113(2):142–7.
40. Cipriani A, Accordini S, Nose M, Purgato M, Girlanda F, Tansella M, et al. Aripiprazole versus haloperidol in combination with clozapine for treatment-resistant schizophrenia: a 12-month, randomized, naturalistic trial. J Clin Psychopharmacol. 2013;33(4):533–7.
41. Bachmann CJ, Lehr D, Theisen FM, Preiss M. Aripiprazole as an adjunct to clozapine therapy in adolescents with early-onset schizophrenia: a retrospective chart review. Pharmacopsychiatry. 2009;42(4):153–7.
42. Mitsonis CI, Dimopoulos NP, Mitropoulos PA, Kararizou EG, Katsa AN, Tsakiris FE, et al. Aripiprazole augmentation in the management of residual symptoms in clozapine-treated outpatients with chronic schizophrenia: an open-label pilot study. Prog Neuro-Psychopharmacol Biol Psychiatry. 2007;31(2):373–7.
43. Karunakaran K, Tungaraza TE, Harborne GC. Is clozapine-aripiprazole combination a useful regime in the management of treatmentresistant schizophrenia? J Psychopharmacol. 2007;21(4):453–6.
44. Ziegenbein M, Wittmann G, Kropp S. Aripiprazole augmentation of clozapine in treatment-resistant schizophrenia: a clinical observation. Clin Drug Investig. 2006;26(3):117–24.
45. De Risio A, Pancheri A, Simonetti G, Giannarelli D, Stefanutto L, Gentile B. Add-on of aripiprazole improves outcome in clozapine-resistant schizophrenia. Prog Neuro-Psychopharmacol Biol Psychiatry. 2011;35(4):1112–6.
46. Muscatello MR, Bruno A, Pandolfo G, Mico U, Scimeca G, Di Nardo F, et al. Effect of aripiprazole augmentation of clozapine in schizophrenia: a double-blind, placebo-controlled study. Schizophr Res. 2011;127(1–3):93–9.
47. Galling B, Roldan A, Hagi K, Rietschel L, Walyzada F, Zheng W, et al. Antipsychotic augmentation vs. monotherapy in schizophrenia: systematic review, meta-analysis and meta-regression analysis. World Psychiatry. 2017;16(1):77–89.

48. McCarthy RH, Terkelsen KG. Risperidone augmentation of clozapine. Pharmacopsychiatry. 1995;28(2):61–3.
49. Raskin S, Katz G, Zislin Z, Knobler HY, Durst R. Clozapine and risperidone: combination/augmentation treatment of refractory schizophrenia: a preliminary observation. Acta Psychiatr Scand. 2000;101(4):334–6.
50. Agarwal V. Risperidone augmentation of clozapine. Indian J Psychiatry. 1999;41(1):86.
51. Morera AL, Barreiro P, Cano-Munoz JL. Risperidone and clozapine combination for the treatment of refractory schizophrenia. Acta Psychiatr Scand. 1999;99(4):305–6.
52. Kontaxakis VP, Ferentinos PP, Havaki-Kontaxaki BJ, Paplos KG, Pappa DA, Christodoulou GN. Risperidone augmentation of clozapine: a critical review. Eur Arch Psychiatry Clin Neurosci. 2006;256(6):350–5.
53. Akdede BB, Anil Yagcioglu AE, Alptekin K, Turgut TI, Tumuklu M, Yazici MK, et al. A double-blind study of combination of clozapine with risperidone in patients with schizophrenia: effects on cognition. J Clin Psychiatry. 2006;67(12):1912–9.
54. Honer WG, Thornton AE, Chen EY, Chan RC, Wong JO, Bergmann A, et al. Clozapine alone versus clozapine and risperidone with refractory schizophrenia. N Engl J Med. 2006;354(5):472–82.
55. Weiner E, Conley RR, Ball MP, Feldman S, Gold JM, Kelly DL, et al. Adjunctive risperidone for partially responsive people with schizophrenia treated with clozapine. Neuropsychopharmacology. 2010;35(11):2274–83.
56. Anil Yagcioglu AE, Kivircik Akdede BB, Turgut TI, Tumuklu M, Yazici MK, Alptekin K, et al. A double-blind controlled study of adjunctive treatment with risperidone in schizophrenic patients partially responsive to clozapine: efficacy and safety. J Clin Psychiatry. 2005;66(1):63–72.
57. Zink M, Kuwilsky A, Krumm B, Dressing H. Efficacy and tolerability of ziprasidone versus risperidone as augmentation in patients partially responsive to clozapine: a randomised controlled clinical trial. J Psychopharmacol. 2009;23(3):305–14.
58. Se Hyun K, Dong Chung J, Yong Min A, Yong SK. The combined use of risperidone long-acting injection and clozapine in patients with schizophrenia non-adherent to clozapine: a case series. J Psychopharmacol. 2010;24(7):981–6.
59. Kaye NS. Ziprasidone augmentation of clozapine in 11 patients. J Clin Psychiatry. 2003;64(2):215–6.
60. Zink M, Mase E, Dressing H. Ziprasidone-augmentation of clozapine. Psychiatr Prax. 2004;31(5):259–61.
61. Kuwilsky A, Krumm B, Englisch S, Dressing H, Zink M. Long-term efficacy and tolerability of clozapine combined with ziprasidone or risperidone. Pharmacopsychiatry. 2010;43(6):216–20.
62. Muscatello MR, Pandolfo G, Mico U, Lamberti Castronuovo E, Abenavoli E, Scimeca G, et al. Augmentation of clozapine with ziprasidone in refractory schizophrenia: a double-blind, placebo-controlled study. J Clin Psychopharmacol. 2014;34(1):129–33.
63. Vieweg WV, Hasnain M. Question regarding ziprasidone and QTc interval prolongation in the ZODIAC study. Am J Psychiatry. 2011;168(6):650–1.
64. Gupta S, Sonnenberg SJ, Frank B. Olanzapine augmentation of clozapine. Ann Clin Psychiatry. 1998;10(3):113–5.
65. Rummel-Kluge C, Komossa K, Schwarz S, Hunger H, Schmid F, Lobos CA, et al. Head-to-head comparisons of metabolic side effects of second generation antipsychotics in the treatment of schizophrenia: a systematic review and meta-analysis. Schizophr Res. 2010;123(2–3):225–33.
66. Nielsen J, Emborg C, Gydesen S, Dybbro J, Aagaard J, Haderup K, et al. Augmenting clozapine with sertindole: a double-blind, randomized, placebo-controlled study. J Clin Psychopharmacol. 2012;32(2):173–8.
67. Kalenderoglu A, Celik M. Augmentation of clozapine with Paliperidone in schizophrenia patients with partial response to treatment: a case series. Turk Psikiyatri Derg. 2016;27(1):57–62.
68. Hou YC. Improvement in psychotic symptoms and social functioning after augmentation of paliperidone with clozapine in a patient with schizoaffective disorder. J Neuropsychiatry Clin Neurosci. 2014;26(1):E26.
69. Maia-de-Oliveira JP, Nunes EA, Ushirohira JM, Machado-de-Sousa JP, Bressan RA, Hallak JE. Paliperidone palmitate for refractory and clozapine-resistant schizophrenia. J Neuropsychiatry Clin Neurosci. 2015;27(1):e14–6.
70. Rajarethinam R, Gilani S, Tancer M, DeQuardo J. Augmentation of clozapine partial responders with conventional antipsychotics. Schizophr Res. 2003;60(1):97–8.
71. Mowerman S, Siris SG. Adjunctive loxapine in a clozapine-resistant cohort of schizophrenic patients. Ann Clin Psychiatry. 1996;8(4):193–7.
72. Mendhekar DN, Gupta D, Lohia D, Jiloha RC. Pimozide augmentation of clozapine in hebephrenic schizophrenia: a case report. Indian J Psychiatry. 2003;45(1):55.
73. Friedman J, Ault K, Powchik P. Pimozide augmentation for the treatment of schizophrenic patients who are partial responders to clozapine. Biol Psychiatry. 1997;42(6):522–3.
74. Friedman JI, Lindenmayer JP, Alcantara F, Bowler S, Parak M, White L, et al. Pimozide augmentation of clozapine inpatients with schizophrenia and schizoaffective disorder unresponsive to clozapine monotherapy. Neuropsychopharmacology. 2011;36(6):1289–95.
75. Gunduz-Bruce H, Oliver S, Gueorguieva R, Forselius-Bielen K, D'Souza DC, Zimolo Z, et al. Efficacy of pimozide augmentation for clozapine partial responders with schizophrenia. Schizophr Res. 2013;143(2–3):344–7.

76. Lu ML, Lane HY, Lin SK, Chen KP, Chang WH. Adjunctive fluvoxamine inhibits clozapine-related weight gain and metabolic disturbances. J Clin Psychiatry. 2004;65(6):766–71.
77. Silver H, Kushnir M, Kaplan A. Fluvoxamine augmentation in clozapine-resistant schizophrenia: an open pilot study. PubMed PMID: 8886304.
78. Wigard ME, van Gool AR, Schulte PF. Addition of fluvoxamine to clozapine: theory and practice. Tijdschr Psychiatr. 2013;55(2):113–21.
79. Lu ML, Lane HY, Chen KP, Jann MW, Su MH, Chang WH. Fluvoxamine reduces the clozapine dosage needed in refractory schizophrenic patients. J Clin Psychiatry. 2000;61(8):594–9.
80. Lu ML, Chen TT, Kuo PH, Hsu CC, Chen CH. Effects of adjunctive fluvoxamine on metabolic parameters and psychopathology in clozapinetreated patients with schizophrenia: a 12-week, randomized, double-blind, placebo-controlled study. Schizophr Res. 2017;193:126–33.
81. Hinze-Selch D, Deuschle M, Weber B, Heuser I, Pollmacher T. Effect of coadministration of clozapine and fluvoxamine versus clozapine monotherapy on blood cell counts, plasma levels of cytokines and body weight. Psychopharmacology. 2000;149(2):163–9.
82. Papetti F, Morel-Pingault V, Buisse V, Maziere L, Banayan M, Thauby S, et al. Clozapine-resistant schizophrenia related to an increased metabolism and benefit of fluvoxamine: four case reports. L'Encéphale. 2007;33(5):811–8.
83. Polcwiartek C, Nielsen J. The clinical potentials of adjunctive fluvoxamine to clozapine treatment: a systematic review. Psychopharmacology. 2016;233(5):741–50.
84. Silver H, Kaplan A, Jahjah N. Fluvoxamine augmentation for clozapine-resistant schizophrenia. Am J Psychiatry. 1995;152(7):1098.
85. Spina E, Avenoso A, Salemi M, Facciola G, Scordo MG, Ancione M, et al. Plasma concentrations of clozapine and its major metabolites during combined treatment with paroxetine or sertraline. Pharmacopsychiatry. 2000;33(6):213–7.
86. Wetzel H, Anghelescu I, Szegedi A, Wiesner J, Weigmann H, Harter S, et al. Pharmacokinetic interactions of clozapine with selective serotonin reuptake inhibitors: differential effects of fluvoxamine and paroxetine in a prospective study. J Clin Psychopharmacol. 1998;18(1):2–9.
87. Buchanan RW, Kirkpatrick B, Bryant N, Ball P, Breier A. Fluoxetine augmentation of clozapine treatment in patients with schizophrenia. Am J Psychiatry. 1996;153(12):1625–7.
88. Rahman MS, Grace JJ, Pato MT, Priest B. Sertraline in the treatment of clozapine-induced obsessive-compulsive behavior. Am J Psychiatry. 1998;155(11):1629–30.
89. Allen L, Tejera C. Treatment of clozapine-induced obsessive-compulsive symptoms with sertraline. Am J Psychiatry. 1994;151(7):1096–7.
90. Taylor D, Ellison Z, Ementon Shaw L, Wickham H, Murray R. Co-administration of citalopram and clozapine: effect on plasma clozapine levels. Int Clin Psychopharmacol. 1998;13(1):19–21.
91. Cupina D, Boulton M. Secondary delusional parasitosis treated successfully with a combination of clozapine and citalopram. Psychosomatics. 2012;53(3):301–2.
92. Gambi F, De Berardis D, Campanella D, Carano A, Sepede G, Salini G, et al. Mirtazapine treatment of generalized anxiety disorder: a fixed dose, open label study. J Psychopharmacol. 2005;19(5):483–7.
93. Gambi F, De Berardis D, Sepede G, Campanella D, Galliani N, Carano A, et al. Effect of mirtazapine on thyroid hormones in adult patients with major depression. Int J Immunopathol Pharmacol. 2005;18(4):737–44.
94. Benjamin S, Doraiswamy PM. Review of the use of mirtazapine in the treatment of depression. Expert Opin Pharmacother. 2011;12(10):1623–32.
95. Zoccali R, Muscatello MR, Torre DL, Malara G, Canale A, Crucitti D, et al. Lack of a pharmacokinetic interaction between mirtazapine and the newer antipsychotics clozapine, risperidone and olanzapine in patients with chronic schizophrenia. Pharmacol Res. 2003;48(4):411–4.
96. Zoccali R, Muscatello MR, Cedro C, Neri P, La Torre D, Spina E, et al. The effect of mirtazapine augmentation of clozapine in the treatment of negative symptoms of schizophrenia: a double-blind, placebo-controlled study. Int Clin Psychopharmacol. 2004;19(2):71–6.
97. Delle Chiaie R, Salviati M, Fiorentini S, Biondi M. Add-on mirtazapine enhances effects on cognition in schizophrenic patients under stabilized treatment with clozapine. Exp Clin Psychopharmacol. 2007;15(6):563–8.
98. Sahli C, Bryois C. Psychotropics and weight gain. Praxis (Bern 1994). 2004;93(35):1393–401.
99. Carano A, De Berardis D, Gambi F, Salerno MR, Campanella D, Castrovilli M, et al. Psychopathologic patterns in obesity. Ann Ital Chir. 2005;76(5):461–4.
100. Repo-Tiihonen E, Eloranta A, Hallikainen T, Tiihonen J. Effects of venlafaxine treatment on clozapine plasma levels in schizophrenic patients. Neuropsychobiology. 2005;51(4):173–6.
101. Mico U, Bruno A, Pandolfo G, Maria Romeo V, Mallamace D, D'Arrigo C, et al. Duloxetine as adjunctive treatment to clozapine in patients with schizophrenia: a randomized, placebo-controlled trial. Int Clin Psychopharmacol. 2011;26(6):303–10.
102. Smith T, Riskin J. Effect of clozapine on plasma nortriptyline concentration. Pharmacopsychiatry. 1994;27(1):41–2.
103. Biondi M, Fedele L, Arcangeli T, Pancheri P. Development of obsessive-compulsive symptoms during clozapine treatment in schizophrenia and its positive response to clomipramine. Psychother Psychosom. 1999;68(2):111–2.

104. Sinha S, Simlai J, Praharaj SK. Very low dose amitriptyline for clozapine-associated Sialorrhea. Curr Drug Saf. 2016;11(3):262–3.
105. Bastiampillai T, Gupta A, Allison S, Chan SK. NICE guidance: why not clozapine for treatment-refractory bipolar disorder? Lancet Psychiatry. 2016;3(6):502–3.
106. Li XB, Tang YL, Wang CY, de Leon J. Clozapine for treatment-resistant bipolar disorder: a systematic review. Bipolar Disord. 2015;17(3):235–47.
107. Chang JS, Ha KS, Young Lee K, Sik Kim Y, Min Ahn Y. The effects of long-term clozapine add-on therapy on the rehospitalization rate and the mood polarity patterns in bipolar disorders. J Clin Psychiatry. 2006;67(3):461–7.
108. Bender S, Linka T, Wolstein J, Gehendges S, Paulus HJ, Schall U, et al. Safety and efficacy of combined clozapine-lithium pharmacotherapy. Int J Neuropsychopharmacol. 2004;7(1):59–63.
109. Dembowski C, Rechlin T. Successful antimanic treatment and mood stabilization with lamotrigine, clozapine, and valproate in a bipolar patient after lithium-induced cerebellar deterioration. A case report. Pharmacopsychiatry. 2003;36(2):83–6.
110. Mattai A, Fung L, Bakalar J, Overman G, Tossell J, Miller R, et al. Adjunctive use of lithium carbonate for the management of neutropenia in clozapine-treated children. Hum Psychopharmacol. 2009;24(7):584–9.
111. Pinninti NR, Houdart MP, Strouse EM. Case report of long-term lithium for treatment and prevention of clozapine-induced neutropenia in an African American male. J Clin Psychopharmacol. 2010;30(2):219–21.
112. Kelly DL, Conley RR, Feldman S, Yu Y, McMahon RP, Richardson CM. Adjunct divalproex or lithium to clozapine in treatment-resistant schizophrenia. Psychiatry Q. 2006;77(1):81–95.
113. Small JG, Klapper MH, Malloy FW, Steadman TM. Tolerability and efficacy of clozapine combined with lithium in schizophrenia and schizoaffective disorder. J Clin Psychopharmacol. 2003;23(3):223–8.
114. Foster R, Olajide D. A case of clozapine-induced tonic-clonic seizures managed with valproate: implications for clinical care. J Psychopharmacol. 2005;19(1):93–6.
115. Balen RM, Procyshyn RM. Valproic acid for seizure prophylaxis during clozapine therapy: where's the evidence? Int J Psychiatry Clin Pract. 1999;3(4):249–51.
116. Suzuki T, Uchida H, Takeuchi H, Nakajima S, Nomura K, Tanabe A, et al. Augmentation of atypical antipsychotics with valproic acid. An open-label study for most difficult patients with schizophrenia. Hum Psychopharmacol. 2009;24(8):628–38.
117. Horowitz E, Bergman LC, Ashkenazy C, Moscona-Hurvitz I, Grinvald-Fogel H, Magnezi R. Off-label use of sodium valproate for schizophrenia. PLoS One. 2014;9(3):e92573.
118. Citrome L, Casey DE, Daniel DG, Wozniak P, Kochan LD, Tracy KA. Adjunctive divalproex and hostility among patients with schizophrenia receiving olanzapine or risperidone. Psychiatr Serv. 2004;55(3):290–4.
119. Centorrino F, Baldessarini RJ, Kando J, Frankenburg FR, Volpicelli SA, Puopolo PR, et al. Serum concentrations of clozapine and its major metabolites: effects of cotreatment with fluoxetine or valproate. Am J Psychiatry. 1994;151(1):123–5.
120. Facciola G, Avenoso A, Scordo MG, Madia AG, Ventimiglia A, Perucca E, et al. Small effects of valproic acid on the plasma concentrations of clozapine and its major metabolites in patients with schizophrenic or affective disorders. Ther Drug Monit. 1999;21(3):341–5.
121. Kando JC, Tohen M, Castillo J, Centorrino F. Concurrent use of clozapine and valproate in affective and psychotic disorders. J Clin Psychiatry. 1994;55(6):255–7.
122. Malik S, Lally J, Ajnakina O, Pritchard M, Krivoy A, Gaughran F, et al. Sodium valproate and clozapine induced neutropenia: a case control study using register data. Schizophr Res. 2018;195:267–73.
123. Pantelis C, Adesanya A. Increased risk of neutropaenia and agranulocytosis with sodium valproate used adjunctively with clozapine. Aust N Z J Psychiatry. 2001;35(4):544–5.
124. De Berardis D, Campanella D, Serroni N, Rapini G, Olivieri L, Fornaro M, et al. Clozapine-related pericarditis during titration phase in a patient with resistant schizophrenia and concomitant valproate treatment: a case report. J Clin Psychopharmacol. 2014;34(5):649–51.
125. Ronaldson KJ, Fitzgerald PB, Taylor AJ, Topliss DJ, Wolfe R, McNeil JJ. Rapid clozapine dose titration and concomitant sodium valproate increase the risk of myocarditis with clozapine: a case-control study. Schizophr Res. 2012;141(2–3):173–8.
126. Migliardi G, D'Arrigo C, Santoro V, Bruno A, Cortese L, Campolo D, et al. Effect of topiramate on plasma concentrations of clozapine, olanzapine, risperidone, and quetiapine in patients with psychotic disorders. Clin Neuropharmacol. 2007;30(2):107–13.
127. Dursun SM, Devarajan S. Clozapine weight gain, plus topiramate weight loss. Can J Psychiatry. 2000;45(2):198.
128. Greg Deardorff O, Syed A, Ames CJ, Yaeger JS. Ranitidine, metformin, and topiramate: managing weight gain in a clozapine-treated patient with schizoaffective disorder. Prim Care Companion CNS Disord. 2014;16(3). PCC.13/01598.
129. Navarro V, Pons A, Romero A, Bernardo M. Topiramate for clozapine-induced seizures. Am J Psychiatry. 2001;158(6):968–9.
130. Hahn MK, Remington G, Bois D, Cohn T. Topiramate augmentation in clozapine-treated patients with schizophrenia: clinical and metabolic effects. J Clin Psychopharmacol. 2010;30(6):706–10.

131. Muscatello MR, Bruno A, Pandolfo G, Mico U, Bellinghieri PM, Scimeca G, et al. Topiramate augmentation of clozapine in schizophrenia: a double-blind, placebo-controlled study. J Psychopharmacol. 2011;25(5):667–74.
132. Goff DC. Review: lamotrigine may be an effective treatment for clozapine resistant schizophrenia. Evid Based Ment Health. 2009;12(4):111.
133. Kalyoncu A, Mirsal H, Pektas O, Unsalan N, Tan D, Beyazyurek M. Use of lamotrigine to augment clozapine in patients with resistant schizophrenia and comorbid alcohol dependence: a potent anti-craving effect? J Psychopharmacol. 2005;19(3):301–5.
134. Tiihonen J, Wahlbeck K, Kiviniemi V. The efficacy of lamotrigine in clozapine-resistant schizophrenia: a systematic review and metaanalysis. Schizophr Res. 2009;109(1–3):10–4.
135. Vayisoglu S, Anil Yagcioglu AE, Yagcioglu S, Karahan S, Karci O, Gurel SC, et al. Lamotrigine augmentation in patients with schizophrenia who show partial response to clozapine treatment. Schizophr Res. 2013;143(1):207–14.
136. Urban AE, Wiglusz MS, Cubala WJ, Landowski J, Krysta K. Rapid-onset agranulocytosis in a patient treated with clozapine and lamotrigine. Psychiatr Danub. 2015;27(Suppl 1):S459–61.
137. Egger C, Muehlbacher M, Grohmann R, Stuppaeck C. Clozapine intoxication in a patient with lamotrigine-induced rash. Pharmacopsychiatry. 2010;43(1):35–6.
138. Tourian L, Margolese HC. Late-onset agranulocytosis in a patient treated with clozapine and lamotrigine. J Clin Psychopharmacol. 2011;31(5):665–7.
139. Risch SC, Horner MD, McGurk SR, Palecko S, Markowitz JS, Nahas Z, et al. Double-blind donepezil-placebo crossover augmentation study of atypical antipsychotics in chronic, stable schizophrenia: a pilot study. Schizophr Res. 2007;93(1–3):131–5.
140. Stryjer R, Strous R, Bar F, Shaked G, Shiloh R, Rozencwaig S, et al. Donepezil augmentation of clozapine monotherapy in schizophrenia patients: a double blind cross-over study. Hum Psychopharmacol. 2004;19(5):343–6.
141. Bora E, Veznedaroglu B, Kayahan B. The effect of galantamine added to clozapine on cognition of five patients with schizophrenia. Clin Neuropharmacol. 2005;28(3):139–41.
142. Kishi T, Matsuda Y, Iwata N. Memantine add-on to antipsychotic treatment for residual negative and cognitive symptoms of schizophrenia: a meta-analysis. Psychopharmacology. 2017;234(14):2113–25.
143. Thomas C, Carroll BT, Maley RT, Jayanti K, Koduri A. Memantine and catatonic schizophrenia. Am J Psychiatry. 2005;162(3):626.
144. Veerman S, Schulte P, de Haan L. Memantine add-on to clozapine treatment for residual negative symptoms of schizophrenia. Psychopharmacology. 2017;234(23–24):3535–6.
145. de Lucena D, Fernandes BS, Berk M, Dodd S, Medeiros DW, Pedrini M, et al. Improvement of negative and positive symptoms in treatment-refractory schizophrenia: a double-blind, randomized, placebo-controlled trial with memantine as add-on therapy to clozapine. J Clin Psychiatry. 2009;70(10):1416–23.
146. Veerman SR, Schulte PF, Smith JD, de Haan L. Memantine augmentation in clozapine-refractory schizophrenia: a randomized, doubleblind, placebo-controlled crossover study. Psychol Med. 2016;46(9):1909–21.
147. Veerman SR, Schulte PF, Deijen JB, de Haan L. Adjunctive memantine in clozapine-treated refractory schizophrenia: an open-label 1-year extension study. Psychol Med. 2017;47(2):363–75.
148. Seddigh R, Azarnik S, Keshavarz-Akhlaghi AA. Levothyroxine augmentation in clozapine resistant schizophrenia: a case report and review. Case Rep Psychiatry. 2015;2015:678040.
149. Lin CH, Lin CH, Chang YC, Huang YJ, Chen PW, Yang HT, et al. Sodium benzoate, a D-amino acid oxidase inhibitor, added to clozapine for the treatment of schizophrenia: a randomized, double-blind, placebo-controlled trial. Biol Psychiatry. 2018;84(6):422–32.
150. Qurashi I, Collins JD, Chaudhry IB, Husain N. Promising use of minocycline augmentation with clozapine in treatment-resistant schizophrenia. J Psychopharmacol. 2014;28(7):707–8.
151. Marini S, De Berardis D, Vellante F, Santacroce R, Orsolini L, Valchera A, et al. Celecoxib adjunctive treatment to antipsychotics in schizophrenia: a review of randomized clinical add-on trials. Mediat Inflamm. 2016;2016:3476240.
152. Muscatello MR, Bruno A, De Fazio P, Segura-Garcia C, Pandolfo G, Zoccali R. Augmentation strategies in partial responder and/or treatment-resistant schizophrenia patients treated with clozapine. Expert Opin Pharmacother. 2014;15(16):2329–45.
153. Behdani F, Roudbaraki SN, Saberi-Karimian M, Tayefi M, Hebrani P, Akhavanrezayat A, et al. Assessment of the efficacy of omega-3 fatty acids on metabolic and inflammatory parameters in patients with schizophrenia taking clozapine and sodium valproate. Psychiatry Res. 2018;261:243–7.
154. Peet M, Horrobin DF. Group EEMS. A dose-ranging exploratory study of the effects of ethyl-eicosapentaenoate in patients with persistent schizophrenic symptoms. J Psychiatr Res. 2002;36(1):7–18.
155. Caniato RN, Alvarenga ME, Garcia-Alcaraz MA. Effect of omega-3 fatty acids on the lipid profile of patients taking clozapine. Aust N Z J Psychiatry. 2006;40(8):691–7.
156. Emsley R, Myburgh C, Oosthuizen P, van Rensburg SJ. Randomized, placebo-controlled study of ethyl-eicosapentaenoic acid as supplemental treatment in schizophrenia. Am J Psychiatry. 2002;159(9):1596–8.

157. Fenton WS, Dickerson F, Boronow J, Hibbeln JR, Knable M. A placebo-controlled trial of omega-3 fatty acid (ethyl eicosapentaenoic acid) supplementation for residual symptoms and cognitive impairment in schizophrenia. Am J Psychiatry. 2001;158(12):2071–4.
158. Zhang L, Zhao J. Profile of minocycline and its potential in the treatment of schizophrenia. Neuropsychiatr Dis Treat. 2014;10:1103–11.
159. Orsolini L, Sarchione F, Vellante F, Fornaro M, Matarazzo I, Martinotti G, et al. Protein-C reactive as biomarker predictor of schizophrenia phases of illness? A systematic review. Curr Neuropharmacol. 2018;16:583–606.
160. Martinotti G, Di Iorio G, Marini S, Ricci V, De Berardis D, Di Giannantonio M. Nerve growth factor and brain-derived neurotrophic factor concentrations in schizophrenia: a review. J Biol Regul Homeost Agents. 2012;26(3):347–56.
161. Kelly DL, Vyas G, Richardson CM, Koola M, McMahon RP, Buchanan RW, et al. Adjunct minocycline to clozapine treated patients with persistent schizophrenia symptoms. Schizophr Res. 2011;133(1–3):257–8.
162. Kelly DL, Sullivan KM, McEvoy JP, McMahon RP, Wehring HJ, Gold JM, et al. Adjunctive minocycline in clozapine-treated schizophrenia patients with persistent symptoms. J Clin Psychopharmacol. 2015;35(4):374–81.
163. Wehring HJ, Elsobky T, McEvoy JP, Vyas G, Richardson CM, McMahon RP, et al. Adjunctive minocycline in clozapine-treated patients with schizophrenia: analyzing the effects of minocycline on clozapine plasma levels. Psychiatry Q. 2018;89(1):73–80.
164. Diaz P, Bhaskara S, Dursun SM, Deakin B. Double-blind, placebo-controlled, crossover trial of clozapine plus glycine in refractory schizophrenia negative results. J Clin Psychopharmacol. 2005;25(3):277–8.
165. Evins AE, Fitzgerald SM, Wine L, Rosselli R, Goff DC. Placebo-controlled trial of glycine added to clozapine in schizophrenia. Am J Psychiatry. 2000;157(5):826–8.
166. Javitt DC, Silipo G, Cienfuegos A, Shelley AM, Bark N, Park M, et al. Adjunctive high-dose glycine in the treatment of schizophrenia. Int J Neuropsychopharmacol. 2001;4(4):385–91.
167. Doruk A, Uzun O, Ozsahin A. A placebo-controlled study of extract of ginkgo biloba added to clozapine in patients with treatment-resistant schizophrenia. Int Clin Psychopharmacol. 2008;23(4):223–7.
168. Sanghani SN, Petrides G, Kellner CH. Electroconvulsive therapy (ECT) in schizophrenia: a review of recent literature. Curr Opin Psychiatry. 2018;31:213–22.
169. Rosenquist PB, Miller B, Pillai A. The antipsychotic effects of ECT: a review of possible mechanisms. J ECT. 2014;30(2):125–31.
170. Ahmed S, Khan AM, Mekala HM, Venigalla H, Ahmed R, Etman A, et al. Combined use of electroconvulsive therapy and antipsychotics (both clozapine and non-clozapine) in treatment resistant schizophrenia: a comparative meta-analysis. Heliyon. 2017;3(11):e00429.
171. Zheng W, Cao XL, Ungvari GS, Xiang YQ, Guo T, Liu ZR, et al. Electroconvulsive therapy added to non-clozapine antipsychotic medication for treatment resistant schizophrenia: meta-analysis of randomized controlled trials. PLoS One. 2016;11(6):e0156510.
172. Klapheke MM. Clozapine, ECT, and schizoaffective disorder, bipolar type. Convuls Ther. 1991;7(1):36–9.
173. Safferman AZ, Munne R. Combining clozapine with ECT. Convuls Ther. 1992;8(2):141–3.
174. Green AI, Zalma A, Berman I, DuRand CJ, Salzman C. Clozapine following ECT: a two-step treatment. J Clin Psychiatry. 1994;55(9):388–90.
175. Benatov R, Sirota P, Megged S. Neuroleptic-resistant schizophrenia treated with clozapine and ECT. Convuls Ther. 1996;12(2):117–21.
176. Grover S, Hazari N, Kate N. Combined use of clozapine and ECT: a review. Acta Neuropsychiatr. 2015;27(3):131–42.
177. Cardwell BA, Nakai B. Seizure activity in combined clozapine and ECT: a retrospective view. Convuls Ther. 1995;11(2):110–3.
178. Tang WK, Ungvari GS. Efficacy of electroconvulsive therapy combined with antipsychotic medication in treatment-resistant schizophrenia: a prospective, open trial. J ECT. 2002;18(2):90–4.
179. Tang WK, Ungvari GS. Efficacy of electroconvulsive therapy in treatment-resistant schizophrenia: a prospective open trial. Prog Neuro-Psychopharmacol Biol Psychiatry. 2003;27(3):373–9.
180. Kho KH, Blansjaar BA, de Vries S, Babuskova D, Zwinderman AH, Linszen DH. Electroconvulsive therapy for the treatment of clozapine nonresponders suffering from schizophrenia – an open label study. Eur Arch Psychiatry Clin Neurosci. 2004;254(6):372–9.
181. Masoudzadeh A, Khalilian AR. Comparative study of clozapine, electroshock and the combination of ECT with clozapine in treatmentresistant schizophrenic patients. Pak J Biol Sci. 2007;10(23): 4287–90.
182. Petrides G, Malur C, Braga RJ, Bailine SH, Schooler NR, Malhotra AK, et al. Electroconvulsive therapy augmentation in clozapine-resistant schizophrenia: a prospective, randomized study. Am J Psychiatry. 2015;172(1):52–8.
183. Kim HS, Kim SH, Lee NY, Youn T, Lee JH, Chung S, et al. Effectiveness of electroconvulsive therapy augmentation on clozapine-resistant schizophrenia. Psychiatry Investig. 2017;14(1):58–62.
184. Cotovio G, Velosa A, Oliveira-Maia AJ, Barahona-Correa B. Clozapine-resistant schizophrenia treated

with ultra-brief pulse, unilateral electroconvulsive therapy. J ECT. 2017;33(1):e3–4.
185. Grover S, Chakrabarti S, Hazari N, Avasthi A. Effectiveness of electroconvulsive therapy in patients with treatment resistant schizophrenia: a retrospective study. Psychiatry Res. 2017;249: 349–53.
186. Kales HC, Dequardo JR, Tandon R. Combined electroconvulsive therapy and clozapine in treatment-resistant schizophrenia. Prog Neuro-Psychopharmacol Biol Psychiatry. 1999;23(3):547–56.
187. Remington G, Saha A, Chong SA, Shammi C. Augmentation strategies in clozapine-resistant schizophrenia. CNS Drugs. 2005;19(10):843–72.
188. Barber S, Olotu U, Corsi M, Cipriani A. Clozapine combined with different antipsychotic drugs for treatment-resistant schizophrenia. Cochrane Database Syst Rev. 2017;3:CD006324.
189. Barnes TR, McEvedy CJ, Nelson HE. Management of treatment resistant schizophrenia unresponsive to clozapine. Br J Psychiatry Suppl. 1996;31: 31–40.

24 Fecal Microbiota Transplantation in the Treatment-Resistant Psychiatric Disorders

Alper Evrensel and Mehmet Emin Ceylan

24.1 Introduction

Humans are not only created by eukaryotic cells. Prokaryotic microorganisms are colonized almost in every part of the human body [1]. These prokaryotes are in a commensal and cooperative relationship with human organ systems [2]. These communities of microorganisms living in various parts of the body are called microbiota [3]. Recent studies have revealed that the brain is also not sterile and there is a living brain microbiota [4]. The microorganism colonization is most commonly found in intestines, and it is called gut microbiota [5]. 3.8×10^{13} (380 trillion) prokaryotic cells live in human intestines. This number is ten times higher than the number of eukaryotic cells in an adult [6]. The intestinal microorganisms are not only numerically superior but also contain 150 times more genes than the number of genes in a human DNA [7].

The bidirectional relationship between gut and brain microbiota has been indicated by numerous preclinical and clinical studies [8]. Commensal microorganisms maintain the health of the human body. Microbial imbalance (dysbiosis) may cause the formation of psychiatric disorders [9]. Dysbiosis can be repaired through dietary regimens, probiotics, prebiotics, and FMT. FMT is made by the transfer of feces from a healthy donor to the intestines of the patient for restoration of gut microbiota composition [10]. Although there are plenty of clinical studies about FMT, we can state that it has possible treatment potential in psychiatric disorders.

24.2 Potential Role of the Gut Microbiota in Psychiatric Disorders

The Nobel Prize-winning Russian scientist Elie Metchnikoff was the first who has mentioned about the importance of gut microbiota for human health [11]. A hundred years after Metchnikoff, today, we have well understood the connection between microbiota and the human body in detail. The immune system plays a key role in this relationship [12].

The effect of microorganisms on the immune system begins in the intrauterine period [13]. Toll-like receptors (TLRs) on the intestinal epithelial cells constitute the first step of cytokine production [14, 15]. Gut microorganisms are in interaction with TLRs [16–18]. When the intestinal permeability is impaired, bacterial lipopolysaccharides leak into the bloodstream. Toll-like receptor stimuli increase the production of inflammatory cytokines [19]. Neuroinflammation may play a role in the etiopathogenesis of depression [20, 21]. The depression caused by inflammatory

A. Evrensel (✉) · M. E. Ceylan
Department of Psychiatry, Uskudar University, Istanbul, Turkey

Y.-K. Kim (ed.), *Treatment Resistance in Psychiatry*, https://doi.org/10.1007/978-981-10-4358-1_24

cytokines can be prevented by antidepressant drugs [22, 23]. Antidepressants have anti-inflammatory activity [24]. Probiotic bacteria, like antidepressants, also exhibit an anti-inflammatory effect by increasing interleukin-10 (IL-10) levels [25]. Injection of Lactobacillus GG (a probiotic bacterium) to experimental animals increases plasma IL-10 levels [26]. The effects of changes in the microbiota composition in the postnatal period may last lifelong [27]. Dendritic cells, which are a group of cells in the immune system of the intestinal tract, absorb the bacteria and their metabolites in the intestinal lumen into its cytoplasm by touching them. Bacterial metabolites and nucleic acids can thus reach the brain via systemic circulation [28].

Intestinal epithelium constitutes the largest mucosa in the body. Its surface area is almost equal to the size of a tennis court (approximately 260–300 m^2) [29]. The intestinal mucosa provides the absorption of nutrients as well as setting a physical barrier between the bacteria and the host. This barrier is formed by tight junction proteins and mucus layer [30]. The change in the microbiota composition can cause micro damages in the intestinal epithelium wall. The leakage of microorganism-derived endotoxins (lipopolysaccharides and peptidoglycans) into the systemic circulation is called "leaky gut" [9, 31].

The leaky gut hypothesis was first expressed by Jakop Fine in 1955, and it has been suspected for long time [32]. It has been later revealed in animal experiments that bacterial-borne endotoxins are passed into the systemic bloodstream as a result of deterioration in intestinal permeability [33]. As a result, an immunological reaction may occur [34].

If the mother gives birth through vaginal route, the baby is colonized with the dominant bacteria in the mother's vaginal flora (*Lactobacillus* and *Prevotella* species) [35]. If the baby is born with Caesarean section, the bacteria living in the mother's skin flora (*Staphylococcus* and *Corynebacterium* species) move to the intestinal microbiota of the newborn [36]. The incidence of allergic diseases is higher in the children born through Caesarean section than the children who are born by vaginal [37].

This situation that the baby is exposed on the first day of life may have a lifelong impact on the infant's health and growth [8]. Intestinal microbiota of the children delivered by Caesarean section can be repaired by application of the mother's vaginal flora into the baby's mouth [35].

Antibiotics are one of the most important factors that change the microbiota composition of the body. Antibiotics use in the first year of life may carry the risk of developing depression in adulthood [38]. In an experiment, it has been observed that anxiety-like behaviors decreased after 7 days of vancomycin application to rats. However, this effect disappears 2 weeks after the intestinal bacterial composition returns to its original state [39]. Yet, the long-term use of broad-spectrum antibiotics leads to a permanent compositional change on the gut microbiota, which may continue for a long time [40].

Depression-like behaviors are observed in germ-free mice [39]. Still, germ-free mice have got lower scores in anxiety tests compared to conventional mice [41]. Microbiota has an effect on amygdala functions and fear response [42]. The presence and absence of gut bacteria and its bacterial composition play a significant role in brain functions from the first day of life [43].

24.3 FMT as a Restorer of Microbiota Dysbiosis

Dysbiosis, which occurs in the microbiota due to the causes such as nutrition, antibiotic use, stress, and aging, can be restored through FMT [44, 45]. The main purpose of FMT is to restore the dysfunction in the intestines with a healthy bacterial flora transplantation [46].

24.3.1 History of FMT

The first known FMT was applied in China 1700 years ago [47]. The feces suspension called "yellow soup" has been orally ingested in cases of diarrhea and food poisoning. We do not know with which knowledge Chinese physician Ge Hong applied this remedy. It may have been used for emetic and purgative purposes in food poisoning [48]. There is no record found in the medical texts about the application of FMT in the following centuries after Ge Hong. Another traditional Chinese physician Li Shizhen applied FMT for the treatment of gastrointestinal complaints such as constipation, diarrhea, and vomiting in the sixteenth century [47]. Two centuries after Li Shizhen, Italian anatomist Fabricius Aquapendente used the fecal suspension with the name of "transfaunation" in the treatment of animals [49]. We know that German soldiers had used camel stool in treatment of bacterial dysentery upon the suggestions of Bedouins during the Second World War in Africa [50].

24.3.2 Main Application Area of FMT

FMT was first applied in modern medicine in 1958. Four cases of pseudomembranous enterocolitis caused by *Clostridium difficile* have been successfully treated by fecal transplantation [51]. Second series of *Clostridium difficile* infection (CDI) cases treated with FMT has been reported in 1981 [52]. Following these publications, an in-depth investigation of FMT was carried out, and its effect mechanism was better understood. Today, we have strong evidence about the effectiveness of FMT in recurrent CDI cases. FMT is effective in treatment of recurrent CDI and inflammatory bowel diseases [53]. There are no randomized controlled studies about the use of FMT in treatment of psychiatric disorders. In this respect, animal experiments are promising [54].

24.3.3 Application of FMT

FMT is applied according to the Amsterdam protocol [50]. Ethical conditions must be fulfilled before its application [55]. In the past, stool sample was used to be taken from a healthy person in the immediate circle of the patient. In the last 5 years, it has been suggested to be taken from a feces bank. Stool banks use fresh feces donated by reliable and healthy donors who often have some medical screenings [56]. Donors should be following a healthy diet, get no medication, and have a healthy lifestyle by paying attention to their physical health [50].

The transfer material should be between 150 and 250 g. Stool should be taken immediately before FMT and should be fresh [50]. FMT may induce defecation reflex by causing irritation in the intestines of the patient. However, for the process to be successful, the transplanted feces must remain in the intestines of the recipient for at least 4 h. For this purpose, an antidiarrheal drug called lopermid is given before FMT [45, 57].

Before FMT, fecal suspension should be prepared. The stool can be diluted with water, physiological saline, or milk. The fecal suspension is cleaned from solid particles through filtering and is transferred to 60 ml syringes [44, 50]. The ideal method of preparing the stool suspension has not yet been specified. When diluted with physiological saline, feces were found to have a lower success rate compared to the dilution with water. It is argued that when the electrical mixer is used, the oxygen that was mixed into the suspension decreases the number of anaerobic bacteria, and thus the effectiveness of the treatment is reduced [50].

The fecal suspension can be applied to the patient in two routes. It can be delivered to the upper gastrointestinal tract via esophagogastroduodenoscopy or nasogastric tube. It can be delivered to the lower gastrointestinal tract by colonoscopy [45]. In 3/4 of the cases, colonoscopy was used, and esophagogastroduodenoscopy was used in 1/4 of the cases [58]. This proportion may be the result of patients' demands because some of the patients do not prefer FMT. Women are more reluctant than men, and young people are more reluctant than old people. Colonoscopy is rather preferred by many patients. A third of the patients think that this operation should be free [59].

FMT may be rarely implemented because of its unlikeable aspects for the patient. In cases when the transfer needs to be urgently done, the donor's health screenings may take time and FMT may be delayed. For this reason, an alternative method to FMT has been tried [60]. The sample of stool was put in the swallowable capsules after it has been centrifuged. Capsules were stored at

−80°. They were administered to the patients through per-oral route 15 times a day for 2 days. In 70% of the cases, complete remission was achieved after 3 days, and the same procedure was repeated once more to the rest of cases [61]. Oral administration is a noninvasive and more comfortable method. It can be predicted that its use will be spread and will be utilized to restore intestinal microbiota after antibiotic treatments in the future [62].

24.4 FMT as a Treatment Method in Treatment-Resistant Psychiatric Disorders

FMT has been searched mostly in CDI. The use of antibiotics can result in dysbiosis and *Clostridium difficile* can become dominant in the microbiota. FMT repairs the damaged bacterial flora [63]. FMT may be a promising method in treatment-resistant psychiatric disorders.

The relationship between depression and microbiota has currently become quite visible [5]. Animal models of depression are obtained through administration of bacterial lipopolysaccharide [64]. Positive changes have been observed in immune parameters after intestinal microbiota repair in many animal experiments. In one of the experiments, the level of IL-10 increased after the supplementation of probiotic bacteria in germ-free mouse [65]. In another experiment with a germ-free mouse, *Bifidobacterium infantis* reduced the anxiety and depression scores [66]. *Bifidobacterium infantis* has been described as a "psychobiotic bacterium" because of its antidepressant-like effect [16]. Probiotic bacteria such as *Bifidobacterium longum* and *Lactobacillus helveticus* have reduced anxiety scores in rats [67]. In a RCT performed on healthy volunteers, experiment subjects were given *Lactobacillus helveticus* and *Bifidobacterium longum* or placebo during a month. Anxiety scores and the levels of anxiety-related blood parameters reduced in the subjects who had taken probiotic bacteria [68]. In an experiment conducted by Bruce-Keller and colleagues. FMT has been administered from the rats fed on a high fat diet to the rats fed on a normal diet. Leaky gut syndrome, neuroinflammation, and behavioral disorders were detected in rats fed on a normal diet following FMT [69].

In an animal experiment, autistic behavior of the rats has been reduced after given *Bacteroides fragilis* (a probiotic bacteria). *Bacteroides fragilis* has repaired the gut and reduced the leakage [70]. In one of the studies conducted on fecal specimens, the stool of autistic children indicated more *Clostridium* species [71, 72]. It has been reported that autistic symptoms retrograded in two children who were applied FMT and in five autistic children who were given bacteroides [58].

In a study comparing the fecal microbiota analysis of 28 cases of first episode psychosis and 16 healthy individuals, a significant difference has been detected between two groups in terms of Lactobacillus levels. This difference also correlates with severity of the symptom and treatment [73]. In another study designed in a similar way, Jiang and colleagues compared the fecal microbiota analysis of 46 depressed patients and 30 healthy individuals. Bacteroides, Proteobacteria, and Actinobacteria levels were higher, and Firmicutes levels were lower in the depressed patients. These results have been interpreted as the increase of harmful bacteria groups and the decrease of beneficial bacteria in depressed patients [74]. In a recently published meta-analysis, it has been concluded that probiotic bacteria are effective in treatment of the depression [75]. The intestinal microbiota composition of depressed patients may be modulated by FMT as well as through probiotics. In the experiment of Zheng et al., FMT was applied to the germ-free mice from depressed patients. Depression-like behaviors were observed in mice after FMT [54]. If the depression can be transmitted through FMT, can the treatment be also transferred? We have hoped to give a positive answer to this question.

The microbiota composition changes with age, and as a result, cognitive inefficiency may arise [11]. The western diet may also disrupt the microbiota composition. The resulting dysbiosis may lead to hippocampal dysfunction and cognitive impairment [76]. *Bifidobacterium longum* 1714 has been found to reduce stress and to have a positive effect on the memory in healthy individuals [77]. However, in a RCT that the same researchers performed on healthy individuals in the following year, the application of *Lactobacillus rhamnosus* (a probiotic bacterium) was not superior to the placebo with regard to its effects on anxiety, stress-related measures, HPA response, and cognitive performance [78]. Nevertheless, the number of publications has been increasing, which suggests that leaky gut and bacterial LPS-induced neuroinflammation are the etiopathogenesis of Alzheimer's disease [79].

Another factor that disrupts the intestinal permeability and cause dysbiosis is the chronic alcohol use. Probiotics may be useful in treatment of alcohol addiction by restoring the intestinal tract [80]. It is also possible to make the same prediction for FMT.

In the light of these studies, the potential use of FMT in treatment resistant psychiatric disorders emerges through the restoration of impaired gut microbiota.

24.5 Reliability and Side Effects

Basic indications for the use of FMT are CDI and inflammatory bowel diseases such as Crohn's disease and ulcerative colitis. Although the overall medical condition of the patients who had stool transplantation is quite bad, FMT is a reliable practice. Diarrhea, constipation, gas, and abdominal pain can be observed in the day of FMT application even though it is rare [50]. In a series of 317 cases, enteritis, bleeding, and peritonitis were reported only in 3 cases [81]. Exacerbation of colitis has been reported in one case [82]. Posttransplant peritonitis has caused the death of a case [83]. Brandt et al. have not reported any side effect in long-term follow-up study [53].

Although the history of the FMT goes seventeen centuries back, its use has increased in the last 30–40 years. For this reason, there are many uncertainties about it [84].

It is not known how and through which illness the gut microbiota composition changes. Even though it is easier and cheaper, it is riskier to take the transplanted stool from the donor. For this reason, the production of probiotic bacteria in culture may be suggested. It is not known whether the feces obtained from the stool bank is different from the fresh stool in terms of activity. The use of water, saline, or milk in dilution of feces may have different consequences on the efficacy of treatment. It may be appropriate to use different diluter for each indication. There is no consensus about how many grams the ideal stool should be. It is necessary to determine whether the transplantation is more effective by oral route or anal route. The changes in the immune and metabolic system in short and long term after FMT should be revealed in detail. No serious risk has been reported in patients with poor physical health. However, possible risks of FMT that may be encountered when it is applied with psychiatric indications are not yet known. Large-scale case series and RCTs are required in order to determine these risks and illuminate the unknown points.

Conclusion

The composition of healthy gut microbiota may change due to nutrition, medications (antibiotics, antidepressants), and stress. Change in the composition of microbiota can lead to various metabolic and immunological problems. The microbiota composition can be restored using FMT and probiotic bacteria. FMT is a life-saving, easily applicable and reliable treatment method for recurrent CDI and inflammatory bowel diseases. Positive results have been reported in the treatment of metabolic, immunologic, and neuropsychiatric disorders that are accompanied by intestinal permeability. In this respect, preclinical studies are promising. It carries the potential to be effective in treatment-resistant disorders that do not respond to the classical psychiatric treatment methods. It seems that this potential will be clearly understood in the next decade.

References

1. Rieder R, Wisniewski PJ, Alderman BL, Campbell SC. Microbes and mental health: a review. Brain Behav Immun. 2017;66:9–17.
2. Dinan TG, Stilling RM, Stanton C, Cryan JF. Collective unconscious: how gut microbes shape human behavior. J Psychiatr Res. 2015;63:1–9.

3. Khanna S, Tosh PK. A clinician's primer on the role of the microbiome in human health and disease. Mayo Clin Proc. 2014;89(1):107–14.
4. Branton WG, Ellestad KK, Maingat F, Wheatley BM, Rud E, Warren RL, et al. Brain microbial populations in HIV/AIDS: α-proteobacteria predominate independent of host immune status. PLoS One. 2013;8(1):e54673.
5. Evrensel A, Ceylan ME. The gut-brain axis: the missing link in depression. Clin Psychopharmacol Neurosci. 2015;13(3):239–44.
6. Sender R, Fuchs S, Milo R. Revised estimates for the number of human and bacteria cells in the body. PLoS Biol. 2016;14(8):e1002533.
7. Lozupone CA, Stombaugh JI, Gordon JI, Jansson JK, Knight R. Diversity, stability and resilience of the human gut microbiota. Nature. 2012;489(7415):220–30.
8. Sharon G, Sampson TR, Geschwind DH, Mazmanian SK. The central nervous system and the gut microbiome. Cell. 2016;167(4):915–32.
9. Evrensel A, Ceylan ME. Microbiome: the missing link in neuropsychiatric disorders. Eur Med J Innov. 2017;1(1):83–8.
10. Xu MQ, Cao HL, Wang WQ, Wang S, Cao XC, Yan F, et al. Fecal microbiota transplantation broadening its application beyond intestinal disorders. World J Gastroenterol. 2015;21(1):102–11.
11. Scott KA, Ida M, Peterson VL, Prenderville JA, Moloney GM, Izumo T, et al. Revisiting Metchnikoff: age-related alterations in microbiota-gut-brain axis in the mouse. Brain Behav Immun. 2017;65:20–32.
12. Sarkar A, Lehto SM, Harty S, Dinan TG, Cryan JF, Burnet PW. Psychobiotics and the manipulation of Bacteria-gut-brain signals. Trends Neurosci. 2016;39(11):763–81.
13. Olszak T, An D, Zeissig S, Vera MP, Richter J, Franke A, et al. Microbial exposure during early life has persistent effects on natural killer T cell function. Science. 2012;336(6080):489–93.
14. McCusker RH, Kelley KW. Immune-neural connections: how the immune system's response to infectious agents influences behavior. J Exp Biol. 2013;216(Pt 1):84–98.
15. McKernan DP, Dennison U, Gaszner G, Cryan JF, Dinan TG. Enhanced peripheral toll-like receptor responses in psychosis: further evidence of a pro-inflammatory phenotype. Transl Psychiatry. 2011;1:e36.
16. Dinan TG, Quigley EM. Probiotics in the treatment of depression: science or science fiction? Aust New Zeland J Psychiatry. 2011;45(12):1023–5.
17. Carvalho FA, Aitken JD, Vijay-Kumar M, Gewirtz AT. Toll-like receptor-gut microbiota interactions: perturb at your own risk. Annu Rev Physiol. 2012;74:177–98.
18. Lucas K, Maes M. Role of the toll like receptor (TLR) radical cyclein chronic inflammation: possible treatments targeting the TLR4 pathway. Mol Neurobiol. 2013;48(1):190–204.
19. Ait-Belgnaoui A, Durand H, Cartier C, Chaumaz G, Eutamene H, Ferrier L, et al. Prevention of gut leakiness by intestinal microbiota modulation leads to attenuated HPA response to an acute psychological stress in rats. Psychoneuroendocrinology. 2012;37(11):1885–95.
20. Jeon SW, Kim YK. Neuroinflammation and cytokine abnormality in major depression: cause or consequence in that illness? World J Psychiatry. 2016;6(3):283–93.
21. Kim YK, Na KS, Myint AM, Leonard BE. The role of pro-inflammatory cytokines in neuroinflammation, neurogenesis and the neuroendocrine system in major depression. Prog Neuro-Psychopharmacol Biol Psychiatry. 2016;64:277–84.
22. Udina M, Castellví P, Moreno-España J, Navinés R, Valdés M, Forns X, et al. Interferon-induced depression in chronic hepatitis C: a systematic review and meta-analysis. J Clin Psychiatry. 2012;73(2):1128–38.
23. McNutt MD, Liu S, Manatunga A, Royster EB, Raison CL, Woolwine BJ, et al. Neurobehavioral effects of interferon-α in patients with hepatitis-C: symptom dimensions and responsiveness to paroxetine. Neuropsychopharmacology. 2012;37(6):1444–54.
24. Maes M, Kenis G, Kubera M, De Baets M, Steinbusch H, Bosmans E. The negative immunoregulatory effects of fluoxetine in relation to the cAMP-dependent PKA pathway. Int Immunopharmacol. 2005;5(3):609–18.
25. Levkovich T, Poutahidis T, Smillie C, Varian BJ, Ibrahim YM, Lakritz JR, et al. Probiotic bacteria induce a 'glow of health'. PLoS One. 2013;8(1):e53867.
26. Kopp MV, Goldstein M, Dietschek A, Sofke J, Heinzmann A, Urbanek R. Lactobacillus GG has in vitro effects on enhanced interleukin-10 and interferon-gamma release of mononuclear cells but no in vivo effects in supplemented mothers and their neonates. Clin Exp Allergy. 2008;38(4):602–10.
27. Costello EK, Stagaman K, Dethlefsen L, Bohannan J, Relman DA. The application of ecological theory toward an understanding of the human microbiome. Science. 2012;336(6086):1255–62.
28. Smythies LE, Smythies JR. Microbiota, the immune system, black moods and the brain melancholia updated. Front Hum Neurosci. 2014;8:720.
29. Helander HF, Fändriks L. Surface area of the digestive tract – revisited. Scand J Gastroenterol. 2014;49(6):681–9.
30. Borre YE, O'keeffe GW, Clarke G, Stanton C, Dinan TG, Cryan JF. Microbiota and neurodevelopmental windows: implications for brain disorders. Trends Mol Med. 2014;20(9):509–18.
31. Maes M, Kubera M, Leunis JC, Berk M. Increased IgA and IgM responses against gut commensals in chronic depression: further evidence for increased bacterial translocation or leaky gut. J Affect Disord. 2012;141(1):55–62.
32. Fink MP. Leaky gut hypothesis: a historical perspective. Crit Care Med. 1990;18(5):579–80.
33. Hornig M. The role of microbes and autoimmunity in the pathogenesis of neuropsychiatric illness. Curr Opin Rheumatol. 2013;25(5):488–95.

34. Fetissov SO, Déchelotte P. The new link between gut–brain axis and neuropsychiatric disorders. Curr Opin Clin Nutr Metab Care. 2011;14(5):477–82.
35. Dominguez-Bello MG, De Jesus-Laboy KM, Shen N, Cox LM, Amir A, Gonzalez A, et al. Partial restoration of the microbiota of cesarean-born infants via vaginal microbial transfer. Nat Med. 2016;22(3):250–3.
36. Bäckhed F, Roswall J, Peng Y, Feng Q, Jia H, Kovatcheva-Datchary P, et al. Dynamics and stabilization of the human gut microbiome during the first year of life. Cell Host Microbe. 2015;17(5):690–703.
37. Bager P, Wohlfahrt J, Westergaard T. Caesarean delivery and risk of atopy and allergic disease: meta-analyses. Clin Exp Allergy. 2008;38(4):634–42.
38. Slykerman RF, Thompson J, Waldie KE, Murphy R, Wall C, Mitchell EA. Antibiotics in the first year of life and subsequent neurocognitive outcomes. Acta Paediatr. 2017;106(1):87–94.
39. Bercik P, Denou E, Collins J, Jackson W, Lu J, Jury J, et al. The intestinal microbiota affect central levels of brain-derived neurotropic factor and behavior in mice. Gastroenterology. 2011;141(2):599–609.
40. Desbonnet L, Clarke G, Traplin A, O'Sullivan O, Crispie F, Moloney RD, et al. Gut microbiota depletion from early adolescence in mice: implications for brain and behavior. Brain Behav Immun. 2015;48:165–73.
41. Neufeld KM, Kang N, Bienenstock J, Foster JA. Reduced anxiety-like behavior and central neurochemical change in germ-free mice. Neurogastroenterol Motil. 2011;23(3):255–64.
42. Hoban AE, Stilling RM, Moloney G, Shanahan F, Dinan TG, Clarke G, et al. The microbiome regulates amygdala-dependent fear recall. Mol Psychiatry. 2017;23(5):1134–44.
43. Macedo D, Filho AJMC, Soares de Sousa CN, Quevedo J, Barichello T, Júnior HVN, et al. Antidepressants, antimicrobials or both? Gut microbiota dysbiosis in depression and possible implications of the antimicrobial effects of antidepressant drugs for antidepressant effectiveness. J Affect Disord. 2017;208:22–32.
44. Evrensel A, Ceylan ME. The role of fecal microbiota transplantation in psychiatric treatment. Anadolu Psikiyatri Derg. 2015;16(5):380.
45. Evrensel A, Ceylan ME. Fecal microbiota transplantation and its usage in neuropsychiatric disorders. Clin Psychopharmacol Neurosci. 2016;14(3):231–7.
46. Vindigni SM, Surawicz CM. Fecal microbiota transplantation. Gastroenterol Clin N Am. 2017;46(1):171–85.
47. Zhang F, Luo W, Shi Y, Fan Z, Ji G. Should we standardize the 1,700-year-old fecal microbiota transplantation? Am J Gastroenterol. 2012;107(11):1755.
48. Jia NA. Misleading reference for fecal microbiota transplant. Am J Gastroenterol. 2015;110(12):1731.
49. Borody TJ, Warren EF, Leis SM, Surace R, Ashman O, Siarakas S. Bacteriotherapy using fecal flora: toying with human motions. J Clin Gastroenterol. 2004;38(6):475–83.
50. Smits LP, Bouter KE, de Vos WM, Borody TJ, Nieuwdorp M. Therapeutic potential of fecal microbiota transplantation. Gastroenterology. 2013;145(5):946–53.
51. Eiseman B, Silen W, Bascom GS, Kauvar AJ. Fecal enema as an adjunct in the treatment of pseudomembranous enterocolitis. Surgery. 1958;44(5):854–9.
52. Bowden TA, Mansberger AR, Lykins LE. Pseudomembranous enterocolitis: mechanism of restoring floral homeostasis. Am Surg. 1981;47(4):178–83.
53. Brandt LJ, Aroniadis OC, Mellow M, Kanatzar A, Kelly C, Park T, et al. Long-term follow-up of colonoscopic fecal microbiota transplantation for recurrent Clostridium difficile infection. Am J Gastroenterol. 2012;107(7):1079–87.
54. Zheng P, Zeng B, Zhou C, Liu M, Fang Z, Xu X, et al. Gut microbiome remodeling induces depressive-like behaviors through a pathway mediated by the host's metabolism. Mol Psychiatry. 2016;21(6):786–96.
55. Ma Y, Liu J, Rhodes C, Nie Y, Zhang F. Ethical issues in fecal microbiota transplantation in practice. Am J Bioeth. 2017;17:34–45.
56. Di Bella S, Drapeau C, García-Almodóvar E, Petrosillo N. Fecal microbiota transplantation: the state of the art. Infect Dis Rep. 2013;5(2):e13.
57. Evrensel A, Ceylan ME. The future of fecal microbiota transplantation method in neuropsychiatric disorders. Turk Psikiyatri Dergisi. 2016;27(1):71–2.
58. Aroniadis OC, Brandt LJ. Fecal microbiota transplantation: past, present and future. Curr Opin Gastroenterol. 2013;29(1):79–84.
59. Brandt LJ, Aroniadis OC. An overview of fecal microbiota transplantation: techniques, indications, and outcomes. Gastrointest Endosc. 2013;78(2):240–9.
60. Youngster I, Gerding DN. Editorial: making fecal microbiota transplantation easier to swallow: freeze-dried preparation for recurrent Clostridium difficile infections. Am J Gastroenterol. 2017;112(6):948–50.
61. Youngster I, Russell GH, Pindar C, Ziv-Baran T, Sauk J, Hohmann EL. Oral, capsulized, frozen fecal microbiota transplantation for relapsing Clostridium difficile infection. JAMA. 2014;312(17):1772–8.
62. Borody TJ, Brandt LJ, Paramsothy S. Therapeutic faecal microbiota transplantation: current status and future developments. Curr Opin Gastroenterol. 2014;30(1):97–105.
63. Bakken JS, Borody T, Brandt LJ, Brill JV, Demarco DC, Franzos MA, et al. Treating Clostridium difficile infection with fecal microbiota transplantation. Clin Gastroenterol Hepatol. 2011;9(12):1044–9.
64. Kubera M, Curzytek K, Duda W, Leskiewicz M, Basta-Kaim A, Budziszewska B, et al. A new animal model of (chronic) depression induced by repeated and intermittent lipopolysaccharide administration for 4 months. Brain Behav Immun. 2013;31:96–104.
65. Macpherson AJ, Uhr T. Gut flora-mechanisms of regulation. Eur J Surg Suppl. 2002;587:3–7.
66. Desbonnet L, Garrett L, Clarke G, Kiely B, Cryan JF, Dinan TG. Effects of the probiotic Bifidobacterium infantis in the maternal separation model of depression. Neuroscience. 2010;170(4):1179–88.

67. Messaoudi M, Lalonde R, Violle N, Javelot H, Desor D, Nejdi A, et al. Assessment of psychotropic-like properties of a probiotic formulation (lactobacillus helveticus R0052 and Bifidobacterium longum R0175) in rats and human subjects. Br J Nutr. 2011;105(5):755–64.
68. Messaoudi M, Violle N, Bisson JF, Desor D, Javelot H, Rougeot C. Beneficial psychological effects of a probiotic formulation (Lactobacillus helveticus R0052 and Bifidobacterium longum R0175) in healthy human volunteers. Gut Microbes. 2011;2(4):256–61.
69. Bruce-Keller AJ, Salbaum JM, Luo M, Blanchard E 4th, Taylor CM, Welsh DA, et al. Obese-type gut microbionta induced neurobehavioral changes in the absence of obesity. Biol Psychiatry. 2015;77(7):607–15.
70. Hsiao EY, McBride SW, Hsien S, Sharon G, Hyde ER, McCue T, et al. Microbiota modulate behavioral and physiological abnormalities associated with neurodevelopmental disorders. Cell. 2013;155(7):1451–63.
71. Finegold SM, Molitoris D, Song Y, Liu C, Vaisanen ML, Bolte E, et al. Gastrointestinal microflora studies in late-onset autism. Clin Infect Dis. 2002;35(Suppl 1):6–16.
72. Song Y, Liu C, Finegold SM. Real-time PCR quantitation of clostridia in feces of autistic children. Appl Environ Microbiol. 2004;70(11):6459–65.
73. Schwarz E, Maukonen J, Hyytiäinen T, Kieseppä T, Orešič M, Sabunciyan S, et al. Analysis of microbiota in first episode psychosis identifies preliminary associations with symptom severity and treatment response. Schizophr Res. 2017;192:398–403.
74. Jiang H, Ling Z, Zhang Y, Mao H, Ma Z, Yin Y, et al. Altered fecal microbiota composition in patients with major depressive disorder. Brain Behav Immun. 2015;48:186–94.
75. Wallace CJK, Milev R. The effects of probiotics on depressive symptoms in humans: a systematic review. Ann General Psychiatry. 2017;16:14.
76. Noble EE, Hsu TM, Kanoski SE. Gut to brain Dysbiosis: mechanisms linking western diet consumption, the microbiome, and cognitive impairment. Front Behav Neurosci. 2017;11:9.
77. Allen AP, Hutch W, Borre YE, Kennedy PJ, Temko A, Boylan G, et al. Bifidobacterium longum 1714 as a translational psychobiotic: modulation of stress, electrophysiology and neurocognition in healthy volunteers. Transl Psychiatry. 2016;6(11):e939.
78. Kelly JR, Allen AP, Temko A, Hutch W, Kennedy PJ, Farid N, et al. Lost in translation? The potential psychobiotic Lactobacillus rhamnosus (JB-1) fails to modulate stress or cognitive performance in healthy male subjects. Brain Behav Immun. 2017;61:50–9.
79. Jiang C, Li G, Huang P, Liu Z, Zhao B. The gut microbiota and Alzheimer's disease. J Alzheimers Dis. 2017;58(1):1–15.
80. Leclercq S, de Timary P, Delzenne NM, Stärkel P. The link between inflammation, bugs, the intestine and the brain in alcohol dependence. Transl Psychiatry. 2017;7(2):e1048.
81. Gough E, Shaikh H, Manges AR. Systematic review of intestinal microbiota transplantation (fecal bacteriotherapy) for recurrent Clostridium difficile infection. Clin Infect Dis. 2011;53(10):994–1002.
82. De Leon LM, Watson JB, Kelly CR. Transient flare of ulcerative colitis after fecal microbiota transplantation for recurrent Clostridium difficile infection. Clin Gastroenterol Hepatol. 2013;11(8):1036–8.
83. Aas J, Gessert CE, Bakken JS. Recurrent Clostridium difficile colitis: case series involving 18 patients treated with donor stool administered via a nasogastric tube. Clin Infect Dis. 2003;36(5):580–5.
84. Vandenplas Y, Pierard D, De Greef E. Fecal microbiota transplantation: just a fancy trend? J Pediatr Gastroenterol Nutr. 2015;61(1):4–7.

Neurosurgical Intervention for Treatment-Resistant Psychiatric Disorders

25

Daniel E. Nijensohn and Teodoro Forcht Dagi

25.1 Introduction

When psychiatric disorders that can be expected to respond to psychotropic medications and other standard therapies become “treatment-resistant,” neurosurgical *intervention*, carried out by a multidisciplinary experienced team with appropriate safeguards, may present an attractive option, delivering clinical improvement with relatively few complications or side effects and at a reasonable cost-benefit ratio. Nevertheless, surgical intervention remains controversial.

Neurosurgery is reemerging as an important therapeutic option for *disabling psychiatric disease*. In this chapter, we will refer to neurosurgery for psychiatric disease synoptically as *psychosurgery*. This is the second time around for psychosurgery. The abuses of the past, including indiscriminate indications, poor patient selection, questionable trials, poor outcome studies, and lack of adequate informed consent, resulted in a pall that continues to darken this field and complicates investigation and practice. The negative ethical and social valence of psychosurgery must be acknowledged and carefully and conscientiously addressed.

Psychosurgery is also referred to as surgery of the psyche, surgery for behavioral disorders, psychiatric surgery, neurosurgery for mental disorders, limbic system surgery, and neurosurgery for disorders of memory, mood, and metabolism. It may involve ablation, stimulation, or disconnection of cerebral targets, always with the objective of altering abnormal affective and behavioral states caused by mental illness. It is classified as *functional neurosurgery* because it attempts to improve or restore function by altering underlying physiology. Not all functional neurosurgery targets psychiatric illness. Other examples include the treatment of epilepsy, Parkinson’s disease, or pain. Dysfunction within motor, mood, memory and cognitive brain circuits appears to be responsible for the signs and symptoms of neurological and psychiatric illnesses. Functional neurosurgery offers the possibility of modulating the activity of these circuits.

The *surgical targets* are varied and may be cortical, nuclear, or connectome related. These

D. E. Nijensohn (✉)
Neurosurgery Department, Yale University School of Medicine, New Haven, CT, USA

Neurosurgery Division, St. Vincent’s Medical Center, Bridgeport, CT, USA

Neurosurgery Section, Bridgeport Hospital, Bridgeport, CT, USA

Yale Gamma Knife Center & Yale New Haven Hospital, New Haven, CT, USA

T. F. Dagi
HLM Venture Partners, Boston, MA, USA

Dentistry and Biomedical Sciences, Queen’s University, Belfast, UK

Anglo Scientific LTD, The Royal Institution of Great Britain, London, UK

Y.-K. Kim (ed.), *Treatment Resistance in Psychiatry*, https://doi.org/10.1007/978-981-10-4358-1_25

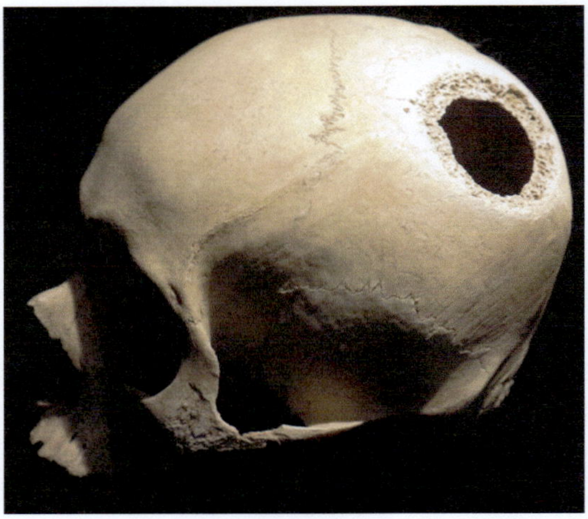

Fig. 25.1 Prehistoric attempt at trepanation (a hole in the skull produced surgically) from Paracas, Peru [135] (*Connecticut medicine*, September 2014)

targets may or may not display physiologic or anatomic abnormalities using currently available diagnostic techniques.

Although psychosurgery has *prehistoric* roots (Fig. 25.1) [135] and was attempted desultorily in the later nineteenth century, its real *history* begins with the idea that psychiatric disease could be explained physiologically by abnormalities of neuronal connection and that interruption of the frontal connections could be used to tame aggression. Based in part on a number of anecdotal clinical observations and in part on *Fulton*'s work in primates at Yale University [51, 52], Moniz [59, 126] and later Freeman and others introduced the operation of *prefrontal leucotomy/lobotomy* in the 1930s [49, 57]. At the time, this operation was felt to represent a very credible and advanced application of basic neuroscience [126, 143, 146, 150]. The procedure was overused. Within two decades, it was largely overtaken by the *psychotropic medications* that were introduced in the early 1950s and by less radical and safer neurosurgical procedures with fewer objectionable cognitive side effects [179]. Nevertheless, psychosurgery as a whole could not overcome the negative publicity promulgated by the anti-psychiatry movement of the 1960s, by the fear that psychosurgery could be used to suppress political and social dissidence, by the idea that psychosurgery should be considered for control of violence, by the proposal to use psychosurgery to reduce the urban rioting of the late 1960s, and by the common lack of voluntary informed consent on the part of the patient. The technical improvements did not suffice to overcome the extent of social opprobrium. In time, in some US jurisdictions like Oregon, psychosurgery without appropriate controls could be prosecuted as a felony [18, 56, 64, 100, 103, 115, 132, 134–136, 146, 151, 163, 179]. The Japanese Society for Psychiatry and Neurology banned the surgical treatment for psychiatric disorders in 1975. In Japan, there has been no neurosurgical treatment for psychiatric disorders since then [79].

More recently, the perception of psychosurgery began to change. Objections diminished. The reasons behind the change include, arguably, a combination of fundamental advances in our understanding of *neuroscience*, the development of more precise *image-guided stereotactic* surgical techniques, and socially responsive changes in emphasis. Newer technologies and *stereotactic* techniques including *MR image-guided high-intensity focused ultrasound* (*MR-HIFU*) lesioning and frame-based or frameless *stereotactic radiosurgery* made the procedure appear more controlled and less risky and contributed to the acceptability of lesioning cerebral targets [66, 83, 85, 152, 172].

The success of *deep brain stimulation* (DBS) for *Parkinson's* disease and other *movement disorders* opened the door to reevaluating functional neurosurgery for other indications. The Parkinson's precedent was important because stereotactic surgery for Parkinson's was initially eclipsed by medications that seemed physiologically ideal: they offered effective dopaminergic proxies and substitutes and, in that sense, were more suitable for that purpose, perhaps, than the psychotropic medications were for psychiatric disease. But like the medications for psychiatric disease, *L-Dopa* did not have a lasting effect, and on the basis of extensive experimental work in the neurosciences, the surgical option was once again considered. The recognition that medical therapy for psychiatric disease had limitations similar to those of Parkinson's was the stimulus that inspired the careful and limited reintroduction of psychosurgery in the USA. The guiding principles were based on guarding against the errors of the past, careful reporting and monitoring, and on highly restricted limited indications.

Regarding DBS, many psychiatrists have agreed with *Insel*, former director of the National Institute of Mental Health, who wrote "if mental disorders are brain circuit disorders, then successful treatments need to tune circuits with precision. Chemicals may be less precise than electrical interventions that target specific circuits" and have proved increasingly willing to reconsider their objections to psychosurgery in general and DBS in particular [72].

Although outcome studies began to reemerge in the mid-1990s and the FDA approved a *humanitarian device exemption* for DBS for severe OCD in 2009 based on a review of data from 26 patients with severe and treatment-resistant disease, long-term data remained elusive. A 2014 *consensus statement* on ethical and scientific guidelines for stereotactic neurosurgery for psychiatric disorders sponsored by the World Society for Stereotactic and Functional Neurosurgery Committee on Neurosurgery for Psychiatric Disorders and authored by a multidisciplinary international consortium of neurosurgeons, neurologists, psychiatrists, neuropsychologists, bioethicists, philosophers, regulatory experts, and legal scholars highlighted, for example, the lack of Level I evidence, even around established procedures such as cingulotomy and capsulotomy for depression and obsessive-compulsive disorder. It emphasized unreservedly the categorical importance of comprehensively collecting credible data around investigational procedures such as DBS [89, 137]. "Credible data" is a difficult but necessary target. *Trial design* must be carefully thought through. The classical randomized controlled trial approach may not be applicable in this field. Recent developments in trial methodology and statistics suggest that alternative designs may be more applicable and, ultimately, more productive [15, 35, 41, 57, 64, 69, 70, 101, 103, 118, 134, 142, 150, 151, 159, 164, 170, 174, 188].

From a historical perspective, *contagious exuberance* appeared unwisely, but not uncommonly after initial improvements in a small number of cases. A large series may not lead to the same conclusions. *St. Jude Medical*, now *Abbott*, abandoned the recent *Broden* trial (*BROdmann Area 25 DEep brain Neuromodulation (DBS) of the subgenual cingulate gyrus for the treatment of major depression*) [120] because under careful monitoring, it proved beneficial in no more than 20% of cases – no better than the 17% of the control group (Holtzheimer et al., *Lancet Psychiatry*, October 2017) [173].

25.1.1 The Proper Ambit of Psychosurgery

The original *indications* for *prefrontal leucotomy* were agitation and violence, indications for which the alternatives in the late 1930s ranged from restraints to ice baths to insulin-induced seizures, to electroshock therapy, and to barbiturates [179]. It could be argued that the induction of seizures and perhaps the use of barbiturates were intended to be therapeutic, but the other treatments were simply ways in which difficult patients were managed by the understaffed institution to which they were relegated. The *side effects* of leucotomy, which included passivity, flattened affect, and blunted cognition, were not necessarily considered objectionable given the objectives, not unlike facial anesthesia after trigeminal rhizotomy for trigeminal neuralgia. Over time, however, as the indications for psychosurgery were uncritically expanded to include far more normal individuals, these side effects were re-adjudicated and judged to be unwanted complications. Until psychosurgery was first effectively abandoned, the goal was more carefully targeted procedures, more carefully performed, using more advanced techniques.

The current ambit of psychosurgery can be divided into two parts. On the one hand, there are strong signals of efficacy in *obsessive-compulsive disorder* (OCD) and in major *affective disorders* including *major depressive disorder* (MDD), *bipolarity*, and severe *anxiety*.

On the other hand, there is interest in developing models and exploring indications for other disabling, treatment-resistant conditions including *anorexia nervosa* (AN) and *morbid obesity*, *post-traumatic stress disorder* (PTSD), and *substance abuse* (SA). Some include treatment for certain residual aspects of *traumatic brain injury* (TBI), *memory and sleep disorders* (i.e., *Alzheimer*'s and *cognitive disorders*), *aggressiveness*, and *Tourette's syndrome* (TS). Whether the objectives of surgery for TBI, TS, and memory and sleep disorders should be classified as psychosurgery remains disputed. Indeed, the entirety of this second category is highly fraught with controversy.

In any case, psychosurgery is reserved for severely incapacitated patients with treatment-refractory illnesses and low quality of life. A history of personality disorder, substance abuse, or other Axis II symptomatology serves as a relative *contraindication*. In rare instances only, patients with severe violent outbursts and potential for serious injury or self-mutilation or severe aggressive disorders – typically on the basis of certain recognized genetic abnormalities – might be considered for *amygdalotomy*, *thalamotomy*, and *hypothalamotomy*.

Schizophrenia has proven to be much more difficult to treat than depression and OCD and is not currently a surgical indication. Some patients with *mixed disorders*, combining symptoms of anxiety, depression, and OCD, remain candidates for surgery [96].

Certain *principles* should govern the *practice of psychosurgery*. All patients must be referred for surgical intervention by the treating psychiatrist, who must be committed to continue caring for the patient, to the evaluation process and to postoperative management. Detailed documentation of the extent, severity, and diagnostic and therapeutic history must be provided. The specifics of pharmacologic trials should include agents used, dose, duration, response, and reason for discontinuation [27].

Although this point should be obvious, it requires frequent restatement. The family must participate in the evaluation and the decision-making process, and patients must not be abandoned once the psychosurgical procedure is completed. The postoperative psychiatric treatment and management program must be in place before any procedure is contemplated. In general, only patients older than 18 years who are able to render voluntary informed consent and participate in the decision-making process should be considered for surgery [27].

Finally, it should be self-evident that the only acceptable goal of psychosurgery is the treatment of illness. It must never be deployed for social or political purposes [117–119, 189].

For social and historical reasons, one should not be surprised to see a higher level of *evidence* required for psychosurgical interventions than for other indications. The answer to the question "what is evidence enough?" cannot be easily answered, nor answered across the board. The elevation of psychosurgery to a standard of care will require both professional and social consensus and a great deal of discussion around criteria for defining costs and for assigning benefits [28].

25.1.2 Identity, the Mind, the Brain

Diffusion MRI is becoming an indispensable tool to investigate a variety of psychiatric disorders such as schizophrenia, major depressive disorder, eating disorders, attention deficit disorder, addictions, and so on. It has shed insightful light on our understanding of neural *connectivity* and how abnormalities in connectivity may contribute to the pathogenesis of *psychiatric illnesses* [174].

While the notion that brain function might be successfully modulated through the ablation or stimulation of specific anatomical targets is rooted in ideas around *cerebral localization*, the *biological basis* of most psychiatric illnesses remains poorly understood, and the direct association of targets, symptoms, and diseases remains elusive. Nevertheless, there is strong support for the idea that signaling within the central nervous system involves *two parallel systems*, one *neuronal and synaptic*, and the other *neurochemical*. In addition, experimental and clinical evidence suggests that a number of psychiatric conditions are open to chemical (pharmacological) *modulation*; the stimulation or ablation of certain anatomical targets in the brain and elsewhere (procedures like *vagal nerve stimulation* will not be discussed here) modulates neuronal and neurochemical signaling and that such modulation may benefit some forms of psychiatric illness [72, 148].

25.1.2.1 Outcome Measures

It is important to develop uniform, standardized, and clinically meaningful *outcome measures*. Many obstacles will have to be overcome including diagnostic ambiguities, existing non-standardized presurgical evaluation tools, center bias, and varied outcome assessment scales [26, 27, 130].

Some existing tools include:

1. The *Yale-Brown Obsessive-Compulsive Scale* (YBOCS) to assess the severity of OCD: a score >20 is enough for candidacy for a psychosurgical procedure.
2. The *Beck Depression Inventory* (BDI): a score >30 confirms the severity of depression.
3. The *Global Assessment of Function* (GAF) to assess disability: a score <50 justifies psychosurgery.
4. The *Pippard Postoperative Rating Scale* (PPRS) assesses outcomes according to five categories: symptom free (A), much improved (B), slightly improved (C), unchanged (D), and worse (E). Although comparisons are imperfect, the PPRS appears to have some clinical validity. For example, if categories A and B are considered satisfactory, then cingulotomy is effective in 56%, subcaudate tractotomy in 50%, limbic leucotomy in 61%, and capsulotomy in 67% of patients with OCD [125]. In patients with major affective disorder, in contrast, cingulotomy is slightly more effective [27]. Capsulotomy patients did better than cingulotomy patients, but transient deterioration in mental status was much more marked [27].

It is helpful to think of outcomes in this domain in the same way one would approach clinical trials: the key is to correlate primary clinical indications and endpoints. Currently, data supporting the overall clinical superiority of any one procedure is not persuasive [147].

25.1.3 Prevalence of Various Procedures

All things being equal and without reference to specific indications, *cingulotomy* is the most prevalent functional operation carried out for psychiatric illness in general in the USA, whereas in Europe, *capsulotomy and limbic leucotomy* are more prevalent. They all appear roughly equivalent therapeutically but in terms of unwanted side effects, cingulotomy appears to be the safest of all procedures currently performed. Regardless of procedures, surgical failures should be investigated, and if the lesion size or location is suboptimal, then consideration should be given to a repeat procedure. At least 45% of patients undergoing cingulotomy require repeat operation with good results being salvaged in half. Repeat surgery in capsulotomy patients has been reported as 20%. The exact size or volume of tissue required for an effective outcome at each of the target sites has yet to be determined. As already noted, surgery should be considered as only one aspect in the overall management of these patients [26, 27].

There is increasing interest in *neuromodulation* over a number of functional indications including memory enhancement in age-related dementia, as well as in psychosurgery for major depression, PTSD, substance abuse, and others [95].

25.2 Neuroanatomy, Targets, Techniques

While the neuroanatomical correlate of psychiatric illness has been associated with the *limbic system* (LS), described by Broca [19], Jakob [78], Papez [29, 141], McLean [122], and others, there is no specific site or set of sites in which psychiatric illness can be rooted. Nevertheless, a large number of sites have been targeted for *stimulation or ablation*. Indeed, some have proposed the term *limbic system surgery* as an alternative to psychosurgery. *Neurosurgical interventions for psychiatric disorders* have been directed at various *targets* within this system and its interconnections with the *cortico-striato-thalamic-cortical circuits* (CSTCC) which appear to play a central role in the pathophysiology of major affective illness, OCD, and other anxiety disorders. Electrical stimulation of specific areas within the LS (e.g., the *anterior cingulum* (AC)) has been shown to alter both autonomic responses and anxiety levels in humans.

Additional interventions have been directed at the anatomical *circuit of Papez* [141], which consists of the *hippocampus-fornix-septum-mammillary bodies-anterior thalamic nuclei-cingulate gyrus-hippocampus*. The term "anatomical" is used because these anatomical connections can be clearly identified, even though their physiological relationships are less convincing. In some reported cases, *the internal capsule, the basal ganglia, and the nucleus accumbens* have also been targeted. Stimulation of the *hypothalamus* produces autonomic, endocrine, and complex motor effects which suggest that it may integrate and coordinate the behavioral expression of emotional states [100, 115]. *Neurochemical models* suggest that affective and anxiety disorders may be mediated via *monoaminergic systems*. Because of the diffuse nature of the monoaminergic projections and their role as neuromodulators, these models are not particularly instructive in terms of functional neuroanatomy and target identification. The *serotonergic system* has received emphasis when relating to OCD. Although the exact neuroanatomical and neurochemical mechanisms underlying OCD, depression, and other anxiety states remain unclear, it is believed that the *basal ganglia, limbic system, and frontal cortex* play a principal role in the pathophysiology of these diseases.

Presentations included in the recent scientific program of the World Society for Stereotactic and Functional Neurosurgery (WSSFN) (June 2017, Berlin meeting) offer a useful sample of the questions that continue to be asked in the field:

- Is surgery for psychiatric disorders really needed?
- DBS for OCD: Why it is not flying like DBS for Parkinson's?
- Two failed trials of DBS for depression: what went wrong?
- What happened to DBS of the *subthalamic nucleus* (STN) for OCD?
- How to proceed? Why is the field stagnating?
- Are psychiatrists averse to psychiatric surgery?
- Why is psychosurgery still "experimental"?
- What are the "ideal requirements" for neurosurgery to become an accepted credible treatment of refractory patients?
- When is a patient with OCD treatment-refractory?
- When is a patient with major depression treatment-refractory?
- How can we image the brain circuitry involved with psychiatric disease?
- Are there good animal models for psychiatric disorders? [41, 159, 185]

25.2.1 Stimulation and Ablation

Early psychosurgery was predicated on the idea that certain circuits should be interrupted and/or nuclei ablated. Superficial and deep stimulating electrodes were used experimentally to stimulate and to study brain tissue in humans since the late 1940s, but it took another half century before they were applied to psychosurgery, even though the technology was well known and *stimulation* had been used for experimental studies in animals since the nineteenth century.

The introduction of *stereotactic techniques* to create well-localized and discrete cerebral lesions in specific target sites in the 1950s represented a major advance in neurosurgery (Fig. 25.2). Stereotactic methods were particularly attractive in psychosurgery and functional neurosurgery because it was thought they would improve the risk-benefit ratio [71, 85, 171, 176,

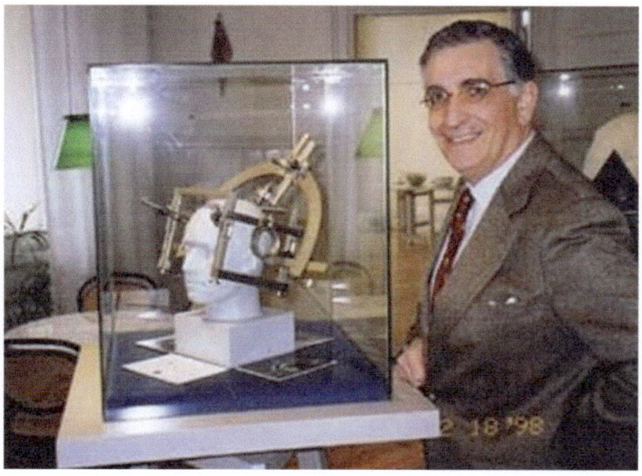

Fig. 25.2 Dr. Nijensohn, next to an early Leksell stereotactic frame in Stockholm, Sweden [99]

178]. Delgado, for example, advanced the idea that implantable intracranial stimulating electrodes could assist in diagnosis and possibly the treatment of schizophrenia and epilepsy [32, 33]. Heath also performed clinical studies with intracranial electrodes to modulate brain activity and to understand and treat intractable psychiatric disorders [66, 67]. Cooper seized on an adverse event arising from an ablation procedure for Parkinson's to identify a *target* for stereotactic intervention. In the course of an ablation procedure for treatment of *Parkinson's disease* (PD), a small *thalamic* stroke ensued and precipitated a halt to the procedure prior to the planned ablation. Upon awaking from anesthesia, the patient was surprisingly freed from tremor and rigidity, without hemiparesis. Cooper had serendipitously discovered the thalamus was a better ablation target that effectively eliminated the hallmark symptoms of Parkinson's disease [25]. He continued to create innovative surgical methods, including implanting *Medtronic* DBS electrodes to electrically stimulate the BG-thalamocortical circuitry to mimic the therapeutic effects of a thalamotomy. The initial developments in *stereotactic functional neurosurgery for movement disorders* were later applied to psychosurgery, reinvigorating it. Cooper's findings influenced *Benabid*, whose seminal paper ushered in modern-day, long-term high-frequency DBS, as an alternative treatment to reduce tremor [12, 25].

Thalamotomy and *Pallidotomy* for PD – used in the 1950s and 1960s – were largely abandoned in the 1970s after the introduction of *levodopa*. But medications proved ineffective in the long term, and stereotactic surgery was revisited. The *globus pallidus* was understood to be "overactive" in PD causing bradykinesia and tremor. Radiofrequency lesioning of the *internal segment of the pallidum* – the output nucleus of the basal ganglia – was extensively researched by De Long et al. at Emory (1990s) for the treatment of involuntary movements [34].

It was also held at the time that the *subthalamic nucleus* (STN) *of Luys* might be a much better target for ablation. The STN was avoided, however, out of concern that a lesion in this vascular structure could cause serious bleeding. As a result, STN became a target for *stimulation* rather than *ablation* [15, 182].

Whereas ablation destroys brain cells, high-frequency DBS activates them via *electrodes* placed in targeted areas and connected to a control device similar to a cardiac pacemaker under the skin (Fig. 25.3). The *programmable stimulator* or *pacemaker* can be externally adjusted to deliver continuous stimulation with control of the rate, amplitude, and duration of the pulses. *Electrodes* have been used experimentally since the late 1940s to stimulate brain tissue in humans and also to produce lesions through thermocoagulation. In anterior cingulotomy, for example, a 10 mm exposed portion of the electrode is heated to 85 °C for 60 s. In the case of DBS, each electrode includes an *anode* and a *cathode*. When an electrical current is applied, the brain tissue between them joins the circuit. Three to five volts are usually applied in DBS, at pulse frequencies above 100/s. At such frequencies brain tissue immediately surrounding the electrodes is deactivated or depolarized. However, just outside that area, volume conduction leads to electrical stimulation of axons, propagated upstream to cell bodies and downstream to synapses, interrupting local brain function while also producing effects more remotely.

Medtronic is currently the primary manufacturer of clinical and investigative DBS systems, although *Boston Scientific* and *St. Jude Medical* (*Abbott*) are releasing similar devices [120, 173].

The Medtronic stimulating electrodes (model 3387 or 3389) are commonly used to deliver long-

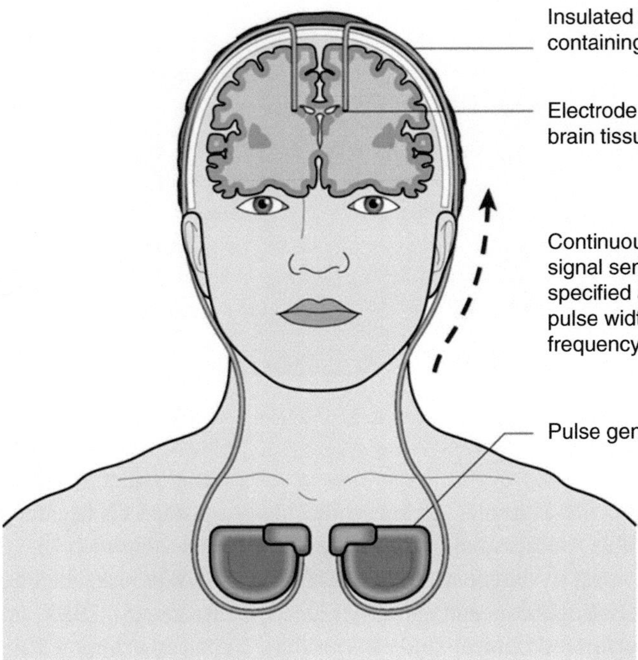

Fig. 25.3 Diagram of deep brain stimulation (DBS) [135] (*Connecticut medicine*, Sept 2014)

term DBS for clinical and investigative purposes. The DBS electrodes are connected via Medtronic lead extenders to their battery-powered IPG (*implantable pulse generator*).

Medtronic Activa™ series of open-loop neurostimulation devices *(Activa SC*™*, Activa PC*™*, and Activa RC*™) are FDA-approved and differ on the basis of dimensions, weight, and battery type. These IPG devices are capable of delivering single- or dual-channel electrical stimulation with a frequency of 2–250 Hz, a pulse width of 60–450 ms, and an amplitude of 0.0–10.5 V [40, 173].

The precise mechanism of action of *DBS* remains controversial. Nevertheless, high-frequency stimulation was noted to act clinically very much like a lesion, appearing to block or override the abnormal activity in the network. As already noted, *DBS* was initially developed by Benabid in France as a less abrasive approach than lesioning for treatment of tremor. It eventually earned a second chance for psychosurgery. Although DBS does not work better than pallidotomy to alleviate the symptoms of PD, it became preferred because it was reversible and adjustable. In 2006 *Benabid* wrote "beware, psychosurgery is back," recommending being vigilant about transparency, and the use of scientific and ethical rigor when treating disorders of the mood and mind [12, 13].

Trials of DBS in treatment-resistant psychiatric disorders began in the late 1990s, initially focusing on OCD, MDD, and TS. Despite serious issues – small participant numbers and a lack of consensus over brain targets – DBS is now trialed in a wide range of psychiatric conditions [2, 3, 6, 34, 35, 41, 48, 50, 57, 60, 61, 66, 69, 78–80, 87, 94–97, 99, 101, 102, 105, 110, 113, 116, 120, 122, 124, 129, 133, 137, 146, 147, 154, 157–160, 162, 164].

The number of *ablative procedures* has also increased. In both stimulation and ablation procedures, a *stereotactic cage-frame* is attached to the head as a means of directing electrodes or energy beams to deep brain locations mapped by MRI, although *frameless* computer-assisted neuro-navigation is emerging. All but three of the psychosurgical procedures in current use involve the insertion of electrodes into the brain. The exceptions are *vagal nerve stimulation* (VNS) [165], made minimally invasive by Ventureyra in Ottawa, as per personal communication, *gamma knife capsulotomy* (through *gamma knife surgery*, where multiple nar-

Table 25.1 2017 psychosurgical cerebral targets

Target	Psychiatric disorder
Deep brain	
Anterior limb of the internal capsule (ALIC)	OCD, *major depressive disorder* (MDD) *depression, anorexia nervosa* (AN)
Nucleus accumbens (NAcc)	OCD, MDD, AN, *addictions*
Subgenual cortex (SG)/area 25	MDD
Globus pallidus (GPi)	*Tourette's syndrome* (TS)
Habenula (Hb)	MDD
Posterior hypothalamus (PH)	*Aggressive behavior* (AB)
Thalamus, centromedian nucleus (CM)	TS
Subthalamic nucleus (STN)	OCD
Inferior thalamic peduncle (iThP)	MDD
Nucleus basalis of Meynert (NBM)	*Alzheimer's disease* (AD)
Basolateral amygdala complex (BLAc)	*Post-traumatic stress disorder* (PTSD)
Cortical	
Dorsolateral frontal	MDD
Orbitofrontal	MDD

Targets and original authors
Gabriels, OCD, *anterior limb of the internal capsule* (ALIC), 2003 [53, 58]
Sturm, OCD, *nucleus accumbens* (NAcc), 2003 [93, 175]
Jiménez, MDD/OCD, *inferior thalamic peduncle* (iThP) 2005/2009 [81]
Mayberg, MDD, *subgenual cortex* (SG)/area 25, 2005 [94, 120]
Visser-Vandewalle, Tourette's, *Inferior thalamic peduncle* (InThP), 2006 [1, 138, 180]
Mallet, OCD, *subthalamic nucleus* (STN), 2008 [112]
Kuhn, Addiction to alcohol/tobacco, *nucleus accumbens* (NAcc), 2007/2009 [109, 129]
Wu, Anorexia, *nucleus accumbens* (NAcc), 2013 [121, 186]
Nuttin, OCD, *Bed nucleus of the stria terminalis* (BNST), 2017 [110]

row beams of gamma radiation intersect at a pre-mapped point in the brain, hence the skull is not opened) [102], and the relatively new and increasingly utilized *MR image-guided high-intensity focused ultrasound (MR-HIFU, MRgFUS)* lesioning [9, 89, 118].

With the explosion in putative *targets* for the alteration of functional neural states (Table 25.1), the roster of potential *tools* for intervention has also expanded. On the engineering side, interventional MRI approaches have emerged for DBS implantation, eliminating the need for awake surgery. In addition, a number of tools for precise lesioning, e.g., implanted *lasers* and focused *ultrasound*, have also emerged.

With respect to psychosurgery specifically, several DBS *targets* have been adopted for certain *specific* conditions. These targets, which were found to produce the most benefit with the fewest adverse effects, were initially chosen in four ways:

1. The *subthalamic nucleus* (STN) became the favored target in *Parkinson's* (PD). Following DBS for Parkinson's, some patients with comorbid OCD experienced a reduction in the severity of those symptoms, hence its selection for trials in OCD.
2. The first DBS trial, in 1999, targeted the *anterior limb of the internal capsule* (ALIC), because lesion surgery to that area had been found in some cases to reduce the symptoms of severe *OCD*. The *anterior cingulate* and *subcaudate areas*, and the *combination* of the two, were chosen for similar reasons, in relation to MDD.
3. fMRI revealed increased metabolic activity in the *subgenual cortex* and *habenula* in some patients with *MDD*. Hence, those areas were targeted based on the hypothesis that such hyperactivity may be causal, rather than simply a manifestation of depression.
4. *Tourette's* occupies a boundary zone between movement and compulsive disorder, contributing to the wide range of brain targets available: *thalamus*, *STN*, *globus pallidus*, *nucleus accumbens*, and *internal capsule* [93, 111, 138].

Several authors have sought to explain the beneficial effects of stimulation-based procedures and lesion surgery on depressed mood and anxiety by referencing to two *cortico-striato-thalamo-cortical* (CSTC) *loops*. Similar loops were previously identified in relation to movement disorders – prior to the introduction of DBS – including *inhibitory (–)* (*GABA*-based) and *excitatory (+)* (*glutamate*-based) pathways. The CSTC-*affective loops*, by contrast, involve a wider range of neurotransmitters and complex interactions that are yet to be defined. Such circuits may explain the variety of targets that seem to produce at least some benefit in psychiatric DBS studies. It seems reasonable to speculate that tapping into and stimulating the loop at many points could influence and modify the whole network.

Currently, DBS therapy is FDA approved for medically refractory PD, essential tremor, dystonia, and OCD; in addition, other disorders under investigation include Tourette's syndrome, treatment-resistant depression, chronic pain, alcohol and drug addiction, cluster headache, and Alzheimer's disease [92, 106, 109, 138, 162].

25.2.1.1 Targets

For some of the main targets and their indications for some psychiatric disorders, see Table 25.1.

25.2.1.2 Techniques

Each procedure has different indications, techniques, results, and complications (see Tables 25.2 and 25.3).

Table 25.2 Psychosurgical techniques

a. Stimulation	*Cerebral cortical stimulation*
	Deep brain stimulation (DBS), *neuromodulation*
	Vagal nerve stimulation (VNS)
b. Ablation-lesioning	
"Open"	*Leucotomy-lobotomy, "modified" lobotomy, topectomy* [145]
"Closed"	
Stereotactic	
Framed or frameless	
Through a burr hole, cortical or subcortical (electrode-mediated)	*Thermocoagulation, cryo-coagulation, radiofrequency,* LASER
Through an intact skull	*MRI image-guided high-intensity focused ultrasound* (MR-HIFU)
	Gamma radiosurgery, like capsulotomy for OCD, and *nucleotomy*, nucleus accumbens *for* addiction

Four main lesioning procedures evolved as the safest and most effective; these all performed bilaterally and under stereotactic conditions to allow for precise lesioning of target structures (see Table 25.3):

1. *Anterior cingulotomy*
2. *Subcaudate tractotomy*
3. *Limbic leucotomy*
4. *Anterior capsulotomy*

Anterior Cingulotomy

Fulton [51] was the first to suggest that the *anterior cingulum* would be an appropriate target for psychosurgical intervention, initially carried out as an open procedure. Foltz and White [46] reported their experience with stereotactic cingulotomy for intractable pain and noted the best results were in those patients with concurrent anxiety-depression. Ballantine [8] in the 1960s subsequently demonstrated the safety and effectiveness of *cingulotomy*, which became the psychosurgical procedure of choice in North America for many decades [26, 153]. Results of bilateral cingulotomy on patients suffering from a variety of psychiatric disorders were reported retrospectively by Ballantine et al. (MGH, Boston, MA) in 1987: 62% of patients with *severe affective disorder* had worthwhile improvement. Cingulotomy was less effective for *OCD* (25–30%) [5, 8, 26, 27, 39, 45, 70, 80, 86, 96].

Surgical indications: treatment-refractory MDD, *chronic anxiety*, or OCD, and occasionally for severe *chronic pain* [26, 53, 97].

Initially these procedures were performed with ventriculography, but over the past several years, this has been replaced by *MRI-guided stereotactic techniques* [170]. *Target coordinates*: a point in the cingulum 7 mm from the midline and 20–25 mm posterior to the tip of the frontal horns. *Lesions* are done by *thermocoagulation.* Intraoperative *stimulation*: not performed routinely. On the day after surgery, a postoperative MRI scan is obtained to document the placement and extent of the lesions and R/O complications [27].

In over 800 cingulotomies performed at the MGH since 1962, there have been no deaths, few

Table 25.3 Lesioning (ablation)

Ablation procedures	Author	Date	Condition
1-Anterior cingulotomy	Foltz and White [46]	1962	MDD, OCD
2-Subcaudate tractotomy	Knight [76]	1964	MDD, OCD
3-Limbic leucotomy	Kelley [85]	1973	OCD
4-Anterior capsulotomy	Talairach [178]	1973	OCD
	Leksell [99]		
Some other procedures			
Hypothalamotomy	Sano [161]	1966–1972	Aggressive behavior (AB)
	Schvarcz [166]	1975	
Bilateral amygdalotomy	Narabayashi [131]	1961–1972	AB
	Balasubramaniam [7]		PTSD

complications, and no infections. An independent analysis demonstrated no significant behavioral or intellectual deficits as a result of the lesions themselves with significant IQ gains postoperatively. This improvement was greatest in patients with chronic pain and depression but negligible in those with the diagnosis of schizophrenia [27].

Subcaudate Tractotomy

Subcaudate tractotomy was introduced by Knight [90] in Great Britain in 1964 as an attempt to restrict the size of the surgical lesion and therefore minimize the side effects seen with standard prefrontal lobotomy. The aim was to interrupt white matter tracts between orbital cortex and subcortical structures by placing a lesion in the region of the *substantia innominata* just below *the head of the caudate nucleus* [10, 27, 55, 74, 107, 147].

In patients with MDD and OCD, improvement with minimal symptoms was clinically observed in two thirds of the patients. The best review of the surgical results for *subcaudate tractotomy* was presented by *Gotekpe* in 1975 [55, 107]. Good results were seen in 68% of patients suffering from depression, 62.5% of patients with anxiety states, and 50% of patients with OCD. *Surgical indications* included MDD, OCD, and anxiety states as well as a variety of other psychiatric diagnoses [27].

The surgical procedure was performed with *stereotactic techniques* using boney landmarks and ventricular outline. The *target coordinates* were 15 mm from the midline and 10–11 mm above the planum sphenoidale at the most anterior part of the sella turcica. Lesions were initially done using *radioactive implantable Yttrium 90 seeds* [27].

Patients with schizophrenia, personality disorder, and drug or alcohol abuse did poorly. Some patients who had only temporary benefit from the initial lesion had second lesions lateral to the first with good results seen in about half [27].

The incidence of *complications* was small but has included postoperative seizures in 2.2% and undesirable personality traits in 6.7%. Transient disinhibition was common. Of the 25 patients that had died at the time of a review, 3 patients had committed suicide. One patient died from inadvertent destruction of the hypothalamus when an yttrium seed migrated off target [27, 100].

Limbic Leucotomy

Limbic leucotomy was introduced by Kelley [85] in 1973, which combines *subcaudate tractotomy* and *anterior cingulotomy*.

This procedure was designed to disconnect orbital-frontal-thalamic pathways with the first lesion and interrupt an important portion of *Papez*'s circuit with the latter, reasoning that these two lesions might lead to a better result for the symptoms of OCD than either lesion alone.

Indications for surgical intervention included OCD, anxiety states, depression, and a variety of other psychiatric diagnoses [27, 30, 35, 125, 127, 129, 148, 154].

Gotekpe found 89% of patients with OCD clinically improved; chronic anxiety, 66%; depression, 78%; and a small number of schizophrenics.

Overall, 80% were improved. It was noted that postoperative symptom improvement was not immediate, with a fluctuating but progressive reduction of symptoms over the first postoperative year [55].

This procedure is carried out *stereotactically*, and three small (6 mm diameter) lesions are placed in the lower medial quadrant of each frontal lobe and two lesions in each cingulate gyrus. Lesions are done with a *cryoprobe* or *thermocoagulation* [27].

Intraoperative stimulation is performed, and if pronounced autonomic responses are observed, it is felt it provides physiologic proof of correct location [27].

Although many patients suffer of lethargy, confusion, and lack of sphincter control in the early postoperative period, persistent complications are rare. No patients developed seizures postoperatively, one patient suffered severe memory loss due to improper lesion placement, and 12% of patients complained of persistent lethargy. Measurements of IQ showed slight improvement postoperatively [27].

Anterior Capsulotomy

Although *Talairach* (France) was the first to describe it in 1973 [176, 178], *Leksell* (Sweden) popularized the procedure for patients with a variety of psychiatric disorders [85, 99]. The aim is to interrupt presumed *fronto-thalamic connections* in the *anterior limb of the internal capsule* as they pass between the *head of the caudate nucleus* and the *putamen*.

Clinical indications of capsulotomy initially include MDD, chronic anxiety states, and OCD [27, 70, 89, 123, 139, 156].

The target coordinates are in the anterior one third of the anterior branch of the internal capsule, 5 mm behind the tip of the frontal horns, and 20 mm lateral to the midline at the level of the intercommissural plane [27].

Intraoperative electrical stimulation has not been helpful in terms of determining optimal placement of lesions within the capsule [27].

Lesions: through *thermocoagulation*, using a bipolar electrode system, and also performed with the *gamma knife* and with *ultrasound* [75, 83, 85, 88, 102, 152].

In a review of all cases of capsulotomy previously reported in the literature, Mindus [123, 124] found sufficient data to categorize 64% to have a satisfactory result. In the first patients operated by Leksell [16, 99], 50% of patients with *OCD* and 48% of depressed patients had a satisfactory response. Only 20% of patients with anxiety neurosis and only 14% of patients with schizophrenia were improved. In this classification system, only patients who were free of symptoms or markedly improved were judged as having a satisfactory response. In another series with *OCD* who underwent *capsulotomy* and were followed prospectively by independent psychiatrists, there was an overall satisfactory result of 70% [27, 102].

Complications of the surgery included transient episodes of confusion with occasional nocturnal incontinence. One patient was noted to have an intracranial hemorrhage without neurological sequelae, and another suffered seizures. One patient committed suicide in the postoperative phase, and eight suffered from depression requiring treatment. Excessive fatigue, poor memory, slovenliness, and weight gain are common after capsulotomy. No evidence of cognitive dysfunction has been reported in 200 capsulotomy patients studied using a variety of psychometric tests. Reoperation was required in two patients who did not achieve a satisfactory result with only one improving after the second operation [27, 139, 156].

25.2.2 Other Less Frequent Ablation Procedures: *Hypothalamotomy, Amygdalotomy, Thalamotomy*

Lateral hypothalamotomy has been performed for *morbid obesity* (MO) [101].

Posteromedial hypothalamotomy has been tried for *aggressive violent behavioral disorders* (*Sano*) [161]. The stereotactic target coordinates are 3 mm inferior to the middle point between the *anterior and posterior commissures* (CMP) and 2 mm lateral to the wall of the third ventricle. Previous to the lesion, stimulation is done to obtain a sympathetic response with arterial hypertension and tachycardia. Schvarcz [166] reported 11 cases treated with this technique, with treatment-resistant hetero or self-aggressiveness. With a follow-up of 6–48 months, 7 patients out of 11 were "cured" reentering society, 3 were controlled with medication, and only 1 failed to improve. This was without endocrine or cognitive post-op complications. Hypersomnia and transient tachycardia have been reported resolving in no more than 10 days. Tourette's is treated with *thalamotomy* [23], and bilateral stereotactic *amygdalotomy* is used in the management of severe aggressive behavioral disorders [7, 131].

For the preferred targets used in the treatment of certain refractory psychiatric disorders, see Table 25.4.

Table 25.4 Preferred cerebral targets

Psychiatric disorder	Preferred target
Obsessive-compulsive disorder (OCD)	*Anterior limb of the internal capsule* (ALIC), *ventral striatum* (VS)
Tourette's syndrome (TS)	*Centromedian-parafascicular complex* (CM-Pf) *of the thalamus*
Major depression (MDD)	*Subgenual cingulate* (SC)/area 25
Addiction, substance abuse	*Nucleus accumbens* (NAcc)
Eating disorders: *anorexia and bulimia*	*Ventral caudate nucleus* (CN) and NAcc
Aggression	*Posterior hypothalamus* (PH)
Schizophrenia	*Modern psychosurgery is ineffective*
Alzheimer's, cognitive disorders	*Fornix* (Fx), *entorhinal cortex* (EC)
	Nucleus basalis of Meynert (NBM)
Bipolar disorders, panic disorders, anxiety disorders, attention deficit disorders	*Several targets, including Amygdala*
Post-traumatic stress disorders (PTSD)	

25.2.2.1 *Obsessive-Compulsive Disorder* (OCD)

Prevalence: 2% of the world's population, with a rate of suicide attempts of 10–27% throughout the patient's life. 10–40% of patients with OCD are treatment-resistant [27].

The *selection* of the stereotactic target to treat patients with OCD takes into account the present knowledge of its physiopathology. The disorder is related to an anomaly in the *cortico-striatal-thalamic-cortical* (CSTC) *pathway* involving flow of information from motivational regions toward cognitive and motor areas. OCD and dysmorphic disorder seem to originate in the *caudate nucleus*. Tourette's and trichotillomania originates in the *putamen*. Spectroscopy shows decrease of N-acetyl aspartate in the caudate in the first case and in the putamen in the latter. Smaller left-sided putamen is seen in patients with trichotillomania. In this as well as in Tourette's, symptoms are mainly motor, while in classical OCD and dysmorphia, symptoms are both cognitive and spatial visual. A theory suggests that there is a possible *imbalance* between the described *direct* and *indirect pathways*, favoring the direct one in the CSTC circuit. This would lead to hyperactivity of the orbitofrontal cortex and the anterior cingulum. It would also lead to a decrease in the flow of information responsible for motivation toward the cognition system and eventually to the motor system carried by the limbic circuit. In OCD, repeated thoughts and motivation to act (*obsessions*) persist, since the motor circuit fails to eliminate both the thoughts and the motivation to carry them out, leading to a stereotyped repetition of motor responses (*compulsions*).

fMRI and PET show hyperactivity of the orbitofrontal cortex, the medial thalamus, the caudate nucleus, and the anterior cingulum in patients with OCD. This hyperactivity decreases with successful treatment with medications. Patients with orbitofrontal hyperactivity respond better to behavioral therapy and less well to SSRIs.

The DBS *targets* for OCD include the VC/VS, NAc, STN, and *inferior thalamic peduncle*

Table 25.5 Neurosurgery for OCD

Ablation
Thermo-capsulotomy
Gamma knife anterior capsulotomy
Cingulotomy
Limbic leucotomy
DBS
Subthalamic nucleus (STN)
Anterior limb of the internal capsule (ALIC)
Electrodes in four different targets produce similar results: nucleus accumbens (NAcc), *anterior limb of the internal capsule* (ALIC), *ventral striatum* (VS), *subthalamic nucleus* (STN)
Stimulation of the inferior thalamic peduncle (InThP) *achieve even better results*
Bed nucleus of the stria terminalis (BNST)

(InThP) (see Table 25.5). Among early outcome reports, Nuttin and colleagues found that three of four patients with OCD benefited from DBS. A study by Greenberg et al. found positive outcomes in 16 of 26 [58]. Interestingly, several studies found that DBS in the region of the *ventral capsule/ventral striatum* (VC/VS) resulted in smiling and laughter during surgery, indicating that this circuitry may be related to mood alteration. Because of these positive results, a *humanitarian device exception* (HDE) from the US FDA was obtained in 2009 for DBS for OCD.

Bilateral DBS appears to be more effective than unilateral.

Parkinson's patients also suffering OCD show OCD improvement with DBS of the *STN*; PET shows decreased metabolism in the left cingulum (areas 24 and 32) and in the left medial frontal gyrus (area 6). At the same time, those with decrease of Y-BOCS with DBS show decreased orbitofrontal cortex and ventromedial prefrontal region metabolism, close to the tract that connects the thalamic nuclei with the cortical orbitofrontal region. This is precisely the tract included in the *subcaudate tractotomy.*

Due to its anatomical location, it is probable that an electrode placed for DBS or for ablation in the *ALIC* will also affect the *NAcc*. It is still not known with exactitude which one of these two targets is responsible for improvement. The *nucleus accumbens* is involved with the processing of reward, motivation, and addiction and is divided into two regions: core and shell. The *core* is located in the lateral part of the nucleus and connects with the extrapyramidal system. The *shell* is located in the *ventromedial* part of the nucleus as well as two thirds caudal, surrounding the core and connecting with the limbic system. The nucleus accumbens receives the *afferent glutamatergic* pathway from the hippocampus, amygdala, thalamus and prefrontal cerebral cortex, and the *dopaminergic* inflow from the substantia nigra. The principal *efferent* flow is *GABAergic* toward the ventral pallidum with projections toward the substantia nigra compacta and to the limbic portions of the subthalamic nucleus. Only the shell of the nucleus accumbens has efferent connections toward the lateral hypothalamus and the amygdala. This portion of the nucleus accumbens is the possible surgical target for DBS in patients with OCD [5, 16, 17, 21, 30, 35, 37, 47, 48, 50, 53, 69, 75, 76, 80, 93, 100, 101, 105, 108, 120, 123, 129, 139, 140, 151, 152, 155, 169, 170, 174, 175].

25.2.2.2 *Tourette's Syndrome* (TS)

TS is a neuropsychiatric disorder which becomes symptomatic in childhood or adolescence and that involves uncontrollable repetitive movements or unwanted sounds, repeatedly blinking of the eyes, shrugging shoulders (tics), or blurting out offensive words.

World *prevalence:* 5 cases every 10,000 people. It is associated with OCD, attention deficit disorder, and hyperactivity. Tourette's is considered malignant when the symptoms become disabling and associated with self-aggression [96, 148].

TS is felt to be a disorder of *cortico-striato-thalamic-cortical loops.*

Cappabianca et al. [23] reported four patients with Tourette's treated with *thalamotomy (dorsomedial* and *interlaminar nuclei).* Treatment was unilateral in three and bilateral in the 4th. There was great improvement in one patient with total resolution of the tics, but in two cases only a transient improvement ensued. Babel et al. published a series of 16 patients with Tourette's treated with a ventrolateral/medial thalamotomy together with a thermoablation of the *zona incerta*, with significant improvement of the tics [4, 62, 138, 162, 163, 181].

DBS of *CM/PF* and *PVS* interrupts the retro-excitatory feed between the *thalamus* and the *striatum. Voi* projects to the region of the face in the premotor area; hence, it is used as target for TS. Since TS is also close to OCD, *NAcc* is also used as a surgical target [82, 93, 116, 138].

DBS of *GPi* is not effective. The reason is unclear since GPi is known to be inhibited by the same physiopathology. Some researchers tried DBS on the postero-ventrolateral part of GPi because of TS tics being considered hyperkinesias similar of the dyskinesias of patients with Parkinson's. One thing to take into account is that the limbic region of GPi is located antero-medially and is not reached by DBS if the electrode is in the postero-ventrolateral region of the nucleus, since it is rather large. So, DBS of GPi for TS requires precise placement of the electrode for the modulation of the circuitry [101, 116, 160]. DBS of *globus pallidus external* (GPe) is based on the hypothesis that this nucleus is hyperactive in TS.

For ablation and/or DBS targets for TS, see Table 25.6.

Surgical *candidates* for DBS for TS:

1. Older than 18 (or even 25) years of age
2. Yale Global Tic Severity Scale (YGTSS) >35/50, for at least 12 months
3. Failure of conventional medical treatment: at least three different α-adrenergic agonists, two dopaminergic antagonists and benzodiazepines, at least for 12 weeks at an adequate therapeutic dose
4. Failure to respond to no less than ten sessions of behavioral modification

Table 25.6 Neurosurgery for Tourette's

Ablation and/or DBS targets for Tourette's (TS)
Thalamus
Intralaminar thalamic nuclei (ILN)
Centromedian-parafascicular thalamic complex (CM-Pf)
Ventral oral internal thalamic nuclei (Voi)
Medial thalamic nuclei – substantia paraventricularis (PVS)
Globus pallidus, internal segment-GPi
Anterior limb of the internal capsule/nucleus accumbens (ALIC/NAcc)
Other: GPe, STN, *zona incerta* (ZI)

The pathophysiology of TS is related to an excessive dopaminergic activity of the *striatum*, with direct stimulation of the *internal part* of the *globus pallidum* (GPI), inhibiting the indirect route [22]. The hypoactivity of the GPI leads to a disinhibition of the thalamocortical pathway, retro-feeding in a positive way the *centromedian-parafascicular complex* (CM-Pf) of the *thalamus*, and the *medial nucleus* of the *thalamus substantia paraventricularis* (PVS) toward the *striatum* where there is also increase activity [111]. All this contributes to maintain the circuit in hyperactivity and the thalamocortical projections disinhibited. CM projects to the motor region of the *putamen*, while PF does it to the associate regions of both the *putamen* and the *caudate*. PVS projects toward the VS (*ventral striatum*). It is probable that in TS, there is an alteration of the D2 inhibitory dopaminergic receptor in the indirect pathway. In summary, both the motor and limbic circuits seem involved in Tourette's with hyperactivity of the thalamus leading to prefrontal cerebral hyperactivity.

Electrical activity recordings of neurons of the *medial thalamus* in patients undergoing DBS show that those that received DBS at low frequency (2–15 Hz) show increased electrical activity, while DBS at high frequency (25–45 Hz) seems to exert a calming effect and is associated with clinical improvement. DBS does not seem to produce permanent and persistent neuroplastic changes [1, 4, 6, 9, 22, 82, 88, 92, 97, 98, 105, 106, 117, 122, 138, 154, 162].

25.2.2.3 *Major Depressive Disorder (MDD)*

Prevalence: 5–10% of the world's population; 20–40%, *refractory* to pharmacological treatment. *Suicide* rate (in refractory depression): 15%. Treatment-resistant/refractory depression *definition*: when patients fail with at least four antidepressants and psychotherapy. To be considered for surgery, depression must be severe: a score bigger than 20 in the *Hamilton Rating Scale for Depression* (HAMD) or equal or bigger than 30 in the *Beck Depression Inventory* (BDI). *Electroconvulsive therapy* (ECT) is no longer a precondition for surgery, since some patients refuse ECT and are afraid of memory loss and general adverse public opinion [69]. *Depression* occurs when there is a loss of emotional homeostasis at stressful situations of life. The *physiopathology* is multidimensional, involving more than one cerebral region and several neurotransmitter systems. The structures that originate this pathology are still elusive. The metabolic findings observed in functional studies could be just a consequence rather than a cause and perhaps only adaptive changes of the circuitry to a certain lesion. There is involvement of the *cortico-striatal-thalamic-cortical* circuit with cognitive, motor, neuroendocrine, and affective involvement and manifestations. At the cortical level, there is a hypoactive "*dorsal* compartment," explaining the "*negative*" motor and cognitive symptoms. This compartment would be comprised by the anterior, dorsal, and lateral prefrontal cortex, the dorsal anterior cingulum, and the parietal and premotor cortex connecting with the dorsal striatum. The "*positive*" affective symptoms can be explained by the hyperactivity of a "*ventral* compartment" including the subgenual cingulum, the orbitofrontal cortex, and the anterior insular region. This compartment connects with the limbic region, and both compartments inhibit each other in a reciprocal fashion. In addition, there are three structures that intervene in the balance of the activity of those two compartments: the *amygdala* (that directs this balance towards the stimulation of the ventral compartment), the *pregenual cingulum* (that inhibits both compartments), and the *hippocampus* (HC). The hippocampus has connections with the amygdala and projects toward the hypothalamus influencing sleep, appetite, and the hypothalamic pituitary adrenal axis. One hypothesis regarding the neuroanatomy of depression involves hyperactivity of the *amygdala* caused by dysfunction of the *hippocampus* [72, 100].

The most commonly used DBS target for depression is the *subgenual cingulum* (SC) (area 25 of Brodmann) (*Mayberg and Lozano*) [108]. The subgenual cingulum shows increased metabolism in depression. PET and fMRI show decreased blood flow in the prefrontal (areas 46 and 9) and premotor cerebral cortex (area 6), anterior dorsal cingulum (area 24), and anterior insula. These findings can be reversed with the use of *SSRIs* and other antidepressants, *ECT* and *transcranial magnetic stimulation* (TMS). For these reasons, the SC was suggested as a possible target to treat depression with high-frequency DBS. After treatment, imaging shows decrease of cerebral blood flow in the SC and an increase in the prefrontal cortex, concomitant with clinical improvement, but as mentioned, the Broden trial by St. Jude's failed [173]. To avoid confusion: the subgenual cingulum is a different target than that used for anterior cingulotomy ablation [2, 3, 31, 62, 64, 72, 75, 89, 108, 113, 114, 120, 148, 149, 158, 164]. Another target used for DBS in depression is the *nucleus accumbens* (NAcc). The most optimal location to place the electrode is in its ventral, caudal, and medial regions. This is where the *reward* system is located, clinically manifested as *anhedonia* [14, 147].

For neurosurgery for depression (MDD), see Table 25.7.

Table 25.7 Neurosurgery for depression (MDD)

Ablative surgery	
	Cingulotomy
	Anterior capsulotomy
	Subcaudate tractotomy
	Limbic leucotomy
Cerebral stimulation	
a-Cortical	*Dorsolateral cerebral cortex*
b-Deep-DBS	*Targets*
	Subgenual cortex cingulum
	Nucleus accumbens (NAcc)
	Ventral striatum (VS)
	Ventral/Anterior limb of the internal capsule (ALIC)
	Inferior thalamic peduncle (InThP)
	Lateral habenula (LHb)
	Medial forebrain bundle (MFB)
	Limbic-Internal globus pallidus (GPi)
Vagal N. STIM (VNS)	*Cervical vagal nerve* (VN)

25.2.2.4 *Aggressive Behavior* (AB) *Disorders*

The constellation of *aggressive behavior disorders* constitutes a family of conditions. Whether individually or as a family, they are challenging to define. Almost all of them have, or invoke by, complex social and political implications [18, 20, 37, 42, 43, 47, 73, 82, 86, 94, 119, 144, 161, 166, 183]. *Aggressive personality traits* are related and relatively common phenomena that do not necessarily meet the criteria for true personality disorders. AB disorders are amorphous conditions. They are defined formally as the "deliberate use or threat of deliberate use of physical force or power against one-self, or another person, or against a group or community, which results or may result in injury, death, psychological harm, mal–development or deprivation" (WHO). The more common clinical definition, "an attack to property, others, or oneself with the deliberate intention of destruction," is only slightly more specific [131].

AB can be associated with organic psychosis, schizophrenia, mental retardation, emotional disorders, dementia, and, as already noted, personality disorders. They occur most frequently in the acute phase of mental illness. Rare genetic syndromes like *Tourette's and Lesch-Nyhan* may also include elements of aggressive behavior. *Aggression*, however, must also be understood as a normal component of mammalian behavior. Two basic types are recognized: a *predatory* kind related to the search for food and a *defensive* or affective kind serving as reaction to threat. In the case of the human beings, social rules establish proper or acceptable limits of aggressive behavior. The etiology of aggressive disorder is very complex. It is multifactorial, influenced by both external (socioeconomic and cultural) and endogenous factors, including, for example, the putative *overactivity* of the *fury circuit of Papez* (comprising the amygdala, thalamus, hypothalamus, insula, ventral striatum, and internal capsule in the limbic system) or the putative *underactivity* of the *orbitofrontal cerebral cortex* – which modulates behavior – and the *anterior cingulum gyrus*. The orbitofrontal cortex has an inhibitory control on aggressive behavior. Put simplistically it evaluates and is associated with the capacity to mitigate the consequences of such behavior. The hypothalamus behaves as a control center receiving many central and peripheral afferent impulses relating to the biologic condition and the context. In the case of affective or defensive aggression activated by a threat, there is great sympathetic discharge, hyperactivity of the posterior medial hypothalamus, amygdala, periaqueductal dorsal gray matter, and minimal cerebral activation. Predatory aggression, in contrast, involves a more significant component of cortical activation as well as involvement of the ventral *periaqueductal grey* and the *lateral hypothalamus*, with scarce sympathetic response. Activation of the *hypothalamus* causes cluster headaches, arterial hypertension, aggression, hypersexuality, insomnia, hyperphagia, and psychomotor excitation. Bilateral destruction of the *amygdala* causes loss of fear. At the same time, a lesion of the amygdala takes away the ability to respond to facial expressions, and patients can experience disinhibited, inappropriate behavior [100, 115, 183]. While society has a clear and logical interest in regulating aggressive behavior, particularly when it verges on the criminal, there are many ethical questions that arise when such behavior – and its management – is medicalized. The medical and surgical approaches to AB must contend with issues of informed consent and conflict of interest. The treatment of aggressive disorders by surgery, whether by ablation or by stimulation, demands extreme caution. The contours of the AB are at least as sociologically and politically defined as they are medical. This warning, therefore, applies not only to researchers and doctors but to society as a whole. The same comments and considerations apply to the medicalized and surgical treatment of *addiction* and *sexual* behavior. The use of medical and surgical approaches to restrict and publish free expression, political resistance, and other forms of politically undesirable behavior has a long and ugly history in totalitarian regimes (e.g., Argentina 1952, Evita's secret lobotomy) [134, 136]. The surgical treatment of AB remains controversial from medical and ethical perspectives [103, 109, 134–136, 140, 163].

For neurosurgery for *aggressive behavior* (AB) disorders, see Table 25.8.

Table 25.8 Neurosurgery for aggressive behavior (AB) disorders

Ablation
Anterior capsulotomy (AC)
Cingulotomy (C)
Subcaudate tractotomy (SCT)
Limbic leucotomy (LL)
Posterior hypothalamotomy (PH)
Amygdalotomy (A)
DBS
Internal globus pallidus (GPi)
Posterior hypothalamus (PH), *thalamus* (T)

Surgical indications are limited to those with chronic and/or progressive AB, treatment-resistant, usually associated with mental retardation and other social/occupational disability. Patients who fall in this category also constitute classical examples of vulnerable individuals. They are generally under special legal protection, and their management is generally subject to special ethical oversight. It is mandatory that family, an ethics committee, and sometimes the court participate fully and actively.

The appropriate modern surgical technique for AB involves *high-frequency* DBS of the *posteromedial hypothalamus* [100, 115, 119, 128]. It has been effective in patients with both violence against others and against themselves. DBS has similar results to *radiofrequency posteromedial hypothalamotomy* with the advantage of reversibility [36]. Surgery of this area bears a significant risk, since this region is eloquent and vascularized, and a deep cerebral hemorrhage can be fatal. DBS of the posterior hypothalamic region was originally introduced to treat *trigeminal autonomic cephalalgias*, thought to result from hyperactivation of the posterior hypothalamic region (pHr) during the painful episodes. Patients experiencing chronic cluster headaches were often found to exhibit aggressive bouts during such episodes. The pHr was used as a lesional target in patients with aggressive behavior and disruptive behavior that could be induced by acute electrical stimulation of the so-called triangle of Sano [161]. The known interconnections between the pHr, the amygdala, and the overall so-called Papez circuit may explain the role of the pHr in the development of disruptive behavior [20, 33, 36, 37, 42, 43, 47, 73, 80, 86, 119, 161, 166].

25.2.2.5 "Reward-Based" Psychiatric Disorders: Drug Addiction/*Substance Dependence* (SD)

Although *DBS* is FDA-approved to treat movement disorders and, through a *humanitarian device exception* (HDE), also OCD, it is not approved for *addiction*. Intermittent bilateral DBS of the *nucleus accumbens* (NAcc) *shell* reduces intravenous methamphetamine intake and seeking in Wistar rats. In humans, there have been case reports of DBS having a beneficial effect on reducing the *consumption of alcohol, nicotine, cocaine, and heroin*, although these were patients receiving DBS for disorders other than addiction (such as *depression*). A recent small case series of five severely alcohol-dependent patients from Lübeck, Germany, in whom bilateral electrodes implanted in the nucleus-accumbens, showed a reduction in craving. In two patients, there was complete abstinence from alcohol. In heroin dependence, a case report of two subjects who received bilateral DBS to the NAcc reported an improvement in depressive symptoms and anxiety and a reduction, though not cessation, in their drug use [102, 109, 129].

25.2.2.6 *Eating Disorders* (ED)

These are severe psychiatric disorders associated with self-driven food refusal and emaciation, altered body perception, and preoccupations with weight. They include *anorexia nervosa* (AN), *bulimia nervosa* (BN), and *eating disorder not otherwise specified* (EDNOS) [63, 121, 169].

AN has high rates of morbidity, comorbidity, and mortality and a chronic course in a considerable percentage of patients. Evidence-based treatment options based on underlying neurobiological mechanisms of the disease are scarce. The *fronto-striatal circuitry*, in particular the *insula*, the *ventral striatum* (VS) and the prefrontal, orbitofrontal, temporal, parietal, and anterior cingulate *cortices* appear to be implicated in the etiopathogenesis of AN. Thus, the areas communicating between the limbic and the cortical systems, such as the *NAcc* and the *cingulate* and *insular cortices*, may be of investigational interest as target areas for future neurosurgical interventions [142].

The reversibility of DBS is a major advantage over ablative surgery. The overlap in symptomatology and the common neural circuitry associated with reward-related disorders like OCD and AN, as well as the established efficacy of *accumbal*-DBS in OCD, has been intriguing. It suggests that DBS of the NAcc and other areas associated with reward might offer an effective treatment for patients with chronic, treatment-refractory AN. The goal is not only to provide weight restoration but also significant and sustained improvement in AN core symptoms and other associated comorbidities and complications [105].

Targets for *DBS* in *anorexia nervosa* (AN) [63, 101] include the *ventral caudate nucleus*, the *anterior limb of the internal capsule*, and the NAcc. Patient BMIs have recovered to normal after 3–6 months of DBS. Comorbid psychiatric conditions such as OCD and anxiety have also been shown to improve. The time course for recovery is slow, but no severe side effects or complications have been reported. Nevertheless, bilateral DBS implantation-stimulation of the NAcc failed to show clinical efficacy in patients with *bulimia nervosa* (BN) 66 and in those with severe coexisting psychological conditions such as *substance misuse*, compulsive hair-tugging or twisting (*trichotillomania*), or self-harm. There is some evidence to indicate that bilateral *anterior capsulotomy* may be a better target approach for these conditions [105]. The same group, led by Lozano in Toronto has tried subcallosal cingulate DBS for treatment refractory anorexia nervosa.

Lateral and *dorsomedial ablative hypothalamotomy* and DBS of the *lateral* and *dorsomedial hypothalamus* have been used for *morbid obesity* (MO) [101].

25.2.2.7 Schizophrenia

Schizophrenia is a chronic, severe, and disabling psychiatric disease characterized by perturbations in cognition, affect, and behavior. Of the many available treatments, pharmaceutical interventions remain the first choice. However, some 20% of patients with schizophrenia exhibit refractory schizophrenia that does not respond well to pharmaceutical intervention. This is a persistent problem that has prevailed for decades. Alternatives have long been sought. Psychosurgery has long been tried as an alternative treatment. Nevertheless, and despite many refinements and innovations, the procedures are ineffective [27].

25.2.2.8 Memory: Alzheimer's

Memory is the ability to recall information, encoded and stored in the brain and retrieved by the brain. There are three types of memory: *immediate or* "working" memory (based in the superior frontal cerebral cortex); *short-term* or "episodic" memory, associated with the circuit of Papez; and *long-term* or "semantic-procedural" memory, which is more complex. There are also three types of *amnesia: transient global* amnesia (TGA), *anterograde* amnesia, and *retrograde* amnesia. The *hippocampus, fornix, entorhinal cortex*, and *nucleus basalis of Meynert* have been targeted in animal models and patients [92].

Memory loss is the salient symptom and sign of *dementia*-related disorders, including the increasingly prevalent and socially pressing *Alzheimer's disease* (AD). To date, pharmacological treatments for AD have had limited and only short-lasting effects. For this reason, other approaches, including DBS, have been suggested, i.e., DBS of the fornix [24, 65]. Additional translational work has focused on the ability of implantable brain or neuromorphic chips to improve brain function, to be tolerated by the cerebral environment, to establish functional connections with neurons, and to improve neurological performance. The mechanisms underlying memory enhancement may include the release of specific neurotransmitters and neuroplasticity. DBS might even be disease-modifying. Nevertheless, it is still premature to conclude that DBS can be used in the treatment of AD, and this will need to wait for the results of ongoing clinical trials (*Lipsman and Lozano*) [90].

Kahana (University of Pennsylvania), under a contract from the *Defense Advanced Research Projects Agency* (DARPA), studies the *hippocam-*

pus, the very seat of memory formation [84]. The importance of the hippocampus emerged from the study of a patient, Henry Molaison, known worldwide as H.M., who had severe seizures until *Scoville* removed the hippocampus from both hemispheres [167]. In 1953, *Milner* of the MNI-McGill showed that without them, H.M. could form no new memories for facts, figures, or faces. This finding, one of the most important in modern brain science, opened the way for direct-recording experiments [38].

Fried (UCLA), also with DARPA, found improved spatial memory by electrically stimulating the *entorhinal cortex.* The subjects played a virtual taxi driver game in which the goal is to drop off passengers as quickly as possible in an unfamiliar city [50].

25.2.2.9 *Post-traumatic Stress Disorder* (PSTD)

Deep brain stimulation (DBS) of the *basolateral amygdala* is tested for management of *treatment-refractory* combat *post-traumatic stress disorder* (PTSD) by Koek et al. (UCLA) [88].

25.2.2.10 Coma

DBS of the *thalamus* has been attempted in patients with severe *traumatic brain injury* (TBI), with the goal of improving arousal and attention in patients relegated to a vegetative or minimally conscious state [168, 187].

25.2.2.11 Closed Loop, WINCS, and MINCS

A number of tools to explore the mechanisms of DBS have been developed. The Wireless Instantaneous Neurotransmitter Concentration System (*WINCS*) (*Lee*, Mayo Clinic (2010)) treats refractory psychiatric illness disrupted-disordered neurocircuitry using *neuromodulation. WINCS* measures levels of *serotonin* – a neurotransmitter with a key role in depression – in real time. It uses *fast-scan cyclic voltammetry*, an electrochemical method. WINCS is miniaturized, wireless, and computer controlled, tried in both animal studies and human patients undergoing DBS [2, 142, 177].

Mayo Investigational Neuromodulation Control System (*MINCS*) is a closed-loop electrochemical feedback system for DBS developed in 2014. It is optically and wirelessly linked to WINCS and implantable for closed-loop dynamic neurochemical control of psychotherapeutic interventions [2, 68, 177].

Lee's closed "smart" loop system is the *WINCS Harmoni (WINCS* plus *MINCS)* [2, 177].

25.2.2.12 Optogenetics: Nanotechnology

The *future* of psychosurgery likely includes sonogenetics, brain augmentation, neuromorphic chips, cyborgs, trans-humanity technologies, the field of brain-machine technologies (carbon nanotubes, nanowires, nanoscale coating), labs-on-a-chip, and other fusion technologies. If the problem of plasticity is solved, the brain-machine interface may result in a humans' analogue to Moore's law. Indeed, were that to be the case, the application of implants will surpass simple memory augmentation. Human cyborgs, linguists may say, will be directly connected to a vast database of information. Progress on this scale will doubtlessly result in tremendous and far reach ethical dilemmas. *Endovascular nanotechnology* may also advance the promise of the *brain-computer interface* (BCI), by leveraging a human's innate capacity to adjust the activity of fields of cortical neurons as new motor tasks are learned or recreated after injury. *Emerging techniques* may also allow for a new means of target selection, modulation, and control, offering specificity of effect and other advantages over current ablation and DBS techniques. In *optogenetics*, genes encoding photoreceptor membrane proteins (channel rhodopsins) are delivered to specifically targeting neurons. Because expression is controlled by cell-specific promoters, only particular cells will bear the photoreceptor. These cells can be activated by specific wavelengths of light, allowing for differential control of neuronal subpopulations in a given target by expressing different channel rhodopsins under the control of various promoters. Control requires an implanted light source, which still carries, however, many of the disadvantages of implanted DBS, including infection and device failure. *Chemogenetics*, like optogenetics, utilizes the delivery of the gene for repair of a defective receptor, sensitive to novel ligands. As such, neuronal subpopulations expressing the relevant channel/receptors could be activated by the administration of a drug. This scenario avoids the need for an implanted device. The pursuit and realization of these technologies and approaches will inevitably invoke pressing and profound ethical issues [35, 44, 118, 134, 142].

Neuroethics

Ethics is the study of moral behavior. It pertains to right and wrong, and how to live well. Neuroethics is the field focused specifically on research in and treatment of neurological and psychiatric conditions. There are a number of models of ethical behavior and a number of approaches to ethical decision-making. One of the best-known approaches is based on the principles of beneficence, non-maleficence, respect for persons and autonomy. Only democracies are capable of guaranteeing independence of ethical oversight entities [28, 54, 91, 104, 105, 140, 150, 163, 184].

Voluntary fully informed consent pertains to a patient's right to be informed about his or her condition and proposed course of treatment and his or her right to provide or withhold consent an agreement [11]. Vulnerable populations, but not restricted to children and adults with limited decision-making capacity or ability to provide consent, need to be specially protected [89, 103].

Conflicts of interest involving researchers, clinicians, and other personnel engaged in patient management and research constitute a special problem [54, 77].

There is a history of ethical problems specific to research and patient management in psychiatry, particularly with respect to voluntary, fully informed consent, competence, and capacity. Involuntary hospitalization and treatment, including such measures as electroshock and psychosurgery, have been deployed abusively by totalitarian regimes such as the USSR, Nazi Germany, and others, to control dissidents and punish free expression. Similar practices were employed in the federal prison system in Atascadero and Vacaville, California, USA, in the 1950s–1960s [134–136, 189].

"Psychosurgery and Mind Control": ethical issues in psychosurgery are many, and they are inseparable from the political order. Psychosurgery can be used for good or evil: as a treatment or a tool for political control. Surgery on the brain for psychiatric indications is aggressive and hazardous. To counter the risk of psychosurgical abuses, societies must be kept informed of the advances, opportunities, and risks in this field with utmost transparency [27, 32, 33, 134–136, 189]. It is necessary to guarantee appropriate professional safeguard based on guidelines that emerged after the *Nuremberg Trial* and are embodied in the *Helsinki Accord*, the *Belmont Report* (Ethical Principles and Guidelines for the Protection of Human Subjects of Research, issued by the National Commission for the Protection of Human Subjects of Biomedical and Behavioral Research, HEW, 1974), and similar documents [132].

References

1. Ackermans L, Kuhn J, Neuner I, et al. Surgery for Tourette syndrome. World Neurosurg. 2012;80(3–4):S29.e15–e22.
2. Anderson RJ, Frye MA, Abulseoud OA, et al. Deep brain stimulation for treatment-resistant depression: efficacy, safety and mechanisms of action. Neurosci Biobehav Rev. 2012;36(8):1920–33.
3. Andrade P, Noblesse LH, Temel Y, et al. Neurostimulatory and ablative treatment options in major depressive disorder: a systematic review. Acta Neurochir. 2010;152(4):565–77.
4. Babel TB, Warnke PC, Ostertag CB. Immediate and long- term outcome after infrathalamic and thalamic lesioning for intractable Tourette's syndrome. J Neurol Neurosurg Psychiatry. 2001;70(5):666–71.
5. Baer L, Rauch SL, Ballantine HT Jr, et al. Cingulotomy for intractable obsessive-compulsive disorder. Prospective long-term follow-up of 18 patients. Arch Gen Psychiatry. 1995;52(5):384–92.
6. Bajwa RJ, de Lotbinière AJ, King RA, et al. Deep brain stimulation in Tourette's syndrome. Mov Disord. 2007;22(9):1346–50.
7. Balasubramaniam V, Ramamurthi B. Stereotactic surgery. Neurol India. 1965;13:93–6.
8. Ballantine HT, Bouckoms AJ, Thomas EK, et al. Treatment of psychiatric illness by stereotactic cingulotomy. Biol Psychiatry. 1987;22:807–19.
9. Barbosa D, Oliveira-Souza R, Monte Santo F, et al. The hypothalamus at the crossroads of psychopathology and neurosurgery. Neurosurg Focus.

2017;43(3):E15. https://doi.org/10.3171/2017.6.FOCUS17256.
10. Barlett JR, Bridges PK. The extended subcaudate tractotomy lesion. In: Sweet WH, Obrador S, Martin-Rodriguez JG, editors. Neurosurgical treatment in psychiatry, pain and epilepsy. Baltimore: University Park Press; 1977. p. 387–98.
11. Beloucif S. Informed consent for special procedures: electroconvulsive therapy and psychosurgery. Curr Opin Anaesthesiol. 2013;26:182–5.
12. Benabid AL, Pollak P, Louveau A, et al. Combined (thalamotomy and stimulation) stereotactic surgery of the VIM thalamic nucleus for bilateral Parkinson disease. Appl Neurophysiol. 1987;50(1–6):344–3.
13. Benabid AL. Attention, la psychochirurgie est de retour! Rev Neurol. 2006;162(8–9):797–9.
14. Bewernick BH, Kayser S, Sturm V, et al. Long-term effects of nucleus accumbens deep brain stimulation in treatment-resistant depression: evidence for sustained efficacy. Neuropsychopharmacology. 2012;37(9):1975–85.
15. Binder DK, Eskandar BJ. Modern neurosurgery for psychiatric disorders. Neurosurgery. 2000;47(1):9–21.
16. Bingley T, Leksell L, Meyerson BA, et al. Long term results of stereotactic capsulotomy in chronic obsessive-compulsive neurosis. In: Sweet WH, Obrador S, Martin-Rodriguez JG, editors. Neurosurgical treatment in psychiatry, pain and epilepsy. Baltimore: University Park Press; 1977. p. 287–9.
17. Blomstedt P, Sjöberg RL, Hansson M, et al. Deep brain stimulation in the treatment of obsessive-compulsive disorder. World Neurosurg. 2012; https://doi.org/10.1016/j.wneu.2012.10.006.
18. Breggin PR. Psychosurgery for the control of violence: a critical review. In: Fields W, Sweet WH, editors. Neural basis of violence and aggression. St. Louis: Warren H. Green; 1975. p. 350–78.
19. Broca P. Anatomie comparée des circonvolutions cerebrales: le grande lobe limbique et la scissure limbique dans la série des mammifères. Rev Anthropol. 1878;1:385–498.
20. Broggi G, Franzini A. Treatment of aggressive behavior. In: Lozano A, Gildenberg P, Tasker R, editors. Textbook of stereotactic and functional neurosurgery. Berlin: Springer; 2009. p. 2971–7.
21. Burzaco J. Stereotactic surgery in the treatment of obsessive compulsive neurosis. In: Perris C, Struwe G, Janssen B, editors. Biological psychiatry. Amsterdam: Elsevier; 1981. p. 1108–9.
22. Cannon E, Silburn P, Coyne T, et al. Deep brain stimulation of anteromedial globus pallidus interna for severe Tourette's syndrome. Am J Psychiatry. 2012;169(8):860–6.
23. Cappabianca P, Spaziante R, Carrabs G, et al. Surgical stereotactic treatment for Gilles de la Tourette's syndrome. Acta Neurol (Napoli). 1987;9(4):273–80.
24. Carey B. Pacemaker' for the brain can help memory. April 20, 2017. New York Times.
25. Cooper IS, Upton AR, Amin I. Reversibility of chronic neurologic deficits: some effects of electrical stimulation of the thalamus and internal capsule in man. Appl Neurophysiol. 1980;43(3–5): 244–58.
26. Corkin S, Twitchell TE, Sullivan EV. Safety and efficacy of cingulotomy for pain and psychiatric disorders. In: Hitchcock ER, Ballantine HT, Myerson BA, editors. Modern concepts in psychiatric surgery. Amsterdam: Elsevier; 1979. p. 253–72.
27. Cosgrove GR, Rauch SL, Eskandar EN. Psychosurgery, Massachusetts General Hospital. Boston: Harvard Medical School; 2017. neurosurgery.mgh.harvard.edu
28. Dagi TF. Psychiatric surgery and the ethics of uncertainty. In: Sweet WH, Obrador S, Martín-Rodríguez JG, editors. Neurosurgical treatment in psychiatry. Baltimore: University Park Press; 1977.
29. Dagi TF, Poletti CE. A reformulation of the circuit of Papez: effect of hippocampal influence on unit responses in cingulate cortex of unsedated squirrel monkeys. Brain Res. 1983;259:229–36.
30. de Koning PP, Figee M, van den Munckhof P, et al. Current status of deep brain stimulation for obsessive-compulsive disorder: a clinical review of different targets. Curr Psychiatry Rep. 2011;13(4):274–82.
31. Delaloye S, Holtzheimer PE. Deep brain stimulation in the treatment of depression. Dialogues Clin Neurosci. 2014;16:83–91.
32. Delgado JM. Physical control of the mind: toward a psychocivilized society. New York: Harper and Row; 1986.
33. Delgado JM, Mark V, Sweet W, et al. Intracerebral radio stimulation and recording in completely free patients. J Nerv Ment Dis. 1968;147:329–40.
34. DeLong MR, Wichmann T. Basal ganglia circuits as targets for neuromodulation in Parkinson disease. JAMA Neurol. 2015;72(11):1354–60.
35. Denys D, Mantione M, Figee M, et al. Deep brain stimulation of the nucleus accumbens for treatment-refractory obsessive-compulsive disorder. Arch Gen Psychiatry. 2010;67(10):1061–8.
36. Diaz Perez G, Chiorino R, Donoso P, et al. Posterior hypothalamotomy using the stereotaxic method in the treatment of erethism and aggressiveness. Neurocirugia. 1968;26:12–8.
37. Dieckmann NG, Hassler R. Treatment of sexual violence by stereotactic hypothalamotomy. In: Sweet WH, Obrador S, Martin-Rodriguez JG, editors. Neurosurgical treatment in psychiatry, pain and epilepsy. Baltimore: University Park Press; 1977. p. 451–62.
38. Dittrich L. Patient H.M.: a story of memory, madness, and family secrets. New York: Random House; 2017.
39. Dougherty DD, Baer L, Cosgrove GR, et al. Prospective long-term follow-up of 44 patients who received cingulotomy for treatment-refractory obsessive-compulsive disorder. Am J Psychiatry. 2002;159(2):269–75.

40. Edwards CA, Kouzani A, Lee KH, et al. Neurostimulation devices for the treatment of neurologic disorders. Mayo Clin Proc. 2017;92(9):1427–44.
41. Eskandar E, re. World Society for Stereotactic and Functional Neurosurgery (WSSFN) Meeting in Berlin, June 26–29, 2017. Massachusetts General Hospital-Harvard. www.wssfn-congress.org/.
42. Espinoza J, Arango G, Gálvez J, et al. Posteromedial hypothalamus deep brain stimulation for impulsive aggression: indications and results. In: Cukiert A, editor. Neuromodulation. Sao Paulo: Alaúde Editorial; 2010. p. 386–98.
43. Faria MA. Violence, mental illness, and the brain—a brief history of psychosurgery: Part I, from trephination to lobotomy. Surg Neurol Int. 2013;4:49. Part 2 of this series: From the limbic system and cingulotomy to deep brain stimulation. Part 3 – From deep brain stimulation to amygdalotomy for violent behavior, seizures, and pathological aggression in humans. Surg Neurol Int 4: 91.
44. Feldman RP, Alterman LR, Goodrich TJ. Contemporary psychosurgery and a look to the future. J Neurosurg. 2001;95:944–56.
45. Fodstad H, Strandman E, Karlsson B, et al. Treatment of obsessive compulsive states with stereotactic anterior capsulotomy or cingulotomy. Acta Neurochir. 1982;62:1–23.
46. Foltz EL, White LE Jr. Pain relief by frontal cingulotomy. J Neurosurg. 1962;19:89–94.
47. Franzini A, Messina G, Cordella R, et al. Deep brain stimulation of the posteromedial hypothalamus: indications, long-term results, and neurophysiological considerations. Neurosurg Focus. 2010;29(2):E13.
48. Franzini A, Messina G, Gambini O, et al. Deep-brain stimulation of the nucleus accumbens in obsessive compulsive disorder: clinical, surgical and electrophysiological considerations in two consecutive patients. Neurol Sci. 2010;31(3):353–9.
49. Freeman W, Watts JW. Prefrontal lobotomy; indications and contraindications. Arch Neurol Psychiatr. 1948;60:97–100.
50. Fried I, Suthana N, Haneef Z, et al. N Engl J Med. 2012;366:502–10.
51. Fulton JE. Frontal lobotomy and affective behavior a neurophysiological analysis. New York: WW Norton; 1951.
52. Fulton JF, Jacobsen CF. Fonctions des lobes frontaux; etude comparee chez l'homme et les singes chimpanzes. In: Proceedings of the international neurological congress. London; 1935. p. 552.
53. Gabriëls L, Cosyns P, Nuttin B, et al. Deep brain stimulation for treatment-refractory obsessive-compulsive disorder: psychopathological and neuropsychological outcome in three cases. Acta Psychiatr Scand. 2003;107(4):275–82.
54. Glannon W. Neuroethics. Bioethics. 2006;20:37–52.
55. Goktepe EO, Young LB, Bridges PK. A further review of the results of stereotactic subcaudate tractotomy. Br J Psychiatry. 1975;126:270–80.
56. Gostin L. Ethical considerations of psychosurgery: the unhappy legacy of the pre-frontal lobotomy. J Med Ethics. 1980;6:149–54.
57. Greenblatt SH, Dagi TF, Epstein M. A history of neurosurgery: in its scientific and professional contexts. Park Ridge: American Association of Neurological Surgeons; 1977.
58. Greenberg BD, Gabriels LA, Malone DA Jr, et al. Deep brain stimulation of the ventral internal capsule/ventral striatum for obsessive-compulsive disorder: worldwide experience. Mol Psychiatry. 2010;15(1):64–79.
59. Gross D, Schafer G. Egas Moniz (1874–1955) and the 'invention' of modern psychosurgery: a historical and ethical reanalysis under special consideration of Portuguese original sources. Neurosurg Focus. 2011;30:E8.
60. Guridi J, Aldave G. Surgical targets in psychiatric disorders. From movement to emotions. Neurocirugia (Astur). 2011;22(1):5–22.
61. Harris M, Blomstedt P, Zrinzo L. Future of brain stimulation: new targets, new indications, new technology. Mov Disord. 2013;28:1784–92.
62. Hassler R, Dieckmann NG. Relief of obsessive compulsive disorders, phobias and tics by stereotactic coagulation of the rostral intralaminar and medial thalamic nuclei. In: Laitinen LV, Livingston KV, editors. Surgical approaches in psychiatry, Proceedings of the 3rd International Congress of Psychosurgery. Baltimore: University Park Press; 1973. p. 206–692.
63. Hernández M, Zarate A, Valencia FJ, et al. El papel actual de la cirugía del sistema límbico, el caso de la anorexia y la bulimia terminales. Arch Neurocien (Méx). 2009;14(1):11–21.
64. Hitchcock ER, Ballantine HT, Meyerson BA, editors. Modern concepts in psychiatric surgery. New York: Elsevier/North Holland Biomedical Press; 1979. p. 111–27.
65. Hardenacke K, Shubina E, Bührle CP, et al. Deep brain stimulation as a tool for improving cognitive functioning in Alzheimer's dementia: a systematic review. Front Psych. 2013;4:1–11.
66. Heath RG. Electrical self-stimulation of the brain in man. Am J Psychiatry. 1963;120:571–7.
67. Heath RG. Modulation of emotion with a brain pacemaker: treatment for intractable psychiatric illness. J Nerv Ment Dis. 1977;165(5):300–17.
68. Hebb AO, Zhang JJ, Mahoor MH, et al. Creating the feedback loop: closed-loop neurostimulation. Neurosurg Clin N Am. 2014;25(1):187–204.
69. Heeramun-Aubeeluck A, Lu Z. Neurosurgery for mental disorders: a review. Afr J Psychiatry (Johannesbg). 2013;16:177–81.
70. Heller AC, Amar AP, Liu CY, et al. Surgery of the mind and mood: a mosaic of issues in time and evolution. Neurosurgery. 2006;59(4):720–33.
71. Henderson J. Stereotactic frame-based vs. frameless for ablation and DBS, USA. Frameless Stereotaxic Navigation Systems: FDA Safety Communication-Navigational Accuracy Errors, FDA announcement. 2017.

72. Henn FA. Circuits, cells, and synapses: toward a new target for deep brain stimulation in depression. Neuropsychopharmacology. 2012;37(1):307–8.
73. Hernando V, Pastor J, Pedrosa M, et al. Low-frequency bilateral hypothalamic stimulation for treatment of drug-resistant aggressiveness in a young man with mental retardation. Stereotact Funct Neurosurg. 2008;86(4):219–23.
74. Hodgkiss AD, Malizia AL, Bartlett JR, et al. Outcome after the psychosurgical operation of stereotactic subcaudate tractotomy, 1979–1991. J Neuropsychiatry Clin Neurosci. 1995;7(2):230–4.
75. Holtzheimer PE, Kelley ME, Gross RE, et al. Subcallosal cingulate deep brain stimulation for treatment-resistant unipolar and bipolar depression. Arch Gen Psychiatry. 2012;69(2):150–8.
76. Huff W, Lenartz D, Schormann M, et al. Unilateral deep brain stimulation of the nucleus accumbens in patients with treatment-resistant obsessive-compulsive disorder: outcomes after one year. Clin Neurol Neurosurg. 2010;112(2):137–43.
77. Insel T. Not being an expert in a particular area like DBS, I would be inclined to accept .... attracting attention for over a decade with her contagious exuberance for DBS. 2016. https://mindthebrain.blog/tag/thomas-insel/.
78. Jakob C. Nueva contribucion a la fisiopatologia de los lobulos frontales. La Semana Med. 1906;13(50):13259.
79. Japanese Society for Psychiatry and Neurology. Resolution denying psychosurgery. Seishin Shinkeigaku Zasshi. 1975;77:541. (Jpn)
80. Jenike MA, Baer L, Ballantine HT, et al. Cingulotomy for refractory obsessive-compulsive disorder. A long-term follow-up of 33 patients. Arch Gen Psychiatry. 1991;48:548–55.
81. Jiménez F, Nicolini H, Lozano AM, et al. Electrical stimulation of the inferior thalamic peduncle in the treatment of major depression and obsessive-compulsive disorders. World Neurosurg. 2013; https://doi.org/10.1016/j.wneu.2012.07.010.
82. Jiménez F, Soto JE, Velasco F, et al. Bilateral cingulotomy and anterior capsulotomy applied to patients with aggressiveness. Stereotact Funct Neurosurg. 2012;90(3):151–60.
83. Jung HH, Kim SJ, Roh D, et al. Bilateral thermal capsulotomy with MR-guided focused ultrasound for patients with treatment-refractory obsessive-compulsive disorder: a proof-of-concept study. Mol Psychiatry. 2015;20(10):1205–11.
84. Kahana MJ. Memory search. In: Byrne JH, editor. Learning and memory: a comprehensive reference. 2nd ed. Oxford: Academic; 2017. p. 181–200. \Bed 2.
85. Kelley D, Richardson A, Mitchell-Heggs N. Stereotactic limbic leucotomy: neurophysiologic aspects and operative technique. Br J Psychiatry. 1973;123:133–40.
86. Kim CH, Chang JW, Koo MS, et al. Anterior cingulotomy for refractory obsessive-compulsive disorder. Acta Psychiatr Scand. 2003;107(4):283–90.
87. Kisely S, Hall K, Siskind D, et al. Deep brain stimulation for obsessive-compulsive disorder: a systematic review and meta-analysis. Psychol Med. 2014; 44:3533–42.
88. Koek RJ, Langevin JP, Krahl SE, et al. Amygdala deep brain stimulation for combat post-traumatic stress disorder. Brain Stimul. 2015;8(2):312.
89. Kondziolka D, Flickinger JC, Hudak R. Results following gamma knife radiosurgical anterior capsulotomies for obsessive compulsive disorder. Neurosurgery. 2011;68(1):28–32.
90. Knight GC. Bifrontal stereotactic tractotomy: an atraumatic operation of value in the treatment of value in the treatment of psychoneurosis. Br J Psychiatry. 1969;115:257–66.
91. Kringelbach ML, Aziz TZ. Neuroethical principles of deep-brain stimulation. World Neurosurg. 2011;76:518–9.
92. Kuhn J, Hardenacke K, Lenartz D, et al. Deep brain stimulation of the nucleus basalis of Meynert in Alzheimer's dementia. Mol Psychiatry. 2015;20(3):353–60.
93. Kuhn J, Lenartz D, Mai JK, Huff W, et al. Deep brain stimulation of the nucleus accumbens and the internal capsule in therapeutically refractory Tourette-syndrome. J Neurol. 2007;254(7):963–5.
94. Kuhn J, Lenartz D, Mai JK, Huff W, et al. Disappearance of self-aggressive behavior in a brain-injured patient after deep brain stimulation of the hypothalamus: technical case report. Neurosurgery. 2008;62(5):E1182.
95. Kuhn J, Bauer R, Pohl S, et al. Observations on unaided smoking cessation after deep brain stimulation of the nucleus accumbens. Eur Addict Res. 2009;15:196–201.
96. Kurlan R, Kersun J, Ballantine HT Jr, et al. Neurosurgical treatment of severe obsessive-compulsive disorder associated with Tourette's syndrome. Mov Disord. 1990;5(2):152–5.
97. Le Beau J. Anterior cingulectomy in man. J Neurosurg. 1954;11:268–76.
98. Leckman JF, de Lotbinière AJ, Marek K, et al. Severe disturbances in speech, swallowing, and gait following stereotactic infrathalamic lesions in Gilles de la Tourette's syndrome. Neurology. 1993;43(5):890–4.
99. Leksell L. Stereotactic radiosurgery. J Neurol Neurosurg Psychiatry. 1983;46:797–803.
100. Leone M, Franzini A, Broggi G, et al. Therapeutic stimulation of the hypothalamus: pathophysiological insights and prerequisites for management. Brain. 2005;128(Pt 8):E35.
101. Lévêque M. Psychosurgery, new techniques for brain disorders. Springer International Publishing. Switzerland; 2014.
102. Lippitz BE, Mindus P, Meyerson BA, et al. Lesion topography and outcome after thermocapsulotomy or gamma knife capsulotomy for obsessive-compulsive disorder: relevance of the right hemisphere. Neurosurgery. 1999;44(3):452–8.
103. Lipsman N, Giacobbe P, Bernstein M, et al. Informed consent for clinical trials of deep brain stimulation in

psychiatric disease: challenges and implications for trial design. J Med Ethics. 2012;38:107–11.
104. Lipsman N, Zener R, Bernstein M. Personal identity, enhancement and neurosurgery: a qualitative study in applied neuroethics. Bioethics. 2009;23:375–83.
105. Lipsman N, Bernstein M, Lozano AM. Criteria for the ethical conduct of psychiatric neurosurgery clinical trials. Neurosurg Focus. 2010;29:E9.
106. Lipsman N, Neimat S, Lozano AM. Deep brain stimulation for treatment-refractory obsessive-compulsive disorder: the search for a valid target. Neurosurgery. 2007;61:1–11.
107. Lovett LM, Crimmins R, Shaw DM. Outcome in unipolar affective disorder after stereotactic tractotomy. Br J Psychiatry. 1989;155:547–50.
108. Lozano AM, Mayberg HS, Giacobbe P, et al. Subcallosal cingulate gyrus deep brain stimulation for treatment-resistant depression. Biol Psychiatry. 2008;64(6):461–7.
109. Luigjes J, van den Brink W, Feenstra M, et al. Deep brain stimulation in addiction: a review of potential brain targets. Mol Psychiatry. 2012;17:572–83.
110. Luyten L, Hendrickx S, Raymaekers S, et al. Electrical stimulation in the bed nucleus of the stria terminalis alleviates severe obsessive-compulsive disorder. Mol Psychiatry. 2016;21(9):1272–80.
111. Maciunas RJ, Maddux BN, Riley DE, et al. Prospective randomized double-blind trial of bilateral thalamic deep brain stimulation in adults with Tourette syndrome. J Neurosurg. 2007;107(5):1004–14.
112. Mallet L, Polosan M, Jaafari N, et al. Subthalamic nucleus stimulation in severe obsessive-compulsive disorder. N Engl J Med. 2008;359(20):2121–34.
113. Malone DA Jr. Use of deep brain stimulation in treatment-resistant depression. Cleve Clin J Med. 2010;77(Suppl 3):S77–80.
114. Malone DA Jr, Dougherty DD, Rezai AR, et al. Deep brain stimulation of the ventral capsule/ventral striatum for treatment-resistant depression. Biol Psychiatry. 2009;65(4):267–75.
115. Mark VH, Ervin FR. Violence and the brain. New York: Harper and Row; 1970. p. 1–174.
116. Martínez-Fernández R, Zrinzo L, Aviles-Olmos I, et al. Deep brain stimulation for Gilles de la Tourette syndrome: a case series targeting subregions of the globus pallidus internus. Mov Disord. 2011;26(10):1922–30.
117. Martinez-Torres I, Hariz MI, Zrinzo L, et al. Improvement of tics after subthalamic nucleus deep brain stimulation. Neurology. 2009;72(20):1787–9.
118. Mashour GA, Walker EE, Martuza RL. Psychosurgery: past, present, and future. Brain Res Rev. 2015;48(3):409.
119. Matera R, Ríos E, Barbosa E, et al. Stereotaxic hypothalamotomy in aggressiveness. Acta Neurol Latinoam. 1972;18:96–9.
120. Mayberg HS, Lozano AM, Voon V, et al. Deep brain stimulation for treatment-resistant depression. Neuron. 2005;45:651–60.
121. McLaughlin NC, Didie ER, Machado AG, et al. Improvements in anorexia symptoms after deep brain stimulation for intractable obsessive-compulsive disorder. Biol Psychiatry. 2013;73(9):e29–31.
122. McLean PD. Some psychiatric implications of physiologic studies on the frontotemporal portion of limbic system. Electroencephalogr Clin Neurophysiol. 1952;4:407–18.
123. Mindus P, Nyman H. Normalization of personality characteristics in patients with incapacitating anxiety disorders after capsulotomy. Acta Psychiatr Scand. 1991;83(4):283–91.
124. Mindus P, Rasmussen SA, Lindquist C. Neurosurgical treatment for refractory obsessive-compulsive disorder: implications for understanding frontal lobe function. J Neuropsychiatry Clin Neurosci. 1994;6(4):467–77.
125. Mitchell-Heggs N, Kelly D, Richardson A. Stereotactic limbic leucotomy—a follow-up at 16 months. Br J Psychiatry. 1976;128:226–40.
126. Moniz E. Prefrontal leucotomy in the treatment of mental disorders. Am J Psychiatry. 1937;93:1379–85.
127. Montoya A, Weiss AP, Price BH, et al. Magnetic resonance imaging-guided stereotactic limbic leukotomy for treatment of intractable psychiatric disease. Neurosurgery. 2002;50(5):1043–9.
128. Mpakopoulou M, Gatos H, Brotis A, et al. Stereotactic amygdalotomy in the management of severe aggressive behavioral disorders. Neurosurg Focus. 2008;225(1):E6.
129. Müller UJ, Voges J, Steiner, et al. Deep brain stimulation of the nucleus accumbens for the treatment of addiction. Ann N Y Acad Sci. 2013;1282:119–28.
130. Nangunoori R, Tomycz ND, Quigley M, et al. Deep brain stimulation for psychiatric diseases: a pooled analysis of published studies employing disease-specific standardized outcome scales. Stereotact Funct Neurosurg. 2013;91:345–54.
131. Narabayashi H, Nagao T, Saito Y, et al. Stereotactic amygdalotomy for behavior disorders. Arch Neurol. 1963;9:1–16.
132. National Commission for the Protection of Human Subjects of Biomedical and Behavioral Research: The Belmont Report. Rockville, MD, United States Department of Health and Human Services, report and recommendations: psychosurgery, Department of Health and Human Services. Pub No (OS) 77-002. Washington, DC: US Government Printing Office; 1979.
133. Neuner I, Podoll K, Lenartz D, et al. Deep brain stimulation in the nucleus accumbens for intractable Tourette's syndrome: follow-up report of 36 months. Biol Psychiatry. 2009;65(4):e5–6.
134. Nijensohn DE, Savastano LE, Kaplan AD, et al. Prefrontal lobotomy in the last months of the illness of Eva Perón. World Neurosurg. 2012;77(3–4):583–90.
135. Nijensohn DE, Goodrich I. Psychosurgery: past, present, and future, including prefrontal lobotomy and Connecticut's contribution. Conn Med. 2014;78(8):453–63.
136. Nijensohn DE. Prefrontal lobotomy on Evita was done for behavior/personality modification, not just for pain control. Neurosurg Focus. 2015;39(1):E12.

137. Nuttin B, Wu H, Mayberg H, et al. Consensus on guidelines for stereotactic neurosurgery for psychiatric disorders. J Neurol Neurosurg Psychiatry. 2014;85:1003–8.
138. Okun MS, Foote KD, Wu SS, et al. A trial of scheduled deep brain stimulation for Tourette syndrome: moving away from continuous deep brain stimulation paradigms. JAMA Neurol. 2013;70(1):85–94.
139. Oliver B, Gascón J, Aparicio A, et al. Bilateral anterior capsulotomy for refractory obsessive-compulsive disorders. Stereotact Funct Neurosurg. 2003;81(1–4):90–5.
140. Oshima H, Katayama Y. Neuroethics of deep brain stimulation for mental disorders: brain stimulation rewards in humans. Neurol Med Chir. 2010;50:845–52.
141. Papez JW. A proposed mechanism of emotion. Arch Neurol Psychiatr. 1937;38:725–43.
142. Piedimonte FC. New trends in psychosurgery. In: Cukiert A, editor. Neuromodulation. Sao Paulo: Alaúde; 2010. p. 405–23.
143. Pool JL. Topectomy: a surgical procedure for the treatment of mental illness. J Nerv Ment Dis. 1949;110:164–73.
144. Poblete M, Zamboni R. Tractotomía mamilotalámica en el tratamiento de Agresividad. Neurocirugía (Chile). 1977;35:279–81.
145. Pool JL, Heath RG, Weber JJ. Topectomy; surgical indications and results. Bull N Y Acad Med. 1949;25:335–44.
146. Poppen JL. Technique of prefrontal lobotomy. J Neurosurg. 1948;5:514–20.
147. Poynton AM, Kartsounis LD, Bridges PK. A prospective clinical study of stereotactic subcaudate tractotomy. Psychol Med. 1995;25(4):763–70.
148. Price BH, Baral I, Cosgrove GR, et al. Improvement in severe self-mutilation following limbic leucotomy: a series of 5 consecutive cases. J Clin Psychiatry. 2001;62(12):925–32.
149. Puigdemont D, Pérez-Egea R, Portella MJ, et al. Deep brain stimulation of the subcallosal cingulate gyrus: further evidence in treatment-resistant major depression. Int J Neuropsychopharmacol. 2011;22:1–13.
150. Rabins P, Appleby BS, Brandt J, et al. Scientific and ethical issues related to deep brain stimulation for disorders of mood, behavior and thought. Arch Gen Psychiatry. 2009;66:931–7.
151. Robison RA, Taghva A, Liu CY, et al. Surgery of the mind, mood and conscious state: an idea in evolution. World Neurosurg. 2012;77(5–6):662–86.
152. Rylander G. Stereotactic radiosurgery in anxiety and obsessive-compulsive states: psychiatric aspects. In: Hitchcock ER, Ballantine HT, Myerson BA, editors. Modern concepts in psychiatric surgery. Amsterdam: Elsevier; 1979. p. 235–40.
153. Richter EO, Davis KD, Hamani C, et al. Cingulotomy for psychiatric disease: microelectrode guidance, a callosal reference system for documenting lesion location, and clinical results. Neurosurgery. 2004;54(3):622–8.
154. Robertson M, Doran M, Trimble M, et al. The treatment of Gilles de la Tourette syndrome by limbic leucotomy. J Neurol Neurosurg Psychiatry. 1990;53(8):691–4.
155. Roh D, Chang WS, Chang JW, et al. Long-term follow-up of deep brain stimulation for refractory obsessive-compulsive disorder. Psychiatry Res. 2012;200(2–3):1067–70.
156. Rück C, Larsson KJ, Mataix-Cols D. Predictors of medium and long-term outcome following capsulotomy for obsessive-compulsive disorder: one site may not fit all. Eur Neuropsychopharmacol. 2012;22(6):406–14.
157. Sturm V, Lenarz D, Koulousakis A, et al. Nucleus accumbens. A target for deep brain stimulation in obsessive-compulsive and anxiety disorders. J Chem Neuroanat. 2003;26:293–9.
158. Sachdev PS, Sachdev J. Long-term outcome of neurosurgery for the treatment of resistant depression. J Neuropsychiatry Clin Neurosci. 2005;17(4):478–85.
159. Saddichha S, Chaturvedi SK. Clinical practice guidelines in psychiatry: more confusion than clarity? A critical review and recommendation of a unified guideline. ISRN Psychiatry. 2014; https://doi.org/10.1155/2014/828917.
160. Saleh C, Gonzalez V, Cif L, et al. Deep brain stimulation of the globus pallidus internus and Gilles de la Tourette syndrome: toward multiple networks modulation. Surg Neurol Int. 2012;3(Suppl 2):S 127–42.
161. Sano K, Mayanagi Y. Posteromedial hypothalamotomy in the treatment of violent, aggressive behaviour. Acta Neurochir Suppl (Wien). 1988;44:145–51.
162. Savica R, Stead M, Mack KJ, et al. Deep brain stimulation in Tourette syndrome: a description of 3 patients with excellent outcome. Mayo Clin Proc. 2012;87(1):59–62.
163. Schermer M. Ethical issues in deep brain stimulation. Front Integr Neurosci. 2011;5:1–5.
164. Schlaepfer TE, Cohen MX, Frick C, et al. Deep brain stimulation to reward circuitry alleviates anhedonia in refractory major depression. Neuropsychopharmacology. 2008;33(2):368–77.
165. Schlaepfer TE, Frick C, Zobel A, et al. Vagus nerve stimulation for depression: efficacy and safety in a European study. Psychol Med. 2008;38(5):651–61.
166. Schvarcz JR, Drollet R, Rios E, et al. Stereotactic hypothalamotomy for behaviour disorders. J Neurol Neurosurg Psychiatry. 1972;35:356–9.
167. Scoville WB. Selective cortical undercutting as a means of modifying and studying frontal lobe function in man; preliminary report of 43 operative cases. J Neurosurg. 1949;6:65–73.
168. Shah SA, Schiff ND. Central thalamic deep brain stimulation for cognitive neuromodulation: a review of proposed mechanisms and investigational studies. Eur J Neurosci. 2010;32(7):1135–44.
169. Sheth SA, Neal J, Tangherlini F, et al. Limbic system surgery for treatment-refractory obsessive-compulsive disorder: a prospective long-term follow-up of 64 patients. J Neurosurg. 2013;118(3):491–7.

170. Spangler WJ, Cosgrove GR, Ballantine HT, et al. Magnetic resonance image-guided stereotactic cingulotomy for intractable psychiatric disease. Neurosurgery. 1996;38:1071.
171. Spiegel EA, Wycis HT. Principles and application of stereoencephalotomy. Brain Nerve. 1952;4:129–37.
172. Steiner L. Gamma knife radiosurgery. In: Schmidek HH, Sweet WH, editors. Operative neurosurgical techniques. New York: Grune & Stratton; 1988. p. 515–29.
173. St. Jude Medical Announces Clinical Study of Deep Brain Stimulation. 2008. https://www.meddeviceonline.com/.../st-jude-medical-announces-clinical-study-of-d-0... Holtzheimer PE et al (2017) Lancet Psychiatry, https://doi.org/10.1016/S2215-0366.(17)30371-1.
174. Sun B, de Salles A. Neurosurgical treatments for psychiatric disorders© 2015. 2015.
175. Sturm V, Lenarz D, Koulousakis A. Nucleus accumbens. A target for deep brain stimulation in obsessive-compulsive and anxiety disorders. J Chem Neuroanat. 2003;26:293–9.
176. Talairach J, Tournoux P. Co-planar stereotaxic atlas of the human brain: 3-dimensional proportional system – an approach to cerebral imaging. New York: Thieme Medical Publishers; 1988.
177. Tye S, Fraye M, Lee KH. DBS, Neuromodulation, WINCS (Wireless Instantaneous Neurotransmitter Concentration Sensory System) in vivo and in real time- Mayo Clinic-2010 disrupting disordered neurocircuitry. Treating refractory psychiatric illness with neuromodulation. J Neurosurg. 2014;120(5):1131–7.
178. Talairach J, Hecaen H, David M. Lobotomie prefrontale limitee par electrocoagulation des fibres thalamo-frontalis leur emergence du bras anterior de la capsule interne. In: Proceedings of the 4th Congress Neurologique Internationale, Masson, Paris. 1949. p. 141.
179. Valenstein ES. Great and desperate cures: the rise and decline of psychosurgery and other radical treatments for mental illness. New York: Basic Books; 1986.
180. Visser-Vandewalle V, Van der Linden C, Ackermans L. Deep brain stimulation in Gilles de la Tourette's syndrome. Guidelines of the Dutch-Flemish Tourette surgery study group. Neurosurgery. 2006;58:E590.
181. Viswanathan A, Jimenez-Shahed J, Baizabal Carvallo JF, et al. Deep brain stimulation for Tourette syndrome: target selection. Stereotact Funct Neurosurg. 2012;90(4):213–24.
182. Wang X, Chang C, Geng N, et al. Long-term effects of bilateral deep brain stimulation of the subthalamic nucleus on depression in patients with Parkinson's disease. Parkinsonism Relat Disord. 2009;15(8):587–91.
183. Williams S. Amygdaloid neurosurgery for aggressive behaviour Sydney, 1967–1977: societal, scientific, ethical and other factors. Australas Psychiatry. 2009;17(5):410–6.
184. Wind JJ, Anderson DE. From prefrontal leukotomy to deep brain stimulation: the historical transformation of psychosurgery and the emergence of neuroethics. Neurosurg Focus. 2008;25:E10.
185. World Society for Stereotactic and Functional Neurosurgery (WSSFN). Surgery for psychiatric disorders, meeting program. June 2017. Berlin; 2017.
186. Wu H, Van Dyck-Lippens PJ, Santegoeds R, et al. World Neurosurg. 2013;80(3–4):S29.e1–10. https://doi.org/10.1016/j.wneu.2012.06.039.
187. Yamamoto T, Katayama Y, Kobayashi K, et al. Deep brain stimulation for the treatment of vegetative state. Eur J Neurosci. 2010;32(7):1145–51.
188. Yampolsky C, Bendersky D. Cirugía de los trastornos del comportamiento: el estado del arte. Revision de la literatura. Rev Argent Neuroc. 2014;28(3):78–98.
189. Young GJ, Bi WL, Smith TR, Brewster R, et al. Evita's lobotomy. J Clin Neurosci. 2015;22(12):1883–8.

Index

A
Aberrant Behavior Checklist–Irritability (ABC-I) scores, 34
Ablative procedures, 384
Absolute risk reduction (ARR), 6
Acceptance and commitment therapy (ACT), 171
Acceptance-facilitating interventions (AFI), 319
Addiction, DLPFC, 330
Adult-onset tics, 237
Aggressive behavior (AB) disorders, 393, 394
Aggressive personality traits, 393
Aggressive violent behavioral disorders, 388
Alcoholism, 39, 40
Alliance-based approach of psychodynamic psychiatry, 296
Allostatic load model, 155, 156
Alzheimer's disease (AD), 395, 396
Amsterdam protocol, 371
Amygdala reactivity, 156
Amygdalotomy, 380
Animal models of binge eating, 255
Animal models of depression
  abnormal behavior simulations, 82
  amphetamine, 81
  apomorphine, 81
  behavioral alterations and serotonergic dysfunction, 82
  behavioral models, 81
  behavioral strategy, 80
  biochemical tests, 80
  biological hypothesis, 81, 83
  chronic mild stress, 81
  directed reproduction of mice, 82
  dopaminergic receptors, 79
  drug co-administration, 83
  forced swimming test, 81
  genetic model, 83
  glutamatergic activity, 84
  glutamatergic modulators, 84
  glutamatergic receptor transcripts, 84
  ketamine, 84
  muricide model, 80, 81
  NMDA receptor antagonist, 84
  noradrenaline deficiency, 83
  olfactory bulbectomy, 81
  oxotremorine, 81
  pharmacological interactions, 81
  physiological mechanisms, 82
  Porsolt forced swimming test, 82
  preclinical research, 79
  psychomotor stimulants, 79
  reserpine, 81
  tail suspension test, 81
  telomeres, 82
  yohimbine, 81
Anorexia nervosa (AN), 253–255, 306
  repetitive transcranial magnetic stimulation, 258
  treatment-resistant model, 254, 255
Anterior capsulotomy, 386, 388
Anterior cingulotomy, 386
Antidepressant-induced synaptic plasticity enhancement, 92
Antidepressants, 6
Antidepressant trials, 15
Antipsychotics, 5, 6
Anxiety disorders, 304
  evidence-based treatments, 207
  machine learning and prediction of treatment response/resistance, 73
  prevalence, 207
  selective serotonin reuptake inhibitors, 207
Apnea-hypopnea index (AHI) in children, 264
Asp40-allele carriers, 39
Attention-deficit/hyperactivity disorder (ADHD), 9, 264
  academic and social functioning and parenting styles, 218
  alpha-2 agonists, 229
  behavioral therapy, 223
  behavioral treatments, 219
  catechol-O-methyltransferase, 36
  cell adhesion, 216
  in childhood, 215
  combined behavioral and medication treatment, 219
  core symptom presentation, 218
  dopamine beta-hydroxylase genes, 36
  dietary treatments, 225

Y.-K. Kim (ed.), *Treatment Resistance in Psychiatry*, https://doi.org/10.1007/978-981-10-4358-1

Attention-deficit/hyperactivity disorder (ADHD) (*cont.*)
differential diagnoses, 218
diffuse tensor imaging studies, 217
dopaminergic and serotonergic signaling, 35
economic and psychosocial costs, 215
eicosapentaenoic acid, 225
etiology, 216
evaluation and treatment, 217
executive dysfunction, 35
fractional anisotropy, 217
frontoparietal network, 217
fronto-striatal-cerebellar circuit in children, 217
gene-environment interactions, 229
goal-directed executive processes and attention, 217
herbal remedies, 226
heritability, 216
hyperactivation and impulsivity, 35, 217
impulsive behaviors, 219
investigational drugs, 226
latrophilin 3 gene, 36
long-term pharmacotherapy, 219
LPHN3 polymorphism, 37
medication and behavioral treatments, 228
methylphenidate, 36, 216, 219
microstructural white matter abnormalities, 217
MRI voxel-based morphometry studies, 217
natural supplements, 226
neurofeedback training, 226–227
neuroimaging, 229
neuroimaging studies, 229
noninvasive brain stimulation, 226
nonpharmacologic
behavior classroom management, 224
behavioral parent training, 223, 224
executive functioning deficits, 224
multimodal treatments, 224
social skills, 224
nutritional and herbal supplements, 226
parent management training, 219
parent-rated symptoms, 219
patient characteristics, 228
perinatal risk factors, 217
pharmacogenetic factors, 228
pharmacogenomics, 229
pharmacologic
agents, 226
evidence-based approach, 223
non-stimulant pharmacologic treatment, 222, 223
stimulants, 219, 222
TMAP algorithm, 223
pharmacotherapy with methylphenidate, 35
polyunsaturated fatty acids, 225
prenatal, perinatal and postnatal environment, 217
psychiatric comorbidities, 218
psychoeducational testing and reports cards, 218
psychosocial risk factors, 217
screening scales, 218
social functioning, 215
substance use disorders, 215
synaptosomal-associated protein 25, 35
treatment, 218, 229
tryptophan hydroxylase 2, 36
resistance, 227, 228
US prevalence, 215
visual, spatial and motor processing, 217
Augmentation strategies, 19
Autism spectrum disorders (ASD)
abnormal neurodevelopment, 34
antipsychotics, 34
impaired social communication, 34
pharmacogenetics
gene polymorphisms, 34
methylphenidate, 35
neurotransmitter genes, 34
risperidone efficacy and safety, 34
risperidone treatment, 35
pharmacogenomic effects of SSRIs, 34
repetitive behaviors, 34
selective serotonin reuptake inhibitors, 34
serotonin transporter gene, 34
stimulant medications
methylphenidate, 34
mixed amphetamine salts, 34
Autism Treatment Evaluation Checklist (ATEC), 34

B
Bacterial metabolites and nucleic acids, 370
Bacteroides fragilis, 372
Beck Depression Inventory (BDI), 381, 392
Beck's cognitive model of depression, 312
Behavioral activation (BA), 311
activity monitoring, 313
activity scheduling, 313
assessment of goals and values, 313
contingency management, 313
for depression, 312
motivational factors, 318
smartphone-delivered treatment, 318
Behavioral explanations for depression, 313
Behavioral parent training, 223, 224
Behavioral surgery, 88
Belmont Report, 397
Bifidobacterium infantis, 372
Bifidobacterium longum, 372
Binge eating disorder, 253, 254, 258, 259
Biological markers, treatment resistance, 17
Biological psychiatry, 306
Biopsychosocial approach, 296, 301, 304, 306
Biopsychosocial assessment, 301
Biopsychosocial model hypothesis, 195, 196
Bipolar depression, 8
Bipolar disorder, 47–49
DBS, 332
ECT, 330, 331
pathophysiology, 139
randomized controlled trial, 330
rTMS, 331
tDCS, 331
treatment-resistance
clinical features, 141
clinical presentation and progression, 140

executive functioning, 145
functional and psychopathological impact, 141
maintenance phase, 145
mood stabilizers, 141
mood states, 140
pathophysiological basis, 141, 142
psychiatric medications, 141
psychosocial interventions, 145
subsyndromal depressive symptoms, 141
vagal nerve stimulation, 331
Blockbuster and stratified medicine approaches, 274
Boredom/stress, 237
Brain augmentation, 396
Brain biomarker-based prediction of treatment response, 73
Brain circuit dysfunction, TRPD, 194
Brain-computer interface (BCI), 396
Brain-derived neurotrophic factor (BDNF), 195
Brain-machine technologies, 396
Brief behavioral activation treatment of depression (BATD), 313
Brief Psychiatric Rating Scale (BPRS), 109
Bulimia nervosa (BN), 253–256, 258, 259
Buprenorphine (BUP)
dosage, 180
opioid-related side effects, 181
respiratory depression, 181

C

Candidate-gene approach, 34
Capsulotomy and limbic leucotomy, 381
Carer anxiety, 255
Cartesian dualism, 297
CGI-improvement scale (CGI-I) score, 190
Chemical imbalance, 87
Chemogenetics, 396
Child Behavior Checklist-Attention Problem (CBCL-AP), 218
Childhood-onset schizophrenia (COS), 116
Childhood sexual abuse and adult depressive symptoms, 90
Childhood trauma, 87
Chronic systemic inflammation, PTSD, 195
Cingulotomy, 381
Circadian sleep-wake cycle, 266
Circuitry neural regions, 156, 157
Classroom management, behavioral strategies, 224
Clinical Antipsychotic Trials of Intervention Effectiveness (CATIE) study, 44, 114
Clinical drug trials, 4
Clinical global impression (CGI) scale, 109, 125, 211
Clinical Global Impressions-Improvement Scale (CGI-I), 34, 166
Clinical Global Impressions Scale-Severity scale (CGI-S) score, 123, 190
Closed loops, 396
Closed-loop dynamic neurochemical control of psychotherapeutic interventions, 396
Clozapine augmentation, 350
with Alzheimer's disease, drug treatments
acetylcholinesterase inhibitors, 357
donepezil, 357
galantamine, 357
memantine, 357, 358
with antidepressants
amitriptyline, 355
melatonergic antidepressant agomelatine, 355
nonadrenergic and specific serotoninergic antidepressants, 354, 355
selective serotonin reuptake inhibitors, 353, 354
serotonin and norepinephrine reuptake inhibitors, 355
tricyclics, 355
first-generation antipsychotics, 353
haloperidol augmentation, 353
intolerability/inefficacy, 359
minocycline, 358
with mood stabilizers/anticonvulsants
lamotrigine, 357
lithium, 355, 356
topiramate, 356
valproic acid, 356
omega-3 fatty acid, 358
second-generation antipsychotics
amisulpride, 351
aripiprazole, 351, 352
paliperidone, 353
risperidone, 352
sertindole, 353
ziprasidone, 352, 353
Clozapine-resistant schizophrenia, 123
adjunctive ECT, 358, 359
augmentation strategies (*see* Clozapine augmentation)
criteria for, 351
refractory, 350
ultra-resistant, 350
Cluster A personality disorders, 45
Cogmed, working memory, 224
Cognition system, 389
Cognitive behavioral therapy (CBT), 8, 91, 147, 165, 170, 183, 298, 311
client-centered second-wave psychological treatment, 312
in group format, 312
in guided self-help format, 312
in individual format, 312
maladaptive cognitions, 312
TS, 240
Cognitive behavioral therapy for insomnia (CBT-I), 263
Cognitive-behavioral treatments, 306
Cognitive bias modification (CBM), ED, 258
Cognitive impairment in euthymic bipolar disorder, 145
Cognitive remediation therapy (CRT) for eating disorders, 257
Cohen's rule, 6
Collaborative care, 301
Coma, 396
Combination strategies, 18
Comorbidity, psychiatric disorder, 16

Conners Abbreviated Symptom Questionnaire (ASQ), 218
Conners' Rating Scale-Revised (CRS), 218
Contingency management, 183, 184
Cortico-striato-thalamic-cortical circuits (CSTCC), 382
Cost Utility of the Latest Antipsychotic Drugs in Schizophrenia Study (CUtLASS), 114
Creative person-centered narrative psychopharmacotherapy, 282
Creative psychopharmacotherapy, 279–281, 283
Creativity and resilience, 289
Cumulative stress exposure, 153, 154
Cyborgs, human, 396

D

Decision-making, 13
Deep brain stimulation (DBS), 147, 329, 330, 340, 341, 379, 384, 386
  for Parkinson's disease, 378
  pulse generator and stimulating electrodes, 329
Delayed-onset disorder, 152, 153
Dementia, 42
Dementia-related disorders, 395
Demographic factors, 17
Depression
  brain MRI measurements, 66
  DBS, 334, 335
  ECT, 332, 333
  rTMS, 333
  tDCS, 334
  TNS, 334
  vagal nerve stimulation, 334
Depression CBT Self-Help Guide, 315, 316
Depression-like behaviors, 370
Depressive and anxiety disorders, 88
Depressive disorder, MRI, 69
Deprexis, 315
Diacetylmorphine, 182
Diagnostic anxiety disorder, 207
Diffusion MRI, 380
Digital CBT/BA Depression Interventions for Research and Practice, 319, 320
Disability-adjusted life years (DALYs), 3
Disease-staging model, 73
Drug addiction, 394
Drug-specific genotype associations, 46
Drug therapies, 183
Drug treatment guidelines, 282, 283
Dysbiosis, 372
Dysfunctional circuitry, 87
Dysmorphic disorder, 389

E

Eating disorders (ED), 253, 305, 394, 395
  behavior, 306
  CRT, 257, 258
  oxytocin, 258
  recovery approach, 256
  staging model, 253, 254
  treatments, 257
    CBM, 258
    clinical management, 257
    cognitive remediation therapy, 257
    neuro-progressive changes, 257
Electroconvulsive therapy (ECT), 122–124, 130, 145–147, 326, 339, 392
  ECT-induced mania, 331
Emotional disorders, 313
Emotional homeostasis, 392
Endocannabinoid (eCB) system, OCD, 172
Endovascular nanotechnology, 396
Environmental factors, 17
  antidepressants, 91
Epigenetic dysregulation, 92
Epigenetic modifiers, 87
Epigenetic regulation, 88, 91, 93
Evidence-based and practice-based COMBOs, 284
Evidence-based internet interventions for depression, 315
Evidence-based medicine, 274
Evidence-based therapies for mood disorders, 301
Expectancy theory, 7
Experimental treatment strategies, 19
Exposure and Ritual (response) Prevention (ERP), 165
  OCD, 168–170
Extended-release naltrexone, 183
Eye movement desensitization and reprocessing (EMDR), 197

F

Face-to-face and digital therapies, 318
Face-to-face care, CBT and BA, 313, 314, 318
Fast-scan cyclic voltammetry, 396
Fatal myocarditis, 117
Favorable therapeutic context, 285, 286
Fecal microbiota transplantation (FMT)
  applications, 371
  in CDI, 372
  donor's health screenings, 371
  ethical conditions, 371
  fecal suspension, 371
  germ-free mice, depression, 372
  history, 370
  indications, 373
  in modern medicine, 371
  reliability and side effects, 373
  in treatment resistant psychiatric disorders, 372, 373
5-HTTLPR polymorphism, 47
Functional recovery, 14

G

Gene-childhood trauma interaction
  bipolar disorder, 89
  depression, 90
  PTSD, 90, 91
  schizophrenia, 89

Gene-environment interactions, 88
Generalized anxiety disorder (GAD), 37, 38
  antipsychotics
    olanzapine, 210
    treatment, 210
  chronic wax and wane course, 209
  cognitive and psychomotor impairments, 210
  dopaminergic and serotonin receptors, 210
  GABA-ergic anticonvulsants, 210
  levetiracetam, 210
  management, 209
Genes and childhood trauma, 87
Genetic biomarkers
  epidemiological (family and twin) studies, 33
  epigenetic approaches, 33
  gene–environment interaction, 33
  genome-wide association (GWA) studies, 33
  molecular (linkage and association) methods, 33
  transcriptional and microRNA analyses, 33
  treatment response-related genetic variability, 33
Genetic polymorphism of serotonin transporter promoter gene, 300
Genetic predispositions, 17
Genetics, 27
Genome-Based Therapeutic Drugs for Depression (GENDEP) project, 47
Genome-wide approach, 34
Glial cells, 102, 103
Global Assessment of Functioning (GAF), 125, 381
Glutamatergic neurotransmission, 101, 102
Goal-oriented utilization of placebo responses, 287
Golden age of psychopharmacology, 89
Gut and brain microbiota, 369
Gut microbiota for human health, 369, 370

H

Hamilton Anxiety Scale (HAM-A), 190
Hamilton Rating Scale for Depression (HAM-D) scoring, 190, 392
Hawthorne effect, 8
HDAC inhibitor-augmented psychotherapy, dysfunctional neural circuits, 92, 93
Human cyborgs, 396
Humanitarian device exception (HDE), 394
Hydromorphone, 182
Hypersomnia, 265
Hypnotics, 263
Hypothalamotomy, 380
Hypothalamus-pituitary-adrenal (HPA) axis dysregulation, 194, 195

I

ICBT programs, 317
Image-guided stereotactic surgical techniques, 378
Imipramine treatment, 15
Impaired executive functioning, 224
Industry-sponsored studies, 5
Inflammatory pathways, 103
Inflammatory processes, 19
Insomnia, 262
  alcohol use disorder, 262
  antidepressants, 262
  brain activation abnormalities, 262
  causes, 262
  indications, 263
  neurotransmitter imbalance, 262
  off-label sedatives, 263
  psychological problems, 262
  psychostimulants, 263
  severe depressive symptoms, 262
  suicidality, 262
Insufficient/negative therapeutic response, 276
Integrated approaches, TRP
  biological markers, 87
  brain stimulation techniques, 88
  electroconvulsive therapy, 87
  environmental factors, 88
  gene expression, 87
  neuroplasticity hypotheses, 88
  non-pharmacological treatment, 88
  psychotherapeutic approaches, 88
International Society for Bipolar Disorders (ISBD) criteria, 140, 141
International Suicide Prevention Trial (Inter SePT), 115
Internet-based and smartphone app-delivered mental health interventions, 314
Internet-based CBT (ICBT), 312
Internet interventions for depression, 315
  uptake and implementation, 318, 319
Interpersonal and social rhythm therapy (IPSRT), 147
Interpersonal psychotherapy, 197
Interpersonal therapy (IPT), 91
Intraoperative stimulation, 388

K

Keaky gut hypothesis, 370
Kindling effect, PTSD, 155

L

Lactobacillus helveticus, 372
Lactobacillus rhamnosus, 373
Lateral and dorsomedial ablative hypothalamotomy, 395
Lateral hypothalamotomy, 388
Learned helplessness and pessimism, 275
Learning disorders, 218
Lesioning (ablation), 387
Light therapy, 265
Limbic leucotomy, 386–388
Lithium, 6
Long-acting injections of antipsychotics (LAIAs), evidence-proved advantages, 276
Long-term psychodynamic psychotherapy (LTPP), 301
Low-frequency TMS (LF-rTMS), 330

M

Machine learning and prediction of treatment response/resistance, 71
Magnetic seizure therapy (MST), 147
Major depressive disorder (MDD), 311
  cortico-striatal-thalamic-cortical circuit, 392
  ECT, 392
  etiology, 99
  neurosurgery, 392
  physiopathology, 392
  prevalence, 391
  subgenual cingulum, 392
  transcranial magnetic stimulation, 392
Mayo Investigational Neuromodulation Control System (MINCS), 396
Measurement-based care, 18
Medical bioinformatics, 73
Medical care, 8
Medical causes of disability, 3, 4
Medical comorbidity, 16
Medication efficacy for somatic disorders, 9, 11
Medtronic stimulating electrodes, 383
Memory loss, 395
Mental and substance use disorders, prevalence, 3, 4
Mental functioning domain-based approach, 73
Mental health medicines, 273
Metabolomics, 27
Metabotropic glutamate receptors (mGlus), 102
Methadone (MET)
  cardiotoxic side effects, 181
  CYP3A4 (demethylation), 180
  dosage, 180
  forms, 180
  induction phase, 180
  respiratory depression, 181
  side effects, 181
mHealth apps for TRD, 315
Microglia cells, 102
Mind-body problem and psychodynamic psychiatry, 297, 298
Mindfulness-based interventions, 147
Mindfulness-based therapy, 197
Mindless psychiatry, 274
Mobile health applications (mHealth apps), 312
Monoaminergic systems, 382
Monotherapy before polytherapy, 284
Montgomery-Åsberg Depression Rating Scale (MADRS), 125
Mood disorders, 301
  baseline EEG measurement markers, 70, 71
  electroencephalography, 68
  machine learning and prediction of treatment response/resistance, 72
  MRI, 69, 70
  and psychotic disorders, 304
MoodGYM, 315
  for depression, 317
Moodivate app, 315, 316
Mood stabilizers, TRS
  lamotrigine, 127
  lithium, 126, 127
  topiramate, 127
  valproate, 125, 126
Mood Tools–Depression Aid, 315
Morphine sulphate, 181
Motivational interviewing, 183
MRI-guided stereotactic techniques, 386
MR image-guided high-intensity focused ultrasound (MR-HIFU) lesioning, 378, 385
Multimodal Treatment Study of Children with ADHD study, 218
Munich Antidepressant Response Signature (MARS) project, 47

N

Naloxone, 182
Naltrexone, 182
National Epidemiological Survey on Alcohol and Related Conditions, 215
Need-adapted (NA) approach, 303
Nested case-control study design in TRP research, 28, 29
Neural plasticity, antidepressants, 91
Neuroanatomical correlate of psychiatric illness, 381
Neurobiological etiology of TRD, 99, 103
Neurobiology and psychopathology, mental disorders, 274
Neurochemical models, 382
Neurodegeneration, 101
Neuroethics, 397
Neurogenesis, 101
Neuroimaging, 27
Neuroinflammation, 101
  in OCD, 172
Neuromodulatory strategies
  adverse effects, 337, 338
  clinical application, psychiatric disorders, 330–337
  DBS, 329, 330, 338
  ECT, 326, 337
  TDCS, 327, 338
  TMS, 326, 338
  TNS, 338
  tVNS, 329
  VNS, 327, 338
Neuromorphic chips, 396
Neuronal functioning, 101
Neuroplasticity hypotheses, 88
Neurosurgery, 377
NICE guidelines, 298
Nigrostriatal deficit, RLS, 264
Non-adherence by psychiatric diagnosis, 13
Non-clozapine antipsychotic combination therapy (NCCAT), 122
Nontreatment-resistant depression, 18
Nucleus accumbens, 390
Nuremberg Trial, 397
Nurses' Observation Scale for Inpatient Evaluation (NOSIE), 109

O

Observer effect, 8
Obsessive–compulsive and related disorders (OCRDs), 38
Obsessive–compulsive disorder (OCD), 9, 335
ablative procedures, 170
in adolescence, 165
anterior limbs of internal capsules, 170
baseline EEG measurement markers, 71
biological predictors, 171
in childhood, 165
clinical trials, 166
cognitive-behavioral therapy, 165
compulsions, 165
DBS target, 389
developmental trajectories, 165
direct and indirect pathways, 389
electroencephalography, 69
endophenotype, 239
ERP
distress-provoking stimuli, 169
patient adherence, 168, 169
predictors of, 168
psychotherapy, 169
residential treatment, 169
treatment response, 169
first-line pharmacotherapy, 165
gamma knife capsulotomy, 170
glutamatergic agents, 172
neurosurgical interventions, 170, 390
neurosurgical lesions, 170
noninvasive neuromodulation, 172
obsessions, 165
pharmacotherapy
antipsychotic medication, 168
aripiprazole, 167
clomipramine, 167
haloperidol, 167, 168
medication adherence, 167
mirtazapine, 168
monotherapy with clomipramine, 167
olanzapine, 167
quetiapine, 167
risperidone, 167, 168
serotonergic medication, 167
SRI response, 166
switching SSRIs, 167
venlafaxine, 168
prevalence rates, 165
randomized controlled trials, 165
repetitive TMS, 170
serotonin reuptake inhibitors, 165
stereotactic target, 389
transcranial magnetic stimulation, 170
OCD, *see* Obsessive–compulsive disorder (OCD)
Opioid dependence
buprenorphine, 179
long-acting depot formulation, 183
oral methadone, 179
oxycodone, 179
pharmacotherapies, 180
prognosis and treatment adherence, 179
psychological and behavioural symptoms, 179
psychosocial therapies, 179
retention and treatment adherence, 183
Opioid-induced QT prolongation or arrhythmias (torsade des pointes), 181
Optimism, 275
Optogenetics, 396
Outcome measures, 14

P

Paediatric autoimmune neuropsychiatric disorders associated with streptococcal infections (PANDAS), 246
Pallidotomy, 383
Panic disorders, 9
and anxiety disorders, 335
brain MRI measurements, 67
clinical guidelines, 189
cognitive domain, 189
prevalence, 189
somatic/physical domain, 189
TRPD (*see* Treatment-resistant panic disorder (TRPD))
World Health Organization survey, 189
Panic Disorder Severity Scale (PDSS) score, 190
Panic disorder with agoraphobia (PDA), 37
Patient adherence, 298
Patient-centered medicine in primary care, 296
Patient management, 275
Periodic limb movement disorder (PLMD), 264
Periodic limb movements during sleep (PLMS), 264, 265
Personalized medicine, 18, 159, 160
Person-centered narratives of therapeutic benefit, 286, 287
Person-centered psychopharmacology, 276
Person-centered psychopharmacotherapy, 289, 290
P-glycoprotein, 17
Pharmacogenetics, 33
cocaine dependence, 41
genetic biomarkers identification, 33
on nicotine dependence, 40, 41
opioid dependence, 41
therapeutic response, 33
treatment algorithms, 33
Pharmacogenomics, 34
Pharmacokinetic factors, 12
Pharmacotherapy to medical interventions, 9
Pharmacotherapy treatment outcomes, 4
Physician-patient relationship, 285
Pippard Postoperative Rating Scale (PPRS), 381
Placebo and nocebo phenomena, 7, 287, 288
Plasma drug concentrations, 12
Plasticity-augmented psychotherapy, 88
Polymorphic alleles for cytochrome P (CYP) 450, 13
Polymorphisms, 13
Polypharmacy, 280
of mental health medicines, 284

Posteromedial hypothalamotomy, 388
Postoperative psychiatric treatment and management program, 380
Posttransplant peritonitis, 373
Post-traumatic stress disorder (PTSD), 38, 39, 305, 336, 396
aetiology in depression and, 157
CBT and cognitive reprocessing treatment, 157
classification, 152
clinical staging strategy, 152
cognitive behavioural interventions, 159
cognitive behavioural school, 152
cognitive deficits, 159
comorbidity, 152
C reactive protein, 159
duration of illness, 157
inflammation in, 159
interpersonal psychotherapy, 160
medications and psychotherapy, 159, 160
minocycline and aspirin, 159
network abnormalities and functional connectivity, 160
neurobiological database, 159
neurofeedback, 160
noradrenergic and serotoninergic neurotransmission, 159
partial remission following treatment, 158
prevalence, 151
psychological and pharmacological treatments, 151
psychopharmacological approaches, 159
relapse rate in patients, 158
social withdrawal and hypervigilance, 160
staging approach, 152, 158, 159
transcranial magnetic stimulation, 160
trauma-focused therapies, 152
Practice of psychosurgery, 380
Prefrontal leucotomy/lobotomy, 378, 379
Prevalence of treatment resistance in mental disorders, 16
Primary outcomes in psychiatric treatments, 6
Primary resilience, 278
Prokaryotic microorganisms, 369
Proteomics, 27
Pseudo-resistance, 12, 113
Psychiatric illnesses, 380
Psychiatric interventions vs. placebo, 10–11
Psychiatric pathology, 295
Psychobiological concept, 277
Psychodynamic approaches, 304
anxiety disorders, 305
genetic and environmental influences, 299
interpersonal interactions and transactions, 305
neuroscience/biological intervention, 296
patient's illness, 296
trauma and childhood adversity, 300
Psychodynamic psychotherapy (PDT), 197, 295, 298, 299
diagnostic comorbidity, 297
patients' emotional states, 297
psychopharmacologic treatment, 297
Psychological and social interventions, 15
Psychological and syndromal complexity, 300
Psychological stress, 300
Psychopharmacologic drugs, 6
Psychosocial interventions, bipolar disorder, 147, 148
Psychosocial therapies, 183
Psychosurgery, 377–379
cerebral targets, 385
techniques, 386
Psychotic disorders, 301–303
Psychotropic drugs, 4, 5
PTSD, *see* Post-traumatic stress disorder (PTSD)
Publication bias, 4, 5

R

Randomized controlled trials (RCTs), 4
Rapid eye movement (REM) sleep latency, 262
Reconsolidation-updating mechanism, 92
Recovery After an Initial Schizophrenia Episode (RAISE) project, 303
Refractoriness, BD, 140, 145
Refractory psychiatric disorders, cerebral targets, 389
Refractory psychiatric illness disrupted-disordered neurocircuitry, 396
Refractory TS, flow chart, 247
Regression, 8
Relapses and recurrences during continued treatment, 15
REM sleep behavior disorder, 266
Repetitive transcranial magnetic stimulation (rTMS), 66
Reporting study methods, 6
Research inadequate response, 14
Resilience, 277–279
and creativity of patients, 289, 290
and salutogenesis, 274
Resistant bipolar depression, 142–144
animal models (*see* Animal models of depression)
antidepressants, 79
definition, 79
management, 79
Respiratory disturbance index (RDI), 264
Restless legs syndrome (RLS), 264, 265
Reversal of thalamic hyperactivity after antidepressant treatment, 67
Risperidone LAI (RLAI), 123

S

Scheduled therapist assistance, 315
Schizophrenia (SCH), 8, 42–44, 65, 336, 350, 380, 395
antipsychotic iloperidone, 44
antipsychotics, 42
baseline EEG measurement markers, 70
BDNF dinucleotide repeat polymorphism, 45
brain MRI measurements, 66
chlorpromazine, 44
clozapine efficacy, 43
clozapine treatment, 43
dopamine D1 and D2 genetic variants, 43

dopamine receptor 3 gene, 45
DRD3 Ser9Gly functional polymorphism, 43
electroencephalography, 68
familial-loading score, 45
5-HTTLPR polymorphism, 44
gene association studies, 45
genome-wide association studies, 44
haloperidol, 44
human leukocyte antigen A1 allele, 45
Kell blood group complex subunit-related family member 4, 44
machine learning and prediction of treatment response/resistance, 71
MRI, 69
negative symptoms, 337
neuronal PAS domain protein 3, 44
olanzapine efficacy, 43
positive symptoms, 336, 337
risperidone
action, 44
efficacy, 43
treatment, 44
Schizophrenia Patient Outcomes Research Team (PORT) report, 302
Schizophrenia spectrum disorders, 45
Secondary resilience, 278
Selective serotonin reuptake inhibitors (SSRIs), 8
Self-rating instruments, 15
Sensitisation and kindling, PTSD, 154
Separate sampling, 27
Sequenced Treatment Alternatives to Relieve Depression (STAR*D) study, 16, 47
Serotonergic system, 382
Severe traumatic brain injury, 396
Sheehan Disability Scale score, 191
Short-term psychodynamic psychotherapy (STPP) for depression, 300
Single nucleotide polymorphisms (SNPs), 302
Sleep and wake problems
in anxiety disorders, 262
disruption of sleep patterns, 261
GAD, 261
hypersomnia, 262
hypnotic use problems, 262
hypothalamic-pituitary-adrenal axis dysregulation, 262
irregular circadian sleep-wake cycle, 262
parasomnia, 262
physician-patient interviews, 262
polysomnographic findings, 262
PTSD, 261
RLS, 262
SAD, 261
sleep apnea, 262
sleepiness, 262
subjective complaints, 261
symptoms, 261, 262
Sleep apnea, 263, 264
Sleep disturbances, 262
Sleepiness and hypersomnia, 265, 266
Sleep medicine, 262
Slow-release oral morphine sulphate, 182
Social anxiety disorder (SAD), 38, 210, 211
brain MRI measurements, 67
electroencephalography, 68
MRI, 70
Social phobia, 38
Social skills training, 224
Sonogenetics, 396
Spirituality and religiosity, 278
Staging models, 15
Standardized mean difference (SMD), treatment improvement, 6
Stereotactic cage-frame, 384
Stereotactic functional neurosurgery for movement disorders, 383
Stereotactic radiosurgery, 378
Stereotactic techniques, 382
Steven-Johnson syndrome, 127
Stimulation and ablation, 382–384
Stimulation-based procedures and lesion surgery, depression, 385
Stress desensitisation, 155
Stress exposures, PTSD, 154
Subcaudate tractotomy, 386, 387, 390
and cingulotomy, 147
Substance dependence (SD), 394
Substance use disorders (SUDs), 39
Subsyndromal PTSD, 154
Superficial and deep stimulating electrodes, 382
Supportive psychodynamic psychotherapy (SPP), 304
Symptomatic factors, treatment resistance, 17
Syndromal episodes, 14
Syndromal recovery, 14
Syndrome-based diagnostic system, 73
Synergistic drug combinations, 274, 283

T

Tardive syndromes, 117
Tavistock Adult Depression Study, 301
Telomeres, 82
Tertiary resilience, 279
Texas Children's Revised Medication Algorithm Project (TMAP), 223
Thalamotomy, 380, 383, 389
Therapeutic pessimism, 274
Therapist-guided self-help interventions, 315
Thermocoagulation, 386, 388
Tic disorders, diagnostic criteria, 238
Tourette syndrome (TS)
anticonvulsant topiramate, 241
antipsychotics, 240
AZD5213, H3R receptor, 243
baclofen, 241
cannabinoids, 242
childhood-onset neurodevelopmental disorder, 237
clinical and genetic definitions, 237

Tourette syndrome (TS) (*cont.*)
comorbid symptoms, 238, 243
conventional treatment, 241–242
cortico-striato-thalamic-cortical loops, 390
DBS of globus pallidus external, 391
deep brain stimulation, 248
deutetrabenazine, 242, 243
developmental time course, 237
differential diagnosis, 247
ecopipam, selective D1/D5 receptor agonist, 242
electrical activity recordings of neurons, 391
epidemiology, 238
heterogeneous aetiology, 239
International databases, 238
isotope neurochemical ligand studies, 239
and Lesch-Nyhan syndromes, 393
management, 240
motor and limbic circuits, 391
neuroleptic drugs, 240
neurosurgery, 391
non-dopaminergic agents, 240
noradrenergic and serotoninergic systems, 239
pathophysiology, 391
pharmacological treatment, 240, 244
prefrontal cerebral hyperactivity, 391
prevalence, 238
with psychiatric comorbidities, 237
quality of life, 239
repetitive transcranial magnetic stimulation, 246
self-injurious behaviour, 239
thalamotomy, 390
treatment response, 243, 245, 246
valbenazine, 242, 243
ventrolateral/medial thalamotomy, 390
VMAT2 inhibitors, 241
Tourette Syndrome Association (TSA), 245
Transcranial direct current stimulation (tDCS), 147, 327, 339
Transcranial magnetic stimulation (TMS), 326, 327, 339
mania, 146
Transcutaneous vagus nerve stimulation (tVNS), 328
Transdisciplinary integrative psychiatry, 274
Trans-humanity technologies, 396
Trauma-focused therapy, 152
Treasure's maintenance model, 254, 255
of bulimia nervosa, 256
Treatment adequacy assessment, 12
Treatment as usual (TAU) for MDD, 311
Treatment failures, 275, 276
management, 276, 277
Treatment of resistant schizophrenia (TRS), 350
Treatment-refractory Tourette syndrome, 243, 245, 246
Treatment related factors, 17
Treatment resistance in anxiety disorder
GAD (*see* Generalized anxiety disorder (GAD))
SAD (*see* Social anxiety disorder (SAD))
Treatment-resistant bipolar depression, 301
Treatment-resistant depression (TRD), 26, 300, 311
acetylsalicylic acid and tetracycline antibiotics, 103
antidepressants, 103
anti-inflammatory agents, 103
brain structural alterations, 100
cyclooxygenase-2 selective nonsteroidal anti-inflammatory medications, 103
DNA methylation and histone modification, 100
functional variants, 100
genetic vulnerability, 99
inflammation, 100
ketamine's treatment effects, 103
Treatment-resistant GAD/SAD
biological mechanisms, 208
cognitive behavior therapy, 208
D-Cycloserine effect, 209
dysfunctional emotion regulation, 208
g-aminobutyric acid (GABA)-ergic anticonvulsants, 209
limbic-medial prefrontal circuit, 208
maladapted behavioral coping strategies, 208
medication treatment, 208
neuropeptides, 209
N-methyl-D-aspartate (NMDA) partial agonist D-cycloserine, 209
non-compliance, 208
pharmacological agents, 209
psychosocial theories, 208
psychotherapeutic modalities, 209
reduced resting-state functional connectivity, 208
serotonin-norepinephrine reuptake inhibitor, 208
treatment compliance, 208
Treatment-resistant mania/hypomania management, 144, 145
Treatment-resistant panic disorder (TRPD)
anxiety sensitivity reduction, 192
biopsychosocial and cognitive model, 196
borderline personality traits, 192
childhood adversities, 193
comorbid psychiatric diseases, 192
definition, 189, 191
ethnic minority, 192
factors associated, 191
medical comorbidities, 193
non-pharmacological intervention
acupuncture, 197
CBT, 197
coping skills and exposure therapy, 197
EMDR, 197
exercise augmentation, 197
fish oil supplements, 197
herbal remedy, 197
interpersonal psychotherapy, 197
light therapy, 197
mindfulness-based therapy, 197
neuro-stimulation therapy, 197
physical symptoms, 198
psychodynamic psychotherapy, 197
repetitive trans-cranial magnetic stimulation, 197
S-adenosylmethionine, 197
transcranial direct current stimulation, 197
tryptophan supplements, 197

vagus nerve stimulation, 197
yoga, 197
pathophysiology
biopsychosocial hypothesis, 195, 196
brain circuit dysfunction, 194
brain derived neurotrophic fator, 195
chronic systemic inflammation, 195
genetic factors, 193, 194
hypothalamus-pituitary-adrenal (HPA) axis dysregulation, 194, 195
monoamine-related neurotransmitter pathway genes, 193
pharmacogenetic studies, 194
stress axis dysregulation, 195
personal demographic characteristics, 192
personality traits, 192
pharmacological intervention, 196
pharmacotherapy, 192
physical and autonomic symptoms, 190
predictors, 191
psychological and behavioral resistance, 192
psychopathology, 190
psychosocial stressors, 193
psychotherapy, 192
remission criteria, 190
self-concepts, 192
sex and ethnicity, 192
social economic status, 192
stressful life events, 193
symptomatic manifestations, 192
traits, 192
treatment, 197
Treatment-resistant patient group, 30
Treatment-resistant psychiatric disorder (TRP)
biological causes, 25
biomarker studies, 25
control group selection, 29
definition, 25
differential measurement bias, 27
experimental study design, 29
management, 25
nested case-control study design, 28
operational intervention (experimental), 29
post hoc experimental study, 26, 28
recruit and enroll patients, 28
risk factors, 25
subject compliance and tolerance, 27
treatment algorithm (observational), 29
treatment approaches, 25
treatment-responsive group, 25
Treatment resistant schizophrenia (TRS)
amisulpride augmentation, 124, 125
antidepressants
fluoxetine, 129
fluvoxamine, 127
low-dose D-cycloserine, 129
memantine, 129
mirtazapine, 129
NMDA/glycine site modulators, 129
aripiprazole, 125
categorical and criteria-based approach, 112
clozapine
adverse effects, 120, 121
aggression and suicidality, 115
with antipsychotics, 126
biological measures, 118
blood dyscrasias, 114
catatonic symptoms, 115
in children and adolescents, 116
clinical outcomes, 118
cognitive symptoms, 115
depressive symptoms, 115
in elderly, 117
hematological monitoring, 119
metabolic parameters, 119
oral dosage and pharmacokinetic factors, 118
with other agents, 128
positive and negative symptoms, 114, 115
in postpartum, 116, 117
during pregnancy, 116, 117
pregnancy and lactation, 114
prescription practice and barrier in usage, 118
pretreatment assessment and monitoring, 119
quality of life, 116
response predictors, 118
with risperidone, 124
tardive syndromes, 117
definitions, 110–112
first generation of antipsychotics, 109
high-dose antipsychotic use, 123
LAI antipsychotics, 122, 123
management, 112, 114
modified Kane's criteria, 112
mood stabilizers (*see* Mood stabilizers, TRS)
NCCAT, 122
non-clozapine antipsychotic and ECT combination, 122
pharmacotherapy, 113
post-clozapine augmentation strategies, 123
ECT, 123, 124
pseudo-resistance, 113
risk factors, 112, 113
second-generation antipsychotic drugs, 109
treatment guidelines, 112
Trial-and-error approach, 65
Tricyclic antidepressants (TCAs), 8
Trier Social Stress Test, 194
Trigeminal nerve stimulation (TNS), 327, 340

U

Unguided ICBT programs, 315
Unipolar depression, 45–47

V

Vagus nerve stimulation (VNS), 146, 328, 340, 384
Vesicular monoamine transporter-2 inhibitors, TS, 241

Videoconferencing psychotherapy (VCP), 315
Vigilance Algorithm Leipzig (VIGILL), 71
Voluntary fully informed consent, 397

W

Wireless Instantaneous Neurotransmitter Concentration System (WINCS), 396
Working memory deficits, 224
Working memory training (WMT), 224
World Society for Stereotactic and Functional Neurosurgery (WSSFN), 382

Y

Yale-Brown Obsessive Compulsive Scale (YBOCS), 165, 381

MIX
Papier aus verantwortungsvollen Quellen
Paper from responsible sources
FSC® C105338

If you have any concerns about our products,
you can contact us on
ProductSafety@springernature.com

In case Publisher is established outside the EU,
the EU authorized representative is:
Springer Nature Customer Service Center GmbH
Europaplatz 3, 69115 Heidelberg, Germany

Printed by Libri Plureos GmbH
in Hamburg, Germany